Stedman's

OPHTHALMOLOGY
WORDS

SECOND EDITION

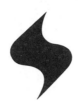

Stedman's
OPHTHALMOLOGY
WORDS

SECOND EDITION

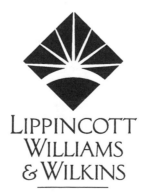

LIPPINCOTT
WILLIAMS
&WILKINS

Series Editor: Beverly Wolpert
Database Content Editor: Jennifer Schmidt
Art Direction: Jonathan Dimes
Art Coordinator: Jennifer Clements
Associate Marketing Manager: John Trader
Production Manager: Tricia Smith
Typesetter: Peirce Graphic Services, Inc.
Printer & Binder: Victor Graphics

Printed in the United States of America

Second Edition, 2000

99 00
1 2 3 4 5 6 7 8 9 10

Contents

Acknowledgments

An important part of our editorial process is the involvement of medical transcriptionists — as advisors, reviewers and/or editors.

We extend special thanks to Sandy Kovacs, CMT, and Patricia White, CMT, for editing the new terms added to *Stedman's Ophthalmology Words, Second Edition*, helping to resolve many difficult content questions, and contributing much of the material for the appendix sections.

We also extend special thanks to Martha Richards, RRA, for reviewing, proofreading, researching, and helping to resolve questions related to the content used from the first edition of *Stedman's Ophthalmology Words*. We are grateful, as well, to our MT Editorial Advisory Board for *Stedman's Ophthalmology Words, Second Edition,* including Annie Becker, Valerie Curtiss, Peggy Gibson, Alice Lazenby, and Carol Scully. These medical transcriptionists served as important contributors, editors, and advisors.

Other important contributors to this edition include Gaylen Wood, CMT, who helped us with the sample reports section of the appendix; and Jeanne Bock, CSR, MT; Betsy Dearborn; Sheila L. Hatch, MT; Renée Hentz; Robin Koza; Sandra Manzo; Kathryn Mason, CMT; Peg Nelson, CMT; LaVerne Randol, CMT; Diana Rezac, CMT; Averill Ring, CMT; Anna Sargent; Laurie Spangler; Judi Walls; Tina Whitecotton, CMT; and Teddy Wright, all of whom participated in our term-gathering process.

Barb Ferretti played an integral role in the process by reviewing the content files for format, updating the database, and providing a final quality check.

As with all our *Stedman's* word references, this resource incorporates the suggestions and expertise of our many contacts in the medical transcriptionist community. Thanks to all of our advisory board participants, reviewers, and editors; AAMT meeting attendees; and others who have written us with requests and comments — keep talking, and we'll keep listening.

Editor's Preface

How many times have you heard, "This is Dr. Jones dictating an ophthalmology consult on. . . ."? Did you immediately reach for your cup of coffee, take a drink, sit back, and think, "Well, this is going to be a long, difficult report"?

The transcription of ophthalmology reports has been a difficult, tedious task for most medical transcriptionists, but none of us can seem to pinpoint why. Good reference books are the key to successfully transcribing difficult technical reports. When asked to edit the second edition of *Stedman's Ophthalmology Words,* I knew this was my opportunity to work with other medical transcriptionists to formulate a reference that would be the first one an MT turns to when transcribing ophthalmology dictation.

The first task was to peruse ophthalmology journals, manufacturer and meeting literature, books, and websites for new terms. In conversations with many colleagues about what they would like to see in this edition, the overwhelming requests were for more intraocular lens implants and surgical equipment. I believe we have achieved these goals.

In this book, you will also find terms relating to thyroid eye disease, diabetic eye disease, oculoplastics, and neuro-ophthalmologic diagnoses and procedures. Sample operative reports have been added, and a section on drugs by indication is new. Accurate anatomic illustrations will aid you in gaining a better understanding of the eye and its surrounding structures.

I am honored that Lippincott Williams & Wilkins asked me to edit this book. It is certainly a privilege to work with a company whose people value the input from the professionals creating excellent quality medical documents on a daily basis. How refreshing! The opportunity to give back to the profession I love is a rare one indeed, and I thank LWW for giving me the chance.

Sandy Kovacs, CMT

Publisher's Preface

Stedman's Ophthalmology Words, Second Edition offers an authoritative assurance of quality and exactness to the wordsmiths of the healthcare professions — medical transcriptionists, medical editors and copy editors, health information management personnel, court reporters, and the many other users and producers of medical documentation.

We have received many requests for updates to *Stedman's Ophthalmology Words*. As the requests continued to accumulate, we realized that medical language professionals needed a comprehensive, current reference for ophthalmology.

Users will find thousands of words encompassing the function and structure of the eye, peripheral muscles, and nerves, along with diseases and disorders of the eye. This collection includes terminology used in ophthalmologic diagnosis and testing, as well as in treatments. Users will also find words for surgical instruments, procedures, and drugs.

This compilation of 60,000 entries, fully cross-indexed for quick access, was built from a base vocabulary of more than 42,000 medical words, phrases, abbreviations and acronyms. The extensive A-Z list was developed from the database of *Stedman's Medical Dictionary* and supplemented by terminology found in current medical literature (please see list of References on page xvii).

We at Lippincott Williams & Wilkins strive to provide you with the most up-to-date and accurate word references available. Your use of this wordbook will prompt new editions, which we will publish as often as updates and revisions justify. We welcome your suggestions for improvements, changes, corrections, and additions — whatever will make this *Stedman's* product more useful to you. Please complete the postpaid card at the back of this book, and send your recommendations care of "Stedman's" at Lippincott Williams & Wilkins.

Explanatory Notes

Medical transcription is an art as well as a science. Both are needed to correctly interpret the dictation of a physician, whose language is a product of education, training, and experience. This variety in medical language means there are several acceptable ways to express certain or similar terms, including jargon. *Stedman's Ophthalmology Words, Second Edition* provides variant spellings and phrasings for many terms. These elements, in addition to complete cross-indexing, make *Stedman's Ophthalmology Words, Second Edition* a valuable resource for determining the validity of terms as they are encountered.

Alphabetical Organization

Alphabetization of main entries is letter-by-letter as spelled, ignoring punctuation, spaces, prefixed numbers, or other characters. For example:

F/M base curve contact lens
FR3
fraction
3M
MacCallan classification
MC-7000

In subentry alphabetization, the abbreviated singular form or the spelled-out plural form of the noun main entry word is ignored.

Subentry terms starting with Greek letters fall under the spelled-out version of the Greek letter, which appears as a main entry with the symbol as a variant. For example:

alpha, α
    a. angle
    a.$_1$-antitrypsin
    a. crystallin

Format and Style

All main entries are in **boldface** to expedite locating a sought-after term, to enhance distinction between main entries and subentries, and to relieve the textual density of the pages.

Irregular plurals and variant spellings are shown on the same line as the singular or preferred form of the word. For example:

lemniscus, pl. lemnisci

heterotropia, heterotropy

Hyphenation

As a rule of style, multiple eponyms (e.g., Mears-Rubash approach) are hyphenated. Also, hyphens have been added between a manufacturer and one or more eponyms (e.g., Vital-Metzenbaum dissecting scissors). Please note that hyphenation is a question of style, not of accuracy, and thus is a matter of choice (as is also the case with the use of apostrophes and the possessive "s" on eponyms, as explained below).

Possessives

Possessive forms with eponyms have been dropped in this reference for the sake of internal consistency, as well as conformance to written guidelines of the American Association for Medical Transcription (AAMT) and the American Medical Association (AMA). Please note, however, that retaining the possessive is a question of style, not of accuracy, and thus is a matter of choice. To form the possessive of a word, simply add the apostrophe or apostrophe "s" to the end of the word.

Cross-indexing

The word list is in an index-like, main entry-subentry format that contains two combined alphabetical listings:

(1) A *noun* main entry-subentry organization is typical of the A-Z section of medical dictionaries like **Stedman's:**

nucleus, pl. nuclei
    accessory n.
    n. lentiform

iridis
    angulus i.
    i. rubeosis

(2) An *adjective* main entry-subentry organization lists words and phrases as you hear them. The main entries are the adjectives or modifiers in a multiword term. The subentries are the nouns around which the terms are constructed and to which the adjectives or modifiers pertain:

nutritional
    n. amblyopia
    n. blindness
    n. deficiency cataract

high
    h. convex
    h. hyperopia
    h. intensity illuminator

This format provides the user with more than one way to locate and identify a multiword term. For example:

nystagmus
    acquired jerk n.

acquired
    a. jerk nystagmus

corneal
    c. abrasion

abrasion
    corneal a.

It also allows the user to see together all terms that contain a particular descriptor, as well as all types, kinds, or variations of a noun entity. For example:

blur
    b. and clear exercise
    optical b.
    b. pattern
    spectacle b.

impression
    basilar i.
    i. cytology
    i. debridement
    i. tonometer

Wherever possible, abbreviations are separately defined and cross-referenced. For example:

POZ
>   posterior optical zone

posterior
>   p. optical zone (POZ)

zone
>   posterior optical z. ({POZ)

References

In addition to the manufacturers' literature we gather at various medical meetings, scientific reports from hospitals, and the lists of our MT Editorial Advisory Board members (from their daily transcription work), we used the following sources for new words for *Stedman's Ophthalmology Words, Second Edition:*

Books

Dorland's illustrated medical dictionary, 28th ed. Philadelphia: Saunders, 1994.

Goldman MA. Pocket guide to the operating room. Philadelphia: F. A. Davis, 1996.

Hoffman J. Quick reference of eyecare terminology, 2nd ed. Thorofare, NJ: SLACK, 1998.

Lance LL. Quick look drug book. Baltimore: Lippincott Williams & Wilkins, 1999.

Lamkin JC. The Massachusetts Eye and Ear Infirmary review manual for ophthalmology. 2nd ed. Philadelphia: Lippincott-Raven, 1998.

Mandell GL, Bennett JE, Dolin R. Principles and practice of infectious diseases, 4th ed. New York: Churchill Livingstone, 1995.

Miller NR, Newman NJ. Clinical neuro-ophthalmology, 5th ed. Baltimore: Lippincott Williams & Wilkins, 1999.

Onofrey BE, Skorin L Jr., Holdeman NR. Ocular therapeutics handbook: a clinical manual. Philadelphia: Lippincott-Raven, 1998.

Pyle V. Current medical terminology, 5th ed. Modesto: Health Professions Institute, 1994.

Rowland LP. Merritt's textbook of neurology. Baltimore: Williams & Wilkins, 1997.

Sloane SB. The medical word book, 3rd ed. Philadelphia: WB Saunders Company, 1991.

Stedman's medical dictionary, 26th ed. Baltimore: Williams & Wilkins, 1995.

Stein HA, Slatt BJ, Stein RM. Ophthalmic terminology: speller and vocabulary builder, 3rd ed. St. Louis: Mosby Year Book, 1992.

Walsh TJ. Neuro-ophthalmology: clinical signs and symptoms, 4th ed. Baltimore: Williams & Wilkins, 1997.

Journals

American Journal of Ophthalmology. New York: Elsevier, 1994–1999.

Archives of Ophthalmology. Chicago: American Medical Association, 1994–1999.

Cornea: The Journal of Cornea and External Disease. Philadelphia: Lippincott Williams & Wilkins, 1998–1999.

Internal Medicine. Montvale, NJ: Medical Economics, 1994–1999.

Journal of the American Association for Medical Transcription. Modesto: American Association for Medical Transcription, 1996–1999.

Journal of Neuro-Ophthalmology [Official Journal of the North American Neuro-Ophthalmology Society]. Philadelphia: Lippincott Williams & Wilkins, 1998–1999.

The Journal of Retinal and Vitreous Diseases. Philadelphia: Lippincott Williams & Wilkins, 1998–1999.

The Latest Word. Philadelphia: WB Saunders Company, 1996–1999.

MT Monthly. Gladstone, MO: Computer Systems Management, 1996–1999.

Ocular Surgery News. Thorofare, NJ: Slack, 1998–1999.

Ophthalmology [American Academy of Ophthalmology, The Eye M.D. Association]. Philadelphia: Lippincott Williams & Wilkins, 1996–1999.

Ophthalmology Times. Cleveland: Advanstar Communications, 1998–1999.

Optomometry and Vision Science [Journal of the American Academy of Optometry]. Baltimore: Lippincott Williams & Wilkins, 1998–1999.

Perspectives on the Medical Transcription Profession. Modesto: Health Professions Institute, 1993–1999.

Retina: The Journal of Retinal and Vitreous Diseases. Philadelphia: Lippincott Williams & Wilkins, 1998–1999.

Wilmer Retina Update [The Wilmer Ophthalmological Institute, Johns Hopkins University School of Medicine]. Baltimore: Lippincott Williams & Wilkins, 1998–1999

Stedman's WordWatcher. Baltimore: Williams & Wilkins, 1995–1999.

Websites

http://www.ajo.com

http://www.djo.harvard.edu/

http://www.hpisum.com

http://www.hsls.pitt.edu/intres/health/ophth.html

http://www.medscape.com

http://www.meei.harvard.edu/web/web.html

http://www.mtmonthly.com/

http://www.nei.nih.gov

http://www.VIRTUALdrugstore.com

http://www.wilmer.jhu.edu/

http://mtdaily.com/

http://odp.od.nih.gov/ods/databases/ibids.html

http://server.nyee.edu/current/current.htm

α (*var. of* alpha)

A

accommodation
  A band
  A Maddox line
  A pattern
  A syndrome

AA

amplitude of accommodation

AACG

acute angle-closure glaucoma

AAMD

atrophic age-related macular
degeneration

AAP

achromatic automated perimetry

Aarskog syndrome

Aase syndrome

ab

  a. externo filtering operation
  a. externo trabeculectomy
  a. interno approach

Abadie sign

abaissement

Abbe refractometer

abducens

  a. facial paralysis
  a. internuclear neuron
  a. nerve
  a. nerve fascicle
  a. nerve palsy
  a. nerve paralysis

abducent nerve (N.VI)

abduct

abduction

  absence of a.
  congenital absence of a.
  a. deficit

abductor muscle

aberrant

  a. degeneration
  a. degeneration of third nerve
  a. regeneration
  a. regeneration of nerve
  a. reinnervation of the
    oculomotor nerve

aberration

  angle of a.
  chromatic lens a.
  color a.

  coma a.
  curvature a.
  dioptric a.
  distantial a.
  distortion a.
  lateral a.
  lens a.
  longitudinal a.
  meridional a.
  monochromatic a.
  newtonian a.
  oblique a.
  optical a.
  regeneration a.
  spherical lens a.

aberrometer

Abex-Turner incision

ability vergence

abiotrophy

  retinal a.

ABK

aphakic bullous keratopathy

ablation

  broad-beam a.
  eccentric a.
  excimer laser a.
  hyperopic a.
  panretinal a.
  peripheral retinal a.
  pituitary a.
  toric a.
  a. zone

ablatio retinae

ablepharia

ablepharon

ablephary

ablepsia, ablepsy

ABMD

anterior basement membrane
dystrophy

Abney effect

abnormal

  a. correspondence
  a. harmonious retinal
    correspondence
  a. nearwork-induced transient
    myopia
  a. staining pattern
  a. unharmonious retinal
    correspondence

abnormality
> angle of a.
> congenital a.
> facial movement a.
> intraretinal microvascular a.
> (IRMA)
> microvascular a.
> retinal a.
> saccadic a.
> skeletal a.
> vascular a.
> vertebrobasilar vascular a.

abortus
> *Brucella* a.

abrader
> cornea a.
> Howard a.

Abraham
> A. iridectomy laser lens
> A. iridotomy
> A. peripheral button iridotomy
> lens
> A. YAG laser lens

abrasio corneae
abrasion
> central a.
> conjunctival a.
> a. of cornea
> corneal a.
> traumatic corneal a.

abrin
abscess, pl. **abscesses**
> cerebral a.
> corneal a.
> fulminant a.
> lacrimal a.
> orbital a.
> psoriatic corneal a.
> retrobulbar a.
> ring a.
> a. ring
> scleral tunnel a.
> subperiosteal a.
> vitreous a.

abscessus siccus corneae
abscission
> corneal a.

absence of abduction
absent guttata
Absidia corymbifera
absolute
> a. accommodation
> a. glaucoma

> a. hemianopsia
> a. hyperopia
> a. intensity threshold acuity
> near point a.
> a. scotoma
> a. strabismus

absolutum
> glaucoma a.

absorbable
> a. gelatin film
> a. suture

Absorbonac ophthalmic
absorptance
> radiant a.

absorption
> fluorescent treponemal
> antibody a.
> a. line

abtorsion
AC
> accommodative convergence
> anterior chamber
> AC eye drops

AC/A
> accommodative
> convergence/accommodation ratio

acanthamebiasis
Acanthamoeba
> A. *castellanii*
> A. *endophthalmitis*
> A. *keratitis*
> A. *mauritaniensis*
> A. *polyphaga*

acanthocytosis
acantholysis
acanthoma
> a. fissuratum

acanthosis
> a. nigricans

acarica
> blepharitis a.

ACC
> anterior central curve

Acc
> accommodation

accelerometer
accessoriae
> glandulae lacrimales a.

accessory
> a. fiber
> a. lacrimal gland
> a. nucleus
> a. organs of eye

accidental
a. image
a. mydriasis
accommodation (A, Acc)
absolute a.
amplitude of a. (AA)
binocular a.
breadth of a.
bright-field a.
convergence a.
a. of crystalline lens
dark-field a.
defective a.
a. disorder
esodeviation a.
esotropia a.
excessive a.
far point of a. (FPA)
fusion with a.
Helmholtz theory of a.
a. insufficiency
iridoplegia a.
near-point a.
near point of a. (NPA)
negative a.
open-loop a.
paralysis of a.
a. paresis
a. phosphene
a. phosphene of Czermak
pinhole a.
position a.
positive a.
punctum proximum of a.
pupils equal, reactive to light and a. (PERLA)
pupils equal, round, reactive to light and a. (PERRLA)
range of a.
reflex a.
a. reflex
relative a.
residual a.
a. response
a. rule
a. spasm
spasm of a.

steady-state a.
subnormal a.
tonic a.
accommodation-convergence ratio
accommodative
a. adaptation
a. amplitude
a. asthenopia
a. convergence (AC)
a. convergence/accommodation ratio (AC/A)
a. cyclophoria
a. effort syndrome
a. esodeviation
a. esophoria
a. esotropia
a. palsy
a. response
a. spasm
a. squint
a. strabismus
a. target
accommodometer
accreta
cataracta membranacea a.
Accugel lens
accumulation
lipid a.
Accurus vitreoretinal surgical system
Accutome black diamond blade
Accuvac smoke evacuation attachment
aceclidine
acellular matrix
acetaldehyde
acetaminophen
a. with oxycodone
acetanilid
acetate
cellulose a.
cortisone a.
Cortone A.
fluorometholone a.
hydrocortisone a.
Hydrocorton A.
medroxyprogesterone a.

NOTES

acetate *(continued)*
    paramethasone a.
    phenylmercuric a.
    potassium a.
    prednisolone a.
    sodium a.
acetazolamide
acetohexamide
acetone
Acetonide
acetoxycyclohexamide (AXM)
acetoxyphenylmercury
aceturate
    diminazene a.
acetylcholine
    a. chloride
    a. receptor deficiency
acetylcholinesterase
    a. deficiency
acetylcysteine
N-**acetyl-β-D-glucosamidase**
ACG
    angle-closure glaucoma
achiasma
achloropsia
achromat
achromate
achromatic
    a. automated perimetry (AAP)
    a. axis
    a. doublet
    a. objective
    a. spectacle lens
    a. threshold
    a. vision
achromatism
achromatopia
achromatopic
achromatopsia, achromatopsy
    atypical a.
    central a.
    cerebral a.
    complete a.
    cone a.
    incomplete a.
    rod a.
    typical a.
    X-linked a.
achromia
Achromycin
    A. Ophthalmic
acid
    boric a.

    a. burn
    a. maltase deficiency
acid-fast bacilli
acidophilic adenoma
acid-resistant penicillin
acinar
    a. dropout
    a. lacrimal gland
Acinetobacter calcoaceticus
acinus, pl. **acini**
    lacrimal gland a.
ACIOL
    anterior chamber intraocular lens
acne
    a. ciliaris
    a. rosacea
    a. rosacea blepharoconjunctivitis
    a. rosacea conjunctivitis
    a. rosacea corneal ulcer
    a. rosacea keratitis
acnes
    Propionibacterium a.
acorea
acorn-shaped eye implant
acoustic
    a. nerve
    a. neuroma
    a. spot
acoustical
    a. shadowing
    a. sonolucent
acquired
    a. abducens nerve lesion
    a. alexia
    a. astigmatism
    a. color defect
    a. distichia
    a. dyschromatopsia
    a. entropion
    a. esotropia
    a. gustolacrimal reflex
    a. Horner syndrome
    a. immune response
    a. immunodeficiency syndrome (AIDS)
    a. jerk nystagmus
    a. melanosis
    a. myopathic ptosis
    a. ocular motor apraxia
    a. pendular nystagmus
    a. retinoschisis
    a. syphilis
    a. toxoplasmosis retinitis

acquisita
epidermolysis bullosa a.

ACR
Clear Eyes ACR

Acremonium

acritochromacy

acrylate
silicone a.

acrylic
a. implant
a. lens

AcrySof
A. foldable intraocular lens
A. MA60 lens

ACS
Alcon Closure System
ACS needle

ACT
alternate cover test

actinic
a. conjunctivitis
a. keratitis
a. keratosis
a. ray ophthalmia
a. retinitis

Actinomadura madurae

Actinomyces

Actinomycetales

actinomycin D

action
mechanism of a.
mode of a.
primary a.
secondary a.

activator
tissue plasminogen a. (tPA)

active pterygium

activity
A.'s of Daily Vision Scale
laser a.

actomyosin ATPase

Acuiometer

acuity
absolute intensity threshold a.
best-corrected visual a.
(BCVA)
binocular visual a.

a. card procedure
central visual a.
detection a.
distance a.
distance visual a. (DVA)
dynamic visual a.
grating a.
identification a.
mean a.
minimum perceptible a.
minimum separable a.
near visual a. (NVA)
numerical visual a.
perceptible a.
potential visual a.
resolution a.
separable a.
Snellen visual a.
spatial a.
stereoscopic a.
Teller visual a.
true visual a. (TVA)
uncorrected visual a. (UCVA,
UNCVA)
Vernier visual a.
visibility a.
visual a. (VA)
a. visual projector

Acular
A. drops
A. Ophthalmic
A. PF

Acuscan Transducer 400

Acuson
A. 128 apparatus
A. ultrasound

acute
a. angle-closure glaucoma
(AACG)
a. atopic conjunctivitis
a. catarrhal conjunctivitis
a. catarrhal rhinitis
a. chalazion
a. chronic glaucoma
a. congestive conjunctivitis
a. congestive glaucoma
a. contagious conjunctivitis

NOTES

5

acute *(continued)*
  a. dacryocystitis
  a. diffuse serous choroiditis
  a. epidemic conjunctivitis
  a. follicular conjunctivitis
  a. hemorrhagic conjunctivitis
  a. idiopathic demyelinating
    optic neuritis
  a. intermittent primary angle-
    closure glaucoma (A/I-PACG)
  a. macular neuroretinopathy
  a. multifocal placoid pigment
    epitheliopathy (AMPPE)
  a. multifocal posterior placoid
    pigment epitheliopathy
  a. posterior multifocal placoid
    pigment epitheliopathy
    (APMPPE)
  a. primary angle-closure
    glaucoma (APACG)
  a. retinal necrosis (ARN)
  a. retinal necrosis syndrome
    (ARN)
  a. spastic entropion
  a. zonal occult outer
    retinopathy (AZOOR)
Acuvue disposable contact lens
acyclic nucleoside analogue
Adams
  A. ectropion
  A. operation
  A. operation for ectropion
Adapettes
Adapt
adaptation
  accommodative a.
  color a.
  dark a.
  light a.
  photopic a.
  retinal a.
  scotopic a.
adapter
  Sheehy-Urban sliding lens a.
  Volk Minus non-contact a.
  Volk retinal scale a.
  Volk ultra field aspherical
    lens a.
  Volk yellow filter a.
  Zeiss cine a.
adaptive immunity
adaptometer
  Collin 140 color a.

color a.
Feldman a.
Goldmann-Weekers dark a.
adaptometry
  dark a.
add
  near a.
  a. power
adduction
  a. impairment
  a. lag
adductor muscle
A-dellen
adenoid cystic carcinoma
adenologaditis
adenoma
  acidophilic a.
  basophilic a.
  chromophobe a.
  endocrine-inactive a.
  Fuchs a.
  invasive a.
  parathyroid a.
  pituitary a.
  pleomorphic a.
  prolactin-secreting a.
  sebaceous a.
  a. sebaceum
adenomectomy
  medical a.
adenophthalmia
adenosine monophosphate (AMP)
adenoviral
  a. keratoconjunctivitis
adenovirus (ADV)
  a. 3
  a. 7
  a. 8
  a. 19
  a. conjunctivitis
adequacy
  blink a.
adherence syndrome
adherens
  leukoma a.
  macula a.
  zonula a.
adherent
  a. cataract
  a. lens
  a. leukoma
adhesion
  cell a.

chorioretinal a.
thermal a.
vitreoretinal a.
adhesive
Brown sterile a.
cyanoacrylate tissue a.
Nexacryl tissue a.
a. syndrome
tissue a.
Adie
A. syndrome
A. tonic pupil
adiposa
cataracta a.
pseudophakia a.
ptosis a.
adipose
a. body
a. tissue
adiposus
arcus a.
aditus orbitae
adjustable suture
adjuster
Serdarevic suture a.
adjustment
early postoperative suture a.
(EPSA)
intraoperative suture a. (ISA)
late postoperative suture a.
(LPSA)
postoperative a.
suture a.
adjuvant microwave thermotherapy
Adler operation
administration
intraocular a.
adnatum
ankyloblepharon filiforme a.
adnexa
ocular a.
a. oculi
adnexal
adolescent cataract
adrenal
a. disorder
a. hypertension

adrenaline
adrenergic drug
Adson forceps
Adsorbocarpine
A. Ophthalmic
Adsorbonac
Adsorbotear
A. Ophthalmic Solution
adtorsion
adult
a. inclusion conjunctivitis
a. medulloepithelioma
adult-onset
a.-o. cataract
a.-o. diabetes mellitus (AODM)
adultorum
blennorrhea a.
ADV
adenovirus
advancement
capsular a.
a. flap
a. procedure
tendon a.
**advancing wave-like epitheliopathy
(AWE)**
Advent pachymeter
adverse reaction
Aebli corneal section scissors
aegypticus
Haemophilus a.
AEO
apraxia of eyelid opening
aerial haze
aerogenes
Enterobacter a.
Aeromonas hydrophila
aerosol keratitis
Aerosporin
aeruginosa
Pseudomonas a.
AES
anti-elevation syndrome
Aesculap
A. argon ophthalmic laser
A. excimer laser

NOTES

Aesculap *(continued)*
    A. Meditec excimer laser
    A. Meditec MEL60 system
aesthesiometer *(var. of*
esthesiometer)
afferent
    a. nerve
    a. pupillary defect (APD)
    a. visual pathway
    a. visual symptom
afocal
    a. optical system
    a. telescope
africanum
    Mycobacterium a.
aftercataract
    a. bur
aftereffect
afterimage
    complementary a.
    negative a.
    positive a.
    a. test
afterimagery
afterperception
aftervision
against motion
against-the-rule astigmatism
agenesis
    colossal a.
ageotropic nystagmus
age-related
    a.-r. cataract
    a.-r. macular degeneration
    (AMD, ARMD)
    a.-r. maculopathy (ARM)
    a.-r. ptosis
    a.-r. retinoschisis
agglutination
    lid a.
    plasmoid a.
agglutinins
aggregate
    cellular a.
aggregation
AGL-400
    Mira AGL-400
aglaucopsia
Agnew
    A. canaliculus knife
    A. canthoplasty
    A. keratome

    A. operation
    A. tattooing needle
Agnew-Verhoeff incision
agnosia
    apperceptive a.
    color a.
    optic a.
    topographic a.
    visual a.
    visual-spatial a.
agonist-antagonist relationship
agonist muscle
Agrikola
    A. lacrimal sac retractor
    A. operation
    A. refractor
    A. tattooing needle
Ahlström syndrome
AHM
    anterior hyaloid membrane
Ahmed
    A. device
    A. drainage seton
    A. glaucoma drainage tube
    A. glaucoma valve
    A. glaucoma valve
    implantation
    A. shunt tube
    A. valve implant
AICA
    anterior inferior cerebellar artery
    AICA syndrome
Aicardi syndrome
aid
    low-vision a.
AIDS
    acquired immunodeficiency
    syndrome
AIDS-related
    A.-r. complex (ARC)
    A.-r. retinitis
aileron
Aimark perimetry
aiming beam
AION
    anterior ischemic optic neuropathy
A/I-PACG
    acute intermittent primary angle-
    closure glaucoma
air
    a. bubble
    a. cell
    a. chamber

a. cystitome
a. injection cannula
intraocular a.
a. rifle
air-block glaucoma
air-fluid exchange
AIRLens contact lens
air-puff
a.-p. contact tonometer
a.-p. noncontact tonometer
Airy
A. cylindric lens
A. disk
AK
astigmatic keratotomy
Akahoshi
A. nucleus sustainer
A. phaco prechopper
A. universal prechopper
Akarpine
A. Ophthalmic
AK Beta
AKBeta
AK-Chlor
A.-C. Ophthalmic
AK-Cide
A.-C. Ophthalmic
AK-Con
A.-C. ophthalmic
AK-Con-A
AK-Dex Ophthalmic
AK-Dilate
A.-D. Ophthalmic Solution
Aker lens pusher
AK-Fluor
AK-Homatropine
A.-H. Ophthalmic
akinesia
Nadbath a.
orbital a.
retrobulbar a.
Scheie a.
supraorbital a.
Van Lint a.
akinesis
pupillary sphincter a.
akinetic

akinetopsia
cerebral a.
AK-Lor
AK-Mycin
AK-NaCl
AK-Nefrin
A.-N. Ophthalmic Solution
AK-Neo-Cort
AK-Neo-Dex
A.-N.-D. Ophthalmic
Akorn
A. Intraoperative Pak
A. OcuCaps
AK-Pentolate
AK-Poly-Bac
A.-P.-B. Ophthalmic
AK-Pred Ophthalmic
AKPro Ophthalmic
AK-Rinse
AK-Spore
A.-S. H.C. Ophthalmic
Ointment
A.-S. H.C. Ophthalmic
Suspension
AK-Sulf
A.-S. Forte
A.-S. Ophthalmic
AK-Taine
AK-Tate
AKTob Ophthalmic
AK-Tracin
A.-T. Ophthalmic
AK-Trol
AK-Vaso-A
AK-Vernacon
Akwa
A. Tears
A. Tears Solution
AK-Zol
AL
axial length
Alabama
A. tying forceps
A. University utility forceps
Alabama-Green
A.-G. clamp
A.-G. needle holder

NOTES

9

alacrima
ala minor ossis sphenoidalis
Aland eye disease
Albalon
    A. Liquifilm
    A. Liquifilm Ophthalmic
Albalon-A
    A.-A. Liquifilm
    A.-A. Ophthalmic
Albamycin
albedo retinae
Albers-Schönberg disease
albescens
    retinitis punctata a.
albicans
    Candida a.
albinism
    autosomal dominant
    oculocutaneous a.
    autosomal recessive ocular a.
    Bergsma-Kaiser-Kupfer
    oculocutaneous a.
    Donaldson-Fitzpatrick
    oculocutaneous a.
    localized a.
    minimal pigment
    oculocutaneous a.
    Nettleship-Falls X-linked
    ocular a.
    ocular a.
    oculocutaneous a.
    partial a.
    punctate oculocutaneous a.
    tyrosinase-negative type
    oculocutaneous a.
    tyrosinase-positive type
    oculocutaneous a.
    yellow-mutant
    oculocutaneous a.
albinoidism
    oculocutaneous a.
    punctate oculocutaneous a.
albinotic
    a. fundus
albipunctalis
    fundus a.
albipunctate fundus
albipunctatus
    fundus a.
albuginea oculi
albuminuric
    a. amaurosis
    a. retinitis

Alcaine
    A. Drop-Tainers
Alclear
alcoholic amblyopia
Alcon
    A. A-OK crescent knife
    A. A-OK ShortCut knife
    A. A-OK slit knife
    A. applanation
    pneumatonograph
    A. aspiration
    A. aspirator
    A. Closure System (ACS)
    A. cryoextractor
    A. cryophake
    A. cryosurgical unit
    A. CU-15 4-mil needle
    A. Digital B 2000 ultrasound
    A. disposable drape
    A. EyeMap EH-290 corneal
    topography system
    A. hand cautery
    A. I-knife
    A. indirect ophthalmoscope
    A. irrigating/aspirating unit
    A. irrigating needle
    A. 20,000 Legacy unit
    A. MA30BA optic Acrysof
    lens
    A. 10,000 Master unit
    A. microsponge
    A. phacoemulsification
    A. phacoemulsification unit
    A. reverse cutting needle
    A. spatula needle
    A. Surgical instrument
    A. suture
    A. taper cut needle
    A. taper point needle
    A. tonometer
    A. ultrasound pachometer
    A. vitrectomy probe
    A. vitrector
Alcon-Biophysic Ophthascan S
Alconefrin
AL/CR ratio
Alder anomaly
Alder-Reilly phenomenon
aldose reductase
Alexander-Ballen retractor
Alexander law
alexia
    acquired a.

A

literal a.
optical a.
pure a.
subcortical a.
alexic
Alezzandrini syndrome
alfa-2a
interferon a.
Alfonso
A. diamond corneal transplant
blade
A. guarded bur
A. pediatric eyelid speculum
Alger
A. brush
A. brush rust ring remover
algera
dysopia a., dysopsia a.
ALGERBRUSH II
Alges bifocal contact lens
algorithm
FASTPAC a.
Lindstrom-Casebeer a.
Swedish interactive
thresholding a. (SITA)
Alhazen theory
Alidase
alignment
ocular a.
primary gaze a.
aliquot
Alizarin Red S dye
ALK
automated lamellar keratoplasty
automated laser keratomileusis
alkali
a. burn
a. burn of cornea
a. burn to eye
alkaline burn
alkaloid
belladonna a.
dissociated a.
ergot a.
miotic a.
undissociated a.
alkaptonuria

ALK-E
automated lamellar keratoplasty-
Excimer
Alkeran
alkyl ether sulfate
allachesthesia
optical a.
allele
Allen
A. cyclodialysis
A. figure
A. operation
A. orbital implant
A. pre-school card
A. stereo separator
Allen-Barkan forceps
Allen-Barker forceps
Allen-Braley
A.-B. forceps
A.-B. implant
Allen-Burian trabeculotome
Allen-ePTFE ocular implant
Allen-Schiötz tonometer
Allen-Thorpe
A.-T. goniolens
A.-T. gonioscopic prism
A.-T. lens
Aller-Chlor
Allerest
A. Eye Drops
Allergan
A. AMO Array S155 lens
A. Humphrey laser
A. Humphrey perimeter
A. Humphrey photokeratoscope
A. Humphrey refractor
A. lensometer
A. lensometer
A. Medical Optics (AMO)
A. Medical Optics
photokeratoscope
allergen
allergic
a. blepharitis
a. blepharoconjunctivitis
a. conjunctivitis
a. eye disease

NOTES

allergic *(continued)*
    a. keratoconjunctivitis
    a. pannus
    a. phlyctenulosis
    a. response
    a. rhinitis
allergica
    iritis recidivans
    staphylococcal a.
AllerMax Oral
Allescheria boydii
allesthesia
    visual a.
alligator scissors
Allis forceps
Alloderm
allograft
    a. corneal rejection
    keratolimbal a. (KLA)
    limbal a.
allokeratoplasty
allopathic keratoplasty
allophthalmia
alloplastic donor material
allopurinol
alloxan diabetes
all-Perspex
    a.-P. CQ lens
    a.-P. Kelman Omnifit lens
all-PMMA intraocular lens
Allport
    A. cutting bur
    A. operation
all-*trans*-retinal
Almocarpine
Almocetamide
Aloe reading unit
Alomide
    A. 0.1%
    A. drops
    A. Ophthalmic
    A. ophthalmic solution
alopecia orbicularis
Alpar implant
Alpern cortex aspirator/hydrodissector
Alpha
    A. Chymar
alpha, α
    a. angle
    a. crystallin
alpha2-adrenergic agonist agent, ophthalmic

alpha-2a
alpha-agonist
alpha-antagonist
alpha₁-antitrypsin
alphabet keratitis
alpha-chymotrypsin
    a.-c. cannula
alpha-chymotrypsin-induced glaucoma
Alphadrol
Alphagan
alpha-methyldopa
alpha-methyl-*p*-tyrosine
ALPI
    argon laser peripheral iridoplasty
Alpidine
Alport syndrome
AL-R
Alrex
    A. ophthalmic suspension
Alström
    A. disease
    A. syndrome
Alström-Hallgren syndrome
Alström-Olsen syndrome
Alsus-Knapp operation
Alsus operation
ALT
    argon laser trabeculopexy
Alternaria alternata
alternata
    Alternaria a.
alternate
    a. cover test (ACT)
    a. cover-uncover test
    a. day esotropia
    a. day strabismus
    a. hyperdeviation
alternating
    a. esotropia
    a. exophoria
    a. exotropia
    a. Horner syndrome
    a. hypertropia
    a. hypotropia
    a. light test
    a. mydriasis
    a. oculomotor hemiplegia
    a. strabismus
    a. sursumduction
    a. tropia
alternation

Alternative
> Soft Mate Enzyme A.

alternocular

altitudinal
> a. field
> a. hemianopia
> a. hemianopsia
> a. scotoma
> a. visual field defect

ALTP
> argon laser trabeculoplasty

aluminum
> a. chloride
> a. eye shield

Alvis
> A. curette
> A. fixation forceps
> A. foreign body spud
> A. operation

Alvis-Lancaster sclerotome

amacrine cell

amaurosis
> albuminuric a.
> Burns a.
> cat's eye a.
> central a.
> a. centralis
> cerebral a.
> congenital a.
> a. congenita of Leber
> diabetic a.
> a. fugax
> gutta a.
> hysteric a.
> intoxification a.
> Leber congenital a.
> a. nystagmus
> a. partialis fugax
> pressure a.
> reflex a.
> saburral a.
> toxic a.
> uremic a.

amaurotic
> a. cat's eye
> a. familial idiocy
> a. idiocy

> a. mydriasis
> a. nystagmus
> a. pupil
> a. pupillary paralysis

ambient

ambiopia

amblyope

amblyopia
> alcoholic a.
> ametropic a.
> anisometric a.
> anisometropic a.
> arsenic a.
> astigmatic a.
> axial a.
> color a.
> a. crapulosa
> crossed a.
> a. cruciata
> deprivation a.
> eclipse a.
> esotropic a.
> ethyl alcohol a.
> ex a.
> a. ex anopia
> a. ex anopsia
> exertional a.
> functional a.
> hysteric a.
> hysterical a.
> index a.
> irreversible a.
> meridional a.
> microstrabismic a.
> nocturnal a.
> nutritional a.
> organic a.
> postmarital a.
> postoperative a.
> quinine a.
> receptor a.
> reflex a.
> refractive a.
> relative a.
> reverse a.
> reversible a.
> sensory a.

NOTES

amblyopia *(continued)*
    strabismal a.
    suppressed a.
    suppression a.
    tobacco a.
    tobacco/alcohol a.
    toxic a.
    traumatic a.
    uremic a.
    West Indian a.
amblyopiatrics
amblyopic
amblyoscope
    major a.
    Worth a.
Ambrose suture forceps
ambulatory vision
AMD
    age-related macular degeneration
amebiasis
amebic keratitis
ameboid
    a. keratitis
    a. ulcer
amelanotic
    a. choroidal melanoma
ameliorate
ameloblastic neurilemoma
Amenabar
    A. capsule forceps
    A. counterpressor
    A. discission hook
    A. iris retractor
    A. lens
    A. lens loupe
America
    Eye Bank Association of A. (EBAA)
American
    A. Academy of Ophthalmology
    A. Hydron instrument
    A. leishmaniasis
    A. Medical Association
    A. Medical Optics
    A. Medical Optics Baron lens
    A. Optical Hardy-Rand-Rittler color plate
    A. Society of Ophthalmic Plastic and Reconstruction Surgery
ametrometer
ametropia
    axial a.
    curvature a.
    index a.
    position a.
    refractive a.
    transient a.
ametropic amblyopia
Amicar
amifloxacin
amikacin
Amikin
amine
    vasoactive a.
aminoaciduria cataract
aminoglutethimide
aminoglycoside
aminophylline
aminopyridine
4-aminoquinoline
aminosteroid
amiodarone
amitriptyline
Ammon
    A. canthoplasty
    A. operation
    A. scleral prominence
ammonia alkali burn
ammonium
    a. hydroxide alkali burn
    a. lactate
amnesic color blindness
amnifocal lens
AMO
    Allergan Medical Optics
    AMO Array foldable intraocular lens
    AMO Array multifocal ultraviolet-absorbing silicone posterior chamber intraocular lens
    AMO Endosol Extra
    AMO HPF 500 pump
    AMO intraocular lens
    AMO IOPTEX Model ACR 360 foldable acrylic lens
    AMO Phacoflex II foldable intraocular lens
    AMO Prestige advanced cataract extraction system
    AMO Prestige Phaco System
    AMO Set-Up
    AMO Vitrax viscoelastic solution
    AMO YAG 100 laser

amobarbital
amodiaquine
Amoils
   A. cryoextractor
   A. cryopencil
   A. cryophake
   A. cryoprobe
   A. cryosurgical unit
   A. refractor
   A. retractor
AMO-PhacoFlex lens and inserter
amorphic lens
amorphous corneal dystrophy
AmoRVitrax
amotio retinae
amoxicillin
AMP
   adenosine monophosphate
amphamphoterodiplopia
amphetamine
amphiphilic drug
amphodiplopia
amphotericin
   a. B
amphoterodiplopia
ampicillin
amplitude
   a. of accommodation (AA)
   accommodative a.
   binocular a.
   b-wave a.
   cone b-wave a.
   convergence a.
   a. of convergence
   divergence a.
   flicker a.
   a. of fusion
   fusional convergence a.
   fusional divergence a.
   fusion with a.
   rod b-wave a.
   rod-cone a.
   vertical fusional vergence a.
AMPPE
   acute multifocal placoid pigment
   epitheliopathy
ampulla, pl. **ampullae**

   a. canaliculi lacrimalis
   a. ductus lacrimalis
   a. of lacrimal canal
   a. of lacrimal duct
amputator
   Smith intraocular capsular a.
Amsler
   A. aqueous transplant needle
   A. chart
   A. corneal graft
   A. grid
   A. grid test
   A. operation
   A. scleral marker
Amsoft lens
Amvisc
   A. Plus
   A. Plus solution
   A. solution
amyloid
   a. cellulitis
   a. corneal degeneration
   a. deposit
   a. P component
   subcutaneous a.
amyloidosis
   conjunctival a.
   localized a.
   orbital a.
   primary familial a.
   secondary a.
   systemic a.
amyltransferase
Amytal
ANA
   antinuclear antibody
Anacel
anaclasis
anaerobic
   a. medium
   a. ocular infection
anagioid disk
anaglyph
   a. test
anagnosasthenia
Anagnostakis operation

NOTES

15

analgesia
  surface a.
analgesic
  opiate a.
analmoscope
  Pickford-Nicholson a.
analog
  prostaglandin a.
  thymidine a.
analogue
  acyclic nucleoside a.
analphalipoproteinemia
analysis
  astigmatic vector a.
  bivariate a.
  corneal topographic a.
  digital-imaging a.
  endothelial cell a.
  Fourier harmonic a.
  image a.
  linkage a.
  logistic discriminant a.
  Neale Reading A.
  pedigree a.
  A. of Radial Keratotomy
    (ARK)
  Topcon noncontact
    morphometric a.
  a. of variance (ANOVA)
  vector a.
  Western immunoblotting a.
analyzer
  Friedmann visual field a.
  GDx nerve fiber a.
  Humphrey field a.
  Humphrey Instruments
    vision a.
  Humphrey lens a.
  Humphrey visual field a.
  nerve fiber layer a.
  Paradigm ocular blood flow a.
  P55 Pachymetric A.
  profile a.
  Tomey retinal function a.
  Vision a.
  ViVa binocular infrared
    vision a.
anamorphosis
anaphoria
anaphylactic
  a. conjunctivitis
  a. reaction
anaphylaxis

anastigmatic
  a. lens
anastomosis, pl. anastomoses
  chorioretinal venous a.
anatomic equator
anatomy
  intracanalicular a.
  intracranial a.
  intraocular a.
  intraorbital a.
  topographic a.
anatropia
anatropic
ANCA
  antineutrophil cytoplasmic antibody
Ancef
anchor
  a. hook
  a. suture
anchor/fixation
  Searcy a.
anchoring suture
Andersen syndrome
Anderson-Kestenbaum procedure
Andosky syndrome
Anectine
Anel
  A. operation
  A. probe
  A. syringe
anemia
  aplastic a.
  macrocytic a.
  Mediterranean a.
  normocytic hypochromic a.
  pernicious a.
  sickle cell a.
anemone cell tumor
anencephaly
Anergan
anergy
anesthesia
  cornea a.
  endotracheal a.
  exam under a. (EUA)
  general a.
  infraorbital a.
  intraorbital a.
  modified Van Lint a.
  O'Brien a.
  orbital a.
  parabulbar a.
  retrobulbar a.

topical a.
Van Lint a.
anesthetic
general a.
inhalation a.
local a.
a. ointment
topical a.
anetoderma
Jadassohn-type a.
aneurysm
arteriovenous a.
basilar artery a.
berry a.
carotid a.
cavernous sinus a.
cerebral artery a.
cirsoid a.
communicating artery a.
fusiform a.
giant a.
intracranial a.
Leber miliary a.
miliary a.
ophthalmic artery a.
a. of orbit
orbital a.
racemose a.
a. of retinal arteriole
retinal artery a.
saccular a.
suprasellar a.
aneurysmal bone cyst
Angelman syndrome
Angelucci
A. operation
A. syndrome
angiitis
angio-Behçet disease
angioblastic meningioma
angiodiathermy
angioedema
angioendotheliomatosis
neoplastic a.
Angiofluor
angiogenesis

angiogram
fluorescein a.
angiography
anterior segment a.
carotid a.
cerebral radionuclide a.
computed tomographic a.
digital subtraction indocyanine
green a. (DS-ICGA)
fluorescein a. (FA)
Heidelberg retinal a.
ICG a.
indocyanine green a. (ICGA)
intravenous fluorescein a.
IV retinal fluorescein a.
magnetic resonance a. (MRA)
orbital a.
retinal a.
vertebral a.
angioid
a. retinal streak
angiokeratoma
a. corporis diffusum
a. corporis diffusum universale
diffuse a.
angioma
cavernous a.
conjunctival a.
episcleral a.
nerve head a.
orbital a.
racemose a.
spider a.
angiomatosis
cerebroretinal a.
encephalofacial a.
encephalotrigeminal a.
meningocutaneous a.
a. of retina
a. retinae
retinal a.
retinocerebellar a.
angiopathia retinae juvenilis
angiopathic retinopathy
angiopathy
cerebral amyloid a.
angiophakomatosis

NOTES

angiosarcoma
    orbital a.
angioscopy
    fluorescein fundus a.
angioscotoma
angioscotometry
angiospasm
angiospastic retinopathy
angiotensin
angle
    a. of aberration
    a. of abnormality
    alpha a.
    anomaly a.
    a. of anomaly
    a. of anterior chamber
    anterior chamber a.
    a. of aperture
    apical a.
    biorbital a.
    cerebellopontine a. (CPA)
    chamber a.
    a. of convergence
    convergence a.
    critical a.
    deformity a.
    a. of deviation
    a. of direction
    disparity a.
    divergent cut a.
    drainage a.
    a. of eccentricity
    elevation a.
    a. of emergence
    filtration a.
    a. of Fuchs
    gamma a.
    a. of incidence
    incident a.
    iridial a.
    iridocorneal a.
    a. of iris
    Jacquart a.
    kappa a.
    lambda a.
    large kappa a.
    lateral a.
    limiting a.
    medial a.
    meter a.
    minimum separable a.
    minimum visible a.
    minimum visual a.

    ocular a.
    optic a.
    pantoscopic a.
    a. of polarization
    posterior a.
    a. recession
    a. of reflection
    a. of refraction
    refraction a.
    space of iridocorneal a.
    a. of squint
    a. squint
    squint a.
    a. structure
    visual a.
    water-contact a.
    wetting a.
    a. width
    zipped a.
angle-closure glaucoma (ACG)
angled
    a. capsule forceps
    a. counterpressor
    a. discission hook
    a. iris hook and IOL dialer
    a. iris retractor
    a. iris spatula
    a. left/right cannula
    a. lens loupe
    a. manipulator
    a. nucleus removal loupe
    a. probe
    a. suction tube
angle-fixated lens
angle-recession glaucoma
angle-supported lens
angling
    pantoscopic a.
angor ocularis
Ångström
    Å. law
    Å. unit
angular
    a. aqueous sinus plexus
    a. blepharitis
    a. blepharoconjunctivitis
    a. conjunctivitis
    a. distance
    a. gyrus
    a. iridocornealis
    a. junction of eyelid
    a. line
    a. vein

angularis
    blepharitis a.
    vena a.
angulated iris spatula
angulation
    haptic a.
angulus
    a. iridis
    a. iridocornealis
    a. oculi lateralis
    a. oculi medialis
anhydrase
    carbonic a.
    a. glycerol
anicteric
aniridia
    sporadic a.
    traumatic a.
Anis
    A. forceps
    A. irrigating vectis
    A. staple lens
aniseikonia
    spectacle-induced a.
aniseikonic lens
anisoaccommodation
anisochromatic
anisochromia
anisocoria
    benign a.
    central a.
    a. contraction
    essential a.
    physiologic a.
    see-saw a.
    simple a.
anisometric amblyopia
anisometrope
anisometropia
    axial a.
    myopic a.
    refractive a.
anisometropic amblyopia
anisophoria
    induced a.
anisopia
anisotropal

anisotropy
ankyloblepharon
    external a.
    a. filiforme adnatum
    a. totale
anlage
    lacrimal duct a.
annular
    a. bifocal contact lens
    a. cataract
    a. corneal graft
    a. corneal graft operation
    a. infiltrate
    a. keratitis
    a. macular dystrophy
    a. plexus
    a. ring
    a. scleritis
    a. scotoma
    a. staphyloma
    a. synechia
    a. ulcer
annulus, anulus
    a. ciliaris
    a. of conjunctiva
    a. iridis major
    a. iridis minor
    a. tendineus communis
    a. of Zinn
    a. zinnii
anomalopia
anomaloscope
    Kamppeter a.
    Nagel a.
anomalous
    a. disk
    a. fixation
    a. retinal correspondence (ARC)
    a. trichromatism
    a. trichromatopsia
    a. vessel
anomaly
    Alder a.
    angle of a.
    a. angle
    Axenfeld a.

NOTES

anomaly *(continued)*
> Axenfeld-Reiger a. (ARA)
> coloboma a.
> coloboma, heart defects, atresia choanae, retarded growth, genital hypoplasia, and ear a.'s (CHARGE)
> congenital a.
> craniofacial a.
> developmental a.
> excavated optic disk a.
> facial a.
> Klippel-Feil a.
> lacrimal angle duct a.
> location a.
> morning glory optic disk a.
> oculocephalic vascular a.
> optical disk a.
> optic disk a.
> osseous a.
> Peters a.
> Rieger a.

anomia
> color a.

anophoria

anophthalmia
> consecutive a.
> primary a.
> secondary a.

anophthalmic socket

anophthalmos
> congenital a.

anophthalmus

anopia
> amblyopia ex a.

anopsia
> amblyopia ex a.
> ex a.

anorthopia

anorthoscope

anotropia

ANOVA
> analysis of variance

anoxia

antagonist
> contralateral a.
> folic acid a.
> inhibitional palsy of contralateral a.
> ipsilateral a.
> thromboxane receptor a.

$_H$**1-antagonist**

antazoline
> naphazoline and a.
> a. phosphate and naphazoline HCl

Antazoline-V Ophthalmic

anteflexion of iris

anterior
> a. axial developmental cataract
> a. axial embryonal cataract
> a. axonal embryonal cataract
> a. basement membrane dystrophy (ABMD)
> camera bulbi a.
> camera oculi a.
> a. capsulectomy
> a. capsule shagreen
> a. capsulotomy
> a. central curve (ACC)
> a. cerebral artery
> a. chamber (AC)
> a. chamber angle
> a. chamber cannula
> a. chamber cleavage syndrome
> a. chamber inflammation
> a. chamber intraocular lens (ACIOL)
> a. chamber irrigating vectis
> a. chamber irrigator
> a. chamber lymphoma
> a. chamber paracentesis
> a. chamber reaction
> a. chamber shallowing
> a. chamber sinus
> a. chamber synechia scissors
> a. chamber tap
> a. chamber trabecula
> a. chamber tube
> a. chamber washout
> a. choroiditis
> a. ciliary artery
> a. ciliary vein
> a. cleavage syndrome
> a. compressive optic neuropathy
> a. conjunctival artery
> a. conjunctival vein
> a. corneal curvature
> a. corneal staphyloma
> a. cylinder
> a. embryotoxon
> a. epithelium corneae
> A. Eye Segment Analysis System

a. focal point
a. hyaloidal fibrovascular proliferation
a. hyaloid membrane (AHM)
a. hydrophthalmia
a. inferior cerebellar artery (AICA)
a. ischemic optic neuritis
a. ischemic optic neuropathy (AION)
a. keratoconus
a. knee of von Willebrandt
lamina elastica a.
a. lens capsule
a. lenticonus
limiting lamina a.
a. limiting lamina
a. limiting ring
a. lip
a. loop traction
a. megalophthalmus
a. membrane dystrophy
a. mosaic crocodile shagreen
a. ocular segment
a. optical zone (AOZ)
a. optic chiasmal syndrome
a. peripheral curve
a. polar cataract
a. pole
a. pole cataract
a. puncture
a. pyramidal cataract
a. scleritis
a. sclerochoroiditis
a. sclerotomy
a. segment
a. segment angiography
a. segment examination
a. segment of eye
a. segment inflammation
a. segment necrosis
a. segment sleeve
a. staphyloma
a. stromal micropuncture
a. symblepharon
a. synechia
a. uveitis

a. visual pathway
a. visual pathway dysfunction
a. vitrectomy
anteriores
limbus palpebrales a.
vena ciliares a.
anterius
foramen lacerum a.
anterograde degeneration
anteroposterior
a. axis
a. axis of Fick
Anthony orbital compressor
anthracis
Bacillus a.
antiacetylcholine
a. receptor antibody
a. receptor antibody assay
anti-Ach receptor antibody
antiadrenergic drug
antibiotic
bacteriocidal a.
bacteriostatic a.
broad-spectrum a.
fluoroquinolone a.
fortified a.
prophylactic a.
Triple A.
antibody, pl. antibodies
antiacetylcholine receptor a.
anti-Ach receptor a.
antilens protein a.
antineutrophil cytoplasmic a. (ANCA)
antinuclear a. (ANA)
antiphospholipid a.
antirecoverin a.
antiretina a.
chromogranin a.
complement-fixing a.
cytokeratin 7 a.
cytokeratin 20 a.
cytotoxic a.
diolipin a.
ELISA a.
glial fibrillary acidic protein a.
HIV-specific a.

NOTES

antibody *(continued)*
    homotropic a.
    indirect fluorescent a.
    Kermix a.
    monoclonal a.
    neurofilament triplets a.
    neuro-specific enolase a.
    pancytokeratin a.
    S-100 protein a.
    stimulatory a.
    synaptophysin a.
    treponemal a.
anticataract drug
anticholinergic drug
anti-elevation syndrome (AES)
antigen
    Australia a.
    early a.
    EBV-associated a.
    EBV nuclear a.
    extractable nuclear a.
    HLA-A29 a.
    HLA-B5 a.
    HLA-B7 a.
    HLA-B15 a.
    HLA-B27 a.
    HLA-DR4 a.
    human leukocyte a.
    ICAM-1 a.
    Kveim a.
    major histocompatibility a.
    nuclear a.
    rheumatoid-associated nuclear a.
    transplantation a.
    viral capsid a.
antigen-presenting cell
antiglaucoma surgery
Antihist-1
antilens protein antibody
Antilirium
antimetropia
antimongoloid slant
antineutrophil cytoplasmic antibody (ANCA)
antinuclear antibody (ANA)
antiophthalmic
antioxidant enzyme
antiphospholipid antibody
antirecoverin antibody
antireflection coating
antiretina antibody
antisuppression exercise
antitonic

antitorque suture
antixerophthalmic
Antley-Bixler syndrome
Anton
    A. symptom
    A. syndrome
Anton-Babinski syndrome
antonina
    facies a.
Antoni pattern
antrophose
anulus *(var. of* annulus)
Anxanil
AO
    AO binocular indirect ophthalmoscope
    AO Ful-Vue diagnostic unit
    AO lens
    AO lensometer
    AO Project-O-Chart
    AO Reichert Instruments
    AO Reichert Instruments applanation tonometer
    AO Reichert Instruments binocular indirect ophthalmoscope
    AO Reichert Instruments Ful-Vue diagnostic unit
    AO Reichert Instruments lensometer
    AO Reichert Instruments Project-O-Chart
    AO rotary prism
    AO Vectographic Project-O-Chart slide
AODM
    adult-onset diabetes mellitus
Aosept
AO-XT 166 lens
AOZ
    anterior optical zone
APACG
    acute primary angle-closure glaucoma
A-pattern
    A.-p. esotropia
    A.-p. exotropia
    A.-p. strabismus
APD
    afferent pupillary defect
Apert syndrome
aperture
    angle of a.

a. disk
numerical a. (NA)
orbital a.
palpebral a.
pupillary a.
a. ratio
apex, pl. **apices**
corneal a.
a. fracture
orbital a.
petrous a.
A. Plus excimer laser
a. of prism
tumor a.
aphacia (*var. of* aphakia)
aphacic (*var. of* aphakic)
aphacos
aphake
aphakia, aphacia
binocular a.
extracapsular a.
monocular a.
aphakic, aphacic
a. bullous keratopathy (ABK)
a. contact lens
a. correction
a. cystoid macular edema
a. detachment
a. eye
a. glaucoma
a. lens
a. pupillary block
a. spectacles
aphasia
Broca a.
optic a.
visual a.
aphose
aphotesthesia
aphotic
apical
a. angle
a. clearance
a. cone
a. radius
a. tumor

a. zone
a. zone of cornea
apices (*pl. of* apex)
aplanatic
a. focus
a. lens
aplanatism
aplasia
lacrimal nucleus a.
macular a.
a. of optic nerve
optic nerve a.
punctum a.
retinal a.
APMPPE
acute posterior multifocal placoid
pigment epitheliopathy
apochromatic
a. lens
a. objective
apocrine gland
Apollo
A. conjunctivitis
A. disease
aponeurosis
aponeurotic ptosis
apoplectic
a. glaucoma
a. retinitis
apoplexy
occipital a.
a. of pituitary
pituitary a.
retinal a.
apoptag
apostilb
apparatus
Acuson 128 a.
ciliary a.
dioptric a.
Frigitronics nitrous oxide
cryosurgery a.
Golgi a.
lacrimal a.
a. lacrimalis
a. suspensorius lentis
Vactro perilimbal suction a.

NOTES

appearance
   beaten-bronze a.
   beaten-copper a.
   beaten-metal a.
   cobblestone a.
   dropped-socket a.
   feathery a.
   fluffy a.
   granular a.
   leonine a.
   mottled a.
   salt-and-pepper a.
   spongy a.
   squashed-tomato a.
appendage of eye
apperceptive
   a. agnosia
   a. prosopagnosia
applanation
   a. pressure
   tension by a. (TAP)
   a. tension (AT)
   a. tonometry
applanometer
applanometry
application
   autologous serum a.
   diathermy a.
   pilot a.
applicator
   beta therapy eye a.
   cotton-tipped a.
   Gass dye a.
   Gifford a.
Appolionio lens
apposition
   central choroidal a. (CCA)
approach
   ab interno a.
   Berke a.
   Caldwell-Luc a.
   fornix a.
   Iliff a.
   limbal a.
   Lynch a.
   pars plana a.
   transcaruncular-
     transconjunctival a.
   transpunctal endocanalicular a.
apraclonidine
   a. HCl
   a. hydrochloride
   a. ophthalmic solution

apraxia
   acquired ocular motor a.
   Cogan congenital
     oculomotor a.
   congenital ocular motor a.
     (COMA)
   constructional a.
   eyelid a.
   a. of eyelid opening (AEO)
   a. of gaze
   ocular motor a.
   oculomotor a.
Apresoline
A-Probe
   Soft-Touch A.-P.
Apt
Aquaflex
   A. contact lens
Aqua-Flow
aqua oculi
Aquasight lens
AquaSite
   A. Ophthalmic Solution
Aquasonic 100 gel
Aqua-Tears
aqueductal stenosis
aqueous
   a. chamber
   fibrinous a.
   a. flare
   a. flow
   a. humor
   a. humor drainage
   a. humor eye
   a. inflow
   a. layer of tear film
   a. misdirected glaucoma
   a. misdirection
   a. outflow
   a. paracentesis
   plasmoid a.
   a. suppressant
   a. tear deficiency (ATD)
   a. tear layer
   a. transplant needle
   a. tube shunt
   a. vein
aqueous-influx phenomenon
aquocapsulitis
aquosus
   humor a.

AR
  autorefraction
  AR 1000 refractor
ARA
  Axenfeld-Reiger anomaly
Arabic eye test
arachnoid
  a. hemorrhage
  a. sheath
arachnoidal cyst
arachnoiditis
  chiasmal a.
  opticochiasmatic a.
  optochiasmatic a.
Aralen Phosphate
arborescent
  a. cataract
  a. keratitis
arborization
  a. pattern
  pattern a.
ARC
  abnormal retinal correspondence
  AIDS-related complex
  anomalous retinal correspondence
    unharmonious ARC
arc
  a. and bowl perimeter
  contact a.
  a. of contact
  nuclear a.
  a. perimeter
  a. perimetry
  a. scotoma
  a. staining
  xenon a.
arcade
  inferior retinal a.
  inferior temporal a.
  inferotemporal a.
  limbal a.
  major a.
  superior vascular a.
  temporal a.
  vascular a.
arc-flash conjunctivitis

arch
  orbital a.
  Salus a.
  superciliary a.
  supraorbital a.
Archer lesion
architecture
  iris a.
  nasal a.
arciform density
Arc-T blade
arcuate
  a. Bjerrum scotoma
  a. commissure
  a. course
  a. field defect
  a. incision
  a. nerve fiber bundle
  a. retinal fold
  a. staining
  a. transverse keratotomy
arcus, gen. and pl. **arcus**
  a. adiposus
  a. corneae
  corneal a.
  a. cornealis
  juvenile a.
  a. juvenilis
  a. lipoides
  a. lipoides corneae
  a. palpebralis inferior
  a. palpebralis superior
  a. parieto-occipitalis
  a. senilis
  a. superciliaris
  unilateral a.
Arden grating
area, pl. **areae, areas**
  aspheric lenticular a.
  Bjerrum a.
  Brodmann a.
  a. centralis
  a. of conscious regard
  a. cribrosa
  a. of critical definition
  fusion a.
  macular a.

NOTES

area *(continued)*
a. Martegiani
medial superior temporal
visual a.
medial temporal visual a.
middle temporal visual a.
mirror a.
MST visual a.
MT visual a.
Panum fusion a.
papillary a.
parastriate a.
pretectal a.
spindle-shaped a.
visual association a.
areflexia
pupillary a.
areolar
a. central choroiditis
a. choroidopathy
ArF excimer laser
argamblyopia
argema
argon
a. blue laser
a. green laser
a. laser coagulator
a. laser endophotocoagulation
a. laser iridectomy
a. laser peripheral iridoplasty
(ALPI)
a. laser photocoagulation
a. laser trabeculopexy (ALT)
a. laser trabeculoplasty (ALTP)
argon-fluoride excimer laser
argon-pumped tunable dye laser
Argyll-Robertson
A.-R. instrument
A.-R. operation
A.-R. pupil
A.-R. pupil sign
argyria
argyriasis
argyrism
Argyrol S.S.
argyrosis
arida
conjunctivitis a.
aridosiliculose cataract
aridosiliquata
cataracta a.
aridosiliquate cataract

Arion
A. operation
A. sling
Aristocort
Aristospan
ARK
Analysis of Radial Keratotomy
Arlt
A. disease
A. epicanthus repair
A. eyelid repair
A. lens
A. lens loupe
A. line
A. operation
A. pterygium
A. scoop
A. sinus
A. trachoma
A. triangle
Arlt-Jaesche
A.-J. excision
A.-J. operation
A.-J. recess
A.-J. sinus
A.-J. trachoma
ARM
age-related maculopathy
arm
Wiltmoser optical a.
Armaly-Drance technique
ARMD
age-related macular degeneration
dry ARMD
wet ARMD
ARN
acute retinal necrosis
acute retinal necrosis syndrome
ARN syndrome
Arnold
zygomatic foramen of A.
Arnold-Chiari malformation
arrachement
array
ordered a.
radial vessel a.
Arrowhead operation
Arrowsmith corneal marker
Arroyo
A. cataract extraction
A. dacryostomy
A. encircling suture
A. expressor

A. forceps
A. implant
A. keratoplasty
A. operation
A. protector
A. sign
A. tenotomy
A. trephine

Arruga
A. capsule forceps
A. cataract extraction
A. dacryostomy
A. elevator retractor
A. encircling suture
A. expressor
A. implant
A. keratoplasty
A. lacrimal trephine
A. lens
A. needle holder
A. operation
A. orbital retractor
A. protector
A. tenotomy

Arruga-Berens operation
Arruga-McCool capsule forceps
Arruga-Moura-Brazil implant
arsenic amblyopia
arterial
a. circle
a. circle of greater iris
a. circle of lesser iris
a. dissection
a. hypertension
a. macroaneurysm
a. occlusive change
a. occlusive disease

arteriogram
carotid a.

arteriography
cerebral a.

arteriola
a. macularis inferior
a. macularis superior
a. medialis retinae
a. nasalis retinae inferior
a. nasalis retinae superior

a. temporalis retinae inferior
a. temporalis retinae superior

arteriolar
a. attenuation
a. narrowing
a. nicking
a. occlusive disease
a. sclerosis
a. sheathing

arteriole
aneurysm of retinal a.
a. communication
copper-wire a.
inferior macular a.
macular a.
narrowed a.
narrowing of retinal a.
perifoveal a.
retinal a.
silver-wire a.
superior macular a.

arteriolovenous crossing
arteriosclerosis
cerebral a.
a. of retina

arteriosclerotic
a. ischemic optic neuropathy
a. retinopathy

arteriosus
arteriovenous (AV)
a. aneurysm
a. communication
a. crossing defect
a. malformation
a. nicking
a. pattern
a. ratio
a. strabismus syndrome

arteritic
a. anterior ischemic optic
neuropathy

arteritis
cranial a.
giant cell a. (GCA)
occlusive retinal a.
pseudotemporal a.
temporal a. (TA)

NOTES

artery
anterior cerebral a.
anterior ciliary a.
anterior conjunctival a.
anterior inferior cerebellar a.
(AICA)
basilar a.
calcarine a.
carotid a.
central a.
central retinal a. (CRA)
cerebellar a.
cerebral a.
ciliary a.
cilioretinal a.
conjunctival a.
copper-wire a.
corkscrew a.
dolichoectatic anterior
cerebral a.
episcleral a.
ethmoidal a.
hyaline a.
hyaloid a.
hypophyseal a.
inferior nasal a.
inferior temporal a.
inferonasal a.
inferotemporal a.
infraorbital a.
internal carotid a.
intracavernous carotid a.
lacrimal a.
long ciliary a.
long posterior ciliary a.
middle cerebral a.
ophthalmic a.
optic a.
parieto-occipital a.
posterior cerebral a.
posterior ciliary a.
posterior conjunctival a.
retinal a.
retrobulbar a.
short ciliary a.
short posterior ciliary a.
superior nasal a.
superior temporal a.
supraorbital a.
tarsal a.
temporal a.
temporo-occipital a.
thrombosed a.

a.-to-vein ratio (A/V)
vertebrobasilar a.
zygomatico-orbital a.
arthrokinetic nystagmus
arthro-ophthalmopathy
hereditary progressive a.-o.
Arthus reaction
articularis
lentis a.
artifact
high-gain a.
artifactiously
artifactual
artificial
a. cornea
a. diabetes
a. divergence procedure
a. divergency surgery
a. eye
a. lens
a. pupil
a. silk keratitis
A. Tears
a. tears
a. UV radiation
a. vision
Artisan lens
Arysoft foldable acrylic lens
A-scan
Cilco Sonometric A-s.
Jedmed A-s.
Jedmed/DGH A-s.
A-s. ultrasonogram
A-s. ultrasonography
Ascaris lumbricoides
Ascher
A. aqueous-influx phenomenon
A. glass-rod phenomenon
A. syndrome
A. vein
Aschner reflex
Asch septal forceps
Ascon instrument
ash leaf spot
ASICO multi-angled diamond knife
AsM
myopic astigmatism
aspartoacylase
aspartylglycosaminuria
aspergillosis
a. uveitis
Aspergillus
A. *flavus*

A. *fumigatus*
A. *terreus*
aspheric
a. cataract lens
a. contact lens
a. cornea
a. lenticular area
a. spectacle lens
aspherical ophthalmoscopic lens
aspheric-viewing lens
aspirate
vitreoretinal a.
aspirating/irrigating vectis
aspiration
Alcon a.
cataract a.
a. of cortex
fine-needle a.
irrigation and a. (I&A)
a. of lens
vitreous a.
aspirator
Alcon a.
Castroviejo orbital a.
Cavitron a.
Cooper a.
Fibra Sonics phaco a.
Fink cataract a.
Kelman a.
Legacy Series 2000
Cavitron/Kelman phaco-
emulsifier a.
Nugent soft cataract a.
Stat a.
aspirator/hydrodissector
Alpern cortex a.
aspirin
assay
antiacetylcholine receptor
antibody a.
enzyme-linked
immunosorbent a. (ELISA)
immunofluorescent a.
Leber hereditary optic atrophy
reverse dot-blot a.
Lowry a.
mucous a.

Raji cell a.
southern blot hybridization a.
urinary GAG a.
urinary glycosaminoglycan
measurement a.
assessment
Hirschberg reflex a.
ocular hemodynamic a.
quantitative haze a.
ASSI
A. cannula
A. IOL inserter forceps
A. universal lens folding
forceps
Associates
Prosthetic Orthotic A.
Association
American Medical A.
A. of Technical Personnel in
Ophthalmology (ATPO)
association
CHARGE a.
teratogenic a.
associative prosopagnosia
Ast
astigmatism
astemizole
asteroid
a. body
a. hyalitis
hyaloid a.
a. hyalosis
asteroides
Nocardia a.
asthenocoria
asthenometer
asthenope
asthenopia
accommodative a.
muscular a.
nervous a.
neurasthenic a.
retinal a.
tarsal a.
asthenopic
astigmagraph
astigmagraphic error

NOTES

astigmatic
    a. amblyopia
    a. axis
    a. clock
    a. dial
    a. dial chart
    a. image
    a. keratotomy (AK)
    a. keratotomy enhancement
    a. lens
    a. marker
    a. refractive error
    a. vector analysis
astigmatism (Ast)
    acquired a.
    against-the-rule a.
    asymmetric a.
    central a.
    compound hyperopic a.
    compound myopic a.
    congenital a.
    corneal a.
    a. correction
    direct a.
    hypermetropic a.
    hyperopic a.
    inverse a.
    irregular a.
    keratometric a.
    lenticular a.
    mixed a.
    myopic a. (AsM)
    oblique a.
    a. of oblique pencils
    penetrating keratoplasty a.
    physiologic a.
    pterygium-induced a.
    radial a.
    radical a.
    refractive a.
    regular a.
    residual a.
    reversed a.
    simple hyperopic a.
    simple myopic a.
    "suture-out" a.
    topographic a.
    total a.
    a. with the rule
    with-the-rule a.
astigmatome
    Terry a.
astigmatometer, astigmometer

astigmatometry, astigmometry
astigmatoscope, astigmoscope
astigmatoscopy, astigmoscopy
astigmia
astigmic
astigmometer (*var. of* astigmatometer)
astigmometry (*var. of* astigmatometry)
astigmoscope (*var. of* astigmatoscope)
astigmoscopy (*var. of* astigmatoscopy)
astrocytic
    a. glioma
    a. hamartoma
astrocytoma
    juvenile pilocytic a.
    pilocytic a.
    retinal a.
asymmetric
    a. astigmatism
    a. papilledema
    a. refractive error
    a. surgery
asymmetry
    chromatic a.
asymptomatic optic neuritis
AT
    applanation tension
    Fluor-I-Strip AT
Atabrine
Atarax
ataxia
    cerebellar a.
    cone dystrophy-cerebellar a.
    familial episodic a.
    familial paroxysmal a.
    Friedreich a.
    hereditary cerebellar a.
    Marie a.
    ocular a.
    optic a.
    Pierre-Marie a.
    spinocerebellar a.
    vestibulocerebellar a.
ataxia-telangiectasia
    a.-t. syndrome
ataxic nystagmus
ATD
    aqueous tear deficiency
atenolol
Athens suture spreader

atheroembolism
atheroma
atherosclerosis
    diffuse a.
    ischemic a.
atherosclerotic ischemic neuritis
athetosis
    pupillary a.
Atkin lid block
Atkinson
    A. block
    A. corneal scissors
    A. 25-G short curved
      cystitome
    A. retrobulbar needle
    A. sclerotome
    A. single-bevel blunt-tip needle
    A. technique
    A. tip peribulbar needle
Atlas-Elite laser
Atlas ophthalmic laser
atonic
    a. ectropion
    a. entropion
    a. epiphora
atopic
    a. cataract
    a. conjunctivitis
    a. eczema keratoconjunctivitis
    a. line
atovaquone
ATPase
    actomyosin ATPase
ATPO
    Association of Technical Personnel
    in Ophthalmology
Atraloc suture
atresia
    a. iridis
    retinal a.
    tilting lens a.
atretoblepharia
atretopsia
Atropa belladonna
Atropair
atrophia
    a. bulbi

    a. bulborum hereditaria
    a. choroideae et retinae
    a. dolorosa
    a. gyrata
atrophic
    a. age-related macular
      degeneration (AAMD)
    a. degenerative maculopathy
    a. excavation
    a. heterochromia
    a. hole
    a. macular degeneration
    a. polychondritis
    a. rhinitis
atrophy
    autosomal-dominant optic a.
    autosomal-recessive optic a.
    band optic a.
    Behr optic a.
    bow-tie optic a.
    bulbous a.
    cavernous optic a.
    central areolar choroidal a.
    central gyrate a.
    cerebral a.
    choriocapillary a.
    chorioretinal a.
    choroidal epithelial a.
    choroidal gyrate a.
    choroidal myopic a.
    choroidal secondary a.
    choroidal vascular a.
    congenital optic a.
    consecutive optic a.
    diabetic optic a.
    diffuse inflammatory eyelid a.
    dominant optic a.
    essential iris a.
    essential progressive a. of iris
    flat chorioretinal a.
    Fuchs a.
    geographic a.
    glaucomatous a.
    gray a.
    growth retardation, alopecia,
      pseudoanodontia, and optic a.
      (GAPO)

NOTES

atrophy *(continued)*
    gyrate a.
    gyrate a. of choroid and
      retina
    helicoid peripapillary a.
    hemifacial a.
    hereditary optic a.
    heredodegenerative a.
    heredofamilial optic a.
    infantile optic a.
    iris a.
    ischemic choroidal a.
    ischemic optic a.
    juvenile optic a.
    Kjer dominant optic a.
    Leber hereditary optic a.
    linear subcutaneous a.
    morning glory optic a.
    myopic choroidal a.
    neuritic a.
    neurogenic iris a.
    nummular a.
    olivopontocerebellar a. (OPCA)
    optic disk a.
    a. of optic nerve
    optic nerve a.
    opticoacoustic nerve a.
    patchy a.
    periorbital fat a.
    peripapillary choroidal a.
    peripheral chorioretinal a.
    pigment a.
    pigmented paravenous
      chorioretinal a.
    pigmented paravenous
      retinochoroidal a.
    postinflammatory a.
    postpapilledema a.
    primary optic a.
    progressive choroidal a.
    progressive encephalopathy with
      edema, hypsarrhythmia and
      optic a. (PEHO)
    progressive hemifacial a.
    progressive optic a.
    retinal pigment epithelial a.
    retinochoroidal a.
    Schnabel optic a.
    secondary optic a.
    segmental iris a.
    senile a.
    sex-linked recessive optic a.
    simple optic a.
    subcutaneous fat a.
    tabetic optic a.
    traumatic a.
    uveal a.

atropine
    A.-Care
    a. conjunctivitis
    Isopto A.
    a. and prednisolone
    prednisolone and a.
    a. sulfate

atropinism

atropinization

Atropisol

attachment
    Accuvac smoke evacuation a.
    desmosomal cellular a.
    MP video endoscopic lens a.
    pathometer a.
    photo-kerato a.
    Planarm Haag Streit a.
    specular a.
    vitreoretinal a.
    zonular a.

attack
    transient ischemic a. (TIA)

attentional dyslexia

attention reflex

attentiveness
    visual a.

attenuation
    arteriolar a.
    focal a.

A-tuck

Atwood loupe

atypical
    a. achromatopsia
    a. coloboma
    a. facial pain
    a. mycobacteria

Aubert phenomenon

audiokinetic nystagmus

auditory
    a. oculogyric reflex
    a. perceptual disability
    a. stimulus

augmentation
    periorbital volume a.

aural
    a. nystagmus
    a. scotoma

Aureomycin

aureus
    methicillin-resistant
      Staphylococcus a.
      Staphylococcus a.
auriasis
auricular glaucoma
Aus Jena-Schiötz tonometer
Australia antigen
Australian Corneal Graft Registry
autofluorescence
autofunduscope
autofunduscopy
autogenous
    a. dermis fat graft
    a. donor material
    a. keratoplasty
autograft
    free conjunctival a.
    free skin a.
    full-thickness a.
    skin a.
    split-thickness a.
autografting
    conjunctival rotation a.
    limbal a.
autoimmune
    a. corneal endotheliopathy
    a. demyelination
autokeratometer
autokeratometry
autokeratoplasty
auto-kerato-refractometer
    KR-7000P a.-k.-r.
    Topcon KR-7500 a.-k.-r.
autokinesis visible light
autokinetic
    a. effect
    a. visible light phenomenon
AutoLensmeter
    Tomey Trooper A.
autologous
    a. chondrocyte transplantation
    a. serum application
autolysis
automated
    a. corneal shaper
    a. hemisphere perimeter

    a. lamellar keratectomy
    a. lamellar keratoplasty (ALK)
    a. lamellar keratoplasty-Excimer
    (ALK-E)
    a. laser keratomileusis (ALK)
    a. microkeratome
    a. refractor
    a. static threshold perimetry
    a. trephine
    a. visual field
automatic
    a. infrared optometer
    a. refractor
    a. tonometry
    a. trephine
    a. twin syringe injector
autonomic
    a. nervous system
    a. nervous system disorder
Autonomous Technologies laser
auto-ophthalmoscope
auto-ophthalmoscopy
autoperimetry
    short wavelength a.
autophagic vacuole
Autophoro-Optimeter
    Clark A.-O.
AutoRef-keratometer
autorefraction (AR)
Autorefractor-7
    Subjective A.-7
autorefractor
    6600 A.
    Hoya AR-570 a.
    Nikon Retinomax K-Plus a.
    Retinomax cordless hand-
    held a.
    Tomey a.
autorefractor/keratometer
    Retinomax K-Plus a.
autoregulation
autosomal
    a. dominant congenital cataract
    a. dominant hereditary optic
    neuropathy
    a. dominant oculocutaneous
    albinism

NOTES

autosomal *(continued)*
    a. dominant retinitis
      pigmentosa
    a. dominant vitelli rupture
    a. recessive hereditary optic
      neuropathy
    a. recessive ocular albinism
autosomal-dominant
    a.-d. ophthalmoplegia
    a.-d. optic atrophy
autosomal-recessive
    a.-r. ophthalmoplegia
    a.-r. optic atrophy
Autoswitch System
autotopographer
    Tomey a.
auxiliary
    a. fiber
    a. lens
auxometer
AV
    arteriovenous
    AV crossing defect
    AV nicking
    AV pattern
    AV strabismus syndrome
A/V
    artery-to-vein ratio
avascular
    a. corneal stroma
    a. keratitis
    a. peripheral retina
    a. plaque
avascularity
Avellino dystrophy
Avit handpiece
avium
    Mycobacterium a.
avulsion
    a. of caruncula lacrimalis
    a. of eyelid
    facial nerve a.
a-wave test
AWE
    advancing wave-like epitheliopathy
awl
    lacrimal a.
    Mustarde a.
axanthopsia
Axenfeld
    A. anomaly
    A. follicular conjunctivitis

    A. nerve loop
    A. syndrome
Axenfeld-Fieger syndrome
Axenfeld-Krukenberg spindle
Axenfeld-Reiger
    A.-R. anomaly (ARA)
    A.-R. syndrome
axes (*pl. of* axis)
axial
    a. amblyopia
    a. ametropia
    a. anisometropia
    a. chamber
    a. cornea
    a. CT scan
    a. curvature map
    a. curvature mapping
    a. embryonal cataract
    a. fusiform developmental
      cataract
    a. hyperopia
    a. illumination
    a. length (AL)
    a. length/corneal radius ratio
      (AL/CR ratio, axial
      length/corneal radius ratio)
    a. length of eye
    a. myopia
    a. partial childhood cataract
    a. point
    a. proptosis
    a. ray of light
    a. tomography
    a. view
axial length/corneal radius ratio
    (*var. of* AL/CR ratio) **(AL/CR**
    ratio, axial length/corneal radius
    ratio)
axillary cataract
axis, pl. **axes**
    achromatic a.
    anteroposterior a.
    astigmatic a.
    a. bulbi externus
    a. bulbi internus
    cylinder a.
    a. of cylindric lens (x)
    Fick a.
    a. of Fick
    a. fixation
    frontal a.
    geometric a.
    hypothalamic-pituitary-thyroid a.

lens a.
a. lentis
longitudinal a.
ocular a.
a. oculi externa
a. oculi interna
optic a.
optical a.
a. opticus
orbital a.
principal optic a.
pupillary a.
red-green a.
sagittal a.
secondary a.
tritan a.
vertical a.
visual a.
Axisonic II ultrasound
AXM
    acetoxycyclohexamide
axometer
axon
    fiber layer of a.
    nerve fiber a.

preganglionic
    parasympathetic a.
retinal a.
axonal loss
axonometer
axoplasm
axoplasmic
    a. flow
    a. stasis
Ayers chalazion forceps
Ayerst instrument
Azar
    A. curved cystitome
    A. lens
    A. lens-holding forceps
    A. lens-manipulating hook
    A. lid speculum
azatadine
azidamfenicol
azithromycin
azlocillin
AZOOR
    acute zonal occult outer retinopathy
Azopt
azotemic retinitis

NOTES

2b
    interferon alfa-2b
baby Barraquer needle holder
Baciguent
bacillary layer
Bacillus
    B. anthracis
    B. cereus
    B. fragilis
    B. pyocyaneus
    B. subtilis
bacillus, pl. **bacilli**
    acid-fast bacilli
    gonococcal b.
    Koch-Weeks b.
    pneumococcal b.
    streptococcal b.
    tubercle b.
    Weeks b.
bacitracin
    b. zinc
    zinc b.
**bacitracin, neomycin, and
    polymyxin B**
**bacitracin, neomycin, polymyxin B,
    and hydrocortisone**
bacitracin and polymyxin B
back
    b. optic zone radius (BOZR)
    b. surface toric contact lens
    b. vertex power (BVP)
background
    b. diabetic retinopathy (BDR)
    b. illumination
    b. luminance
    tigroid b.
Backhaus
    B. clamp
    B. syndrome
backscattering
bacteria
    gram-negative b.
    gram-positive b.
    saprophytic b.
bacterial
    b. blepharitis
    b. blepharoconjunctivitis
    b. collagenase
    b. conjunctivitis
    b. contamination

    b. corneal binding
    b. culture
    b. endophthalmitis
    b. infection
    b. infectious corneal infiltrate
    b. infectious corneal ulcer
    b. keratitis
    b. superinfection
    b. uveitis
bacteriocidal antibiotic
bacteriostatic antibiotic
Bacteroides melaninogenicus
Bacticort
Bactrim
Badal
    B. Lensmeter
    B. operation
    B. stimulus system
Baer nystagmus
Baerveldt
    B. filtering procedure
    B. glaucoma implant
    B. glaucoma implant tube
    B. seton implant
    B. shunt
    B. shunt tube
bag
    capsular b.
    palpebral adipose b.
baggy eyelid
Bagley-Wilmer expressor
Bagolini
    B. lens
    B. striated glasses test
Bahn spud
Baikoff lens
Bailey
    B. chalazion forceps
    B. foreign body remover
    B. lacrimal cannula
Bailey-Lovie
    B.-L. logMar chart
    B.-L. Near Test
    B.-L. visual acuity chart
Bailliart
    B. goniometer
    B. ophthalmodynamometer
    B. ophthalmoscope
Baird chalazion forceps

B

Baker equation (corneal aspheric measurement)
balance
    Humphriss binocular b.
    meridional b.
    muscular b.
balanced
    b. saline solution
    b. salt solution (BSS)
Baldex
balding the limbus
Balint syndrome
ball
    ice b.
    Pinky b.
    retinal ice b.
    Super Pinky b.
ballast
    prism b.
    b. prism
ballasted contact lens
Ballen-Alexander
    B.-A. forceps
    B.-A. orbital retractor
Baller-Gerold syndrome
Ballet
    B. disease
    B. sign
balloon
    b. buckle
    endocapsular b.
    Honan b.
    Lincoff b.
ballottement
    ocular b.
Balo
    concentric sclerosis of B.
balsam
    Canada b.
Baltimore Eye Survey
Bamatter syndrome
band
    #40 b.
    A b.
    cellophane-like b.
    ciliary body b.
    circling b.
    encircling b.
    fascia b.
    H b.
    keratitis b.
    b. keratitis
    b. keratopathy

    M b.
    Mach b.
    b. optic atrophy
    retinal demarcation b.
    scleral b.
    silicone b.
    Storz b.
    traction b.
    Watzke b.
    Z b.
    zonular b.
bandage
    binocle b.
    binocular b.
    Borsch b.
    Elastoplast b.
    monocular b.
    pressure b.
    b. scissors
    b. soft contact lens
bandelette
    keratitis b.
bandpass function
band-shaped
    b.-s. keratitis
    b.-s. keratopathy
Bangerter
    B. iris spatula
    B. method of pleoptics
    B. muscle forceps
    B. pterygium operation
Bangla Joy conjunctivitis
bank
    eye b.
    b. keratitis
    Lions Doheny Eye and Tissue Transplant B.
    New England Eye B.
banking
    venule b.
Bannayan syndrome
Banner
    B. enucleation snare
    B. forceps
    B. snare enucleator
Banophen Oral
Baquacil
bar
    Berens prism b.
    horizontal prism b.
    b. prism
    prism b.

b. reader
skiascopy b.
Bárány
  B. caloric test
  B. sign
barbital
Bardelli lid ptosis operation
Bardet-Biedl syndrome
Bard-Parker
  #15 B.-P. blade
  B.-P. blade
  B.-P. forceps
  B.-P. keratome
  B.-P. knife
  B.-P. razor
  B.-P. trephine
Bard sign
bare
  b. lymphocyte syndrome
  b. scleral technique
bared sclera
bare-sclera excision
baring
  b. of blind spot
  b. of sclera
Barkan
  B. double cyclodialysis operation
  B. goniolens
  B. gonioscopic lens
  B. goniotomy knife
  B. goniotomy lens
  B. goniotomy operation
  B. infant implant
  B. iris forceps
  B. light
  B. membrane
  B. theory
Barkan-Cordes linear cataract operation
Barlow syndrome
Barnes-Hind
  B.-H. contact lens cleaning and soaking solution
  B.-H. wetting solution
Baron-Bietti syndrome
Baron lens

barrage
  double-row diathermy b.
Barraquer
  B. applanation tonometer
  B. cannula
  B. cilia forceps
  B. conjunctival forceps
  B. corneal dissector
  B. corneal utility forceps
  B. cryolathe
  B. curved holder
  B. enzymatic zonulolysis operation
  B. erysiphake
  B. eye shield
  B. hemostatic mosquito forceps
  B. implant
  B. iris scissors
  B. irrigator spatula
  B. keratomileusis operation
  B. keratoplasty knife
  B. lens
  B. method
  B. microkeratome
  B. needle
  B. needle carrier
  B. needle holder
  B. needle holder clamp
  B. operating room tonometer
  B. razor bladebreaker
  B. sable brush
  B. sweep
  B. trephine
  B. vitreous strand scissors
  B. wire speculum
  B. zonulolysis
Barraquer-Carriazo microkeratome
Barraquer-Colibri speculum
Barraquer-DeWecker scissors
Barraquer-Krumeich
  B.-K. Swinger refractor
  B.-K. test
Barraquer-Krumeich-Swinger retractor
Barraquer-Vogt needle
Barraquer-von Mandach capsule forceps

NOTES

Barr body
barred distortion
barrel distortion
Barré sign
Barrett hydrodelineation cannula
Barrie-Jones
   canaliculodacryorhinostomy
   operation
barrier
   blood b.
   blood-aqueous b.
   blood-ocular b.
   blood-optic nerve b.
   blood-retinal b.
   B. drape
   epithelial b.
   ocular b.
   B. Phaco Extracapsular Pack
   posterior capsular zonular b.
   B. sheet
Barrio operation
Barron
   B. donor corneal punch
   B. epikeratophakia trephine
   B. radial vacuum trephine
Barron-Hessburg corneal trephine
Bartel spectacles
Bartholin syndrome
Bartonella henselae
bartonellosis
   ocular b.
basal
   b. cell
   b. cell carcinoma
   b. cell carcinoma of eyelid
   b. cell nevus
   b. cell nevus syndrome
   b. choroid
   b. ciliary body
   b. coil
   b. encephalocele
   b. epithelial nerve
   b. ganglia disease
   b. ganglia lesion
   b. ganglion
   b. iridectomy
   b. junction
   b. lamina
   b. lamina of choroid
   b. lamina of ciliary body
   b. laminar deposit (BLD)
   b. laminar drusen
   b. layer

   b. ophthalmoplegia
   b. phoria
   b. tear secretion
basalis
   b. choroideae lamina
   b. corporis ciliaris lamina
base in (BI)
base
   cilia b.
   b. curve
   b. plate
   sloughing b.
   vitreous b.
baseball lens
Basedow disease
base-down prism (BD)
base-in
   b.-i. prism
   b.-i. reserve
basement
   b. membrane (BM)
   b. membrane disorder
   b. membrane dystrophy
base out (BO)
base-out
   b.-o. prism
   b.-o. reserve
   4Δ b.-o. test
base up, base-up prism
basic
   b. esotropia
   b. exotropia
   b. secretion test
basilar
   b. artery
   b. artery aneurysm
   b. impression
   b. migraine
basin of inferior orbital fissure
basket
   Schultz fiber b.
basket-style scleral supporter
   speculum
Basol-S
basophilic
   b. adenoma
   b. intranuclear inclusion body
   b. reaction
Bassen-Kornzweig syndrome
Basterra operation
BAT
   Brightness Acuity Test
bathomorphic

Batten
- B. disease
- B. syndrome

Batten-Mayou
- B.-M. disease
- B.-M. syndrome

Battle sign
Baumgarten gland
Bausch
- B. & Lomb manual keratometer
- B. & Lomb Optima lens
- B. & Lomb Surgical L161U lens

Bausch-Lomb-Thorpe slit lamp
bay
- junctional b.
- lacrimal b.

Bayadi lens
Baylisascaris procyonis
bayonet forceps
BB shot forceps
BC
- 8.4 BC disposable lens

BCVA
- best-corrected visual acuity

BD
- base-down prism

B-D needle
BDR
- background diabetic retinopathy

bead
- glass b.

beading
- retinal venous b.
- venous b.

beaked forceps
Béal
- B. conjunctivitis
- B. syndrome

beam
- aiming b.
- convergent b.
- divergent b.
- helium neon b.
- He-Ne b.

- proton b.
- b. scatter

Beard
- B. knife
- B. operation

Beard-Cutler operation
beaten-bronze appearance
beaten-copper appearance
beaten-metal appearance
Beaupre cilia forceps
Beaver
- B. blade
- 5435 B. blade
- B. cataract cryoextractor
- B. Dam Eye Study
- B. discission blade
- B. eye blade
- B. goniotomy needle knife
- B. handle
- B. keratome
- B. Ocu-1 curved cystitome
- B. Optimum blade
- B. scleral Lundsgaard blade
- B. Xstar knife

Beaver-Lundsgaard blade
Beaver-Okamura blade
Beaver-Ziegler
- B.-Z. needle blade

BEB
- benign essential blepharospasm

Bechert
- B. 7-mm lens
- B. nucleus rotator

Bechert-Kratz cannulated nucleus retractor
Bechert-McPherson angled tying forceps
Becker
- B. corneal section spatulated scissors
- B. goniogram
- B. gonioscopic prism

Becker-Park speculum
Beckerscope binocular microscope
bed
- capillary b.
- corneal stromal b.

NOTES

B

bed *(continued)*
    recipient b.
    retinal capillary b.
    stromal b.
bedewing
    b. of cornea
    corneal b.
    epithelial b.
    b. to wet
Beebe
    B. lens
    B. loupe
Beer
    B. blade
    B. canaliculus knife
    B. cataract knife
    B. Collyrium
    B. law
    B. operation
Behçet
    B. disease
    B. skin puncture test
    B. syndrome
    B. uveitis
Behr
    B. disease
    B. optic atrophy
    B. pupil
    B. syndrome
Behren rule
Bekhterev
    B. nystagmus
    B. reflex
    B. sign
Belin double-ended needle holder
Belix Oral
Bell
    B. erysiphake
    B. palsy
    B. phenomenon
    B. reflex
belladonna
    b. alkaloid
    Atropa b.
Bellows
    B. cryoextractor
    B. cryophake
belly
    b. of muscle
    muscle b.
    b. of pterygium
belonoskiascopy *(var. of*
  velonoskiascopy)

Belz lacrimal sac rongeur
Benadryl Oral
Benazol
bench
    optical b.
bendazac
bender
    Watt stave b.
bending power
Benedict orbit operation
Benedikt syndrome
benign
    b. anisocoria
    b. concentric annular macular
      dystrophy
    b. dyskeratosis
    b. essential blepharospasm
      (BEB)
    b. mucosal pemphigoid
    b. paroxysmal positional
      vertigo (BPPV)
    b. retinal vasculitis
    b. tumor
Bennett
    B. cilia forceps
benoxinate
    b. hydrochloride
Benson disease
bent
    b. blunt blade
    b. blunt needle
    b. 22-gauge needle
Benton Facial Recognition Test
benzalkonium
    b. chloride
Béraud valve
Bercovici wire lid speculum
**Beren pterygium transplant
operation**
Berens
    B. blade
    B. cataract knife
    B. conical implant
    B. corneal dissector
    B. corneal transplant forceps
    B. corneal transplant scissors
    B. corneoscleral punch
    B. dilator
    B. electrode
    B. expressor
    B. glaucoma knife
    B. iridocapsulotomy scissors
    B. keratoplasty knife

B

B. lens loupe
B. lid everter
B. lid retractor
B. marking calipers
B. muscle clamp
B. muscle forceps
B. orbital compressor
B. partial keratome
B. pinhole and dominance test
B. prism
B. prism bar
B. ptosis forceps
B. ptosis knife
B. pyramidal implant
B. refractor
B. scleral hook
B. sclerectomy operation
B. spatula
B. speculum
B. sterilizing case
B. suturing forceps
B. test object
B. three-character test
B. tonometer
Berens-Rosa scleral implant
Berens-Smith
B.-S. cul-de-sac restoration
B.-S. operation
Berens-Tolman ocular hypertension indicator
Berger
B. sign
B. space
B. symptom
Bergland-Warshawski phaco/cortex kit
Bergmeister
papilla of B.
B. papilla
Bergsma-Kaiser-Kupfer oculocutaneous albinism
Berke
B. approach
B. clamp
B. lid everter
B. operation

B. ptosis
B. ptosis forceps
Berke-Krönlein orbitotomy
Berkeley
B. Bioengineering bipolar cautery
B. Bioengineering brass scleral plug
B. Bioengineering infusion terminal port
B. Bioengineering mechanized scissors
B. Bioengineering ocutome
B. Bioengineering ptosis forceps
B. Bioengineering stiletto
Berke-Motais operation
Berlin
B. disease
B. edema
Berman
B. foreign body locator
B. localizer
Bernard-Horner syndrome
Bernard syndrome
Bernell
B. grid
B. tangent screen
Bernheimer fibers
berry
b. aneurysm
B. circle
Bertel position
besiclometer
Best
B. degeneration
B. disease
B. vitelliform macular dystrophy
best-corrected
b.-c. vision
b.-c. visual acuity (BCVA)
beta
AK B.
b. carotene
b. crystallin

NOTES

beta *(continued)*
    b. radiation
    b. therapy eye applicator
Betadine
Betagan
    B. Liquifilm
Betagen
betamethasone
    b. phosphate eye drops
betaxolol
    b. HCl
    b. hydrochloride
Bethke
    B. iridectomy
    B. operation
Betimol
    B. Ophthalmic
Betoptic
    B. Ophthalmic
    B. S Ophthalmic
Betoptic S
Bettman-Noyes fixation forceps
beveled-edge lens
Bezold-Brücke phenomenon
BFVW
    blood flow velocity waveform
BI
    base in
Bianchi
    B. sign
    B. valve
Biber-Haab-Dimmer
    B.-H.-D. corneal dystrophy
    B.-H.-D. degeneration
bibrocathol
bibrocatol-cincain
bicanalicular tubing
bicarbonate
    sodium b.
bicentric
    b. grinding
    b. spectacle lens
Bick procedure
biconcave
    b. contact lens
biconvex lens
bicoronal scalp flap
bicurve contact lens
bicylindrical lens
Bidwell ghost
Bielschowsky
    B. disease
    B. operation

    B. phenomenon
    B. sign
    B. strabismus
    B. three-step, head-tilt test
Bielschowsky-Jansky
    B.-J. disease
    B.-J. syndrome
Bielschowsky-Lutz-Cogan syndrome
Bielschowsky-Parks head-tilt three-step test
Biemond syndrome
Bietti
    B. crystalline corneoretinal dystrophy
    B. keratopathy
    B. lens
    B. syndrome
    B. tapetoretinal degeneration
bifermentans
    Clostridium b.
Bifidobacterium
bifixation
bifocal, pl. **bifocals**
    b. cement
    cement b.
    b. contact lens
    curved-top b.
    Emerson one-piece segment b.
    executive b.
    b. fixation
    flat top b.
    Franklin b.
    Ful-Vue b.
    b. glasses
    high-add bifocals
    b. intracorneal lens
    invisible b.
    Kryptok b.
    Morck cement b.
    Nokrome b.
    one-piece b.
    Panoptic b.
    plastic b.
    progressive-add b.
    round top b.
    Schnaitmann b.
    b. segment
    b. spectacle lens
    b. spectacles
    straight-line b.
    Ultex b.
    Univis b.
bifoveal fixation

B

bifurcation
big blind spot syndrome
Bigliano tonometer
biguanide
    polyhexamethylene b.
    tropical polyhexamethylene b.
bilaminar membrane
bilateral
    b. altitudinal field defect
    b. hemianopia
    b. homonymous altitudinal
      defect
    b. homonymous hemianopsia
    b. hypotony
    b. keratoconjunctivitis
    b. occipital lobe lesion
    b. sporadic retinoblastoma
    b. strabismus
    b. uveal effusion syndrome
    b. uveitis
    b. visual field defect
bimedial recession
binasal
    b. field defect
    b. hemianopsia
    b. quadrant field
binding
    bacterial corneal b.
Binkhorst
    B. collar stud lens implant
    B. four-loop iris-fixated
      implant
    B. four-loop iris-fixated lens
    B. intraocular lens
    B. iridocapsular lens
    B. irrigating cannula
    B. tip
    B. two-loop intraocular lens
      implant
    B. two-loop lens
Binkhorst-Fyodorov lens
BINO
    binocular internuclear
    ophthalmoplegia
binocle
    b. bandage
    b. dressing

binocular
    b. accommodation
    b. amplitude
    b. aphakia
    b. bandage
    b. depth perception
    b. diplopia
    b. disparity
    b. dressing
    b. eye patch
    b. field
    b. fixation
    b. fixation forceps
    b. function
    b. fusion
    b. hemianopsia
    b. heterochromia
    b. imbalance
    b. indirect ophthalmoscope
    b. indirect ophthalmoscopy
    b. internuclear ophthalmoplegia
      (BINO)
    b. loupe
    b. luster
    b. ophthalmoscope
    b. parallax
    b. perimetry
    b. polyopia
    b. rivalry
    b. single vision (BSV)
    b. strabismus
    b. visual acuity
    B. Visual Acuity Test
binocularity
binoculus
binophthalmoscope
binoscope
biochrome test
bioconvex optic
Bio-Eye ocular implant
biofilm
Biogel Sensor surgical glove
Biohist-LA
BioLon
    B. 1% solution
BioMask
Biomatrix ocular implant

NOTES

45

Biometer
  Ophthasonic Ultrasonic B.
biometric ruler
biometry
  B-scan b.
  b. test
biomicroscope
  high-frequency ultrasound b.
  Nikon FS-3 photo slit
  lamp B.
  b. slit lamp
biomicroscopic indirect lens
biomicroscopy
  contact lens b.
  laser b.
  slit-lamp b.
  ultrasound b. (UBM)
Biomydrin
Bion
  B. Tears
  B. Tears eye drops
  B. Tears Solution
Bio-Optics
  B.-O. Bambi Cell Analysis
  System
  B.-O. Bambi fixed-frame
  method
  B.-O. Bambi image analysis
  system
  B.-O. camera
  B.-O. specular microscope
  B.-O. telescope system
Bio-Pen
  B.-P. biometric ruler
biophotometer
Biophysic
  B. Medical YAG laser
  B. Ophthascan S instrument
Biopore membrane
biopsy
  corneal b.
  greater superficial temporal
  artery b.
  temporal artery b.
  vitreous aspiration b.
biopter test
bioptic amorphic lens system
biorbital angle
Biotic-O
biperiden
biphasic curve
bipolar
  b. cautery

b. cone
b. diathermy adapter clip
b. forceps
b. horizontal interaction
b. retinal cell
b. rod
biprism applanation tonometer
biprong muscle marker
Birbeck granule
Birch-Harman irrigator
Birch-Hirschfeld
  B.-H. entropion operation
  B.-H. lamp
Birch lamp
birdshot
  b. chorioretinitis
  b. chorioretinopathy
  b. choroiditis
  b. retinochoroiditis
  b. retinochoroidopathy
  b. retinopathy
  b. spot
birefractive
birefringence
  corneal b.
birefringent
Birkhauser test chart
Birks
  B. Mark II Colibri forceps
  B. Mark II grooved forceps
  B. Mark II hook
  B. Mark II instrument
  B. Mark II Instruments micro
  trabeculectomy scissors
  B. Mark II micro cross-action
  holder
  B. Mark II micro lock-type
  needle holder
  B. Mark II microneedle-holder
  forceps
  B. Mark II micro push/pull
  spatula
  B. Mark II microspatula
  B. Mark II needle holder
  B. Mark II straight forceps
  B. Mark II suture-tying
  forceps
  B. Mark II toothed forceps
Birks-Mathelone microforceps
Bishop-Harman
  B.-H. anterior chamber cannula
  B.-H. anterior chamber irrigator
  B.-H. bladebreaker

B.-H. foreign body forceps
B.-H. irrigating/aspirating unit
B.-H. knife
B.-H. Superblade
B.-H. tissue forceps
Bishop-Peter tendon tucker
Bishop tendon tucker
Bi-Soft lens
bispherical lens
Bistouri blade
bitartrate
    epinephrine b.
bite
    16-b. nylon suture
bitemporal
    b. disparity
    b. field defect
    b. fugax hemianopsia
    b. hemianopic scotoma
biting rongeur
bitoric contact lens
Bitot
    B. patch
    B. spot
Bitumi monobjective microscope
bivariate analysis
Bjerrum
    B. area
    B. scope
    B. scotoma
    B. scotometer
    B. screen
    B. sign
BKS Refractive System
BK virus
black
    b. braided nylon suture
    b. braided silk suture
    b. cataract
    b. cornea
    b. dot sign
    b. eye
    b. reflex
    b. silk sling suture
    b. sunburst
    b. sunburst sign
black-ball hyphema

blackout
    visual b.
black/white occluder
blade
    #15 b.
    Accutome black diamond b.
    Alfonso diamond corneal
      transplant b.
    Arc-T b.
    #15 Bard-Parker b.
    Bard-Parker b.
    Beaver b.
    5435 Beaver b.
    Beaver discission b.
    Beaver eye b.
    Beaver-Lundsgaard b.
    Beaver-Okamura b.
    Beaver Optimum b.
    Beaver scleral Lundsgaard b.
    Beaver-Ziegler needle b.
    Beer b.
    bent blunt b.
    Berens b.
    Bistouri b.
    broken razor b.
    Castroviejo razor b.
    circular b.
    Cooper Surgeon-Plus
      Ultrathin b.
    CooperVision Surgeon-Plus
      Ultrathin b.
    crescent b.
    Curdy b.
    Curdy-Hebra b.
    Davidoff b.
    Dean b.
    diamond b.
    diamond-dusted knife b.
    Duotrak b.
    b. gauge
    Genesis diamond b.
    Gill b.
    Gill-Hess b.
    Grieshaber b.
    GS-9 b.
    GSA-9 b.
    Hebra b.

B

NOTES

blade *(continued)*
Hoskins razor fragment b.
Katena double-edged
  sapphire b.
Keeler retractable b.
Kellan sutureless incision b.
Knapp b.
b. knife
Lange b.
Martinez corneal trephine b.
Mastel trifaceted diamond b.
McPherson-Wheeler b.
M4-400 freedom b.
Micra double-edged
  diamond b.
Micro-Sharp b.
microvitreoretinal b.
miniature b.
MVB b.
MVR b.
Myocure b.
myringotomy b.
Optimum b.
orbit b.
Orca surgical b.
Planar b.
razor b.
rectangular b.
replaceable b.
Rhein 3-D trapezoid
  diamond b.
ScalpelTec phaco keratome
  slit b.
ScalpelTec wound-
  enlargement b.
Scheie b.
scleral b.
Sharpoint spoon b.
Sharpoint V-lance b.
Sichel b.
slimcut b.
Sputnik Russian razor b.
Stealth DBO diamond b.
Superblade No. 75 b.
Surgistar ophthalmic b.
Thornton arcuate b.
Thornton tri-square b.
trephine b.
UltraThin surgical b.
V-lance b.
Wheeler b.
Ziegler b.

bladebreaker
Barraquer razor b.
Bishop-Harman b.
Castroviejo b.
Castroviejo-style mini b.
I-tech Castroviejo b.
b. knife
razor b.
Swiss b.
Troutman b.
Vari b.
blade/knife
V-lance b./k.
Blair
B. epicanthus repair
B. head drape
B. operation
B. retractor
B. stiletto
Blairex
B. sterile saline
B. System
bland ophthalmic ointment
blank
blocking of lens b.
contact lens b.
semifinished b.
b. spot
Blasius lid flap operation
Blaskovics
B. canthoplasty operation
B. dacryostomy operation
B. flap
B. inversion of tarsus
  operation
B. lid operation
B. tarsectomy
Blaskovics-Berke ptosis
blastoma
pineal b.
Blastomyces
  B. dermatitidis
Blatt operation
Blaydes
B. corneal forceps
B. lens-holding forceps
BLD
basal laminar deposit
bleb
conjunctival b.
b. cup
b. disorder of the cornea
encapsulated b.

endothelial b.
epithelial b.
filtering b.
iron-leaking b.
leaking filtering b.
b. migration
nonleaking b.
postcataract b.
bleb-associated endophthalmitis
blebitis
bleed
  subarachnoid b.
  vitreal b.
bleeding
  intraretinal b.
  limbal b.
Blefcon
Blenderm
  B. tape
  B. tape dressing
blennophthalmia
blennorrhagica
  keratoderma b.
blennorrhea
  b. adultorum
  b. conjunctivalis
  inclusion b.
  neonatal inclusion b.
  b. neonatorum
blennorrheal conjunctivitis
Bleph
Bleph-10
  B.-10 Liquifilm
  B.-10 Ophthalmic
  B.-10 S.O.P.
Blephamide
  B. Ophthalmic
  B. S.O.P.
blepharadenitis
blepharal
blepharectomy
blepharedema
blepharelosis
blepharism
blepharitis
  b. acarica
  allergic b.

angular b.
b. angularis
bacterial b.
chlamydial b.
chronic b. (CB)
b. ciliaris
ciliary b.
clostridial b.
coliform b.
b. conjunctivitis
contact b.
demodectic b.
diplobacillary b.
eczematoid b.
b. follicularis
fungal b.
herpes simplex b.
marginal b.
b. marginalis
meibomian b.
nonulcerative b.
b. oleosa
parasitic b.
b. parasitica
pediculous b.
b. phthiriatica
pustular b.
rickettsial b.
b. rosacea
seborrheic b.
b. sicca
b. squamosa
squamous seborrheic b.
staphylococcal b.
streptococcal b.
b. ulcerosa
viral b.
blepharoadenitis
blepharoadenoma
blepharoatheroma
blepharochalasis
  b. forceps
  Kreiker b.
  b. repair
blepharochromidrosis
blepharoclonus
blepharocoloboma

B

NOTES

blepharoconjunctivitis
    acne rosacea b.
    allergic b.
    angular b.
    bacterial b.
    chronic b.
    herpes simplex b.
    b. rosacea
    staphylococcal b.
    b. vaccinia
blepharodiastasis
blepharokeratoconjunctivitis
blepharomelasma
blepharoncus
blepharopachynsis
blepharophimosis
    epicanthus b.
    b. inversus
    b. ptosis syndrome
blepharophyma
blepharoplast
blepharoplastic
blepharoplasty
    Davis-Geck b.
    transconjunctival lower
      eyelid b.
blepharoplegia
blepharoptosis, blepharoptosia
    b. adiposa
    false b.
    involutional b.
    b. repair
blepharopyorrhea
blepharorrhaphy
    Elschnig b.
blepharospasm, blepharospasmus
    benign essential b. (BEB)
    essential b.
    hemifacial b.
    nonorganic b.
    ocular b.
    primary infantile glaucoma b.
    reflex b.
    symptomatic b.
blepharospasm-oromandibular
    b.-o. dystonia
    b.-o. dystonia syndrome
blepharosphincterectomy
blepharostat
    McNeill-Goldmann b.
blepharostenosis
blepharosynechia
blepharotomy

blepharoxysis
Blessig
    B. cyst
    B. groove
    B. lacuna
Blessig-Iwanoff
    B.-I. cyst
    B.-I. microcyst
blind
    color b.
    legally b.
    b. spot
    b. spot enlargement
    b. spot of Mariotte
    b. spot reflex
    b. spot syndrome
blinding
    b. disease
    b. glare
blindness
    amnesic color b.
    blue b.
    Bright b.
    cerebral b.
    color b.
    concussion b.
    cortical psychic b.
    day b.
    deuton color b.
    eclipse b.
    electric light b.
    epidemic b.
    factitious b.
    flash b.
    flight b.
    functional b.
    green b.
    hysterical b.
    Ishihara test for color b.
    legal b.
    letter b.
    mind b.
    miner's b.
    moon b.
    night b.
    note b.
    nutritional b.
    object b.
    postoperative b.
    protan color b.
    psychic b.
    red b.
    red-green b.

B

river b.
snow b.
solar b.
soul b.
stationary night b.
syllabic b.
b. test
text b.
total b.
transient b.
twilight b.
word b.
X-linked congenital night b.
yellow b.
blindsight
blind-spot projection technique
blink
b. adequacy
b. inadequacy
b. reflex
blinking
Blink-N-Clean
Blinx
Bloch-Stauffer syndrome
Bloch-Sulzberger syndrome
block
aphakic pupillary b.
Atkin lid b.
Atkinson b.
ciliary b.
ciliolenticular b.
ciliovitreal b.
ciliovitrectomy b.
cocaine b.
corneal b.
facial b.
Fine folding b.
lid b.
modified Van Lint b.
Nadbath facial b.
b. nerve
nerve b.
O'Brien lid b.
phakic pupillary b.
posterior peribulbar b.
punch b.
pupil b.

pupillary b.
regional b.
retrobulbar lid b.
reverse pupillary b.
Smith modification of Van
Lint lid b.
Spaeth b.
Stahl caliper b.
Tanne corneal cutting b.
Teflon b.
Van Lint b.
Van Lint-Atkinson lid
akinetic b.
vitreous b.
blockade
nasolacrimal b.
pharmacological b.
blockage nystagmus
blocking of lens blank
blond fundus
blood
b. barrier
b. cyst
b. flow velocity waveform
(BFVW)
b. loss
retinal b.
b. staining of cornea
subhyaloid b.
vitreous b.
blood-and-thunder retinopathy
blood-aqueous
b.-a. barrier
b.-a. barrier breakdown
blood-influx phenomenon
blood-ocular barrier
blood-optic nerve barrier
blood-retinal barrier
bloodshot
blood staining
bloody tears
Bloomberg
B. SuperNumb anesthetic ring
B. trabeculotome set
blooming
b. of lens
b. spectacle lens

NOTES

blot-and-dot hemorrhage
blotchy positive staining
blot hemorrhage
"blown pupil"
blow-out
    b.-o. fracture
    b.-o. fracture of orbit
blue
    b. blindness
    b. cataract
    b. cone
    b. cone monochromasy
    b. cone monochromatism
    B. core PMMA
    b. flash stimulus
    b. limbus
    b. line
    B. Mountain Eye Study
    b. nevus
    b. rubber bleb nevus syndrome
    b. sclera
    b. spike
    b. spot
    b. vision
    B. Vista
blue-dot cataract
blue-field entoptic phenomenon
blue-green argon laser
Blumenthal
    B. anterior chamber maintainer
    B. irrigating cystitome
blunt
    b. needle
    b. trauma
blur
    b. and clear exercise
    optical b.
    b. pattern
    b. point
    spectacle b.
    b. spot
    b. zone
blurred vision
blurring of vision
BM
    basement membrane
B-mode handpiece
BO
    base out
boat hook
bobbing
    converse b.
    inverse ocular b.

    ocular b.
    reverse b.
Boberg-Ans
    B.-A. lens
    B.-A. lens implant
Bodian
    B. lacrimal pigtail probe
    B. mini lacrimal probe
Bodkin thread holder
body, pl. **bodies**
    adipose b.
    asteroid b.
    Barr b.
    basal ciliary b.
    basal lamina of ciliary b.
    basophilic intranuclear
      inclusion b.
    cellular inclusion b.
    ciliary b.
    colloid b.
    conjunctival foreign b.
    copper foreign b.
    cystoid b.
    cytoid b.
    cytoplasmic b.
    Dutcher b.
    electromagnetic removal of
      foreign b.
    Elschnig b.
    embryonal medulloepithelioma
      of ciliary b.
    eosinophilic intranuclear
      inclusion b.
    external geniculate b.
    foreign b. (FB)
    geniculate b.
    Goldmann-Larson foreign b.
    Guarnieri inclusion b.
    Halberstaedter-Prowazek
      inclusion b.
    Hassall b.
    Hassall-Henle b.
    Henderson-Patterson
      inclusion b.
    Henle b.
    Hensen b.
    hyaline b.
    hyaloid b.
    inclusion b.
    intracytoplasmic inclusion b.
    intranuclear eosinophilic
      inclusion b.
    intraocular foreign b.

intraorbital foreign b.
Landolt b.
lateral geniculate b. (LGB)
Leishman-Donovan b.
lenticular b.
lenticular fossa of vitreous b.
Lewy b.
Lipschütz inclusion b.
multivesicular b.
nigroid b.
occult annular ciliary b.
pigmented layer of ciliary b.
pituitary b.
Prowazek-Greeff b.
Prowazek-Halberstaedter b.
Prowazek inclusion b.
psammoma b.
racquet b.
refractile b.
removal of foreign b.
Rosenmüller b.
Rucker b.
Russell b.
Schaumann inclusion b.
sclerotomy removal of
  foreign b.
subconjunctival foreign b.
synaptic b.
trachoma b.
vitreous foreign b.
wartlike b.
Weibel-Palade b.
body-referenced stimulus
Boeck sarcoid
boggy edema
Böhm operation
Bohr model
Boil-n-Soak
bolus dressing
bombé
  b. configuration
  iris b.
Bonaccolto
  B. fragment forceps
  B. jeweler forceps
  B. magnet tip forceps
  B. monoplex orbital implant

B. scleral ring
B. trephine
B. utility forceps
Bonaccolto-Flieringa
  B.-F. scleral ring
  B.-F. scleral ring operation
  B.-F. vitreous operation
Bondek suture
bone
  b. cutter
  ethmoid b.
  foramen of sphenoid b.
  frontal b.
  glandular fossa of frontal b.
  b. graft
  lacrimal b.
  lacrimal sulcus of lacrimal b.
  maxillary b.
  orbital b.
  orbital arch of frontal b.
  orbital border of sphenoid b.
  orbital plane of frontal b.
  orbital plate of ethmoid b.
  orbital plate of frontal b.
  orbital sulci of frontal b.
  orbital wing of sphenoid b.
  palatine b.
  petrous b.
  b. punch
  b. rongeur
  sphenoid b.
  supraorbital arch of frontal b.
  supraorbital margin of
    frontal b.
  temporal b.
  b. trephine
  uncinate process of lacrimal b.
  zygomatic b.
bone-biting
  b.-b. forceps
  b.-b. punch
  b.-b. trephine
Bonn
  B. iris forceps
  B. iris scissors
  B. microiris hook
  B. suturing forceps

B

NOTES

Bonnet
- B. capsule
- B. enucleation operation
- B. sign

Bonnet-DeChaume-Blanc syndrome
Bonnier syndrome
bony cataract
Bonzel
- B. blood staining of cornea
- B. operation

boomerang-shaped lesion
borate
- epinephrine b.
- epinephryl b.
- sodium b.

border
- brushfire b.
- corneoscleral b.
- rolled-up epithelium with wavy b.
- scalloped b.
- b. tissue of Jacoby

Bordetella pertussis
Bores
- B. axis marker
- B. twist fixation ring

boric
- b. acid
- b. acid solution

boring pain
Borrelia
- *B. burgdorferi*
- *B. novyi*
- *B. recurrentis*

Borsch
- B. bandage
- B. dressing

Borthen iridotasis operation
Boruchoff forceps
Bossalino blepharoplasty operation
Boston
- B. Advance cleaner
- B. Advance conditioning solution
- B. Advance reconditioning drops
- B. conditioning solution
- B. contact lens
- B. Envision lens
- B. reconditioning drops
- B. sign
- B. trephine

Botox

bottlemaker's cataract
botulinum
- b. A toxin
- b. injection
- b. toxin A (BTA)

botulism-induced
- b.-i. blurred vision
- b.-i. ptosis

botulismotoxin
Botvin-Bradford enucleator
Botvin iris forceps
bouche de tapir
bound-down muscle
bounding
- b. mydriasis
- b. pupil

bouquet of Rochon-Duvigneaud
boutons
- b. en passant
- b. terminaux

Bovie
- B. electrocautery unit
- B. electrosurgical unit
- B. retinal detachment unit
- B. wet-field cautery

bovied
bovina
- facies b.

bovis
- *Moraxella b.*
- *Mycobacterium b.*

Bower disease
bowl
- Ganzfield b.
- lenticular b.

Bowling lens
Bowman
- B. cataract needle
- B. lacrimal probe
- B. lamina
- B. layer
- B. membrane
- B. muscle
- B. needle stop
- B. operation
- B. stop needle
- B. tube
- B. zone

bowstring
bow-tie
- b.-t. hypoplasia
- b.-t. knot

b.-t. optic atrophy
b.-t. stitch
boxcarring
box measurement
Boyce needle holder
Boyd
B. operation
B. orbital implant
B. zone
Boyden chamber technique
boydii
Allescheria b.
Petriellidum b.
Pseudallescheria b.
Boynton needle holder
Boys-Smith laser lens
BOZR
back optic zone radius
Bozzi foramen
BPPV
benign paroxysmal positional vertigo
BQ
Slit Lamp 900 B.
brachial
b. arch syndrome
b. plexus palsy
brachium
conjunctival b.
b. conjunctivum
brachymetropia
brachymetropic
brachytherapy
orbital plaque b.
palladium 103 ophthalmic
plaque b.
radioactive plaque b.
radon ring b.
Bracken
B. anterior chamber cannula
B. effect
B. fixation forceps
B. iris forceps
B. irrigating/aspirating unit
Bradford snare enucleator
bradykinin

Braid
B. effect
B. strabismus
braided
b. silk suture
b. Vicryl suture
Brailey operation
braille
brailler
Perkins b.
brain
b. cortex
b. damage
b. dysfunction
b. stem
b. tumor
b. tumor headache
brainstem, brain stem
b. dysfunction
b. lesion
b. motor nucleus
Braley sign
branch
b. retinal artery occlusion
(BRAO)
b. retinal vein occlusion
(BRVO)
brancher enzyme deficiency
branching
b. dendrite
b. filament
b. infiltration
b. lesion
Branhamella catarrhalis
BRAO
branch retinal artery occlusion
brasiliensis
Nocardia b.
brass scleral plug
Brawley
B. refractor
B. retractor
Brawner orbital implant
brawny
b. edema
b. scleritis

NOTES

brawny *(continued)*
  b. tenonitis
  b. trachoma
Brayley
  polymorphic macular
    degeneration of B.
Brazilian ophthalmia
breadth of accommodation
break
  conjunctival b.
  giant retinal b.
  iatrogenic retinal b.
  b. phenomenon
  b. point
  retinal b.
  b. in retinal integrity
breakdown
  blood-aqueous barrier b.
  optical b.
  surface b.
breakpoint
  fusion b.
breakthrough
  vitreous hemorrhage b.
breakup
  b. phenomenon
  b. time (BUT)
  b. time of tear
  b. time test
breves
  nervi ciliares b.
Brevital
Brickner sign
bridge
  b. coloboma
  comfort b.
  keyhole b.
  B. operation
  b. pedicle flap
  b. pedicle flap operation
  saddle b.
  b. of spectacles
  b. suture
bridle suture
Brierley nucleus splitter
Briggs strabismus operation
bright
  B. blindness
  b. empty field
  B. eye
  b. staining
bright-field accommodation

brightness
  B. Acuity Test (BAT)
  b. comparison
  b. difference threshold
bright-sense
bright-white flash stimulus
brimonidine
  b. tartrate ophthalmic solution
    0.2%
brinzolamide
  b. ophthalmic suspension
British
  B. N system
  B. Standards Institution
    optotype set
Britt
  B. argon/krypton laser
  B. argon pulsed laser
  B. BL-12 laser
  B. krypton laser
  B. pulsed argon laser
brittle
  b. cornea syndrome
  b. diabetes
broad-beam ablation
broad-spectrum
  b.-s. antibiotic
  b.-s. heater (BSH)
Broca
  B. aphasia
  B. visual plane
Brockhurst technique
Broders grading
Brodmann area
broken razor blade
Brolene
Bromarest
Brombach perimeter
Brombay
bromhexine
bromide
  demecarium b.
  pancuronium b.
Bromley foreign body operation
bromocriptine
Bromphen
brompheniramine
bromvinyldeoxyuridine (BVDU)
Bronson foreign body removal
  operation
Bronson-Magnion
  B.-M. eye magnet
  B.-M. forceps

B

Bronson-Park speculum
Bronson-Turner foreign body
  locator
Bronson-Turtz
  B.-T. refractor
  B.-T. retractor
bronze diabetes
bronzing
  nuclear b.
Brooke tumor
brow
  b. fixation
  b. tape
brown
  b. cataract
  B. sterile adhesive
  B. syndrome
  B. tendon
  B. tendon sheath syndrome
  B. vertical retraction syndrome
Brown-Beard technique
Brown-Dohlman Silastic corneal
  implant
Brown-McLean syndrome
Brown-Pusey corneal trephine
broxyquinoline
Brucella
  B. abortus
  B. suis
Bruch
  B. gland
  B. layer
  B. membrane
Bruchner test
Brücke
  B. fiber
  B. lens
  B. muscle
Brücke-Bartley phenomenon
Brückner reflex testing
Brueghel syndrome
Bruening forceps
brunescens
  cataracta b.
brunescent cataract
Bruns nystagmus

Brunsting-Perry cicatricial
  pemphigoid
brush
  Alger b.
  Barraquer sable b.
  5139 flexible retinal b.
  rotating b.
  Thomas b.
Brushfield spot
Brushfield-Wyatt syndrome
brushfire border
BRVO
  branch retinal vein occlusion
B-scan
  B.-s. biometry
  Humphrey B.-s.
  B.-s. ultrasonogram
  B.-s. ultrasonography
BSH
  broad-spectrum heater
BSS
  balanced salt solution
  BSS sterile irrigating solution
BSV
  binocular single vision
BTA
  botulinum toxin A
BU
  base-up prism
bubble
  air b.
  Chamber sterile adhesive b.
  gas b.
  intraocular gas b.
buckle
  balloon b.
  choroid b.
  encircling band for scleral b.
  encircling silicone b.
  b. height
  prominent b.
  scleral b.
  temporary balloon b.
Bücklers
  B. I dystrophy
  B. II dystrophy
  B. III dystrophy

NOTES

buckling
  b. choroid
  Custodis scleral b.
  b. sclera
  scleral b.
budding yeast cell
Budge
  ciliospinal center of B.
Budinger blepharoplasty operation
**Buedding squeegee cortex extractor
  and polisher**
Buettner-Parel vitreous cutter
buffy coat
bufilcon A
build-up implant
bulb
  b. of eye
  terminal b.
bulbar
  b. conjunctiva
  b. conjunctival scarring
  b. cyanosis
  b. fascia
  b. paralysis
  b. sheath
bulbi (*gen. and pl. of* bulbus) (*See
  also* bulbus)
bulbocapnine
bulbous atrophy
bulbus, gen. and pl. **bulbi**
  atrophia bulbi
  camera vitrea bulbi
  capsula bulbi
  cholesterosis bulbi
  cyanosis bulbi
  endothelium camerae anterioris
    bulbi
  essential phthisis bulbi
  fascia bulbi
  fascia lata musculares bulbi
  fascia musculares bulbi
  hemosiderosis bulbi
  lacertus musculi recti lateralis
    bulbi
  melanosis bulbi
  musculi bulbi
  musculus obliquus inferior
    bulbi
  musculus obliquus superior
    bulbi
  musculus rectus inferior bulbi
  musculus rectus lateralis bulbi
  musculus rectus medialis bulbi

  b. oculi
  phthisis bulbi
  siderosis bulbi
  Tenon fascia bulbi
  trochlea musculi obliqui
    superioris bulbi
  tunica fibrosa bulbi
  tunica interna bulbi
  tunica sensoria bulbi
  tunica vasculosa bulbi
  xanthelasmatosis bulbi
  xanthomatosis bulbi
bulge
  vitreous b.
bulla, pl. **bullae**
  epithelial b.
  ethmoid b.
  b. ethmoidalis cavinasi
  b. ethmoidalis ossis
  b. ossea
bulldog clamp
Buller eye shield
bullosa
  concha b.
  epidermolysis b.
  keratitis b.
  recessive dystrophic
    epidermolysis b.
bullosum
  erythema multiforme b.
bullous
  b. detachment
  b. disorder
  b. keratopathy
  b. pemphigoid
  b. retinoschisis
bull's
  b. eye
  b. eye macular lesion
  b. eye maculopathy
  b. eye retinopathy
bullular canal
Bumke pupil
bundle
  arcuate nerve fiber b.
  b. of Drualt
  Drualt b.
  inferior arcuate b.
  maculopapillary b.
  maculopapular b.
  nerve fiber b.
  papillomacular nerve fiber b.

paracentral nerve fiber b.
superior arcuate b.
Bunge evisceration spoon
Bunker implant
Bunsen grease spot photometer
Bunsen-Roscoe law
buphthalmia, buphthalmos,
 buphthalmus
bupivacaine
bupranolol
bur, burr, burr
 aftercataract b.
 Alfonso guarded b.
 Allport cutting b.
 Burwell b.
 corneal foreign body b.
 cutting b.
 diamond b.
 foreign body b.
 lacrimal sac b.
 Storz corneal b.
 Worst corneal b.
 Yazujian b.
Buratto
 B. irrigating cannula
 B. ophthalmic forceps
Burch
 B. calipers
 B. eye evisceration operation
 B. pick
Burch-Greenwood
 B.-G. tendon tucker
 B.-G. tucker
Burch-Lester speculum
burgdorferi
 Borrelia b.
Burian-Allen
 B.-A. contact lens
 B.-A. contact lens electrode
buried
 b. disk drusen
 b. suture
burn
 acid b.
 alkali b.
 alkaline b.
 ammonia alkali b.

ammonium hydroxide alkali b.
chemical b.
corneal b.
corneal alkali b.
foveal b.
laser b.
light argon laser b.
radiation b.
retinal b.
solar b.
b. spot size
thermal b.
ultraviolet b.
burnetii
 Coxiella b.
Burns amaurosis
Burow flap operation
Burr
 B. butterfly needle
 B. cornea
 B. corneal ring
 B. silicone button
burr (*var. of* bur)
burst
 laser b.
Burton lamp
Burwell bur
Busacca nodule
BUT
 breakup time
butacaine
Butazolidin
Butcher conjunctivitis
butterfly
 b. macular dystrophy
 b. needle
 b. needle infusion port
 b. pattern steepening of the
 cornea
 b. test
butterfly-shaped pigment epithelial
 dystrophy
button
 Burr silicone b.
 collar b.
 corneal b.
 corneoscleral b.

B

NOTES

button *(continued)*
    Graether collar b.
    penetrating keratoplasty b.
    silicone b.
buttonhole
    b. incision
    b. iridectomy
button-tip manipulator
butyl
    b. cyanoacrylate
    b. cyanoacrylate glue
butyrate
    cellulose b.
    cellulose acetate b. (CAB)

Buzard Diamond Barraqueratome Microkeratome System
Buzzi operation
BV100 needle
BVDU
    bromvinyldeoxyuridine
BVP
    back vertex power
b wave
b-wave amplitude
Byrne expulsive hemorrhage lens
Byron
    B. Smith ectropion operation
    B. Smith lazy T correction

C
contraction
cylinder
cylindrical lens
C loop
C value
CAB
cellulose acetate butyrate
cable temple
cabufocon A
CA/C ratio
caecum
punctum c.
caecutiens
Onchocerca c.
Caenorhabditis elegans
caerulea
cataracta c.
caespitosum
Streptomyces c.
caespitosus
Streptomyces c.
Cairns
C. operation
C. procedure
C. trabeculectomy
Cajal
interstitial nucleus of C.
calcareous
c. cataract
c. conjunctivitis
c. degeneration
c. degeneration of cornea
c. deposit
calcarine
c. artery
c. cortex
c. fissure
calciferol
calcific
c. band keratopathy
c. phacolysis
calcification
conjunctival c.
lamellar c.
optic disk drusen c.
sellar c.
calcinosis cutis, Raynaud
phenomenon, esophageal motility

disorder, sclerodactyly, and
telangiectasia (CREST)
calcitriol
calcium
c. alginate swab
c. deposition
c. hydroxide
calcium-containing opacity
calcoaceticus
Acinetobacter c.
calcofluor white
calculation
lens power c.
power c.
calculus, gen. and pl. **calculi**
lacrimal c.
Caldwell-Luc approach
Caldwell view
Caldwell-Waters view
Calendar monthly disposable
contact lens
Calhoun-Hagler
C.-H. lens extraction operation
C.-H. lens needle
Calhoun-Merz needle
Calhoun needle
Calibri forceps
caliculus ophthalmicus
caligation
caligo
c. corneae
c. lentis
c. pupilla
calipers
Berens marking c.
Burch c.
Castroviejo c.
Green c.
Jameson c.
John Green c.
Machemer c.
Stahl c.
Storz c.
surgical c.
Thomas c.
Thorpe c.
Thorpe-Castroviejo c.
Callahan
C. fixation forceps

Callahan *(continued)*
   C. lens loupe
   C. operation
Callender
   C. cell type classification
callipaeda
   Thelazia c.
callosum
   corpus c.
   splenium of corpus c.
Calmette ophthalmoreaction
caloric
   c. irrigation test
   c. nystagmus
caloric-induced nystagmus
calotte
calvaria
Cambridge
   C. acuity card
   C. low-contrast grating
camera, pl. **camerae, cameras**
   Bio-Optics c.
   c. bulbi anterior
   c. bulbi posterior
   Canon CF-60U fundus c.
   Canon CF-60Z fundus c.
   Carl Zeiss fundus c.
   Carl Zeiss Jena Retinophot
     fundus c.
   Coburn c.
   CooperVision c.
   Cr6-45NMf retinal c.
   Docustar fundus c.
   Donaldson fundus c.
   Eyecor c.
   fundus c.
   Garcia-Ibanez c.
   hand-held fundus c.
   Handy non-mydriatic video
     fundus c.
   Holofax Oxford
     retroillumination cataract c.
   House-Urban-Pentax c.
   Kowa PRO II retinal c.
   Kowa RC-XV fundus c.
   c. lucida
   Neitz CT-R cataract c.
   Nidek 3Dx stereodisk c.
   Nikon Retinopan fundus c.
   c. obscura
   c. oculi
   c. oculi anterior
   c. oculi posterior

   Olympus fundus c.
   RC-2 fundus c.
   Reichert c.
   retinal c.
   Retinopan 45 c.
   telecentric fundus c.
   Topcon 50IA c.
   Topcon TRC-50VT retinal c.
   Topcon TRC-50X retinal c.
   Topcon TRV-50VT fundus c.
   TRC-50IX ICG-capable
     fundus c.
   TRC-SS2 stereoscopic
     fundus c.
   c. vitrea bulbi
   Zeiss fundus c.
   Zeiss-Nordenson fundus c.
cAMP
   c. final common pathway
   c. mediated mechanism
Campbell
   iris retraction syndrome of C.
   C. refractor
   C. retractor
   C. slit lamp
campimeter
campimetry
Campodonico
   C. canal
   C. operation
CAM stimulator
Canada balsam
canal
   ampulla of lacrimal c.
   bullular c.
   Campodonico c.
   central c.
   ciliary c.
   Cloquet c.
   Dorello c.
   emissarial c.
   ethmoid c.
   Ferrein c.
   Fontana c.
   Hannover c.
   Hovius c.
   hyaloid c.
   infraorbital c.
   lacrimal c.
   Lauth c.
   nasal c.
   nasolacrimal c.
   c. of Nuck

optic c.
orbital c.
Petit c.
ruffed c.
Schlemm c.
c. of Schlemm
scleral c.
scleroticochoroidal c.
semicircular c.
Sondermann c.
c. of Stilling
supraciliary c.
supraoptic c.
supraorbital c.
tarsal c.
zygomaticofacial c.
zygomaticotemporal c.
canalicular
c. disorder
c. duct
c. laceration
c. pathway
c. route
c. scissors
canaliculi (*pl. of* canaliculus)
canaliculitis
canaliculodacryocystostomy
canaliculodacryorhinostomy
canaliculorhinostomy
canaliculum
canaliculus, pl. **canaliculi**
common c.
inferior c.
c. infraorbitalis opticus
lacrimal c.
c. lacrimalis
c. rod and suture
stenosis c.
superior c.
upper c.
canalis
c. hyaloideus
c. opticus
Canavan disease
cancer-associated retinopathy (CAR, CAR syndrome)

cancrum nasi
candela (cd)
c. laser
c. laser lithotriptor
C. videoimaging system
candela/m²
candela-sec/m²
Candida
C. *albicans*
C. *glabrata*
C. *krusei*
C. *parapsilosis*
C. *tropicalis*
candidal
c. conjunctivitis
c. endophthalmitis
c. keratitis
c. uveitis
candidiasis conjunctivitis
candle
German Hefner c.
candle-meter
candle-power
cannula
air injection c.
alpha-chymotrypsin c.
angled left/right c.
anterior chamber c.
ASSI c.
Bailey lacrimal c.
Barraquer c.
Barrett hydrodelineation c.
Binkhorst irrigating c.
Bishop-Harman anterior
    chamber c.
Bracken anterior chamber c.
Buratto irrigating c.
Castroviejo cyclodialysis c.
cortical cleaving
    hydrodissector c.
Corydon hydroexpression c.
cyclodialysis c.
De LaVega vitreous
    aspirating c.
double irrigating/aspirating c.
Drews irrigating c.
Fasanella lacrimal c.

NOTES

C

cannula *(continued)*
Feaster K7-5460
hydrodissecting c.
Galt aspirating c.
Gans cyclodialysis c.
Gass cataract aspirating c.
Gass vitreous aspirating c.
Ghormley double c.
Gills double irrigating-
aspirating c.
Gills double Luer-Lok c.
Gills irrigating-aspirating c.
Gills-Welsh aspirating c.
Gills-Welsh double-barreled
irrigating-aspirating c.
Gills-Welsh irrigating-
aspirating c.
Gills-Welsh olive-tip c.
Girard irrigating c.
Goldstein c.
goniotomy knife c.
Healon c.
Heyner double c.
Hilton self-retaining infusion c.
Hilton sutureless infusion c.
Hoffer forward-cutting knife c.
infusion c.
iris hook c.
irrigating c.
irrigating/aspirating c.
I-tech c.
Jensen-Thomas irrigating-
aspirating c.
Johnson double c.
J-shaped irrigating/aspirating c.
Kara cataract-aspirating c.
Karickhoff double c.
Keeler-Keislar lacrimal c.
Kelman cyclodialysis c.
Klein curved c.
Kraff cortex c.
lacrimal irrigating c.
Lewicky threaded infusion c.
liquid vitreous-aspirating c.
Look I/A coaxial c.
Maumenee goniotomy knife c.
Maumenee knife goniotomy c.
McIntyre-Binkhorst irrigating c.
McIntyre coaxial c.
Moehle c.
Moncrieff c.
Nichamin hydrodissection c.
Oaks double straight c.

Oaks straight c.
O'Gawa cataract-aspirating c.
O'Gawa two-way aspirating c.
olive-tip c.
O'Malley-Heintz infusion c.
Packo pars plana c.
Pautler infusion c.
Peacekeeper c.
Pearce coaxial
irrigating/aspirating c.
Peczon I/A c.
Pierce coaxial
irrigating/aspirating c.
Pierce I/A c.
Randolph cyclodialysis c.
reel aspiration c.
Roper alpha-chymotrypsin c.
Rowsey fixation c.
Rycroft c.
Scheie anterior chamber c.
Scheie cataract-aspirating c.
self-retaining infusion c.
self-retaining irrigating c.
Shepard incision irrigating c.
Shepard radial keratotomy
irrigating c.
side-port c.
sidewall infusion c.
Simcoe double c.
Simcoe II PC double c.
Simcoe reverse aperture c.
Simcoe reverse irrigating-
aspirating c.
smooth c.
soft-tipped c.
Steriseal disposable c.
sub-Tenon anesthesia c.
Swets goniotomy knife c.
Tenner lacrimal c.
Thomas irrigating-aspirating c.
Thurmond nucleus-irrigating c.
Tri-Port sub-tenon anesthesia c.
Troutman c.
TruPro lacrimal c.
Tulevech c.
two-way cataract-aspirating c.
Ulanday double c.
Veirs c.
Visco expression c.
Viscoflow c.
Visitec irrigating/aspirating c.
vitreous-aspirating c.
Weil lacrimal c.

Weiss self-retaining c.
Welsh cortex stripper c.
Welsh flat olive-tip double c.
Welsh olive-tip c.
Wergeland double c.
West lacrimal c.

Canon
C. Autokeratometer K1
C. Autoref R1
C. auto refraction keratometer
C. auto refractometer
C. CF-60U fundus camera
C. CF-60Z fundus camera
C. perimeter
C. refractor

can opener capsulotomy
Cantelli sign
canthal
c. hypertelorism
c. keratinization
c. ligament
c. raphe
c. recess
c. tendon

canthaxanthin
canthaxanthine crystalline retinopathy
canthectomy
canthi (*pl. of* canthus)
canthitis
cantholysis
canthomeatal
canthopexy
canthoplasty
Agnew c.
Ammon c.
Imre lateral c.

canthorrhaphy
Elschnig c.

canthorum
dystopia c.

canthotomy
external c.
lateral c.

canthus, pl. canthi
inner c.
lateral c.

medial c.
outer c.

cap
compliance c.
corneal c.
Gelfilm c.
SupraCAPS quarter-globe c.

capillaritis
retinal c.

capillary
c. bed
c. closure
c. hemangioma
c. hemangioma of eyelid
c. lumen
nonfenestrated c.
c. nonperfusion
c. perfusion
c. plexus
c. scaffolding

capitis
dolor c.

caplet
TripTone C.'s

capsitis
capsula
c. bulbi
c. lentis

capsular
c. advancement
c. bag
c. cataract
c. debris
c. exfoliation syndrome
c. fixation
c. glaucoma
c. support

capsular-zonular
capsulatum
Histoplasma c.

capsule
anterior lens c.
Bonnet c.
c. contraction syndrome
crystalline c.
curling of c.
exfoliation of lens c.

NOTES

C

capsule *(continued)*
 c. forceps technique
 c. fragment forceps
 c. fragment spatula
 leaves of c.
 c. of lens
 lens c.
 ocular c.
 c. polisher
 pseudoexfoliation of lens c.
 Tenon c.
capsulectomy
 anterior c.
capsulitis
capsulolenticular cataract
capsulorrhexis
 c. capsulotomy
 continuous circular c.
 continuous curvilinear c.
 c. forceps
 Kraff-Utrata c.
 minicircular c.
capsulotome
 Darling c.
capsulotomy
 anterior c.
 can opener c.
 capsulorrhexis c.
 Castroviejo c.
 circular tear c.
 Darling c.
 posterior c.
 c. scissors
 triangular c.
 Vannas c.
 Verhoeff-Chandler c.
capture
 iris c.
 pupillary c.
CAR, CAR syndrome
 cancer-associated retinopathy
Carbacel
carbachol
 Isopto C.
carbacholine
Carbastat Ophthalmic
carbenicillin
carbinoxamine and pseudoephedrine
Carbiset
 C. Tablet
 C.-TR Tablet
Carbocaine

Carbodec
 C. Syrup
 C. Tablet
 C. TR Tablet
carbomycin
carbon
 c. arc lamp
 c. dioxide laser
 c. monoxide retinopathy
carbonic anhydrase
Carboptic Ophthalmic
carboxymethylcellulose sodium
carboxy termini
Carcholin
carcinoid tumor
carcinoma
 adenoid cystic c.
 basal cell c.
 embryonal c.
 epidermoid c.
 c. of eyelid
 meibomian gland c.
 metastatic c.
 radiation-induced c.
 sebaceous cell c.
 signet-ring c.
 squamous cell c.
carcinomatosis
 meningeal c.
carcinomatous meningitis
card
 Allen pre-school c.
 Cambridge acuity c.
 digital acuity c.
 flash picture c.
 illuminated near c. (INC)
 Jaeger acuity c.
 microendoscopic test c.
 reading c.
 reduced Snellen c.
 Rosenbaum c.
 Sherman c.
 Sloan reading c.
 Snellen reading c.
 standard near c.
 stigmatometric test c.
 Teller acuity c.
 test c.
Cardec-S Syrup
cardinal
 c. direction of gaze
 c. field test
 c. ocular movement

c. position
c. position of gaze
c. suture
Cardio-Green dye
Cardona
C. corneal prosthesis forceps
C. corneal prosthesis trephine
C. fiberoptic diagnostic lens
C. focalizing fundus lens implant
C. goniofocalizing implant
C. laser
C. threading forceps
Cardrase
Carl
C. Zeiss fundus camera
C. Zeiss instrument
C. Zeiss Jena Retinophot fundus camera
C. Zeiss lens
C. Zeiss lensometer
C. Zeiss tonometer
C. Zeiss YAG laser
Carlo Traverso maneuver (CTM)
carnitine deficiency
carnosus
pannus c.
carotene
beta c.
carotid
c. aneurysm
c. angiography
c. arteriogram
c. artery
c. artery occlusion
c. artery stenosis
c. artery thrombosis
c. cavernous sinus fistula
c. ischemia
c. obstruction
c. occlusive disease retinopathy
Carpenter syndrome
Carpine
E C.
Isopto C.
P.V. C.

carrier
Barraquer needle c.
minus c.
obligate c.
CAR syndrome (*var. of* CAR)
Cartella eye shield
carteolol
c. HCl
c. hydrochloride
Carter
C. operation
C. sphere
C. sphere introducer
cartilage
central c.
ciliary c.
palpebral c.
tarsal c.
Cartman lens insertion forceps
Cartrol
C. Oral
caruncle
epicanthus c.
lacrimal c.
caruncula, pl. **carunculae**
lacrimal c.
c. lacrimalis
trichosis carunculae
caruncular papilloma
CAS
congenital anterior staphyloma
Casanellas lacrimal operation
cascade
phototransduction c.
case
Berens sterilizing c.
Contique contact lens c.
Fine corneal carrying c.
index c.
trial c.
caseating
c. orbital granuloma
c. tubercle
Casebeer keratorefractive planning program
Casebeer-Lindstrom nomogram
case-control study

NOTES

caseosa
rhinitis c.
caseous necrosis
Cases
Per-Protocol-Observed C.
Casey operation
Caspar
C. ring
C. ring opacity
cast
c. molding
c. resin lens
Castallo
C. refractor
C. retractor
C. speculum
castellanii
Acanthamoeba c.
Castroviejo
C. acrylic implant
C. angled keratome
C. anterior synechia
C. anterior synechia scissors
C. bladebreaker
C. blade holder
C. calipers
C. capsule forceps
C. capsulotomy
C. clip-applying forceps
C. compressor
C. corneal dissector
C. corneal-holding forceps
C. corneal scissors with inside stop
C. corneal section scissors
C. corneal transplant marker
C. corneal transplant scissors
C. corneal transplant trephine
C. corneoscleral forceps
C. corneoscleral punch
C. cyclodialysis cannula
C. cyclodialysis spatula
C. discission knife
C. double-ended spatula
C. electrokeratotome
C. enucleation snare
C. erysiphake
C. fixation forceps
C. improved trephine
C. iridectomy
C. iridocapsulotomy scissors
C. keratectomy
C. keratoplasty scissors

C. lacrimal dilator
C. lacrimal sac probe
C. lens loupe
C. lens spoon
C. lid clamp
C. lid forceps
C. lid retractor
C. mini-keratoplasty
C. mucotome
C. needle holder
C. needle holder clamp
C. operation
C. orbital aspirator
C. radial iridotomy
C. razor blade
C. refractor
C. scleral fold forceps
C. scleral marker
C. scleral shortening clip
C. sclerotome
C. snare enucleator
C. speculum
C. suture forceps
C. suturing forceps
C. synechia scissors
C. synechia spatula
C. twin knife
C. tying forceps
C. vitreous aspirating needle
C. wide grip handle forceps
Castroviejo-Arruga forceps
Castroviejo-Barraquer needle holder
Castroviejo-Colibri forceps
Castroviejo-Galezowski dilator
Castroviejo-Kalt needle holder
Castroviejo-Scheie
C.-S. cyclodiathermy
C.-S. cyclodiathermy operation
Castroviejo-style mini bladebreaker
Castroviejo-Vannas capsulotomy scissors
catadioptric
Catalano
C. corneoscleral forceps
C. intubation set
C. muscle hook
C. tying forceps
catalase
Catalin
Catalyst machine
catamenialis
iritis c.

cataphoria
  mature c.
cataplexy
Catapres
cataract
  adherent c.
  adolescent c.
  adult-onset c.
  age-related c.
  aminoaciduria c.
  annular c.
  anterior axial developmental c.
  anterior axial embryonal c.
  anterior axonal embryonal c.
  anterior polar c.
  anterior pole c.
  anterior pyramidal c.
  arborescent c.
  aridosiliculose c.
  aridosiliquate c.
  c. aspiration
  atopic c.
  autosomal dominant
    congenital c.
  axial embryonal c.
  axial fusiform developmental c.
  axial partial childhood c.
  axillary c.
  black c.
  blue c.
  blue-dot c.
  bony c.
  bottlemaker's c.
  brown c.
  brunescent c.
  calcareous c.
  capsular c.
  capsulolenticular c.
  central c.
  cerulean c.
  cheesy c.
  choroidal c.
  Christmas tree c.
  complete congenital c.
  complicated c.
  concussion c.
  congenital c.

  contusion c.
  copper c.
  Coppock c.
  coralliform c.
  coronary c.
  cortical spokes c.
  corticosteroid-induced c.
  c. couching
  couching of c.
  crystalline c.
  cuneiform c.
  cupuliform c.
  cystic c.
  dendritic c.
  dermatogenic c.
  developmental c.
  diabetic c.
  diabetic-osmotic c.
  diffuse c.
  dilacerated c.
  disk-shaped c.
  drug-induced c.
  dry-shelled c.
  early mature c.
  electric shock c.
  embryonal nuclear c.
  embryonic c.
  embryopathic c.
  evolutional c.
  extracapsular extraction of c.
  c. extraction (CE)
  extraction of extracapsular c.
  extraction of intracapsular c.
  c. extraction operation
  fibrinous c.
  fibroid c.
  flap operation c.
  Fleischer c.
  floriform c.
  fluid c.
  furnacemen's c.
  fusiform c.
  galactose c.
  galactosemia c.
  general c.
  glassblower's c.
  c. glasses

C

NOTES

cataract *(continued)*
 glassworker's c.
 glaucomatous c.
 global c.
 gray c.
 Green c.
 green c.
 hard c.
 heat-generated c.
 heat-ray c.
 hedger c.
 heterochromic c.
 hook-shaped c.
 hypermature c.
 hypocalcemic c.
 hypoglycemic c.
 immature c.
 incipient c.
 infantile c.
 infrared c.
 intracapsular extraction of c.
 intumescent c.
 c. irradiation
 irradiation c.
 juvenile developmental c.
 c. knife
 c. knife guard
 Koby c.
 lacteal c.
 lamellar developmental c.
 lamellar zonular perinuclear c.
 c. lens
 lenticular c.
 life-belt c.
 lightning c.
 c. mask ring
 c. mask shield
 mature c.
 membranous c.
 metabolic syndrome c.
 milky c.
 mixed c.
 Morgagni c.
 morgagnian c.
 myotonic dystrophy c.
 naphthalinic c.
 c. needle
 nuclear developmental c.
 nutritional deficiency c.
 O'Brien c.
 osmotic c.
 overripe c.
 partial c.

 pear c.
 c. pencil
 perinuclear c.
 peripheral c.
 pisciform c.
 poikiloderma atrophicans
  and c.
 poisoning degenerative c.
 polar c.
 posterior polar c.
 posterior subcapsular c. (PSC)
 postinflammatory c.
 postvitrectomy c.
 C. PPO project
 c. of prematurity
 presenile c.
 primary c.
 probe c.
 progressive c.
 puddler's c.
 punctate c.
 pyramidal c.
 radiation c.
 reduplicated c.
 reduplication c.
 ring-form congenital c.
 ring-shaped c.
 ripe c.
 rubella c.
 sanguineous c.
 saucer-shaped c.
 sclerotic c.
 secondary c.
 sedimentary c.
 senescent cortical
  degenerative c.
 senescent nuclear
  degenerative c.
 senile c.
 senile nuclear sclerotic c.
 senile sclerotic c.
 c. senilis
 shaped c.
 siderosis c.
 siderotic c.
 siliculose c.
 snowflake c.
 snowstorm c.
 Soemmering ring c.
 soft c.
 spear developmental c.
 c. spectacles
 c. spindle

spindle c.
spirochetiform c.
spoke-like sutural c.
c. spoon
spurious c.
stationary c.
stellate c.
steroid-induced c.
subcapsular c.
sugar c.
sugar-induced c.
sunflower c.
supranuclear c.
c. surgery
sutural developmental c.
syndermatotic c.
syphilitic c.
tetany c.
thermal c.
total c.
toxic c.
traumatic degenerative c.
tremulous c.
umbilicated c.
vascular c.
Vogt c.
c. with Down syndrome
x-ray-induced c.
zonular pulverulent c.

cataracta
c. accreta
c. adiposa
c. aridosiliquata
c. brunescens
c. caerulea
c. centralis pulverulenta
c. cerulea
c. complicata
c. congenita membranacea
c. coronaria
c. dermatogenes
c. electrica
c. fibrosa
c. membranacea accreta
c. neurodermatica
c. nigra
c. nodiformis

c. ossea
c. zonularis pulverulenta
cataract-aspirating needle
cataractogenesis
cataractogenic drug
cataractous
Catarase
Catarex
C. cataract removal system
C. technology
catarrh
sinus c.
spring c.
vernal c.
catarrhal
c. conjunctivitis
c. corneal ulcer
c. marginal ulceration
c. ophthalmia
c. ulcerative keratitis
catarrhalis
Branhamella c.
Moraxella c.
catatonic pupil
catatropic image
caterpillar-hair ophthalmia
caterpillar ophthalmia
Catford visual acuity test
catgut suture
catheter
C-flex c.
French c.
Lacricath lacrimal duct c.
lacrimal balloon c.
Lincoff balloon c.
red rubber c.
Teflon injection c.
catheterization
c. of lacrimal duct
c. of lacrimonasal duct
catoptric
catoptroscope
cat's
c. eye
c. eye amaurosis
c. eye effect
c. eye pupil

C

NOTES

cat's *(continued)*
    c. eye reflex
    c. eye syndrome
cat scratch disease neuroretinitis
CAU
    chronic anterior uveitis
caudate hemorrhage
cautery
    Alcon hand c.
    Berkeley Bioengineering
      bipolar c.
    bipolar c.
    Bovie wet-field c.
    Codman wet-field c.
    Colorado c.
    Concept disposable c.
    Concept hand-held c.
    disposable c.
    Eraser c.
    Fine micropoint c.
    Geiger c.
    Gonin c.
    Hildreth c.
    Ishihara I-Temp c.
    I-Temp c.
    Khosia c.
    Mentor wet-field c.
    Mira c.
    Mueller c.
    NeoKnife c.
    c. operation
    ophthalmic c.
    Op-Temp disposable c.
    Parker-Heath c.
    pencil c.
    phacoemulsification c.
    Prince c.
    punctal c.
    Rommel c.
    Rommel-Hildreth c.
    Scheie ophthalmic c.
    scleral c.
    Todd c.
    ValleyLab c.
    von Graefe c.
    Wadsworth-Todd c.
    wet-field c.
    Wills c.
    Ziegler c.
cavern
    Schnabel c.
cavernous
    c. angioma

    c. hemangioma
    c. optic atrophy
    c. portion of the oculomotor
      nerve
    c. sinus
    c. sinus aneurysm
    c. sinus fistula
    c. sinus syndrome
    c. sinus thrombosis
caviae
    Nocardia c.
cavinasi
    bulla ethmoidalis c.
cavitary uveal melanoma
cavitation
Cavitron
    C. aspirator
    C. I/A handpiece
    C. irrigating/aspirating unit
    C. irrigation/aspiration system
Cavitron-Kelman
    C.-K. irrigating/aspirating unit
    C.-K. irrigation/aspiration
      system
cavity
    laser c.
    opening of orbital c.
    optic papilla c.
    orbital c.
    schisis c.
    vitreous c.
CB
    chronic blepharitis
cc
    with correction
CCA
    central choroidal apposition
CCD
    choriocapillaris degeneration
CCF
    critical corresponding frequency
c̄cl
    with contact lenses
CCT
    central corneal thickness
C/D
    cup-to-disk ratio
cd
    candela
CD-5 needle
CD8 cell
CDCR
    conjunctivodacryocystorhinostomy

CE
    cataract extraction
Ceclor
cecocentral
    c. depression
    c. scotoma
cecum
    punctum c.
CeeNU
CeeOn
    C. foldable lens
    C. intraocular lens
cefaclor
cefadroxil
cefamandole
    c. sodium
cefazaflur
cefazolin
cefmenoxime
cefoperazone
ceforanide
cefotaxime
cefsulodin
ceftazidime
ceftizoxime
ceftriaxone
cefuroxime
Celestone
Celita
    C. elite knife
    C. sapphire knife
cell
    c. adhesion
    air c.
    amacrine c.
    antigen-presenting c.
    B c.
    basal c.
    bipolar retinal c.
    budding yeast c.
    CD8 c.
    chick lens c.
    clump c.
    cluster of retinoblastoma c.'s
    collagen c.
    cone c.
    conjunctival epithelial c.

conjunctival goblet c.
corneal c.
cytoxic T c.
c. density
endoneural c.
endothelial c.
epithelial c.
epithelioid c.
fat c.
fiber c.
c. and flare (C&F)
flare and c.
foam c.
foreign body c.
ganglion c.
ghost c.
giant epithelial c.
goblet c.
granulomatous inflammatory c.
helper/inducer T c.
heterogeneous c.
horizontal c.'s
inflammatory c.
interplexiform c.
killer c.
Leber c.
leukemic c.
limbal stem c.
lipid c.
c. lysis
M c.
magnocellular c.
mast c.
membrane lipid c.
meningeal c.
metaplastic epithelial c.
c.'s of Mueller
Müller c.
multinucleated giant
  epithelial c.
mural c.
myoepithelial c.
myoid visual c.
nests and strands of c.'s
neural crest c.
paracentral c.
parvocellular c.

C

NOTES

cell *(continued)*
    perineural c.
    perivascular stromal c.
    photoreceptor c.
    pigment c.
    plasma c.
    polygonal pigmented c.
    polyhedral c.'s
    Reed-Sternberg c.
    reticulum c.
    retinal visual c.
    retinoblastoma c.
    rod c.
    satellite c.
    Schwann c.
    sebaceous c.
    secretory epithelial c.
    somatic c.
    spillover c.
    spindle c.
    spindle-shaped c.
    squamous c.
    stem c. (SC)
    suppressor T c.
    Touton giant c.
    vascular endothelial c.
    visual c.
    vitreal c.
    vitreous c.
    water c.
    Wedl c.
    wet c.
    white c.
    wing c.
    X c.
    Y c.
cell-mediated immunity
cellophane
    crinkled c.
    c. macular reflex
    c. maculopathy
    c. retinopathy
cellophane-like band
Cellufluor
Cellufresh
    C. Formula
cellula, cellulae, pl. **cellulae**
    cellulae lentis
cellular
    c. aggregate
    c. debris
    c. inclusion body
cellularity

cellulitis
    amyloid c.
    herpes simplex c.
    orbital c.
    periorbital c.
    preseptal c.
celluloid frame
cellulosa
    tela c.
cellulose
    c. acetate
    c. acetate butyrate (CAB)
    c. acetate butyrate contact lens
    c. acetate frame
    c. butyrate
    hydroxyethyl c.
    c. nitrate
    c. nitrate frame
    c. surgical sponge
Celluvisc
Celsus
    C. lid
    C. spasmodic entropion
      operation
Celsus-Hotz
    C.-H. entropion
    C.-H. operation
cement
    bifocal c.
    c. bifocal
    Morck c.
center
    distance between c.'s (DBC)
    Dutch Ophthalmic Research C.
      (DORC)
    foveal c.
    gaze c.
    geometric c.
    horizontal gaze c.
    Lions Low Vision C.
    optic c.
    optical c.
    pontine gaze c. (PGC)
    pupillary c.
    rotation c.
    c. of rotation
    c. of rotation distance
    vertical gaze c.
    W.K. Kellogg Eye C.
centering ring
Centra-Flex lens
central
    c. abrasion

c. achromatopsia
c. amaurosis
c. angioplastic retinitis
c. angioplastic retinopathy
c. angiospastic retinitis
c. angiospastic retinopathy
c. anisocoria
c. areolar choroidal atrophy
c. areolar choroidal dystrophy
c. areolar choroidal sclerosis
c. areolar pigment epithelial dystrophy
c. artery
c. astigmatism
c. canal
c. cartilage
c. cataract
c. chorioretinitis
c. choroidal apposition (CCA)
c. choroidal sclerosis
c. choroiditis
c. cloudy corneal dystrophy
c. cloudy dystrophy of François
c. cloudy parenchymatous dystrophy
c. corneal thickness (CCT)
c. corneal ulcer
c. crystalline dystrophy
c. defect
c. disk-shaped retinopathy
c. dyslexia
c. edema
c. edema of cornea
c. endothelial photography
c. field
c. fixation
c. fovea
c. fovea of retina
c. fusion
c. gyrate atrophy
c. illumination
c. iridectomy
c. island
c. island of vision
c. keyhole of vision
c. light

c. nervous system (CNS)
c. pigmentary retinal dystrophy
c. posterior curve (CPC)
c. posterior curve of contact lens
c. reflex stripe
c. retina
c. retinal artery (CRA)
c. retinal artery occlusion (CRAO)
c. retinal degeneration
c. retinal lens
c. retinal vein (CRV)
c. retinal vein occlusion (CRVO, nonischemic CRVO)
c. scotoma
c. scotoma syndrome
c. serous chorioretinopathy
c. serous choroidopathy
c. serous retinitis
c. serous retinochoroidopathy
c. serous retinopathy (CSR)
c. speckled corneal dystrophy
c. steep zone
c. stellate laceration
c. striate keratopathy
c. stromal infiltrate
c. suppression
c. thickness of contact lens
c. vestibular imbalance
c. vestibular nystagmus
c. visual acuity
c. yellow point

centralis
  amaurosis c.
  area c.
  fovea c.
centrally-fixing eye
central, steady and maintained fixation (CSM)
centration
  optical zone c.
centrifugal incision
centripetal
  c. incision
  c. nystagmus

NOTES

centrocecal
  c. defect
  c. scotoma
centronuclear myopathy
centrophose
Centurion syndrome
cepacia
  Pseudomonas c.
cephalexin
cephalgia
cephalic
cephalo-orbital
cephalosporin
Cephalosporium
cephalothin
ceratectomy
cerclage operation
cerebellar
  c. artery
  c. astrocytoma tumor
  c. ataxia
  c. ataxia-cone dystrophy
  c. cortex
  c. dysfunction
  c. eye sign
  c. flocculus
  c. hemisphere
  c. hemorrhage
  c. lesion
  c. notch
  c. tonsil
  c. vermis
cerebellomedullary
cerebellopontine
  c. angle (CPA)
  c. angle lesion
  c. angle tumor
cerebelloretinal
cerebellospinal
cerebellotegmental
cerebellothalamic
cerebellum
cerebral
  c. abscess
  c. achromatopsia
  c. akinetopsia
  c. amaurosis
  c. amyloid angiopathy
  c. arteriography
  c. arteriosclerosis
  c. artery
  c. artery aneurysm
  c. atrophy

  c. blindness
  c. cortex
  c. cortex reflex
  c. diplopia
  c. dyschromatopsia
  c. edema
  c. hemisphere lesion
  c. heterotopia
  c. infarction
  c. layer of retina
  c. metamorphopsia
  c. micropsia
  c. palsy
  c. phycomycosis
  c. polyopia
  c. ptosis
  c. radionuclide angiography
  c. stratum of retina
  c. tunnel vision
  c. venous drainage
  c. ventricle
cerebri
  pseudotumor c. (PTC)
cerebritis
cerebrohepatorenal syndrome
cerebro-ocular
cerebro-opthalmic
cerebropupillary reflex
cerebroretinal angiomatosis
cerebrospinal fluid (CSF)
cerebrotendinous xanthomatosis
cerebrum
cereus
  Bacillus c.
cerulea
  cataracta c.
ceruleae
  maculae c.
cerulean cataract
cervical
  c. ganglion
  c. lesion
  c. nystagmus
cervico-ocular reflex (COR)
cervico-oculo-acoustic syndrome
Cestan-Chenais syndrome
Cestan syndrome
Cetamide O
  Isopto C.
  C. ophthalmic
Cetapred
  Isopto C.
  C. ophthalmic

Cetazol
cetylpyridinium chloride
CF
    counting fingers
C3F8
    perfluoropropane gas
        C3F8 gas
C&F
    cell and flare
C-flex catheter
CFTD
    congenital fiber-type disproportion
chafing
      iris c.
chagrin
      peau de c.
chain
      collagen alpha c.
      fenestrated c.
      sialylated c.
chalazion, pl. chalazia
      acute c.
      c. clamp
      collar-stud c.
      c. curette
      Desmarres c.
      c. forceps
      Meyhoeffer c.
      c. trephine
chalcosis
      cornea c.
      c. lentis
chalkitis
Challenger digital applanation
  tonometer
chamber
      air c.
      c. angle
      angle of anterior c.
      anterior c. (AC)
      aqueous c.
      axial c.
      closed c.
      c. collapse
      depth of c.
      eye c.
      flat anterior c.

      hydrometric c.
      moisture c.
      parallel-plate flow c.
      post c.
      posterior c. (PC)
      quiet c.
      reformation of c.
      shallow c.
      shallowing of c.
      C. sterile adhesive bubble
      sterile adhesive bubble c.
      vitreous c.
chamber-deepening glaucoma
chancre of conjunctiva
chancroid
Chandler
      C. iridectomy
      C. iris forceps
      C. syndrome
      C. vitreous operation
Chandler-Verhoeff
      C.-V. lens extraction
      C.-V. operation
change
      arterial occlusive c.
      cortical c.
      fatty c.
      Keith-Wagener c. (KW)
      KW c.
      nuclear c.
      pigment c.
      senile choroidal c.
      skin c.
      surgically induced refractive c.
      trophic c.
changer
      Galilean magnification c.
      Littmann Galilean
        magnification c.
channel
      c. dissector
      lamellar c.
      scleral c.
Charcot
      C. sign
      C. triad

C

NOTES

CHARGE
coloboma, heart defects, atresia
choanae, retarded growth, genital
hypoplasia, and ear anomalies
CHARGE association
CHARGE syndrome
Charleaux
C. oil droplet reflex
C. oil droplet sign
Charles
C. anterior segment sleeve
C. flute needle
C. infusion sleeve
C. intraocular lens
C. irrigating/aspirating unit
C. irrigating contact lens
C. lensectomy
C. vacuuming needle
C. vitrector with sleeve
Charles-Bonnet syndrome
Charlin syndrome
chart
Amsler c.
astigmatic dial c.
Bailey-Lovie logMar c.
Bailey-Lovie visual acuity c.
Birkhauser test c.
color c.
contemporary nearpoint c.
cross-Polaroid projection c.
Donders c.
Duane accommodation c.
E c.
eye c.
Ferris c.
Guibor c.
Illiterate E c.
Illiterate eye c.
kindergarten eye c.
Konig bar c.
Lancaster-Regan dial 1 c.
Lancaster-Regan dial 2 c.
Landolt broken-ring c.
Landolt C acuity c.
Lea Symbol c.
Lebensohn reading c.
Lebensohn visual acuity c.
Lighthouse ET-DRS acuity c.
logMAR c.
pedigree c.
Pelli-Robson contrast
sensitivity c.
Pelli-Robson letter c.

picture c.
Randot c.
reading c.
Regan low-contrast acuity c.
Reuss color c.
Snellen c.
sunburst dial c.
Turtle c.
University of Waterloo c.
vectograph c.
Vistech wall c.
charting
EyeSys c.
Chavasse glass
Chayet corneal marker
ChBFlow
choroidal blood flow
ChBVol
choroidal blood volume
checkerboard
c. hemianopia
c. visual field
check ligament
Chédiak-Higashi syndrome
cheek
c. clamp
c. flap
cheese wire
cheesewiring of sutures
cheesy cataract
chelonei
Mycobacterium c.
chemical
c. burn
c. conjunctivitis
c. diabetes
c. injury
chemically treated spectacle lens
chemofluorescent dye
chemosis
conjunctival c.
chemotic
cherry-red
c.-r. spot
c.-r. spot in macula
c.-r. spot myoclonus syndrome
chevron incision
Cheyne nystagmus
chi, χ
Chiari malformation
chiasm
glioma of optic c.

c. lesion
optic c.
chiasma
c. opticum
c. syndrome
chiasmal
c. arachnoiditis
c. compression
c. disease
c. dysplasia
c. glioma
c. lesion
c. metastasis
post c.
c. sulcus
c. syndrome
c. visual field loss
chiasmapexy
chiasmatic
c. cisterna
c. field defect
c. syndrome
chiasmometer
Chiba eye needle
Chibroxin
chick lens cell
chief fiber
Chievitz
fiber layer of C.
C. fiber layer
transient layer of C.
chip-and-flip phacoemulsification technique
Chiroflex C11UB lens
Chiron
C. ACS microkeratome
C. automated corneal shaper
C. hansatome
chiroscope
chisel
cornea c.
Freer c.
lacrimal sac c.
West lacrimal sac c.
chi-squared test

Chlamydia
C. psittaci
C. trachomatis
chlamydial
c. blepharitis
c. inclusion conjunctivitis
c. infection
Chlo-Amine
Chloracol
chlorambucil
chloramphenicol
c. and prednisolone
chloramphenicol, polymyxin B, and hydrocortisone
Chlorate
chlordecone
chlordiazepoxide
chlorhexidine
chloride
acetylcholine c.
aluminum c.
benzalkonium c.
cetylpyridinium c.
edrophonium c.
hexamethonium c.
methacholine c.
quaternary ammonium c.
sodium c.
tetraethylammonium c.
chlorisondamine
chloroacetophenone
chlorobutanol
Chlorofair
chloroform
chlorolabe
chloroma
Chloromycetin/Hydrocortisone
Chloromyxin
chlorophane
chloropia
chloroprocaine
chloropsia
Chloroptic
C. Ophthalmic
C. S.O.P.
Chloroptic-P Ophthalmic

NOTES

C

chloroquine
 c. keratopathy
 c. retinopathy
chloroquine/hydroxychloroquine retinopathy
Chlorphed
chlorpheniramine
 c. maleate
chlorphentermine
Chlor-Pro
chlorpromazine
chlorpropamide
chlorprothixene
chlortetracycline
chlorthalidone
Chlor-Trimeton
choked
 c. optic disk
 c. reflex
cholesterinosis
cholesterol
 c. emboli of retina
 c. granuloma
 c. plaque
cholesterolosis
cholesterosis
 c. bulbi
cholinergic
 c. drug
 c. mechanism
 c. neuron
 c. pupil
chondrodystrophia calcificans congenita punctata
chondrodystrophic myotonia
chondroitin
 hyaluronate sodium with c.
 c. sulfate
 c. sulfate medium
chondroitinase
chopper
 Davidoff ambidextrous nucleus c.
 Koch c.
 Nagahara karate c.
 Nichamin triple c.
 Nichamin vertical c.
 Olson phaco c.
 Seibel nucleus c.
 Steinert double-ended claw c.
 Sung reverse nucleus c.
chord
 c. diameter

 c. incision
 c. length
choriocapillaris
 c. degeneration (CCD)
 lamina c.
 membrana c.
 c. vascular network
choriocapillary
 c. atrophy
 c. layer
choriocele
chorioid
chorioidea
chorionic vesicle
chorioretinal (C/R)
 c. adhesion
 c. atrophic spot
 c. atrophy
 c. coloboma
 c. degeneration
 c. granuloma
 c. lesion
 c. venous anastomosis
chorioretinitis
 birdshot c.
 central c.
 luetic c.
 peripheral multifocal c. (PMC)
 sclerosing panencephalitis c.
 c. sclopetaria
 senile c.
 syphilitic c.
 Toxoplasma c.
 toxoplasmosis c.
 vitiliginous c.
chorioretinopathy
 birdshot c.
 central serous c.
 disciform c.
 idiopathic central serous c. (ICSC)
 serous c.
choristoma
 epibulbar limbal dermoid c.
 episcleral osteocartilaginous c.
 limbal c.
 osseous c.
 phakomatous c.
 c. tumor
choroid
 basal c.
 basal lamina of c.
 c. buckle

buckling c.
coloboma of c.
c. coloboma
contusion of c.
crescent c.
c. fissure
knuckle of c.
malignant melanoma of the c.
peripapillary c.
reattachment of c.
vascular lamina of c.
c. vein
choroidal
c. blood flow (ChBFlow)
c. blood volume (ChBVol)
c. cataract
c. coloboma
c. detachment
c. dystrophy
c. edema
c. effusion
c. epithelial atrophy
c. filling
c. flush
c. fold
c. granuloma
c. gyrate atrophy
c. hemangioma
c. hemorrhage
c. hyperfluorescence
c. infarct
c. infiltration
c. ischemia
c. lesion
c. mass
c. melanocytic tumor
c. melanoma
c. metastasis
c. myopic atrophy
c. neoplasm
c. neovascularization (CNV)
c. neovascular membrane
  (CNVM)
c. nevus
c. osteoma
c. primary sclerosis
c. pulse

c. ring
c. rupture
c. scan
c. secondary atrophy
c. tap
c. thinning
c. vascular atrophy
c. vascular occlusion
c. vasculature
c. vessel
c. watershed zone
choroidea
choroideae
complexus basalis c.
lamina vasculosa c.
tapetum c.
choroidectomy
choroideremia
choroiditis
acute diffuse serous c.
anterior c.
areolar central c.
birdshot c.
central c.
diffuse c.
disseminated c.
Douvas honeycombed c.
Doyne familial
  honeycombed c.
exudative c.
focal c.
Förster c.
geographic peripapillary c.
c. guttata senilis
histoplasmic c.
Holthouse-Batten superficial c.
Hutchinson-Tays central
  guttate c.
Jensen juxtapapillary c.
juxtapupillary c.
macular c.
metastatic c.
multifocal c.
c. myopia
nongranulomatous c.
posterior c.
proliferative c.

NOTES

choroiditis *(continued)*
    punctate inner c.
    recurrent c.
    senescent macular exudative c.
    senile macular exudative c.
    c. serosa
    serosa c.
    serpiginous c.
    suppurative c.
    syphilitic c.
    Tay c.
    toxoplasmic c.
    traumatic c.
    unifocal helioid c.
choroidocapillaris
    lamina c.
choroidocyclitis
choroidoiritis
choroidopathy
    areolar c.
    central serous c.
    Doyne honeycombed c.
    geographic helicoid
      peripapillary c.
    guttate c.
    helicoid c.
    inner punctate c.
    myopic c.
    peripapillary central serous c.
    senile guttate c.
    serpiginous c.
choroidoretinal dystrophy
choroidoretinitis
choroidosis
choroidovaginal vein
choroidovitreal neovascularization
Choyce
    C. implant
    C. intraocular lens
    C. lens-inserting forceps
    C. Mark VIII implant
    C. Mark VIII lens
Christmas tree cataract
chromatic
    c. asymmetry
    c. dispersion
    c. lens aberration
    c. perimetry
    c. spectrum
    c. vision
chromatism
chromatometer
chromatopsia

chromatoptometer
chromatoptometry
chromatoskiameter
chromic
    c. catgut suture
    c. collagen suture
    c. gut suture
    c. myopia
chromodacryorrhea
chromogranin antibody
chromometer
chromophane
chromophobe adenoma
chromophore
chromoretinopathy
chromoscope
chromoscopy
Chromos imager system
chromostereopsis
chronic
    c. actinic keratopathy
    c. angle-closure glaucoma
    c. anterior uveitis (CAU)
    c. blepharitis (CB)
    c. blepharoconjunctivitis
    c. catarrhal conjunctivitis
    c. catarrhal rhinitis
    c. cyclitis
    c. dacryocystitis
    c. demyelinating optic neuritis
    c. endophthalmitis
    c. follicular conjunctivitis
    c. narrow-angle glaucoma
    c. open-angle glaucoma
      (COAG)
    c. optic disk swelling
    c. optic nerve compression
    c. papilledema
    c. primary angle-closure
      glaucoma (C-PACG)
    c. progressive external
      ophthalmoplegia (CPEO)
    c. serpiginous ulcer
    c. simple glaucoma
    c. superficial keratitis
chrysiasis
chrysoderma
Chu cutter
Churg-Strauss syndrome
Chvostek sign
Chymar
    Alpha C.
chymotrypsin

CI
   convergence insufficiency
Ciaccio gland
Cibasoft contact lens
Cibathin lens
Cibis
   C. conjunctivitis
   C. ectropion
   C. electrode
   C. entropion
   C. liquid silicone procedure
   C. operation
   C. pemphigoid
   C. ski needle
cibisotome
cicatrices (*pl. of* cicatrix)
cicatriceum
   ectropion c.
   entropion c.
cicatricial
   c. conjunctivitis
   c. ectropion
   c. entropion
   c. mass
   c. pemphigoid
   c. retinopathy of prematurity
   c. retrolental fibroplasia
   c. strabismus
cicatrix, pl. cicatrices
   cystoid c.
   filtering c.
cicatrization
cicatrizing
   c. conjunctivitis
   c. trachoma
cidofovir
   c. eye drops
   c. therapy
CIF4 needle
CIGTS
   Collaborative Initial Glaucoma
   Treatment Study
Cilco
   C. argon laser
   C. Frigitronics
   C. Frigitronics laser
   C. Hoffer Laseridge

   C. Hoffer Laseridge laser
   C. intraocular lens
   C. krypton laser
   C. lens forceps
   C. MonoFlex multi-piece
   PMMA intraocular lens
   C. perimeter
   C. Sonometric A-scan
   C. Ultrasound unit
   C. vitrector
   C. YAG laser
Cilco/Lasertek
   C. A/K laser
   C. argon laser
   C. krypton laser
Cilco-Simcoe II lens
Cilco-Sonometrics lens
cilia (*var. of* cilium) (*pl. of*
  cilium)
ciliare
   corpus c.
ciliares
   plicae c.
   processus c.
ciliaris
   acne c.
   annulus c.
   blepharitis c.
   corona c.
   corpus c.
   fibrae circulares musculi c.
   fibrae longitudinales musculi c.
   fibrae meridionales musculi c.
   fibrae radiales musculi c.
   gangliosus c.
   musculus c.
   orbicularis c.
   pars plana corporis c.
   pars plicata corporis c.
   radix oculomotoria ganglii c.
   radix sympathica ganglii c.
   striae c.
   tylosis c.
   zona c.
   zonula c.
ciliariscope
ciliarotomy

NOTES

ciliary
- c. apparatus
- c. artery
- c. blepharitis
- c. block
- c. block glaucoma
- c. body
- c. body band
- c. body coloboma
- c. body inflammation
- c. canal
- c. cartilage
- c. crown
- c. disk
- c. epithelium
- c. flush
- c. fold
- c. ganglion
- c. ganglionic plexus
- c. gland
- c. hyperemia
- c. injection
- c. ligament
- c. margin
- c. margin of iris
- c. muscle
- c. nerve
- c. procedure
- c. process
- c. reflex
- c. region
- c. ring
- c. spasm
- c. staphyloma
- c. sulcus
- c. vein
- c. vessel
- c. zone
- c. zonule

ciliate
ciliectomy
ciliochoroidal
- c. detachment
- c. effusion
- c. melanoma

ciliodestructive surgery
cilioequatorial fiber
ciliogenesis
ciliolenticular block
cilioposterocapsular fiber
cilioretinal
- c. artery
- c. collateral
- c. vein

ciIioscleral
ciliosis
ciliospinal
- c. center of Budge
- c. reflex

ciliotomy
ciliovitreal block
ciliovitrectomy
- c. block

cilium, cilia, pl. **cilia**
- cilia base
- cilia ectopia
- cilia follicle
- cilia forceps
- intraocular cilia

cillo
cillosis
Ciloxan
- C. Ophthalmic

CIMA*flex* 411 foldable silicone lens
CIN
- conjunctival intraepithelial neoplasia

cinching
- c. operation

cinema eye
cine-magnetic resonance imaging
Cine-Microscope
ciprofloxacin
- c. hydrochloride

circadian heterotropia
circinata
- retinitis c.

circinate
- c. exudate
- retinal c.
- c. retinitis
- c. retinopathy

circle
- arterial c.
- Berry c.
- c. of confusion
- c. diffusion
- c. of dispersion
- c. dissipation
- episcleral arterial c.
- c. of greater iris
- c. of Haller
- Hovius c.
- c. of least confusion
- least diffusion c.
- c. of lesser iris

Minsky c.
Randot c.
Vieth-Mueller c.
c. of Willis
Wort c.
Zinn c.
Zinn-Haller arterial c.
circlet
Zinn c.
Circline magnifier
circling band
circular
c. blade
c. ciliary muscle
c. ciliary muscle fiber
c. dichroism
c. nystagmus
c. synechia
c. tear capsulotomy
circularvection
circulating immune complex
circulation
conjunctival c.
episcleral c.
foveolar choroidal c.
perilimbic c.
retinal c.
sludging of c.
circulus
c. arteriosus halleri
c. arteriosus iridis major
c. arteriosus iridis minor
c. vasculosus nervi optici
c. zinnii
circumbulbar
circumciliary flush
circumcorneal injection
circumduction
c. hyperphoria
circumferential
c. vascular plexus of the limbus
circumlental space
circumocular
circumorbital
circumpapillary
c. light reflex

c. telangiectatic microangiopathy
circumscribed episcleritis
canities circumscripta
circus senilis
cirsoid aneurysm
cirsophthalmia
cirsophthalmus
cisterna
chiasmatic c.
cisternography
CIT
corneal impression test
Citelli rongeur
CL
contact lens
Cladosporium
clamp
Alabama-Green c.
Backhaus c.
Barraquer needle holder c.
Berens muscle c.
Berke c.
bulldog c.
Castroviejo lid c.
Castroviejo needle holder c.
chalazion c.
cheek c.
cross-action towel c.
curved mosquito c.
Desmarres lid c.
Erhardt c.
Gladstone-Putterman entropion c.
Gladstone-Putterman transmarginal rotation entropion c.
Halsted curved mosquito c.
Halsted straight mosquito c.
Hartmann c.
Jones towel c.
Kalt needle holder c.
King c.
Moria-France dacryocystorhinostomy c.
mosquito c.
muscle c.

NOTES

clamp *(continued)*
   needle holder c.
   Prince muscle c.
   Putterman levator resection c.
   Putterman-Mueller
     blepharoptosis c.
   Putterman ptosis c.
   Robin chalazion c.
   Schaedel cross-action towel c.
   Schnidt c.
   serrefine c.
   straight mosquito c.
CLARE
   contact lens-induced acute red eye
Clarithromycin
Claritin
clarity
   corneal c.
   optical c.
Clark
   C. Autophoro-Optimeter
   C. capsule fragment forceps
   C. speculum
Clark-Verhoeff capsule forceps
classic
   c. choroidal neovascularization
   c. dendritic keratitis
   c. flower petal pattern
classical congenital esophoria
classification
   Callender cell type c.
   Duane c.
   Gass macular hole c.
   Keith-Wagener-Barker c.
   Leishman c.
   MacCallan c.
   Reese-Ellsworth c.
   Retina Society c.
   Scheie c.
   Shaffer-Weiss c.
   tear secretion c.
   Tessier c.
   Wagener-Clay-Gipner c.
Claude
   C. Bernard syndrome
   C. syndrome
Claude-Bernard-Horner syndrome
Clayman
   C. guide
   C. intraocular lens
   C. lens-holding forceps
   C. lens implant forceps

   C. lens-inserting forceps
   C. posterior chamber lens
Clayman-Knolle irrigating lens loop
Clean
   Gel C.
   Sila C.
cleaner
   Boston Advance c.
   enzymatic c.
   enzyme c.
   gas-permeable daily c.
   Lens Plus daily c.
   Opti-Zyme enzymatic c.
   ProFree/GP weekly
     enzymatic c.
   ReNu Effervescent
     enzymatic c.
   ReNu Thermal enzymatic c.
   Sensitive Eyes daily c.
   Soflens enzymatic contact
     lens c.
   Soft Mate Enzyme Plus c.
   Soft Mate Hands Off daily c.
   Ultrazyme enzymatic c.
   Vision Care enzymatic c.
Clean-N-Soak
Clean-N-Stow
cleanup
   cortical c.
Clear
   C. Eyes
   C. Eyes ACR
   C. Image III
   Lens C.
clear
   c. corneal step incision
   c. corneal tunnel incision
   c. crystalline lens
   c. keratin sleeve
   c. lensectomy
   c. lid vesicle
   c. window
clearance
   apical c.
clearing
   media c.
Cleasby
   C. iridectomy operation
   C. spatula
   C. spatulated needle
cleavage syndrome
cleaver
   Haefliger c.

cleft
corneal c.
cortical c.
cyclodialysis c.
excessive cyclodialysis c.
facial c.
sonolucent c.
c. syndrome
clefting
cortical c.
Tessier c.
CLEK
Collaborative Longitudinal
Evaluation of Keratoconus
clemastine
Clens
Clerf needle holder
clerical spectacles
Clerz 2
click phenomenon
climatic
c. droplet keratopathy
c. proteoglycan stromal
keratopathy
c. stromal keratopathy
clindamycin
clinical trial
Clinitex
C. Charles endophotocoagulator
probe
C. photocoagulator
C. photomydriasis
clinometer
clinoscope
clioquinol
clip
bipolar diathermy adapter c.
Castroviejo scleral
shortening c.
double tantalum c.
Federov four-loop iris c.
Friedman tantalum c.
Halberg trial c.
holding c.
Janelli c.
lens c.
Platina c.

scleral shortening c.
tantalum c.
trial c.
two-way towel c.
clip-applying forceps
clip-on/tie-on occluder
clivus
clobetasol propionate
clock
astigmatic c.
c. dial
clock-mechanism esotropia
clofazimine
C-loop
C.-l. intraocular lens
C.-l. posterior chamber lens
Cloquet canal
closed
c. chamber
eyelids sutured c.
c. loop
c. surgery on eye
closed-angle glaucoma
closed-dissection technique
closed-eye surgery
closed-funnel vitreoretinopathy
closed-loop system
closed-system pars plana vitrectomy
clostridial
c. blepharitis
c. panophthalmitis
Clostridium
C. bifermentans
C. difficile
C. histolyticum
C. perfringens
C. subterminale
C. tetani
C. welchii
closure
capillary c.
crow-foot c.
forced-eye c.
hallucination with eye c.
insufficiency of eyelid c.
synechial c.
wound c.

NOTES

clotrimazole
clouding
    corneal c.
    feathery c.
    hyaloid c.
    vitreous c.
cloudy cornea
clove-hitch suture
cloxacillin
clump
    c. cell
    vortex-like c.
clumped
    c. pigmentation
    c. retinal pigment
clumping
    pigment c.
    pigmentary rarefaction and c.
cluster
    c. headache
    macular c.
    c. of pigmented spots
    c. of retinoblastoma cells
CMAP
    compound muscle action potential
CMD
    cystoid macular degeneration
CME
    cystoid macular edema
CMS AccuProbe 450 system
CMV
    cytomegalovirus
    macular CMV
    CMV retinopathy
CN
    cranial nerve
CNS
    central nervous system
CNV
    choroidal neovascularization
CNVM
    choroidal neovascular membrane
CO$_2$
    C. laser
    C. Sharplan laser
COAG
    chronic open-angle glaucoma
coagulate
coagulating electrode
coagulation
    disseminated intravascular c.
    light c.
    Meyer-Schwickerath light c.

coagulator
    argon laser c.
    Evergreen Lasertek c.
    Grieshaber micro-bipolar c.
    Laserflex c.
    Meyer-Schwickerath c.
    Walker c.
coagulopathy
coalescent mass
coal-mining lensectomy
coaptation bipolar forceps
coarse punctate staining
coastal erysipelas
coast erosion
coat
    buffy c.
    C.'s disease
    C.'s retinitis
    sclerotic c.
    C.'s syndrome
    uveal c.
    C.'s white ring
coated Vicryl suture
coater
    Polaron sputter c.
coating
    antireflection c.
    color c.
    edge c.
    c. of lens
    c. material
    mirror c.
    proteinaceous c.
    RLX c.
    c. for spectacle lens
coaxial illumination
coaxially sighted corneal reflex
cobalt
    c. blue filter
    c. blue light
    c. therapy
cobblestone
    c. appearance
    c. conjunctivitis
    c. papilla
    c. retinal degeneration
Coburn
    C. camera
    C. intraocular lens
    C. irrigation/aspiration system
    C. irrigation/aspiration unit
    C. lensometer

C. refractor
C. tonometer
Coburn-Rodenstock slit lamp
cocaine
    c. block
    c. hydrochloride
    c. methylphenidate
    c. test
cocci
    gram-positive c.
Coccidioides immitis
coccidioidomycosis
    c. immitis
    intraocular c.
Cochet-Bonnet esthesiometer
cochleopupillary reflex
Cockayne syndrome
co-contraction syndrome
codeine
Codman wet-field cautery
coefficient
    c. of facility of outflow
    c. of variation
Coerens tumor
Coffin-Lowry syndrome
Cogan
    C. congenital oculomotor
    apraxia
    C. disease
    C. interstitial keratitis
    C. lid twitch
    C. lid-twitch sign
    C. microcystic corneal
    epithelial dystrophy
    C. microcystic epithelial
    corneal dystrophy
    C. patch
    C. sign
    C. syndrome
Cogan-Boberg-Ans lens implant
Cogan-Reese syndrome
cogwheel
    c. ocular movement
    c. pupil
    c. pursuit
    c. pursuit movement
Cohan-Barraquer microscope

Cohan-Vannas iris scissors
Cohan-Westcott scissors
Cohen
    C. corneal forceps
    C. needle holder
    C. syndrome
Coherent
    C. 920 argon/dye laser
    C. 900 argon laser
    C. 920 argon laser
    C. dye laser
    C. EPIC laser
    C. krypton laser
    C. 7910 laser
    C. LaserLink slit lamp
    C. Medical YAG laser
    C. Novus Omni
    multiwavelength laser
    C. photocoagulator
    C. radiation argon/krypton laser
    C. radiation argon model 800
    laser
    C. radiation Fluorotron
    C. Selecta 7000 laser
cohort study
coil
    basal c.
    electromagnetic scleral
    search c.
    scleral search c.
coin gauge
cold-opposite, warm-same (COWS)
Coleman retractor
Coleman-Taylor IOL forceps
colforsin
coli
    Escherichia c.
Colibri
    C. forceps
    C. microforceps
coliform
    c. blepharitis
    c. organism
colistin
Collaborative
    C. Initial Glaucoma Treatment
    Study (CIGTS)

C

NOTES

Collaborative *(continued)*
  C. Longitudinal Evaluation of
    Keratoconus (CLEK)
collagen
  c. alpha chain
  c. bandage lens
  c. cell
  c. fiber
  c. fibril
  c. fibril interweaving
  c. lamella
  c. plug
  c. and rheumatoid-related
    disease
  c. shield
  c. vascular disease
collagenase
  bacterial c.
collagenolysis
collagenolytic trabecular ring
collagenous trabecular ring
collapse
  chamber c.
collar button
collarette
collar-stud chalazion
collateral
  cilioretinal c.
  c. vessel
colliculus
  superior c.
Collier
  C. sign
  tucked lid of C.
Collin-Beard operation
Collin 140 color adaptometer
Collins syndrome
colliquation
  discrete c.
colliquative
  discrete c.
collision tumor
collodion dressing
colloid
  c. body
  c. cyst
  c. deposit
collyrium, pl. **collyria**
  Beer C.
  C. eye drops
  C. Oresh ophthalmic
Colmascope
coloboma, pl. **colobomata**

c. anomaly
atypical c.
bridge c.
chorioretinal c.
c. of choroid
choroid c.
choroidal c.
ciliary body c.
complete c.
congenital optic nerve c.
dysplastic c.
eyelid c.
fissure c.
Fuchs inferior c.
Fuchs spot c.
c. of fundus
c. iridis
iris c.
c. of iris
c. of lens
c. lentis
c. lobuli
macular c.
ocular c.
optic c.
c. of optic nerve
optic nerve c.
c. palpebrale
peripapillary c.
c. of retina
c. retinae
retinochoroidal c.
typical c.
c. of vitreous
vitreous c.
coloboma, heart defects, atresia
  choanae, retarded growth, genital
  hypoplasia, and ear anomalies
  (CHARGE)
colobomatous
  c. cyst
  c. microphthalmia
  c. optic disk
color
  c. aberration
  c. adaptation
  c. adaptometer
  c. agnosia
  c. amblyopia
  c. anomia
  C. Bar Schirmer strip
  c. bar Schirmer tear test
  c. blind

c. blindness
c. chart
c. coating
c. comparison
c. comparison test
complementary c.
confusion c.
c. confusion
c. constancy
c. contrast
c. defect
deviant c.
c. discrimination
c. disk
c. Doppler imaging
end-point c.
eye c.
c. fusion
incidental c.
metameric c.
c. mixing
Munsell c.
c. naming
opponent c.
c. perception
c. perimetry
primary c.
pure c.
reflected c.
saturated c.
c. saturation
c. scotoma
C. Screening Inventory
c. sense
simple c.
solid c.
c. spectrum
c. theory
c. triangle
c. vision
c. vision test
c. washout
Colorado
 C. cautery
 C. needle
ColorChecker
 Macbeth C.

color-contrast
 c.-c. sensitivity measurement
 c.-c. threshold
colorimeter
colossal agenesis
column
 ocular dominance c.
columnar layer
Colvard pupillometer
Coly-Mycin S
COMA
 congenital ocular motor apraxia
coma
 c. aberration
 eyes-open c.
 metabolic c.
Comberg
 C. contact lens
 C. foreign body operation
 C. localization
Combiline System
combined
 c. dystrophy of Fuchs
 c. fracture
 c. trabeculotomy-trabeculectomy
combined-mechanism glaucoma
comedo pattern
comet scotoma
comfort
 c. bridge
 C. drops
 C. Ophthalmic
 C. Tears
 C. Tears Solution
ComfortKone lens
comitance
comitant
 c. exodeviation
 c. exophoria
 c. exotropia
 c. heterotropia
 c. squint
 c. strabismus
 c. vertical deviation
comminuted orbital fracture
commissura, commissurae,
 pl. **commissurae**

NOTES

commissura *(continued)*
    commissurae opticae
    c. palpebrarum lateralis
    c. palpebrarum medialis
    c. palpebrarum nasalis
    c. palpebrarum temporalis
commissure
    arcuate c.
    c. of Gudden
    Gudden c.
    interthalamic c.
    Meynert c.
    nucleus of posterior c.
    optic c.
    palpebral c.
    posterior chiasmatic c.
    supraoptic c.
common
    c. canaliculus
    c. tendinous ring
commotio retinae
communicating artery aneurysm
communication
    arteriole c.
    arteriovenous c.
communis
    annulus tendineus c.
community-acquired corneal ulcer
Compak-200 mini-excimer
Company
    Neitz Instruments C.
comparison
    brightness c.
    color c.
    c. eyepiece
compass
    Mastel diamond c.
compensated
    c. glaucoma
    c. segment
compensating eyepiece
competition swimmer's eyelid syndrome
complement
    c. component
    c. fixation test
    c. system
complementary
    c. afterimage
    c. color
complement-fixing antibody
complete
    c. achromatopsia

    c. blood count
    c. but pupil-sparing oculomotor nerve paresis
    c. coloboma
    c. congenital cataract
    c. hemianopsia
    c. iridectomy
    c. iridoplegia
    c. palsy
complex
    AIDS-related c. (ARC)
    circulating immune c.
    c. ectropion
    Golgi c.
    immune c.
    major histocompatibility c.
    c. motion tomography
    c. retinal detachment
    triple symptom c.
    tuberous sclerosis c. (TSC)
complexus basalis choroideae
compliance cap
complicata
    cataracta c.
complicated cataract
component
    amyloid P c.
    complement c.
    quick left/right c.
composition of spectacle lens
compound
    c. eye
    Hurler-Scheie c.
    c. hyperopic astigmatism
    c. lens
    c. muscle action potential (CMAP)
    c. myopic astigmatism
    c. nevus
    quaternary ammonium c.
    silver c.
    c. spectacles
    c. vesicle
compression
    chiasmal c.
    chronic optic nerve c.
    c. cyanosis
    c. dressing
    c. gonioscopy
    limbal c.
    c. molding
    optic tract c.
    prechiasmal c.

c. retinopathy
c. suture
compressive
c. nystagmus
c. optic nerve defect
c. optic neuropathy
compressor
Anthony orbital c.
Berens orbital c.
Castroviejo c.
orbital enucleation c.
compulsive eye opening
Compuscan-P pachymeter
computed
C. Anatomy Corneal Modeling System
c. perimetry
c. tomographic angiography
c. tomography (CT)
c. tomography scan
computer-assisted
c.-a. corneal topography
c.-a. videokeratoscope
computerized
c. corneal topography
c. corneal videokeratography
c. photokeratoscope
c. videokeratography (CVK)
computer vision syndrome (CVS)
Computon Microtonometer
concave
c. cylinder
c. mirror
c. reflecting surface
c. spectacle lens
concavity
iris c.
concavoconcave lens
concavoconvex lens
concentration deficit
concentric
c. constriction
c. fold
c. lesion
c. sclerosis of Balo
c. stria

concentrica
encephalitis periaxialis c.
concentrically
Concentrix Fluidics
Concept
C. disposable cautery
C. hand-held cautery
concha bullosa
conclination
concomitance
concomitant
c. exophoria
c. heterotropia
c. strabismus
concretion
conjunctival c.
concussion
c. blindness
c. cataract
c. injury
c. of the retina
condensation
vitreoretinal c.
condensing lens
condition
conjunctival cell c.
null c.
predisposing c.
conditioning film
cone
c. achromatopsia
apical c.
bipolar c.
blue c.
c. b-wave amplitude
c. b-wave implicit time electroretinogram
c. cell
c. degeneration
c. dysfunction
c. dystrophy
c. dystrophy-cerebellar ataxia
c. electroretinogram
c. fiber
c. function
c. granule
layer of rods and c.'s

C

NOTES

cone *(continued)*
 McIntyre truncated c.
 c. monochromat
 monochromatic c.
 c. monochromatism
 muscle c.
 ocular c.
 c. opsin
 pedicle c.
 c. photopigment
 c. response
 retinal c.
 Rochon-Duvigneaud bouquet
  of c.'s
 rods and c.'s
 triad of retinal c.
 twin c.
 c. vision
 visual c.
 X-linked c.
cone-rod
 c.-r. degeneration
 c.-r. dystrophy (CRD)
configuration
 bombé c.
 Kratz-Sinskey loop c.
 plateau iris c.
 vacuolar c.
 whorl-like c.
confluent
 c. defect
 c. drusen
confocal
 c. laser scanning
  ophthalmoscope
 c. laser scanning topography
 c. microscope
 c. microscopy
 c. microscopy identification of
  Acanthamoeba keratitis
 c. optics
 c. scanning laser Doppler
  flowmetry
 c. scanning laser
  ophthalmoscope
 c. scanning laser
  ophthalmoscopy
 c. scanning laser polarimeter
 c. scanning laser tomography
conformer
 eye implant c.
 Fox c.
 McGuire c.

 silicone c.
 Universal c.
confrontation
 c. field defect
 c. method
 c. visual field
 c. visual field test
 c. visual field testing
confusion
 circle of c.
 circle of least c.
 color c.
 c. color
 congenital c.
 visual c.
congenita
 dyskeratosis c.
 ectopia pupillae c.
 myotonia c.
 paramyotonia c.
congenital
 c. abducens facial paralysis
 c. abducens nerve lesion
 c. abducens nerve palsy
 c. abduction paralysis
 c. abnormality
 c. absence of abduction
 c. adduction palsy with
  synergistic divergence
 c. adherence syndrome
 c. amaurosis
 c. anomaly
 c. anophthalmos
 c. anterior staphyloma (CAS)
 c. anterior synechia
 c. astigmatism
 c. brain malformation
 c. bulbar paralysis
 c. cataract
 c. cleft of iris
 c. confusion
 c. conus
 c. crescent
 c. dacryocele
 c. dacryocystitis
 c. dermoid of limbus
 c. dichromatism
 c. dyschromatopsia
 c. dyskeratosis
 c. dystrophic ptosis
 c. dysversion
 c. ectropion
 c. entropion

c. esophoria
c. esotropia
c. facial diplegia
c. fiber-type disproportion (CFTD)
c. fibrosis
c. fibrous syndrome
c. glaucoma
c. hemianopsia
c. hereditary corneal dystrophy
c. hereditary endothelial corneal dystrophy
c. heterochromia
c. Horner syndrome
c. ichthyosis
c. impatency
c. juxtafoveolar syndrome
c. lens dislocation
c. lens opacity
c. leukopathia
c. limbal corneal dermoid
c. limbal corneal dermoid tumor
c. macrodisc
c. macular degeneration
c. medullated optic nerve fiber
c. melanosis oculi
c. miosis
c. muscular dystrophy
c. mydriasis
c. myopathic eyelid retraction
c. myopathic ptosis
c. myopathy
c. myotonic dystrophy
c. nasolacrimal duct obstruction
c. nystagmus
c. ocular melanocytosis
c. ocular motor apraxia (COMA)
c. oculodermal melanocytosis
c. oculofacial paralysis
c. oculomotor nerve palsy
c. oculopalpebral synkinesia
c. optic atrophy
c. optic disk pigmentation
c. optic nerve coloboma
c. optic nerve pit

c. paradoxic gustolacrimal reflex
c. pterygium
c. retinal fold
c. retinoschisis
c. rubella syndrome
c. superior oblique underaction
c. syphilis
c. syphilitic conjunctivitis
c. tilted disk syndrome
c. toxoplasmosis
congenitale
poikiloderma c.
congenitum
corestenoma c.
congested vessel
congestion
c. of conjunctiva
deep c.
superficial c.
transient c.
vascular c.
venous c.
congestive glaucoma
congruent point
congruity
congruous
c. field defect
c. hemianopsia
c. homonymous hemianopic scotoma
c. homonymous horizontal sectoranopia
c. homonymous quadruple sectoranopia
coni (*pl. of* conus)
conical
c. cornea
c. implant
c. protrusion
conjugacy
object/image c.
conjugate
c. disparity
c. focus
c. gaze
c. gaze palsy

NOTES

conjugate *(continued)*
   c. horizontal deviation
   c. horizontal eye movement
   c. movement of eyes
   c. nystagmus
   c. ocular movement
   c. paralysis
   c. point
conjugately
conjunctiva, gen. and pl. **conjunctivae**
   annulus of c.
   bulbar c.
   chancre of c.
   congestion of c.
   emphysema of c.
   epitheliosis desquamativa
     conjunctivae
   c. forceps
   Förster c.
   glandulae mucosae conjunctivae
   leptotrichosis conjunctivae
   lithiasis conjunctivae
   palpebral c.
   plica semilunaris conjunctivae
   c. retractor
   saccus conjunctivae
   sebaceous gland of c.
   semilunar folds of c.
   siderosis conjunctivae
   c. spreader
   tarsal c.
   tela c.
   temporal bulbar c.
   tunica c.
   tyloma conjunctivae
   upper tarsal c.
   xerosis conjunctivae
**conjunctiva-associated lymphoid
  tissue**
conjunctival
   c. abrasion
   c. amyloidosis
   c. angioma
   c. artery
   c. bleb
   c. brachium
   c. break
   c. calcification
   c. cell condition
   c. chemosis
   c. ciliary injection
   c. circulation
   c. concretion

c. contusion
c. crystal
c. cul-de-sac
c. cyst
c. deposit
c. dermoid
c. discharge
c. dysplasia
c. edema
c. epithelial cell
c. exudate
c. flap
c. follicle
c. foreign body
c. gland
c. goblet cell
c. goblet cell density
c. granuloma
c. hemangioma
c. hemorrhage
c. hyperemia
c. impression cytology
c. incision
c. intraepithelial neoplasia
  (CIN)
c. laceration
c. limbus
c. lipodermoid
c. lithiasis
c. lymphangioma
c. lymphoid proliferation
c. lymphoid tumor
c. melanoma
c. melanotic lesion
c. membrane
c. metaplasia
c. necrosis
c. nodule
c. papilla
c. papilloma
c. patch graft
c. phlyctenulosis
c. pigmented nevus
c. pseudomembrane
c. pterygium
c. reaction
c. recession
c. reflex
c. ring
c. rotation autografting
c. sac
c. scarring
c. scissors

c. scraping
c. semilunar fold
c. slough
c. smear
c. squamous cell neoplasia
c. staining
c. tear
c. ulcer
c. varix
c. vascular engorgement
c. vascularization
c. vein
c. vessel
c. xerosis
conjunctivales
glandulae c.
glandulae ciliares c.
glandulae sebaceae c.
venae c.
venae anteriores c.
venae posteriores c.
conjunctivalis
nodulus c.
saccus c.
conjunctiva-Mueller muscle excision
conjunctiviplasty (*var. of*
conjunctivoplasty)
conjunctivitis
acne rosacea c.
actinic c.
acute atopic c.
acute catarrhal c.
acute congestive c.
acute contagious c.
acute epidemic c.
acute follicular c.
acute hemorrhagic c.
adenovirus c.
adult inclusion c.
allergic c.
anaphylactic c.
angular c.
Apollo c.
arc-flash c.
c. arida
atopic c.
atropine c.

Axenfeld follicular c.
bacterial c.
Bangla Joy c.
Béal c.
blennorrheal c.
blepharitis c.
Butcher c.
calcareous c.
candidal c.
candidiasis c.
catarrhal c.
chemical c.
chlamydial inclusion c.
chronic catarrhal c.
chronic follicular c.
Cibis c.
cicatricial c.
cicatrizing c.
cobblestone c.
congenital syphilitic c.
contact c.
contagious granular c.
croupous c.
diphtheritic c.
diplobacillary c.
drug-induced cicatricial c.
(DICC)
drug-induced cicatrizing c.
eczematous c.
Egyptian c.
Elschnig c.
epidemic c.
erythema multiforme c.
exanthematous c.
factitious c.
follicular c.
giant papillary c. (GPC)
gonococcal c.
gonorrheal c.
gout c.
granular c.
hay fever c.
hemorrhagic c.
herpes simplex c.
herpes zoster c.
hyperacute c.
immunological c.

C

NOTES

conjunctivitis *(continued)*
inclusion c.
infantile purulent c.
infectious c.
Koch-Weeks c.
lacrimal c.
lagophthalmia c.
larval c.
c. ligneous
ligneous c.
lithiasis c.
Lymphogranuloma venereum c.
c. medicamentosa
meibomian c.
membranous c.
meningococcus c.
microbiallergic c.
molluscum c.
c. molluscum
Morax-Axenfeld c.
mucopurulent c.
c. necroticans infectiosus
necrotic infectious c.
neisserial c.
neonatal inclusion c.
newborn c.
c. nodosa
nodular c.
nonatopic allergic c.
ocular vaccinial c.
oculoglandular c.
papillary c.
Parinaud oculoglandular c.
Pascheff c.
c. petrificans
phlegmatous c.
phlyctenular c.
pink eye c.
pneumococcal c.
prairie c.
pseudomembranous c.
pseudovernal c.
purulent c.
Reiter c.
rubeola c.
Samoan c.
Sanyal c.
scrofulous c.
shipyard c.
simple acute c.
Singapore epidemic c.
snow c.
spring c.

springtime c.
squirrel plague c.
staphylococcal c.
swimming pool c.
Thygeson chronic follicular c.
toxic follicular c.
toxicogenic c.
trachoma inclusion c.
trachomatous c.
tuberculosis c.
tularemic c.
c. tularensis
unilateral c.
uratic c.
vernal c.
viral c.
Wegener granulomatosis c.
welder's c.
Widmark c.
Wucherer c.
c. xeroderma pigmentosum
conjunctivochalasis
conjunctivodacryocystorhinosto my (CDCR)
conjunctivodacryocystostomy
conjunctivoma
conjunctivoplasty, conjunctiviplasty
conjunctivorhinostomy
conjunctivotarsal
conjunctivo-Tenon flap
conjunctivum
brachium c.
Con-Lish polishing method
connection
Luer c.
synaptic c.
connective
c. tissue
c. tissue membrane
connector
McIntyre nylon cannula c.
Connor wand
Conn syndrome
conoid
c. lens
c. of Sturm
Sturm c.
conomyoidin
conophthalmus
conotruncal anomalies face syndrome
Conradi syndrome

Conrad orbital blowout fracture operation
consecutive
    c. anophthalmia
    c. esotropia
    c. exotropia
    c. optic atrophy
consensual
    c. light reflex
    c. light response
    c. pupillary response
    c. reaction
Consept
    Soft Mate C.
constancy
    color c.
constant
    c. esotropia
    c. exophoria
    c. hypertropia
    c. hypotropia
    c. monocular tropia
    c. nystagmus
    c. strabismus
constricted pupil
constriction
    concentric c.
    focal c.
constructional
    c. ability contact lens
    c. apraxia
consummatum
    glaucoma c.
ContaClair multi-purpose contact lens solution
contact
    arc of c.
    c. arc
    C. A-scan
    c. bandage lens
    c. blepharitis
    C. B-scan
    c. B-scan ultrasonography
    c. burns of globe
    c. conjunctivitis
    c. dermatoconjunctivitis
    eye c.

    c. glasses
    haptic c.
    c. illumination
    iridociliary process c.
    iridolenticular c.
    iridozonular c.
    c. lens (CL)
    c. lens biomicroscopy
    c. lens blank
    c. lens chord diameter
    c. lens curve
    c. lens height
    c. lens-induced acute red eye (CLARE)
    c. lens-induced keratopathy
    c. lens-induced warpage
    c. lens overwearing syndrome
    c. lens-related microbial keratitis
    c. lens thickness
    c. lens training mirror
    c. lens vertex power
    c. low-vacuum lens
    c. method
contact lens (CL) (*See also* lens)
    AIRLens c. l.
    annular bifocal c. l.
    aphakic c. l.
    aspheric c. l.
    c. l. blank
    cellulose acetate butyrate c. l.
    contour c. l.
    decentration of c. l.
    disposable c. l.
    double slab-off c. l.
    Dyer nomogram system of ordering c. l.
    extended-wear c. l. (EWCL)
    finished c. l.
    c. l. flat
    flexible-wear c. l.
    fluorocarbon in c. l.
    gas-permeable c. l.
    Korb c. l.
    lenticular c. l.
    lenticular-cut c. l.
    loose c. l.

C

NOTES

contact lens *(continued)*
    microthin c. l.
    minus carrier c. l.
    polymethyl methacrylate c. l.
    prism ballast c. l.
    prolonged-wear c. l.
    rigid gas-permeable c. l.
    (RGP)
    scratched c. l.
    semifinished c. l.
    silicone acrylate c. l.
    single-cut c. l.
    Soper cone c. l.
    steep c. l.
    thickness of c. l.
    tight c. l.
    toric c. l.
    toroidal c. l.
    wetting angle of c. l.
    X chrom c. l.
    zone of c. l.
contactologist
contactology
contactoscope
contagiosa
    impetigo c.
contagiosum
    ecthyma c.
    keratitis molluscum c.
    molluscum c.
contagious granular conjunctivitis
contaminant
    wind-blown c.
contamination
    bacterial c.
contemporary nearpoint chart
content
    orbital c.
    water c.
contiguous
    c. fibers
    c. pattern
Contino
    C. epithelioma
    C. glaucoma
continuous
    c. circular capsulorrhexis
    c. curvilinear capsulorrhexis
    c. fiber
    c. laser
continuous-wave
    c.-w. argon laser
    c.-w. diode laser

Contique contact lens case
contour
    c. contact lens
    corneal c.
    edge c.
    eyelid c.
    c. interaction
    c. lens
    scalloped c.'s
    c. stereo test
contracted socket
contraction (C)
    anisocoria c.
    c. of cyclitic membrane
    c. and liquefaction
    c. of pupil
    pupillary sphincter c.
    vermiform c.
    vitreous c.
contracture
    socket c.
    spastic paretic facial c.
contralateral
    c. antagonist
    c. eye
contrapulsion
    saccadic c.
contrast
    color c.
    c. discrimination
    gallium citrate c.
    long-scale c.
    low c.
    c. material
    c. medium
    c. sensitivity
    c. sensitivity test
    short-scale c.
    simultaneous c.
    successive c.
    c. threshold for motion
      perception (CTMP)
    c. visualization
contrecoup injury
control
    Integrated Light C. (ILC)
    supranuclear c.
contusion
    c. angle glaucoma
    c. cataract
    c. of choroid
    conjunctival c.
    corneal c.

c. of eye
c. of globe
c. of orbit
vitreoretinal c.
conular
conus, pl. **coni**
congenital c.
distraction c.
c. distraction
inferior c.
lateral oblique c.
myopic c.
c. of optic disk
c. shell type eye implant
supertraction c.
c. supertraction
underlying c.
conventional
c. outflow
c. shell implant
converge
convergence
c. accommodation
c. accommodation ratio (CA/C ratio)
accommodative c. (AC)
c. amplitude
amplitude of c.
c. angle
c. excess
c. excess esotropia
excess esotropia c.
far-point c.
far point of c.
fusional c.
c. insufficiency (CI)
c. insufficiency exotropia
near point of c. (NPC)
negative c.
c. paralysis
c. point
point of c.
c. position
positive c.
proximal c.
punctum proximum of c. (PP)
range of c.

relative c.
c. retraction nystagmus
c. spasm
tonic c.
unit of ocular c.
voluntary c.
convergence-accommodative micropsia
convergence-evoked nystagmus
convergency
c. reflex
voluntary c.
convergent
c. beam
c. deviation
c. exercise
c. light
c. ray
c. squint
c. strabismus
c. wavefront
convergent-divergent pendular oscillation
converging
c. meniscus
c. meniscus lens
c. ray
convergiometer
converse
c. bobbing
Converse double-ended alar retractor
convex
high c.
c. lens
low c.
c. mirror
c. plano lens
c. reflecting surface
c. spectacle lens
convexity
convexoconcave lens
convexoconvex lens
Conway lid retractor
Cook speculum
Cool Touch laser

NOTES

C

Cooper
  C. aspirator
  C. blade fragment
  C. I&A unit
  C. implant
  C. irrigating/aspirating unit
  C. 2000 laser
  C. 2500 laser
  C. Laser Sonics laser
  C. operation
  C. Surgeon-Plus Ultrathin
    blade
CooperVision
  C. argon laser
  C. balanced salt solution
  C. camera
  C. Diagnostic Imaging refractor
  C. Fragmatome
  C. I/A machine
  C. imaging perimeter
  C. irrigating/aspirating unit
  C. irrigating needle
  C. irrigation/aspiration unit
  C. microscope
  C. ocutome
  C. PMMA-ACL Flex lens
  C. refractive surgery
    photokeratoscope
  C. spatulated needle
  C. Surgeon-Plus Ultrathin
    blade
  C. ultrasonography
  C. ultrasound
  C. vitrector
  C. YAG laser
Copeland
  C. implant
  C. panchamber lens
  C. radial panchamber
    intraocular lens
  C. radial panchamber UV lens
  C. retinoscopy
  C. streak retinoscope
Cophene-B
copiopia
copper
  c. cataract
  c. deposition
  c. foreign body
  c. wiring
copper-wire
  c.-w. arteriole
  c.-w. artery

  c.-w. effect
  c.-w. reflex
Coppock cataract
coquille plano lens
COR
  cervico-ocular reflex
Coracin
coralliform cataract
Corbett spud
Corboy
  C. hemostat
  C. needle holder
cordless monocular indirect
  ophthalmoscope
cords of Schwann
core
  nerve c.
  c. vitrectomy
  c. vitreous
corecleisis, coreclisis
corectasia, corectasis
corectome
corectomedialysis
corectomy
corectopia
  midbrain c.
coredialysis
corediastasis
corelysis
coremorphosis
corenclisis
coreometer
coreometry
coreoplasty
corepexy
corepraxy
corestenoma
  c. congenitum
coretomedialysis
coretomy
corkscrew
  c. artery
  c. visual field defect
cornea, gen. corneae
  c. abrader
  abrasio corneae
  abrasion of c.
  abscessus siccus corneae
  alkali burn of c.
  c. anesthesia
  anterior epithelium corneae
  apical zone of c.
  arcus corneae

arcus lipoides corneae
artificial c.
aspheric c.
axial c.
bedewing of c.
black c.
bleb disorder of the c.
blood staining of c.
Bonzel blood staining of c.
Burr c.
butterfly pattern steepening of the c.
calcareous degeneration of c.
caligo corneae
central edema of c.
c. chalcosis
c. chisel
cloudy c.
conical c.
c. curvature (K)
degeneration of c.
deturgescence of c.
diameter of c.
donor c.
dystrophia adiposa corneae
dystrophia endothelialis corneae
dystrophia epithelialis corneae
dystrophy of c.
ectatic c.
edema of c.
endothelial cell surface of c.
epithelium anterius corneae
epithelium posterius corneae
facies anterior corneae
facies posterior corneae
c. farinata
fistula of c.
flat c.
floury c.
c. globosa
c. guttata
guttata of c.
c. guttate lesion
herpes corneae
ichthyosis c.
indolent ulceration of the c.
inferior c.

infiltrate in c.
keratoconus c.
keratoglobus c.
lamina limitans anterior corneae
lamina limitans posterior corneae
lash abrasion of c.
lattice dystrophy of c.
lead incrustation of c.
leukoma corneae
ligamentum circulare corneae
limbus of c.
lipoidosis corneae
liquor corneae
macula corneae
marginal degeneration of c.
marginal ring ulcer of c.
meridian of c.
metaherpetic ulceration of the c.
c. opaca
opalescent c.
oval c.
c. pachymetry
phthisis c.
pigmented line of c.
c. plana
c. plana congenita familiares
posterior conical c.
posterior epithelium of c.
recurrent erosion of c.
ring ulcer of c.
rust ring of c.
c. sensitivity
serpent ulcer of c.
spherical c.
substantia propria corneae
sugar-loaf c.
superficial line of c.
superior c.
transparent ulcer of the c.
transplantation of c.
trepanation of c.
trophic ulceration of the c.
ulceration of c.
ulcus serpens corneae

C

NOTES

cornea *(continued)*
  c. urica
  c. verticillata
  c. vesicle
  Vogt c.
  white ring of c.
  xerosis of c.
cornea-holding forceps
corneal
  c. ablation plumes
  c. abrasion
  c. abscess
  c. abscission
  c. alkali burn
  c. apex
  c. arcus
  c. astigmatism
  c. bedewing
  c. biopsy
  c. birefringence
  c. block
  c. blood staining
  c. burn
  c. button
  c. cap
  c. cell
  c. clarity
  c. cleft
  c. clouding
  c. conjunctival intraepithelial
    neoplasia
  c. contact lens
  c. contour
  c. contusion
  c. corpuscle
  c. crystal
  c. curette
  c. curvature
  c. cylinder
  c. cyst
  c. debrider
  c. decompensation
  c. deep opacity
  c. dehydration
  c. dellen
  c. dendrite
  c. denervation
  c. deposit
  c. deturgescence
  c. diameter
  c. distortion
  c. dysgenesis
  c. dysplasia

  c. dystrophy of Waardenburg-
    Jonkers
  c. ectasia
  c. edema
  c. endothelial guttate dystrophy
  c. endothelial pigmentary
    dispersion
  c. endothelial touch
  c. endothelium
  c. enlargement
  c. epithelial barrier function
  c. epithelial scraping
  c. epithelium
  c. erosion
  c. erysiphake
  c. facet
  c. fascia lata spatula
  c. filament
  c. fissure
  c. fistula
  c. fixation forceps
  c. foreign body bur
  c. furrow degeneration
  c. graft
  c. graft operation
  c. graft spatula
  c. graft step
  c. guttata
  c. guttate dystrophy
  c. guttering
  c. haze
  c. hook
  c. hypoesthesia
  c. implant
  c. impression test (CIT)
  c. incision
  c. inferior limbus
  c. inlay
  c. intercept
  c. iron line
  c. keratitis
  c. knife
  c. knife dissector
  c. laceration
  c. lamella
  c. lamellar groove
  c. leakage
  c. leukoma
  c. light reflex
  c. light shield
  c. luster
  c. marginal furrow
  c. melt

c. meridian
c. microscope
C. Modeling System
c. mushroom
c. nebula
c. needle
c. neovascularization
c. nerve
c. nerve inflammation
c. opacification
c. optical density
c. pachometer
c. pachymeter
c. pannus
c. paracentesis track
c. pellucid
c. perforation
c. phlyctenule
c. phlyctenulosis
c. pocket
c. prosthesis forceps
c. prosthesis trephine
c. protrusion
c. punch
c. punctate infiltrate
c. punctate lesion
c. reflection
c. scar
c. scarring
c. section spatulated scissors
c. sensation
c. sensitivity
C. Shaper microkeratome
c. spatulated scissors
c. splinter forceps
c. spot
c. staining
c. staining test
c. staphyloma
c. steepening
c. storage medium
c. stria
c. stroma
c. stromal bed
c. stromal disease
c. stromal dystrophy
c. stromal remodeling

c. substance
c. superinfection
c. surgery
c. swelling
c. thinning
c. topographic analysis
c. topography
c. topography system (CTS)
c. transparency
c. transplant
c. transplantation
c. transplant centering ring
c. transplant marker
c. trauma
c. trepanation
c. tube
c. ulcer
c. vascularization
c. velum
c. verticillata
c. vortex dystrophy
c. warpage
c. xerosis
cornealis
    arcus c.
    rima c.
Corneascope
    C. nine-ring photokeratoscope
CorneaSparing LTK system
corneitis
Cornelia de Lange syndrome
corneoblepharon
corneodysgenesis
Corneo-Gage PachKnife
corneoiritis
corneolenticular
corneolimbal ring graft
corneomandibular reflex
corneomental reflex
corneopterygoid reflex
corneosclera
corneoscleral
    c. border
    c. button
    c. forceps
    c. groove
    c. incision

NOTES

corneoscleral *(continued)*
  c. junction
  c. laceration
  c. lamella
  c. limbus
  c. melt
  c. punch
  c. right/left hand scissors
  c. sulcus
  c. trabeculum
corneoscleralis
  pars c.
corneoscope
  IDI c.
corners method
cornpicker's pupil
corona
  c. ciliaris
  c. radiata
  Zinn c.
coronal
  c. CT scan
  c. view
coronaria
  cataracta c.
coronary cataract
coroparelcysis
coroplasty
coroscopy
Cor-Oticin
corotomy
corpus
  c. adiposum orbitae
  c. callosum
  c. callosum lesion
  c. ciliare
  c. ciliaris
  vitreum c.
  c. vitreum
corpuscle
  corneal c.
  hyaloid c.
  Toynbee c.
  Virchow c.
corrected
  c. pattern standard deviation
  c. spectacle lens
correction
  aphakic c.
  astigmatism c.
  Byron Smith lazy T c.
  dioptric c.
  distance c.

epicanthal c.
optical c.
spectacle c.
with c. (cc)
without c. (s̄c)
corrective movement
correspondence
  abnormal c.
  abnormal harmonious retinal c.
  abnormal retinal c. (ARC)
  abnormal unharmonious
    retinal c.
  anomalous retinal c. (ARC)
  dysharmonious c.
  harmonious abnormal retinal c.
  harmonious retinal c.
  Hering law of motor c.
  normal retinal c. (NRC)
  c. point
  retinal c.
  sensory c.
corresponding
  c. retinal point
corridor incision
corrugans
  fibrosis choroideae c.
corrugated retinal detachment
corrugator
  c. muscle
Cort-Dome
Cortef
  Delta C.
  Neo-C.
cortex, pl. cortices
  aspiration of c.
  brain c.
  calcarine c.
  cerebellar c.
  cerebral c.
  c. lentis
  occipital c.
  peristriate visual c.
  primary visual c.
  residual c.
  striate visual c.
  vestibular c.
  visual c.
cortical
  c. change
  c. cleanup
  c. cleaving hydrodissection
  c. cleaving hydrodissector

c. cleaving hydrodissector cannula
c. cleft
c. clefting
c. opacification
c. opacity
c. psychic blindness
c. ptosis
c. spokes cataract
c. stripping
c. substance of lens
c. vacuole
c. visual impairment
c. visual insufficiency
c. vitreous
corticolysis
corticonuclear fiber
corticopupillary reflex
corticose vein
corticosteroid
c. drops
ophthalmic c.
c. therapy
corticosteroid-induced
c.-i. cataract
c.-i. glaucoma
corticotropin
cortisol
cortisone
c. acetate
Cortisporin
C. Ophthalmic Ointment
C. Ophthalmic Suspension
Cortone
C. Acetate
coruscation
Corydon hydroexpression cannula
corymbifera
Absidia c.
Corynebacterium
C. *diphtheriae*
C. *keratitis*
C. *pseudodiphtheriticum*
C. *xerosis*
Cosmegen
cosmesis

cosmetic
c. contact shell implant
c. defect
c. iris
c. shell contact lens
Cosopt
C. ophthalmic solution
Costenbader incision spreader
Coston-Trent iris retractor
cotton
C. effect
C. thread tear test
cottonoid
cotton-tipped applicator
cotton-wool
c.-w. exudate
c.-w. patch
c.-w. spot (CWS)
couching
cataract c.
c. of cataract
c. needle
cough headache
count
complete blood c.
endothelial cell c.
finger c.
Kestenbaum capillary c.
counterpressor
Amenabar c.
angled c.
Gill c.
counter rolling
countertorsion
static c.
counting
finger c.
c. fingers (CF)
coup injury
course
arcuate c.
extramedullary c.
cover
Expo Bubble eye c.
Eye-Pak II c.
c. test
cover-uncover test

NOTES

C

Cowen sign
COWS
cold-opposite, warm-same
Coxiella burnetii
Cox II ocular laser shield
Coxsackie virus
Cozean-McPherson tying forceps
CPA
cerebellopontine angle
CPA lesion ·
C-PACG
chronic primary angle-closure
glaucoma
CPC
central posterior curve
CPEO
chronic progressive external
ophthalmoplegia
CR
cycloplegic refraction
C/R
chorioretinal
CR-39 lens
Cr6-45NMf retinal camera
CRA
central retinal artery
crack-and-flip phacoemulsification technique
cracked windshield stromal lesion
cracker
Ernest nucleus c.
Newsom side port nucleus c.
nucleus c.
cranial
c. arteritis
c. foramen
c. nerve (CN)
c. nerve palsy
c. nerve testing
c. stenosis syndrome
craniocervical junction
craniofacial
c. anomaly
c. fibro-osseous tumor
c. syndrome
cranio-orbital surgery
craniopharyngioma
craniostenosis, pl. **craniostenoses**
craniosynostosis
craniotabes
craniotomy
frontal c.

CRAO
central retinal artery occlusion
crapulosa
amblyopia c.
crassus
pannus c.
Crawford
C. fascia
C. fascial stripper
C. forceps
C. hook
C. lacrimal set
C. method
C. needle
C. sling operation
C. technique
C. tube
CRD
cone-rod dystrophy
cream
Drysol c.
crease
eyelid c.
lid c.
superior eyelid c.
Credé
C. method
C. prophylaxis
crepe bandage dressing
crescent
c. blade
c. choroid
congenital c.
c. corneal graft
homonymous c.
monocular temporal c.
c. myopia
myopic c.
c. operation
scleral c.
temporal c.
c. tonofilm
crescentic
c. circumpapillary light reflex
CREST
calcinosis cutis, Raynaud
phenomenon, esophageal motility
disorder, sclerodactyly, and
telangiectasia
CREST syndrome
crest
lacrimal anterior c.
lacrimal posterior c.

neural c.
orbital c.
cretinism
Creutzfeldt-Jakob disease
cribra
 c. orbitalia
 c. orbitalis of Welcker
cribriform
 c. field
 c. ligament
 c. spot
cribrosa
 area c.
 lamina c.
 scleral lamina c.
cri du chat syndrome
Crile needle holder
crinkled cellophane
crisis, pl. **crises**
 glaucomatocyclitic c.
 myasthenic c.
 ocular c.
 oculogyric c.
 Pel c.
cristallinus
 humor c.
Critchett operation
criterion-free measurement
criterion shift
critical
 c. angle
 c. corresponding frequency (CCF)
 c. flicker fusion frequency
 c. illumination
Crock encircling operation
crocodile
 c. lens
 c. shagreen
 c. tear
crofilcon A
Crolom
 C. Ophthalmic Solution
cromoglycate
 sodium c.
cromolyn
 c. sodium

c. sodium 46
c. sodium ophthalmic solution
Cronassial
Crookes
 C. glass
 C. lens
cross
 c. cover test
 c. cylinder
 c. fixation
 Lancaster C.
 optical c.
cross-action
 c.-a. capsule forceps
 c.-a. towel clamp
crossed
 c. amblyopia
 c. cylinder
 c. diplopia
 c. eyes
 c. fixation
 c. hemianopsia
 c. lens
 c. parallax
 c. reflex
cross-eyed
cross-fixation
crossing
 arteriolovenous c.
crosslinked poly (HEMA) glaucoma filtration device
cross-polarization photography
cross-Polaroid projection chart
cross-vector A-scan
croupous
 c. conjunctivitis
 c. rhinitis
Crouzon
 C. disease
 C. syndrome
crowding phenomenon
crow-foot closure
crown
 ciliary c.
 c. glass
 c. glass lens
 spectacle c.

NOTES

cruciata
amblyopia c.
crusher
Lieberman phaco c.
crusting
eyelid c.
lid c.
c. lid
crutch glasses
CRV
central retinal vein
CRVO
central retinal vein occlusion
nonischemic CRVO
central retinal vein occlusion
cryoablation
cryoapplication
Cryo-Barrages vitreous implant
cryocoagulation
cryoedema
cryoenucleator
Gallie c.
cryoextraction
open-sky c.
c. operation
cryoextractor
Alcon c.
Amoils c.
Beaver cataract c.
Bellows c.
Keeler c.
Kelman c.
Rubinstein c.
Thomas c.
cryolathe
Barraquer c.
cryopencil
Amoils c.
Mira endovitreal c.
cryopexy
double freeze-thaw c.
c. probe
retinal c.
transconjunctival c.
transscleral c.
cryophake
Alcon c.
Amoils c.
Bellows c.
Keeler c.
Kelman c.
Rubinstein c.
cryopreservation

cryoprobe
Amoils c.
cryoptor c.
Rubinstein c.
Thomas c.
cryoptor
c. cryoprobe
Thomas c.
cryoretinopexy
cryoretractor
Thomas c.
cryostat
cryostylet, cryostylette
C. 2000
cryosurgery
cryosurgical unit
Cryosystem
Keeler-Amoils Ophthalmic C.
cryotherapy
double freeze-thaw c.
freeze-thaw c.
c. operation
c. probe
retinal c.
transscleral c.
crypt
Fuchs c.
iris c.
cryptochrome
cryptococcal meningitis
cryptococcosis
Cryptococcus
C. laurentii
C. laurentii keratitis
C. neoformans
cryptoglioma
cryptophthalmus, cryptophthalmia, cryptophthalmos
crystal
conjunctival c.
corneal c.
cystine c.
refractile c.
retinal c.
crystallin
alpha c.
beta c.
gamma c.
crystallina
lens c.
crystalline
c. capsule
c. cataract

c. corneal dystrophy
c. deposit
c. humor
c. infiltrate
c. keratopathy
c. lens
c. lens equator
c. opacity
c. retinopathy
crystallitis
Csapody orbital repair operation
C-Scan
C.-S. corneal topography system
TechnoMed C.-S.
CSF
cerebrospinal fluid
CSI lens
CSM
central, steady and maintained fixation
CSR
central serous retinopathy
CT
computed tomography
CT scan of orbit
CTM
Carlo Traverso maneuver
CTMP
contrast threshold for motion perception
CTS
corneal topography system
CU-8 needle
CUA needle
Cuban epidemic optic neuropathy
cube
tumbling E c.
cuboidal
cuff
fibrous tissue c.
Honan c.
opacified c.
subretinal fluid c.
Watzke c.

Cuignet
C. method
C. test
cul-de-sac
conjunctival c. d.-s.
glaucomatous c.-d.-s.
c.-d.-s. irrigating vectis
c.-d.-s. irrigation T-tube
c.-d.-s. irrigator
ocular c.-d.-s.
ophthalmic c.-d.-s.
optic c.-d.-s.
Culler
C. fixation forceps
C. iris spatula
C. lens spoon
C. muscle hook
C. speculum
culture
bacterial c.
c. medium
organ c.
vitreous c.
culturette
Mini-tip c.
cuneate-shaped scotoma
cuneiform cataract
cup
bleb c.
eye c.
flat c.
Galin bleb c.
glaucomatous c.
large physiologic c.
ocular c.
ophthalmic c.
optic c.
perilimbal suction c.
physiologic c.
slit-lamp c.
cup-disk ratio
cupped disk
Cupper-Faden operation
Cüppers
C. method of pleoptics
C. Visuscope

C

NOTES

cupping
    glaucomatous c.
    optic disk c.
    c. of optic disk
    c. of optic nerve
    optic nerve c.
    pathologic c.
cup-to-disk ratio (C/D)
cupuliform cataract
cupulolithiasis
curb tenotomy
Curdy
    C. blade
    C. sclerotome
Curdy-Hebra blade
curette, curet
    Alvis c.
    chalazion c.
    corneal c.
    Fink c.
    Gifford corneal c.
    Gills-Welsh c.
    Green c.
    Heath chalazion c.
    Hebra c.
    Heyner c.
    Kraff capsule polisher c.
    Meyhoeffer chalazion c.
    Skeele c.
    Spratt mastoid c.
    Visitec capsule polisher c.
curlback shell implant
curling of capsule
curl temple
Curran knife needle
curvature
    c. aberration
    c. ametropia
    anterior corneal c.
    cornea c. (K)
    corneal c.
    c. hyperopia
    c. of lens
    c. myopia
    radius of c.
curve
    anterior central c. (ACC)
    anterior peripheral c.
    base c.
    bell-shaped c.
    biphasic c.
    central posterior c. (CPC)
    contact lens c.

    intermediate posterior c. (IPC)
    luminosity c.
    peripheral posterior c. (PPC)
    posterior central c.
    posterior intermediate c.
    posterior peripheral c.
    c. response
    Steiger c.
    Stromberg c.
    visibility c.
    c. width
curved
    c. iris forceps
    c. iris scissors
    c. mosquito clamp
    c. needle eye spud
    c. reflecting surface
    c. retinal probe
    c. scleral-limbal incision of
      Flieringa
    c. tenotomy scissors
    c. tying forceps
curved-top bifocal
curves of spectacle lens
Curvularia
Cushing syndrome
Cusick
    C. goniotomy knife
    C. operation
Cusick-Sarrail ptosis operation
Custodis
    C. nondraining procedure
    C. operation
    C. scleral buckling
    C. sponge
    C. suture
cut
    field c.
    sector c.
cutaneomucouveal syndrome
cutaneous
    c. horn
    c. melanoma
    c. myiasis
    c. pupillary reflex
    c. tissue
cutdown incision
Cuterebra
    C. ophthalmomyiasis
cuticular
    c. layer
    c. stitch

Cutler
   C. implant
   C. lens spoon
   C. operation
Cutler-Beard
   C.-B. bridge flap
   C.-B. operation
cutter
   bone c.
   Buettner-Parel vitreous c.
   Chu c.
   Douvas vitreous c.
   guillotine-type c.
   infusion suction cutter
      vitreous c.
   Kloti vitreous c.
   Machemer vitreous c.
   Maguire-Harvey vitreous c.
   O'Malley-Heintz vitreous c.
   Parel-Crock vitreous c.
   Premiere vitreous c.
   rotating-type c.
   Tolentino vitreous c.
   Utrata c.
   vitreoretinal infusion c.
   vitreous c.
   vitreous infusion suction c.
      (VISC)
cutting bur
CVK
   computerized videokeratography
CVS
   computer vision syndrome
CWS
   cotton-wool spot
cyanoacrylate
   butyl c.
   ethyl c.
   c. retinopexy
   c. tissue adhesive
cyanographic contrast material
cyanographin contrast material
cyanolabe
cyan opacification
cyanopia
cyanopsia
   c. retinae

cyanopsin
cyanosis
   bulbar c.
   c. bulbi
   compression c.
   retina c.
   c. retinae
cycle
   visual c.
cyclectomy
cyclic
   c. adenosine monophosphate
   c. esotropia
   c. guanidine monophosphate
   c. guanosine monophosphate
   c. ocular motor spasm
   c. oculomotor paresis
   c. strabismus
cyclicotomy
cyclitic membrane
cyclitis
   chronic c.
   Fuchs heterochromic c. (FHC)
   heterochromic Fuchs c.
   c. in pars planitis
   plastic c.
   pure c.
   purulent c.
   serous c.
cycloceratitis
cyclochoroiditis
cyclocoagulation
cyclocongestive glaucoma
cyclocryopexy
cyclocryotherapy
   YAG c.
cyclodamia
cyclodestructive procedure
cyclodeviation
cyclodialysis
   Allen c.
   c. cannula
   c. cleft
   Heine c.
   c. spatula
cyclodiathermy
   Castroviejo-Scheie c.

C

NOTES

cyclodiathermy *(continued)*
   c. electrode
   c. operation
cyclodiplopia
cycloduction
cycloelectrolysis
cyclofilcon A
cyclofusion
cyclogram
Cyclogyl
cyclohexylpiperidine
cyclokeratitis
Cyclomydril Ophthalmic
cyclopea
cyclopean eye
cyclopentolate
   c. hydrochloride
cyclophoria
   accommodative c.
   minus c.
   c. minus
   plus c.
   c. plus
   position c.
   c. positive
cyclophorometer
cyclophosphamide
cyclophotocoagulation
   laser transscleral c.
   Nd:YAG c.
   Nd:YAG laser c.
   transpupillary c.
   transscleral laser c.
cyclopia
cycloplegia
cycloplegic
   c. refraction (CR)
   topical c.
cycloplegios suppressant
cyclorotary muscle
cycloscope
cycloscopy
cycloserine
cyclospasm
cyclotherapy
   laser c.
cyclotome
cyclotomy
cyclotorsion
cyclotropia
   minus c.
   c. minus

   c. plus
   c. positive
cyclovergence
cycloversion
cyclovertical muscle
Cyl, cyl.
   cylinder
cylinder (C, Cyl, cyl.)
   anterior c.
   c. axis
   concave c.
   corneal c.
   cross c.
   crossed c.
   Jackson cross c.
   minus c.
   c. retinoscopy
   c. spectacle lens
cylindric, cylindrical
   c. refraction
Cylindrocarpon
cylindroma
CYP1B1 gene
cyproheptadine
cyst
   aneurysmal bone c.
   arachnoidal c.
   Blessig c.
   Blessig-Iwanoff c.
   blood c.
   colloid c.
   colobomatous c.
   conjunctival c.
   corneal c.
   c. degeneration
   dermoid c.
   echinococcus c.
   epibulbar dermoid c.
   epidermal inclusion c.
   epidermoid c.
   epithelial implantation c.
   epithelial inclusion c.
   c. fibrosis
   foveal c.
   hematic c.
   inclusion c.
   infundibular c.
   intracorneal c.
   intraepithelial c.
   iris c.
   Iwanoff c.
   lacrimal ductal c.
   meibomian c.

Naegleria c.
orbital c.
pearl c.
proteinaceous c.
pupillary iris c.
Rathke cleft c.
retinal c.
scleral c.
sebaceous c.
serous c.
spontaneous congenital iris c.
subconjunctival c.
sudoriferous c.
tarsal c.
traumatic corneal c.
traumatic scleral c.
Vahlkampfia c.

cystadenoma
Moll gland c.

cystic
c. amelanotic nevus
c. cataract
c. eye
c. fibrosis
c. hydrocystoma tumor
c. microphthalmia
c. retinal tuft

cysticerci (*pl. of* cysticercus)
cysticercoid
cysticercosis
cysticercus, pl. **cysticerci**
intraocular c.

cysticum
epithelioma adenoides c.

cystine crystal
cystinosis
nephropathic c.

cystitome, cystotome
air c.
Atkinson 25-G short curved c.
Azar curved c.
Beaver Ocu-1 curved c.
Blumenthal irrigating c.
double-cutting sharp c.
Drews angled c.
Graefe c.
irrigating c.

Kelman air c.
kibisitome c.
Knolle-Kelman cannulated c.
Kratz angled c.
Lewicky formed c.
Lieppman c.
Look c.
McIntyre reverse c.
Mendez c.
Neuhann c.
Nevyas double sharp c.
Visitec double-cutting c.
von Graefe c.
Wheeler c.
Wilder c.

cystitomy
cystoid
c. body
c. cicatrix
c. cicatrix of limbus
c. macular degeneration (CMD)
c. macular dystrophy
c. macular edema (CME)
c. macular hole
c. maculopathy
c. retinal degeneration

cystotome (*var. of* cystitome)
CytoFluor II fluorometer
cytoid body
cytokeratin
c. 7 antibody
c. 20 antibody

cytokine therapy
cytologic examination
cytology
conjunctival impression c.
impression c.

cytomegalic inclusion virus
cytomegalovirus (CMV)
macular c.
c. retinitis

cytophotocoagulation
cytoplasmic body
cytotoxic antibody
Cytoxan
C. Injection
C. Oral

C

NOTES

cytoxic T cell
Czapski microscope
Czermak
    accommodation phosphene
    of C.

C. keratome
C. pterygium operation

D
dexter
diopter
  D chromosome ring syndrome
  3D i-Scan ophthalmic
    ultrasound
  D trisomy syndrome
D-15
  D. Hue Desaturated Panel test
  D. test
Dacriose
Dacron suture
dacryadenalgia
dacryadenitis
dacryadenoscirrhus
dacryagogatresia
dacryagogic
dacryagogue
dacrycystalgia
dacrycystitis
dacryelcosis
dacryoadenalgia
dacryoadenectomy operation
dacryoadenitis
  infectious d.
dacryoblennorrhea
dacryocanaliculitis
dacryocele
  congenital d.
dacryocyst
dacryocystalgia
dacryocystectasia
dacryocystectomy operation
dacryocystis
  phlegmonous d.
  syphilitic d.
  trachomatous d.
  tuberculous d.
dacryocystitis
  acute d.
  chronic d.
  congenital d.
  phlegmonous d.
  syphilitic d.
  trachomatous d.
  tuberculous d.
dacryocystoblennorrhea
dacryocystocele
dacryocystoethmoidostomy
dacryocystogram

dacryocystography
dacryocystoptosis, dacryocystoptosia
dacryocystorhinostenosis
dacryocystorhinostomy (DCR)
  endonasal laser d. (ENL-DCR)
  external d. (EXT-DCR)
dacryocystorhinotomy operation
dacryocystostenosis
dacryocystostomy operation
dacryocystotome
dacryocystotomy operation
dacryogenic
dacryogram
dacryohelcosis
dacryohemorrhea
dacryolin
dacryolith
  Desmarres d.
dacryolithiasis
dacryoma
dacryon
dacryops
dacryopyorrhea
dacryopyosis
dacryorhinocystotomy
dacryorrhea
dacryoscintigraphy
dacryosinusitis
dacryosolenitis
dacryostenosis
dacryostomy
  Arroyo d.
  Arruga d.
  Dupuy-Dutemps d.
  Kuhnt d.
dacryosyrinx
dactinomycin
DAF syndrome
Dailey operation
Dailies contact lens
Daily cataract needle
daily-wear contact lens (DWCL)
Daisy irrigation-aspiration
  instrument
Dakrina Ophthalmic Solution
Dalalone
Dalcaine
Dalen-Fuchs nodule
Dalgleish operation
Dallas lens-inserting forceps

Dalrymple
  D. disease
  D. sign
daltonian
daltonism
damage
  brain d.
  dorsal rostral d.
  glaucomatous optic nerve d.
    (GOND)
  optic tract d.
  solar d.
dammini
  Ixodes d.
Danberg iris forceps
Dan chalazion forceps
dancing eye
Dan-Gradle cilia forceps
Dannheim eye implant
dantrolene sodium
dapiprazole
  d. HCl
  d. hydrochloride
DAPS
  dark-adapted pupil size
Daranide
Darin lens
dark
  d. adaptation
  d. adaptometry
  d. disk
  d. empty field
  d. event
  d. retinoscopy
dark-adapted
  d.-a. eye
  d.-a. pupil size (DAPS)
dark-field
  d.-f. accommodation
  d.-f. examination
  d.-f. illumination
dark-ground illumination
dark-room
  d.-r. test
  d.-r. testing
Darling
  D. capsulotome
  D. capsulotomy
Dartmouth Eye Institute
DaSilva dermatome
Daubenton plane

Davidoff
  D. ambidextrous nucleus
  chopper
  D. blade
Daviel
  D. lens spoon
  D. operation
  D. scoop
Davis
  D. forceps
  D. knife needle
  D. spud
  D. trephine
Davis-Geck
  D.-G. blepharoplasty
  D.-G. suture
day
  d. blindness
  90-d. glaucoma
  d. sight
  d. vision
dazzle reflex
dazzling glare
DBC
  distance between centers
DBL
  distance between nasal lines
DCR
  dacryocystorhinostomy
DD
  disk diffusion
DDHT
  dissociated double hypertropia
DDT
  dye disappearance test
de
  d. Grandmont operation
  D. Klair operation
  d. Lange syndrome
  d. Lapersonne operation
  D. LaVega lens pusher
  D. LaVega vitreous aspirating
  cannula
  d. Morsier syndrome
  d. Vincentiis operation
deafness
  diabetes insipidus, diabetes
  mellitus, optic atrophy,
  and d. (DIDMOAD)
  lentigines, electrocardiogram
  abnormalities, ocular
  hypertelorism, pulmonary
  stenosis, abnormal genitalia,

retardation of growth, and d.
(LEOPARD)

Dean
D. blade
D. iris knife
D. knife holder
D. knife needle

death-to-preservation time
debrancher enzyme deficiency
debridement
epithelial d.
impression d.
wipe d.

debrider
corneal d.
Sauer corneal d.

debris
capsular d.
cellular d.
desquamated epithelial d.
epithelial d.
phagocytosed cellular d.
tear film d.

debris-laden tear film
Decadron
D. Phosphate

decalvans
keratosis follicularis
spinulosa d.

decenter
decentered
d. lens
d. spectacles

decentration
d. of contact lens
lens d.
d. of lens

declination
decolorize
decompensated phoria
decompensation
corneal d.
endothelial d.

decompression
Dickson-Wright orbit d.
extracranial optic nerve d.
intracranial optic nerve d.

lateral orbital d.
microvascular d.
optic nerve sheath d. (ONSD)
orbital d.
d. of orbit operation
d. surgery
three-wall d.
transantral d.

decompressive surgery
decrease
visual acuity d.

decreased corneal sensation
decreasing vision
decussation
oculomotor d.
optic d.

deep
d. blunt rake retractor
d. congestion
d. corneal stromal opacity
d. dyslexia
d. filiform dystrophy
d. lamellar keratoplasty (DLK)
d. parenchymatous dystrophy
d. punctate keratitis
d. pustular keratitis
d. retina
d. scleritis
d. sclerotomy

defect
acquired color d.
afferent pupillary d. (APD)
altitudinal visual field d.
arcuate field d.
arteriovenous crossing d.
AV crossing d.
bilateral altitudinal field d.
bilateral homonymous
altitudinal d.
bilateral visual field d.
binasal field d.
bitemporal field d.
central d.
centrocecal d.
chiasmatic field d.
color d.
compressive optic nerve d.

D

NOTES

defect *(continued)*
confluent d.
confrontation field d.
congruous field d.
corkscrew visual field d.
cosmetic d.
directional d.
enzyme d.
epithelial d.
field d.
functional d.
glaucoma field d.
gun-barrel field d.
homonymous field d.
hyperfluorescent window d.
incongruous field d.
inferior altitudinal d.
iris transillumination d.
levator aponeurosis d.
Marcus Gunn relative
    afferent d.
monocular field d.
nasal step d.
nerve fiber bundle d.
paracentral d.
parietal lobe field d.
patchy window d.
persistent epithelial d.
pie-in-the-sky d.
pie-on-the-floor d.
punctate corneal epithelial d.
quadrantic d.
radial transillumination d.
relative afferent pupillary d.
    (RAPD)
retinal pigment epithelial d.
retrochiasmal visual field d.
sector d.
sector-shaped d.
superior homonymous
    quadrantic d.
temporal lobe field d.
trophic d.
vascular filling d.
visual corkscrew d.
visual field d.
window d.
defective accommodation
deficiency
acetylcholine receptor d.
acetylcholinesterase d.
acid maltase d.
aqueous tear d. (ATD)

brancher enzyme d.
carnitine d.
debrancher enzyme d.
familial lecithin:cholesterol
    acyltransferase d.
familial lipoprotein d.
folic acid d.
iatrogenic limbal stem cell d.
limbal stem-cell d.
primary acetylcholine
    receptor d.
supranuclear d.
vitamin A d.
deficit
abduction d.
concentration d.
hemisensory d.
neurologic d.
definition
area of critical d.
deflection
defocus
deformans
osteitis d.
deformity angle
degeneratio
d. hyaloidea granuliformis
d. hyaloideoretinae hereditaria
d. spherularis elaioides
degeneration
aberrant d.
age-related macular d. (AMD,
    ARMD)
amyloid corneal d.
anterograde d.
atrophic age-related macular d.
    (AAMD)
atrophic macular d.
Best d.
Biber-Haab-Dimmer d.
Bietti tapetoretinal d.
calcareous d.
central retinal d.
choriocapillaris d. (CCD)
chorioretinal d.
cobblestone retinal d.
cone d.
cone-rod d.
congenital macular d.
d. of cornea
corneal furrow d.
cyst d.
cystoid macular d. (CMD)

cystoid retinal d.
diabetic macular d.
disciform macular d.
Doyne familial colloid d.
Doyne honeycombed d.
dry senile macular d.
ectatic marginal d.
elastoid d.
equatorial d.
familial colloid d.
familial pseudoinflammatory
  macular d.
fine fibrillar vitreal d.
furrow d.
hepatolenticular d.
hereditary d.
heredomacular d.
hyaline d.
hyaloideoretinal d.
hydropic d.
juvenile macular d.
keratinoid d.
Kozlowski d.
Kuhnt-Junius macular d.
lattice retinal d.
lenticular d.
lipid d.
macular disciform d.
marginal corneal d.
marginal furrow d.
myopic retinal d.
nodular corneal d.
non-neovascular age-related
  macular d.
opticocochleodentate d.
paraneoplastic cerebellar d.
paving-stone d.
pellucid marginal corneal d.
pellucid marginal retinal d.
peripheral cystoid d.
peripheral tapetochoroidal d.
pigmentary perivenous
  chorioretinal d.
primary pigmentary d.
progressive cone d.
progressive myopic d.
red cone d.

reticular cystoid d.
retinal lattice d.
retrograde transsynaptic d.
rod-cone d.
Salzmann nodular corneal d.
scleral d.
senescent disciform macular d.
senile disciform macular d.
senile exudative macular d.
senile furrow d.
senile macular d. (SMD)
Sorsby pseudoinflammatory
  macular d.
spheroid d.
spinocerebellar d.
striatal nigral d.
tapetochoroidal d.
tapetoretinal d.
Terrien marginal d.
tractional retinal d.
transneuronal d.
transsynaptic d.
trophic retinal d.
vitelliform macular d.
vitelline macular d.
vitelliruptive d.
vitreoretinal d.
Vogt d.
Wagner hereditary
  vitreoretinal d.
Wagner hyaloid retinal d.
Wallerian d.
Wilson d.
xerotic d.
degenerative
  d. cerebellar disease
  d. myopia
  d. ocular disease
  d. pannus
  d. retinal disease
  d. retinoschisis
degenerativus
  pannus d.
Degest 2 Ophthalmic
Degos syndrome
degradation
  image d.

NOTES

degree
    45-d. bent reform implant
    prism d.
DeGrouchy syndrome
dehisced
dehiscence
    iris d.
    retinal d.
    wound d.
    Zuckerkandl d.
dehiscent
dehiscing
dehydration
    corneal d.
Dehydrex
dehydrogenase
    glucose 6-phosphate d.
    lactate d.
dehydroretinol
deinsertion
Deiter operation
Dejean syndrome
Deknatel silk suture
delacrimation
delayed
    d. massive suprachoroidal
    hemorrhage
    d. rectifier
    d. visual maturation
deletion mapping
delicate serrated straight dressing
    forceps
delimiting keratotomy
delivery system
Dell astigmatism marker
dellen
    corneal d.
    d. of Fuchs
Deller modification
Delta Cortef
Deltasone
Del Toro operation
DEM
    Developmental Eye Movement
    DEM test
demarcated detachment
demarcation line of retina
demecarium
    d. bromide
demeclocycline
Demerol
demodectic blepharitis
Demodex folliculorum

demonstration
    d. eyepiece
    d. ophthalmoscope
demonstrator
    halo d.
DeMosier syndrome
demyelinating
    d. disease
    d. optic neuropathy
    d. plaque
demyelination
    autoimmune d.
    nystagmus with d.
demyelinative disease
demyelinization
demyelinizing
Dendrid
dendriform
    d. corneal lesion
    d. epithelial lesion
    d. keratitis
    d. ulcer
dendrite
    branching d.
    corneal d.
    epithelial d.
    fragmented d.
    VZV d.
dendritic
    d. cataract
    d. epithelial lesion
    d. epitheliopathy
    d. ghost
    d. herpes simplex corneal
    ulcer
    d. herpes zoster keratitis
    d. keratitis
    d. keratopathy
dendritiform
denervate
denervation
    corneal d.
    d. supersensitivity test
Dennie-Morgan fold
densa
    lamina d.
dense
    d. brunescent nucleus
    d. core granule
    d. opacity
    d. vitreitis
densitometer

density
    arciform d.
    cell d.
    conjunctival goblet cell d.
    corneal optical d.
    endothelial cell d.
    Fas receptor d.
denudation
deorsumduction
deorsumvergence
    left d.
    right d.
deorsumversion
depigmentation
    periocular d.
depigmented spot
Depo-Medrol
deposit
    amyloid d.
    basal laminar d. (BLD)
    calcareous d.
    colloid d.
    conjunctival d.
    corneal d.
    crystalline d.
    fibrillogranular d.
    intraretinal lipid d.
    iron d.
    lipid d.
    mutton-fat d.
    protein d.
    refractile d.
    tear protein d.
deposition
    calcium d.
    copper d.
    epithelial adrenochrome d.
    iron d.
    pigment d.
depressed fracture
depression
    cecocentral d.
    foveal d.
    d. of orbital floor
    posterior corneal d.
    scleral d.

depressor
    muscle d.
    O'Connor d.
    orbital d.
    Schepens scleral d.
    Schepens thimble d.
    Schocket scleral d.
    scleral d.
    Wilder scleral d.
deprimens oculi
deprivation
    d. amblyopia
    stimulus d.
depth
    d. of chamber
    d. of field
    focal d.
    d. of focus
    d. gauge
    d. perception
    d. plate
    sagittal d.
derangement
    pigment d.
Derby operation
Derf needle holder
derma
    epithelial d.
    stromal d.
Derma-K laser
dermal
    d. amyloid infiltration
    d. nevus
Dermalon suture
dermatan sulfate
dermatitidis
    Blastomyces d.
dermatoblepharitis
dermatochalasis
    eyelid d.
dermatoconjunctivitis
    contact d.
dermatogenes
    cataracta d.
dermatogenic cataract
dermatolysis
    d. palpebrarum

D

NOTES

dermatome
    DaSilva d.
    Hall d.
dermatomyositis
dermato-ophthalmitis
dermis
    d. fat graft
    d. patch graft
dermochondral corneal dystrophy of
    François
dermoid
    congenital limbal corneal d.
    conjunctival d.
    d. cyst
    limbal d.
    d. of orbit
    orbital d.
    d. tumor
dermolipoma
Dermostat implant
desaturation
    red d.
Descartes law
Descemet
    D. fold
    D. membrane
    D. membrane detachment
    D. membrane punch
descemetitis
descemetocele
descemetolysis
descemetopexy
    gas-exchange d.
desiccant
desiccate
desiccation keratitis
Desmarres
    D. chalazion
    D. chalazion forceps
    D. corneal dissector
    D. dacryolith
    D. fixation pick
    D. knife
    D. law
    D. lid clamp
    D. lid elevator
    D. lid retractor
    D. marker
    D. operation
    D. refractor
    D. scarifier
desmopressin
desmosomal cellular attachment

desmosome
desquamated epithelial debris
detached
    d. iris
    d. retina
    d. vitreous
detachment
    aphakic d.
    bullous d.
    choroidal d.
    ciliochoroidal d.
    complex retinal d.
    corrugated retinal d.
    demarcated d.
    Descemet membrane d.
    disciform retinal d.
    extrafoveal retinal d.
    exudative serous retinal d.
    foveal retinal d.
    foveolar retinal d.
    funnel-shaped retinal d.
    hyaloid membrane d.
    late phase d.
    macula-off rhegmatogenous
        retinal d.
    macular d.
    matogenous retinal d.
    morning glory retinal d.
    neurosensory retinal d.
    nonrhegmatogenous retinal d.
    open-funnel d.
    pigment epithelial d. (PED)
    d. pocket
    posterior vitreal d. (PVD)
    pseudophakic d.
    d. of retina
    retinal d. (RD)
    retinal pigment epithelium
    serous d.
    rhegmatogenous retinal d.
        (RRD)
    schisis-related d.
    sensory d.
    serous macular d.
    serous pigment epithelial d.
    shallow d.
    tear-induced retinal d.
    tractional retinal d. (TRD)
    traction macular d.
    Trbinger d.
    vitreal d.
    vitreous d.
detamide

detectable focus
detection acuity
deterenol
    d. HCl
deturgescence
    d. of cornea
    corneal d.
deturgescent state
deutan
deuteranoma
deuteranomalopia
deuteranomalous
deuteranomaly
deuteranope
deuteranopia
deuteranopic
deuton color blindness
Deutschman cataract knife
devascularization
development
    visual d.
developmental
    d. anomaly
    d. cataract
    D. Eye Movement (DEM)
    D. Eye Movement test
    d. prosopagnosia
    d. ptosis
deviant color
deviating eye
deviation
    angle of d.
    comitant vertical d.
    conjugate horizontal d.
    convergent d.
    corrected pattern standard d.
    dissociated vertical d.
    downward d.
    forced downward d.
    Hering-Hellebrand d.
    heterotropic d.
    horizontal d.
    incomitant vertical d.
    intermittent d.
    latent d.
    manifest d.
    minimum d.

    periodic alternating gaze d.
    primary d.
    right d.
    Roth-Bielschowsky d.
    secondary d.
    skew d.
    d. squint
    squint d.
    standard d.
    strabismal d.
    supranuclear d.
    tonic downward d.
    tonic upward d.
    torsional d.
    tropia d.
    tropic d.
    vertical comitant d.
deviational nystagmus
Devic disease
device
    Ahmed d.
    crosslinked poly (HEMA)
      glaucoma filtration d.
    doubling d.
    glaucoma drainage d. (GDD)
    Joseph d.
    Keratolux fixation d.
    Krupin d.
    laser-argon d.
    laser-ruby d.
    Look micropuncture d.
    Microjet-based cutting and
      debriding d.
    oblique prism d.
    Ocusert d.
    OptiMed d.
    Putterman-Chaflin ocular
      asymmetry d.
    retrieval d.
    Seton drainage d.
    Tano d.
    Venturi aspiration
      vitrectomy d.
    Welch four-drop d.
DeVilbiss irrigating/aspirating unit
deviometer
devitalized epithelium

D

NOTES

DeWecker
  D. anterior sclerotomy
  D. iris scissors
  D. operation
DeWecker-Pritikin scissors
Dexacidin
Dexair
dexamethasone
  neomycin and d.
  neomycin, polymyxin B,
    and d.
  d. sodium phosphate
  d. solution
  tobramycin and d.
Dexasone
  D. L.A.
Dexasporin
Dexchlor
dexchlorpheniramine
Dexone
  D. LA
Dexon suture
Dexsol
Dexsone
dexter (D)
  oculus d. (right eye)
dextra
  tension oculus d. (tension of
    right eye) (TOD)
  visio oculus d. (vision of
    right eye) (VOD)
dextran
  d. medium
dextroclination
dextrocular
dextrocularity
dextrocycloduction
dextrocycloversion
dextrodepression
dextroduction
dextrogyration
dextrotorsion
dextroversion
Dey-Drop Ophthalmic Solution
Dey-Lube
DFP
  diisopropyl fluorophosphate
DGH-500 Pachette
D&I
  dilation and irrigation
diabetes
  alloxan d.
  artificial d.

brittle d.
bronze d.
chemical d.
D. Control and Complications
  Trial
experimental d.
gestational d.
gouty d.
growth-onset d.
d. innocens
d. inositus
d. insipidus
d. insipidus, diabetes mellitus,
  optic atrophy, and deafness
  (DIDMOAD)
insulin-deficient d.
juvenile d.
ketosis-prone d.
ketosis-resistant d.
Lancereaux d.
latent d.
lipoatrophic d.
lipoplethoric d.
lipuric d.
masked d.
maturity-onset d.
d. mellitus (DM)
Mosler d.
overflow d.
overt d.
pancreatic d.
phlorhizin d.
phosphate d.
piqûre d.
puncture d.
renal d.
skin d.
steroid d.
steroidogenic d.
subclinical d.
temporary d.
toxic d.
type 1 d.
type 2 d.
diabetic
  d. amaurosis
  d. Argyll-Robertson pupil
  d. cataract
  d. iritis
  d. macular degeneration
  d. macular edema (DME)
  d. macular heterotopia
  d. maculopathy

d. melanosis
d. membrane
d. optic atrophy
d. papillopathy
d. retinitis
d. retinopathy (DR)
d. traction
diabetica
    rubeosis iridis d.
diabetic-osmotic cataract
diabeticus
    fundus d.
diagnosis
    neuro-ophthalmologic d.
    nonorganic disorder d.
diagnostic
    d. contact lens
    d. fiberoptic lens
    d. fitting set
    d. positions of gaze
    d. program
dial
    astigmatic d.
    clock d.
    Mendez astigmatism d.
    Regan-Lancaster d.
    sunburst d.
dialer
    angled iris hook and IOL d.
    intraocular lens d.
    Lester lens d.
    Visitec intraocular lens d.
dialysis
    d. retinae
    retinal d.
Diamatrix trapezoidal diamond knife
diameter
    chord d.
    contact lens chord d.
    d. of cornea
    corneal d.
    disk d.
    effective d.
    iris d.
    minimal effective d. (MED)

optical zone d.
visible iris d. (VID)
Diamine T.D.
3,4-diaminopyridine
diamond
    d. blade
    d. blade knife
    d. bur
    D. Dye
    d. micrometer
    d. phaco knife
diamond-bur polishing
diamond-dusted
    d.-d. knife
    d.-d. knife blade
Diamontek knife
Diamox
    D. Sequels
Dianoux operation
diaphanoscopy
DiaPhine trephine
diaphragm
    iris-lens d.
    lens-iris d.
    Potter-Bucky d.
diapositive
    stereo-optic disk d.
diaschisis
diastasis
    iris d.
diathermocoagulator
diathermy
    d. application
    d. electrode
    Mira d.
    d. operation
    d. point
    d. puncture
    d. tip
    d. unit
    wet-field d.
dibromopropamidine
    d. isethionate
DICC
    drug-induced cicatricial conjunctivitis
dichlorphenamide

D

NOTES

127

dichroic
dichroism
   circular d.
dichromasy
dichromat
dichromatic
   d. light
   d. vision
dichromatism
   congenital d.
dichromatopsia
dichromic
Dickey-Fox operation
Dickey operation
Dickson-Wright
   D.-W. operation
   D.-W. orbit decompression
diclofenac sodium
dicloxacillin
dicoria
dictyoma (*var. of* diktyoma)
DIDMOAD
   diabetes insipidus, diabetes mellitus,
   optic atrophy, and deafness
   DIDMOAD syndrome
Dieffenbach
   D. operation
   D. serrefine
diencephalic
   d. lesion
   d. syndrome
diencephalon
Difei glasses
difference
   light d.
difficile
   Clostridium d.
diffraction
   Fraunhofer d.
diffusa
   encephalitis periaxialis d.
diffuse
   d. angiokeratoma
   d. anterior scleritis
   d. atherosclerosis
   d. cataract
   d. choroidal sclerosis
   d. choroiditis
   d. deep keratitis
   d. drusen
   d. endotheliitis
   d. granuloma
   d. inflammatory eyelid atrophy

   d. lamellar keratitis
   d. Lewy body disease
   d. unilateral subacute
     neuroretinitis (DUSN)
diffusion
   circle d.
   disk d. (DD)
diffusum
   angiokeratoma corporis d.
DiGeorge syndrome
Digilab
   D. perimeter
   D. tonometer
digital
   d. acuity card
   D. B System
   D. B System ultrascan
   D. fundus imager
   d. pressure
   D.-slit lamp imager
   d. subtraction indocyanine
     green angiography (DS-ICGA)
   d. subtraction photokeratoscopy
   d. tonometry
digital-imaging analysis
Digitalis purpurea
digito-ocular sign
diisopropyl fluorophosphate (DFP)
diktyoma, dictyoma
dilacerated cataract
dilaceration
Dilatair
dilate
dilated
   d. pupil
   d. retinal examination
   d. stereoscopic fundus
     examination
dilation
   ectatic d.
   d. and irrigation (D&I)
   d. lag
   lag d.
   pharmacological d.
   d. of punctum
   d. of punctum operation
   pupil d.
   transient unilateral d.
dilator
   Berens d.
   Castroviejo-Galezowski d.
   Castroviejo lacrimal d.
   French lacrimal d.

Galezowski lacrimal d.
Heath d.
Heyner d.
Hosford lacrimal d.
House lacrimal d.
iris d.
Jones punctum d.
lacrimal d.
Muldoon lacrimal d.
muscle d.
d. muscle
d. muscle of pupil
Nettleship-Wilder d.
punctal d.
punctum d.
pupil d.
Rolf d.
Ruedemann lacrimal d.
Weiss gold d.
Wilder lacrimal d.
Ziegler lacrimal d.
dilution
pigmentary d.
dimefilcon A
dimenhydrinate
Dimetabs Oral
Dimetane Extentabs
dimethylaminoethanol
dimethylpolysiloxane
dimethyl sulfate
diminazene aceturate
Dimitry
D. chalazion trephine
D. erysiphake
Dimitry-Bell erysiphake
Dimitry-Thomas erysiphake
Dimmer nummular keratitis
dimness of vision
dimple
Fuchs d.
d. veil
dimpling of eyeball
Dine digital scanner
diode
d. endolaser
d. endophotocoagulation
d. laser

d. laser trabeculoplasty (DLT)
light-emitting d. (LED)
diolipin antibody
DIOP
Ocutome D.
diopsimeter
diopter, dioptre (D)
66-d. iridectomy laser lens
prism d.
d. prism
d. sphere (DS)
Dioptimum System
dioptometer, dioptrometer
dioptometry
dioptoscope
dioptoscopy
dioptre (*var. of* diopter)
dioptric
d. aberration
d. apparatus
d. correction
d. medium
d. power
d. system
dioptrometer (*var. of* dioptometer)
dioptrometry
Dioptron
D. Nova
D. Ultima
dioptroscope
dioptroscopy
dioptry
Diphenhist
diphenhydramine hydrochloride
diphtheriae
Corynebacterium d.
diphtheritic conjunctivitis
diphtheroid
dipivalyl epinephrine
dipivefrin
d. HCl
diplegia
congenital facial d.
diplexia
diplobacillary
d. blepharitis
d. conjunctivitis

D

NOTES

129

diplocoria
diplopia
    binocular d.
    cerebral d.
    crossed d.
    direct d.
    heteronymous d.
    homonymous d.
    horizontal d.
    monocular d.
    paradoxical d.
    simple d.
    stereoscopic d.
    torsional d.
    uncrossed d.
    vertical d.
diplopiometer
diploscope
dipping
    ocular d.
    reverse d.
Diprivan
direct
    d. astigmatism
    d. diplopia
    d. glare
    d. gonioscopic lens
    d. illumination
    d. image
    d. method
    d. ophthalmoscope
    d. ophthalmoscopy
    d. parallax
    d. pupillary light reaction
    d. pupillary response
    d. reflex
    d. vision
direction
    angle of d.
    line of d.
    principal line of d.
    principal visual d.
    visual d.
directional
    d. defect
    d. preponderance
direct-light
    d.-l. reflex
    d.-l. refraction
    d.-l. response
director
    grooved d.
Dirofilaria repens

disability
    auditory perceptual d.
    glare d. (GD)
    motor-output d.
disappearance
disc (*var. of* disk)
discharge
    conjunctival d.
    mucoid d.
    mucous d.
    socket d.
    watery d.
disci (*pl. of* discus)
DisCide Disinfecting Toweletts
disciform
    d. chorioretinopathy
    d. degeneration of retina
    d. endotheliitis
    d. herpes simplex keratitis
    d. macular degeneration
    d. macular scar
    d. opacity
    d. process
    d. retinal detachment
disciformans
    retinitis d.
disciformis
    keratitis d.
discission
    d. hook
    d. knife
    d. of lens operation
    Moncrieff d.
    d. needle
    posterior d.
discitis
disclination
discoloration
disconjugate
    d. gaze
    d. roving eye movement
discontinuity
    zone of d.
discoria
discrete
    d. colliquation
    d. colliquative
    d. granuloma
discrimination
    color d.
    contrast d.
    light d.
    spatial d.

two-light d.
visual d.
discus, pl. **disci**
excavatio disci
d. nervi optici
d. opticus
discussion pallor
disease
Aland eye d.
Albers-Schönberg d.
allergic eye d.
Alström d.
angio-Behçet d.
Apollo d.
Arlt d.
arterial occlusive d.
arteriolar occlusive d.
Ballet d.
basal ganglia d.
Basedow d.
Batten d.
Batten-Mayou d.
Behçet d.
Behr d.
Benson d.
Berlin d.
Best d.
Bielschowsky d.
Bielschowsky-Jansky d.
blinding d.
Bower d.
Canavan d.
chiasmal d.
Coats d.
Cogan d.
collagen and rheumatoid-
related d.
collagen vascular d.
corneal stromal d.
Creutzfeldt-Jakob d.
Crouzon d.
Dalrymple d.
degenerative cerebellar d.
degenerative ocular d.
degenerative retinal d.
demyelinating d.
demyelinative d.

Devic d.
diffuse Lewy body d.
Dyggve d.
Eales d.
entero-Behçet d.
epithelial basement
membrane d.
epithelial herpetic d.
Erdheim-Chester d.
exogenous d.
extraorbital d.
Faber d.
Flajani d.
Flatau-Schilder d.
flecked retina d.
Förster d.
Franceschetti d.
Gerstmann-Straussler-
Scheinker d.
Gierke d.
Goldmann-Favre d.
Graefe d.
graft-versus-host d.
Graves d.
Harada d.
helminthic d.
herpetic ocular d.
Hippel d.
HSV ocular d.
HSV stromal d.
Hurler d.
infantile Refsum d.
infectious d.
inflammatory meibomian
gland d.
Jansky-Bielschowsky d.
Jensen d.
Kimmelstiel-Wilson d.
Kjer d.
Koeppe d.
Krill d.
Kuhnt-Junius d.
Kyrle d.
Lauber d.
Leber d.
Leigh d.
Lindau d.

D

NOTES

131

disease *(continued)*
Lindau-von Hippel d.
Machado-Joseph d.
macular d.
Masuda-Kitahara d.
medullary cystic d.
medullary optic d.
meibomian d.
midbrain d.
Mikulicz d.
miner's d.
mitochondrial d.
Möbius d.
multicore d.
multifactorial d.
multifocal chorioretinal d.
muscle-eye-brain d.
mycobacterial d.
neuro-Behçet d.
neuropathic d.
Norrie d.
occlusive vascular d.
ocular surface d. (OSD)
ocular syphilitic d.
oculoglandular d.
Oguchi d.
optic nerve d.
pancreatic d.
Parry d.
plus d.
primary demyelinating d.
primary ocular d.
pulseless d.
Purtscher d.
Recklinghausen d.
Reese-Ellsworth group Va d.
Reese-Ellsworth group Vb d.
Refsum d.
Reis-Bücklers d.
Reiter d.
retinal d.
Sanders d.
shipyard d.
Sichel d.
Sjögren d.
Spielmeyer-Sjögren d.
Spielmeyer-Stock d.
Spielmeyer-Vogt d.
Stargardt d.
Stargardt and Best d.
Steele-Richardson-Olszewski d.
stromal d.
Sturge-Weber d.

syphilitic ocular d.
Tangier d.
Tay d.
Tay-Sachs d.
Thygeson d.
thyroid eye d.
toxic-nutritional d.
van der Hoeve d.
vascular cerebellar d.
vascular occlusive d.
venous occlusive d.
viral ocular d.
visual pathway d.
Vogt d.
Vogt-Koyanagi-Harada d.
Vogt-Spielmeyer d.
von Gierke d.
von Hippel d.
von Hippel-Lindau d.
von Recklinghausen d.
Wagner d.
Werdnig-Hoffmann d.
Westphal-Strümpell d.
Whipple d.
Wilson d.
zone 1 d.
disequilibrium
disinfecting solution
disinserted
d. muscle
d. retina
disinsertion
levator aponeurosis d.
d. of retina
disjugate
d. movement
d. movement of eyes
disjunctive
d. movement
d. nystagmus
disk, disc
Airy d.
anagioid d.
anomalous d.
aperture d.
choked optic d.
ciliary d.
colobomatous optic d.
color d.
conus of optic d.
cupped d.
cupping of optic d.
dark d.

d. diameter
d. diffusion (DD)
doubling of the optic d.
dragged d.
d. drusen
d. drusen hemorrhage
d. edema
edema of optic d.
d. elevation
excavation of optic d.
d. forceps
gelatin d.
hypoplastic d.
ischemic d.
Krill d.
Krupin eye d.
leukemic infiltration of the
  optic d.
micrometer d.
morning glory d.
nasal border of optic d.
neovascularization of d. (NVD)
d. neovascularization
d. neurovascular vessel
Newton d.
d. new vessel
new vessel d.
optic d.
pale optic d.
pallor of d., pallor of d.
d. pallor
pinhole d.
pink eye d.
Placido d.
planoconvex-shaped d.
posterior lamellar d.
Rekoss d.
stenopaic d.
stenopeic d.
stroboscopic d.
swelling of d.
tilted d.
d. vasculature
Whipple d.
disk-fovea distance
disk-shaped cataract
dislocated lens

dislocation
congenital lens d.
intraocular lens d.
d. of lens
lens d.
posterior d.
dislocator
Kirby lens d.
disodium hydrogen phosphate
disorder
accommodation d.
adrenal d.
autonomic nervous system d.
basement membrane d.
bullous d.
canalicular d.
epithelial bleb d.
extraocular muscle d.
d. of eye
eyelid d.
eye movement d.
hemorrhagic d.
histiocytic d.
hyperkeratotic d.
infranuclear d.
lacrimation d.
motion perception d.
myelin d.
myopathic d.
neurologic d.
neuromuscular d.
ocular motility d.
oculodermal d.
oculomotor d.
ophthalmic d.
optic nerve d.
outflow d.
parathyroid d.
postsynaptic congenital
  myasthenic d.
prechiasmal d.
presynaptic congenital
  myasthenic d.
pupil d.
pupillary d.
retinal d.
Sanders d.

D

NOTES

disorder *(continued)*
   sensorimotor d.
   spatial perception d.
   supranuclear d.
   tear film d.
   thyroid gland d.
   vascular d.
   visuospatial d.
   vitreoretinal d.
disorganized globe
disorientation
   topographic d.
disparate retinal point
disparity, pl. **disparities**
   d. angle
   binocular d.
   bitemporal d.
   conjugate d.
   fixation d.
   horizontal retinal d.
   retinal d.
dispenser
   DropTainer d.
dispersing lens
dispersion
   chromatic d.
   circle of d.
   corneal endothelial
    pigmentary d.
   pigment d.
   point of d.
   d. prism
   d. syndrome
displacement
   image d.
   macular d.
   object d.
   d. threshold
disposable
   d. cautery
   d. contact lens
   d. ocutome
   d. trephine
disproportion
   congenital fiber-type d.
   (CFTD)
disruption
   posterior capsular zonular d.
   YAG laser d.
dissecting scissors
dissection
   arterial d.
   open-sky d.

dissector
   Barraquer corneal d.
   Berens corneal d.
   Castroviejo corneal d.
   channel d.
   corneal knife d.
   Desmarres corneal d.
   Green corneal d.
   d. knife
   Martinez d.
   Troutman corneal d.
   Troutman lamellar d.
disseminated
   d. asymptomatic unilateral
    neovascularization
   d. choroiditis
   d. intravascular coagulation
   d. nonosteolytic myelomatosis
dissimilar
   d. image test
   d. segment
   d. target test
dissipation
   circle d.
dissociated
   d. alkaloid
   d. double hypertropia (DDHT)
   d. hyperdeviation
   d. position
   d. vertical deviation
   d. vertical divergence (DVD)
   d. vertical nystagmus
dissociation
   light-near d.
   perception d.
   d. of visual perception
dissociative state
distal
   d. optic nerve syndrome
   d. optic neuropathy
distance
   angular d.
   d. between centers (DBC)
   d. between nasal lines (DBL)
   center of rotation d.
   d. correction
   disk-fovea d.
   egocentric fixation d.
   equivalent d.
   focal d.
   infinite d.
   intercanthal d. (ICD)
   interpupillary d. (IPD)

intraocular d.
marginal reflex d. (MRD)
d. and near (D&N)
object d.
pupillary d. (PD)
vertex of d.
d. visual acuity (DVA)
distant
d. direct ophthalmoscopy
d. gaze
distantial aberration
distichia, distichiasis
acquired d.
distometer
Haag-Streit d.
distortion
d. aberration
barred d.
barrel d.
corneal d.
d. of lens
pin cushion d.
d. of vision
Xeroscope grid d.
distraction
conus d.
d. conus
distribution
gaussian d.
normal d.
districhiasis
disturbance
equilibrium d.
sensation d.
tear-film d.
visual d.
diurnal
d. fluctuation
d. intraocular pressure
measurement
variation d.
d. variation
DIVA test
divergence
d. amplitude
congenital adduction palsy with
synergistic d.

dissociated vertical d. (DVD)
d. excess
excess d.
d. excess exotropia
fusional d.
d. insufficiency
d. insufficiency exotropia
negative vertical d.
d. nystagmus
d. paralysis
point of d.
positive vertical d.
relative d.
d. reserve
strabismus d.
synergistic d.
vertical d.
divergent
d. beam
d. cut angle
d. light
d. ray
d. squint
d. strabismus
diverging
d. meniscus
d. meniscus lens
divers' spectacles
diverticulum of lacrimal sac
divide-and-conquer
d.-a.-c. method
d.-a.-c. technique
divided spectacles
Dix foreign body spud
Dix-Hallpike test
Dixon-Thorpe vitreous foreign body
forceps
DK value
DLK
deep lamellar keratoplasty
DLT
diode laser trabeculoplasty
DM
diabetes mellitus
DME
diabetic macular edema
DMV II contact lens remover

D

NOTES

135

D&N
distance and near
Docustar fundus camera
Dodick
D. lens-holding forceps
D. photolysis
D. photolysis probe
Doherty
D. sphere
D. sphere implant
Dohlman plug
dolichoectatic anterior cerebral artery
Döllinger tendinous ring
doll's
d. eye
d. eye maneuver
d. eye reflex
d. eye sign
d. head maneuver
d. head phenomenon
dolor capitis
dolorosa
atrophia d.
D'ombrain operation
Domeboro solution
dome receptacle
dominance
ocular d.
dominant
d. cystoid macular dystrophy
d. eye
d. gene
d. optic atrophy
d. progressive foveal dystrophy
d. slowly progressive macular dystrophy
Donaldson
D. eye patch
D. fundus camera
D. stereoviewer
Donaldson-Fitzpatrick oculocutaneous albinism
Donders
D. chart
D. glaucoma
D. law
D. line
D. procedure
D. ring
donor
d. cornea
d. eye

d. graft
d. material
d. tissue
donut-cut flap
donut-shaped flap
Doppler
Hadeco intraoperative D.
Siemens Quantum 2000 Color D.
D. ultrasonogram
D. ultrasonography
D. velocimeter
Doran pattern stimulator ophthalmoscope
DORC
Dutch Ophthalmic Research Center
DORC backflush instrument
DORC fast freeze cryosurgical system
DORC handle
DORC microforceps and microscissors
DORC subretinal instrument set
Dorello canal
Dorsacaine
dorsal
d. midbrain syndrome
d. rostral damage
d. vermis
dorsalis
tabes d.
Doryl
dorzolamide
d. hydrochloride
d. hydrochloride ophthalmic solution
d. hydrochloride-timolol maleate ophthalmic solution
dose
Lacrivisc unit d.
mean episcleral heat d.
dot
d. dystrophy
Gunn d.
d. hemorrhage
Horner-Trantas d.
lamina d.
Marcus Gunn d.
d. method
Mittendorf d.
Morgan d.

Trantas d.
white d.
dot-and-blot hemorrhage
dot-like lens
double
    d. arcuate scotoma
    d. concave lens
    d. convex lens
    d. dissociated hypertropia
    d. elevator palsy
    d. freeze-thaw cryopexy
    d. freeze-thaw cryotherapy
    d. homonymous hemianopsia
    d. irrigating/aspirating cannula
    d. lid eversion
    d. lower lid fold
    d. Maddox rod test
    d. refraction
    d. slab-off contact lens
    d. spatula
    d. tantalum clip
    d. vision
double-armed suture
double-contrast visualization
double-cutting sharp cystitome
double-pronged forceps
double-row diathermy barrage
double-running penetrating
  keratoplasty suture
doublet
    achromatic d.
    Wollaston d.
doubling
    d. device
    d. of the optic disk
Doubra lens
Dougherty irrigating/aspirating unit
Douglas cilia forceps
douloureux
    tic d.
Douvas
    D. honeycombed choroiditis
    D. rotoextractor
    D. vitreous cutter
Douvas-Barraquer speculum

down
    endothelial cell side d.
    d. to finger-counting
downbeat nystagmus
down-gaze
downgrowth
    epithelial d.
downward
    d. deviation
    d. gaze
    d. squint
Doyne
    D. familial colloid degeneration
    D. familial honeycombed
      choroiditis
    D. guttate iritis
    D. honeycombed choroidopathy
    D. honeycombed degeneration
    D. honeycombed dystrophy
    D. syndrome
DR
    diabetic retinopathy
Draeger
    D. forceps
    D. high vacuum erysiphake
    D. modified keratome
    D. tonometer
dragged
    d. disk
    d. macula
    d. retina
dragging
    macular d.
    optic disk d.
    retinal d.
drain
    Mentor pre-cut d.
    Penrose d.
drainage
    d. angle
    aqueous humor d.
    cerebral venous d.
    indirect argon laser d.
    lacrimal d.
    d. of lacrimal gland
    d. of lacrimal gland operation
    d. of lacrimal sac

D

NOTES

137

drainage *(continued)*
 d. of lacrimal sac operation
 lymphatic d.
 quadrantic sclerectomy with
  internal d.
 sclerotomy with d.
 subretinal fluid d.
 tear d.
 uveovertex d.
drape
 1021 d.
 Alcon disposable d.
 Barrier d.
 Blair head d.
 Eye-Pak II d.
 Hough d.
 miniophthalmic d.
 3M Steri-Drape d.
 Opraflex d.
 Pro-Ophtha d.
 Steri-Drape d.
 Surgikos disposable d.
 Visi-Drape Elite ophthalmic d.
 Visi-Drape mini aperture d.
 Visi-Drape mini incise d.
 Visiflex d.
Drechslera
dressing
 binocle d.
 binocular d.
 Blenderm tape d.
 bolus d.
 Borsch d.
 collodion d.
 compression d.
 crepe bandage d.
 Elastoplast d.
 Expo Bubble d.
 eye pad d.
 fluff d.
 fluffed gauze d.
 d. forceps
 Harman eye d.
 lens d.
 moistened fine mesh gauze d.
 monocular d.
 pressure patch d.
 Pro-Ophtha d.
 ribbon gauze d.
 saline-saturated wool d.
 sterile adhesive bubble d.
 Telfa plastic film d.
 tie-over Sellotape d.

 tulle gras d.
 wet d.
 wool saturated in saline d.
Drews
 D. angled cystitome
 D. capsule polisher
 D. cataract needle
 D. cilia forceps
 D. inclined prism
 D. irrigating/aspirating unit
 D. irrigating cannula
 D. lens
 D. syndrome
Drews-Knolle reverse irrigating vectis
Drews-Rosenbaum
 D.-R. iris retractor
 D.-R. irrigating/aspirating unit
Drews-Sato
 D.-S. suture-pickup hook
 D.-S. suture-pickup spatula
 D.-S. tying forceps
drift
 d. movement
 post saccadic d.
droop
 lid d.
drooping
 d. of eyelid
droopy lid
droperidol
dropout
 acinar d.
 nerve fiber layer d.
 pigmentary d.
 retinal pigment epithelium d.
dropped-socket appearance
dropper
 eye d.
 undine d.
drops
 AC eye d.
 Acular d.
 Allerest Eye D.
 Alomide d.
 betamethasone phosphate
  eye d.
 Bion Tears eye d.
 Boston reconditioning d.
 Boston Advance
  reconditioning d.
 cidofovir eye d.
 Collyrium eye d.

Comfort d.
corticosteroid d.
eye d.
GenTeal lubricant eye d.
hypertonic d.
Lens Plus rewetting d.
lubricating d.
Mallazine Eye D.
Moisture Ophthalmic D.
Neosporin d.
placebo eye d.
poparacaine ophthalmic d.
Refresh Plus lubricant eye d.
Refresh Tears eye d.
Rondec D.
Sensitive Eyes d.
trifluridine eye d.
Twenty/Twenty d.
DropTainer dispenser
droxifilcon A
Drualt
    bundle of D.
    D. bundle
drug
    d. abuse retinopathy
    adrenergic d.
    amphiphilic d.
    antiadrenergic d.
    anticataract d.
    anticholinergic d.
    cataractogenic d.
    cholinergic d.
    immunosuppressive d.
    d. interaction
    neuroloptic d.
    neuromuscular blocking d.
    neuromuscular disorder-
      causing d.
    nonsteroidal anti-
      inflammatory d.
    ophthalmic d.
    parasympatholytic d.
    parasympathomimetic d.
    sulfa d.
    sympatholytic d.
    systemic d.
    topical d.

drug-induced
    d.-i. cataract
    d.-i. cicatricial conjunctivitis
      (DICC)
    d.-i. cicatrizing conjunctivitis
    d.-i. glaucoma
    d.-i. nystagmus
    d.-i. ptosis
drum
    optokinetic d.
drusen
    basal laminar d.
    buried disk d.
    confluent d.
    diffuse d.
    disk d.
    equatorial d.
    familial d.
    giant d.
    hard d.
    intrapapillary d.
    macular d.
    nerve head d.
    optic disk d.
    optic nerve d.
    d. of optic papilla
    soft d.
    visible d.
dry
    d. ARMD
    D. Eyes
    D. Eyes Solution
    d. eye syndrome
    D. Eye Therapy Solution
    d. fold
    d. senile degenerative
      maculopathy
    d. senile macular degeneration
    d. spot
Drysdale nucleus manipulator
dry-shelled cataract
Drysol cream
DS
    diopter sphere
DS-9 needle
D-shaped keratometric reflection

D

NOTES

DS-ICGA
  digital subtraction indocyanine green
    angiography
dual lens
Dualoop
Dual-Wet
Duane
  D. accommodation chart
  D. classification
  D. classification of squint
  D. retraction syndrome
  D. retractor
duboisii
  Histoplasma d.
Duchenne dystrophy
duct
  ampulla of lacrimal d.
  canalicular d.
  catheterization of lacrimal d.
  catheterization of
    lacrimonasal d.
  excretory d.
  lacrimal d.
  lacrimonasal d.
  meibomian d.
  nasal d.
  nasolacrimal d. (NLD)
  probing lacrimonasal d.
  stenon d.
  tear d.
  d. T-tube lacrimal
ductal orifice obliteration
duction
  forced d.
  full versions and d.'s
  ocular d.
  passive d.
  d. test
  versions and d.'s
  d.'s and versions (D&V)
  vertical d.
ductional
ductus
  d. lacrimales
  d. nasolacrimalis
Duddell membrane
Duke-Elder
  D.-E. lamp
  D.-E. operation
Dulaney lens
Dunnington operation
duochrome test
Duo-Flow

Duolube
Duotrak blade
DuoVisc viscoelastic system
duplex scan
duplicity theory of vision
Dupuy-Dutemps
  D.-D. dacryocystorhinostomy
    dye test
  D.-D. dacryostomy
  D.-D. operation
dura
DURAcare
DURAcare II
dural
  d. arteriovenous malformation
  d. cavernous sinus fistula
  d. sheath
  d. shunt
  d. shunt syndrome
Duralone
Duramist Plus
Duranest
  D. HCl
  D. HCl with epinephrine
Durasoft 2 contact lens
Duratears Naturale
Dura-T lens
Durazyme
Duredge knife
Durette external laser shield
Durham tonometer
Duricef
Durr operation
DUSN
  diffuse unilateral subacute
    neuroretinitis
dusting
  fibrin d.
  iris pigment d.
dust-like opacity
Dutcher body
Dutch Ophthalmic Research Center
  (DORC)
Duverger-Velter operation
D&V
  ductions and versions
DVA
  distance visual acuity
DVD
  dissociated vertical divergence
DWCL
  daily-wear contact lens
Dwelle Ophthalmic Solution

dyclonine
dye
    Alizarin Red S d.
    Cardio-Green d.
    chemofluorescent d.
    Diamond D.
    d. disappearance test (DDT)
    fluorescein d.
    Haag-Streit fluorescein d.
    indocyanine green d.
    materials primary d.
    pooling of d.
    vital d.
    d. yellow laser
Dyer
    D. nomogram system of lens
      ordering
    D. nomogram system of
      ordering contact lens
dyflos
Dyggve disease
Dymadon
dynamic
    d. accommodation insufficiency
    d. refraction
    d. scanning laser
      ophthalmoscopy
    d. strabismus
    d. visual acuity
dynopter
Dynosol
Dyonics syringe injector
dysadaptation
dysaptation
dysautonomia
    familial autonomic d.
dyscephalic
    d. syndrome
    d. syndrome of François
dyschromasia
dyschromatopsia
    acquired d.
    cerebral d.
    congenital d.
dysconjugate gaze
dyscoria
dyscrinic rhinitis

dysfunction
    anterior visual pathway d.
    brain d.
    brainstem d.
    cerebellar d.
    cone d.
    familial autonomic d.
    foveal outer retinal d.
    intraorbital nerve d.
    isolated oculomotor nerve d.
    minimal brain d.
    neurologic d.
    oblique d.
    oculosympathetic d.
    optic nerve d.
    photoreceptor d.
    pontomesencephalic d.
    primary cone d.
    rod-cone d.
dysgenesis
    corneal d.
    iridocorneal mesodermal d.
    mesenchymal d.
    mesodermal d.
    posterior amorphous corneal d.
dysharmonious correspondence
dyskeratosis
    benign d.
    d. congenita
    congenital d.
    hereditary benign
      intraepithelial d.
    intraepithelial d.
    malignant d.
dyslexia
    attentional d.
    central d.
    deep d.
    endogenous d.
    hemianopic d.
    neglect d.
    surface d.
dysmegalopsia
dysmetria
    ocular d.
    saccadic d.
dysmetropsia

D

NOTES

141

dysmorphopsia
dysopia algera
dysopsia algera
dysoric retinopathy
dysplasia
    chiasmal d.
    conjunctival d.
    corneal d.
    encephalo-ophthalmic d.
    fibrous d.
    forebrain d.
    hereditary renal-retinal d.
    macular d.
    oculoauricular d.
    oculoauriculovertebral d.
    oculodentodigital d.
    oculovertebral d.
    ophthalmomandibulomelic d.
    optic disk d.
    optic nerve d.
    orodigitofacial d.
    retinal d.
    septo-optic d.
    vitreoretinal d.
dysplastic
    d. coloboma
    d. retina
Dysport
dysproteinemic retinopathy
dysthyroid
    d. ophthalmopathy
    d. optic neuropathy
    d. orbitopathy
dysthyroidism
dystonia
    blepharospasm-oromandibular d.
    focal d.
dystopia
    d. canthorum
    foveal d.
    orbital d.
dystrophia
    d. adiposa corneae
    d. endothelialis corneae
    d. epithelialis corneae
dystrophica
    elastosis d.
    myotonia d.
dystrophy
    amorphous corneal d.
    annular macular d.
    anterior basement membrane d.
    (ABMD)

anterior membrane d.
Avellino d.
basement membrane d.
benign concentric annular
    macular d.
Best vitelliform macular d.
Biber-Haab-Dimmer corneal d.
Bietti crystalline
    corneoretinal d.
Bücklers I d.
Bücklers II d.
Bücklers III d.
butterfly macular d.
butterfly-shaped pigment
    epithelial d.
central areolar choroidal d.
central areolar pigment
    epithelial d.
central cloudy corneal d.
central cloudy
    parenchymatous d.
central crystalline d.
central pigmentary retinal d.
central speckled corneal d.
cerebellar ataxia-cone d.
choroidal d.
choroidoretinal d.
Cogan microcystic corneal
    epithelial d.
Cogan microcystic epithelial
    corneal d.
cone d.
cone-rod d. (CRD)
congenital hereditary corneal d.
congenital hereditary endothelial
    corneal d.
congenital muscular d.
congenital myotonic d.
d. of cornea
corneal endothelial guttate d.
corneal guttate d.
corneal stromal d.
corneal vortex d.
crystalline corneal d.
cystoid macular d.
deep filiform d.
deep parenchymatous d.
dominant cystoid macular d.
dominant progressive foveal d.
dominant slowly progressive
    macular d.
dot d.
Doyne honeycombed d.

Duchenne d.
ectatic corneal d.
endothelial cell d.
epithelial basement
  membrane d.
Favre d.
Fehr macular d.
fenestrated sheen macular d.
filiform d.
fingerprint corneal d.
flecked corneal d.
Fleischer d.
foveomacular vitelliform d.
Franceschetti d.
François d.
Fuchs combined corneal d.
Fuchs endothelial corneal d.
Fuchs endothelial-epithelial d.
Fuchs epithelial corneal d.
Fuchs epithelial-endothelial d.
furrow d.
gelatinous d.
Goldmann-Favre d.
granular corneal d.
Grayson-Wilbrandt anterior
  corneal d.
Groenouw corneal d.
Groenouw type I d.
Groenouw type II d.
gutter d.
hereditary anterior
  membrane d.
hereditary epithelial corneal d.
hereditary hemorrhagic
  macular d.
hereditary macular d.
hereditary vitelliform d.
honeycomb d.
infantile neuroaxonal d.
  (INAD)
juvenile corneal epithelial d.
juvenile epithelial d.
keratoconus d.
lattice corneal d.
Lefler-Wadsworth-Sidbury
  foveal d.
macroreticular d.

macular corneal d.
Maeder-Danis d.
map d.
map-dot corneal d.
map-dot-fingerprint corneal
  epithelial d.
marginal crystalline d.
Meesman epithelial corneal d.
Meesman juvenile epithelial d.
microcystic corneal d.
microcystic epithelial d.
muscular d.
myotonic d.
North Carolina macular d.
oculocerebrorenal d.
oculopharyngeal d.
ophthalmoplegic muscular d.
parenchymatous corneal d.
pattern d.
pattern d. of pigment
  epithelium of Byers and
  Marmor
pericentral rod-cone d.
pigment epithelial d.
Pillat d.
polymorphous d.
posterior amorphous corneal d.
posterior polymorphic d.
posterior polymorphous
  corneal d.
progressive cone d.
progressive cone-rod d.
progressive foveal d.
progressive macular d.
progressive tapetochoroidal d.
pseudoinflammatory macular d.
Reis-Bücklers ring-shaped d.
Reis-Bücklers superficial
  corneal d.
reticular d.
retinal cone d.
retinal pigmentary d.
ring-like corneal d.
ring-shaped d.
rod and cone d.
rod-cone d.
Salzmann nodular corneal d.

D

NOTES

dystrophy *(continued)*
Schlichting d.
Schnyder crystalline corneal d.
sheen d.
Sjögren reticular d.
Sorsby pseudoinflammatory
macular d.
speckled corneal d.
Stargardt d.
Stocker-Holt d.
Stocker-Holt-Schneider d.

stromal corneal d.
tapetochoroidal d.
vitelliform d.
vitelliruptive macular d.
vitreo-tapetoretinal d.
vortex corneal d.
d. of Waardenburg-Jonkers
Wagner vitreoretinal d.
X-linked cone d.
dysversion
congenital d.

E
esophoria
  E Carpine
  E chart
  E game
  E syndrome
  E test
EA-290
  Toctron EA-290
EaglePlug tapered-shaft punctum plug
EagleVision Freeman punctum plug
Eales disease
early
  e. antigen
  e. lens opacity
  e. mature cataract
  e. postoperative suture adjustment (EPSA)
  E. receptor potential
  e. receptor potential mottling
  E. Treatment Diabetic Retinopathy Study (ETDRS)
early-onset
  e.-o. myope
  e.-o. myopia
EAS-1000 anterior eye segment analysis system
Easterman visual function
EasyClean/GP
Easy Eyes
Eaton-Lambert syndrome
EBAA
  Eye Bank Association of America
Eber needle-holder forceps
EBV
  Epstein-Barr virus
  EBV nuclear antigen
EBV-associated antigen
EC-5000 excimer laser
ECCE
  extracapsular cataract extraction
eccentric
  e. ablation
  e. fixation
  e. gaze
  e. gaze-holding
  e. limitation
  e. photorefraction
  e. vision

eccentricity
  angle of e.
ecchymosis of eyelid
echinococcus
  e. cyst
Echinococcus granulosus
echinophthalmia
Echodide
echography
  kinetic e.
  ocular e.
  orbital e.
  quantitative e.
  topographic e.
echo-ophthalmogram
echo-ophthalmography
EchoScan by Nidek
echothiophate
  e. iodide
  E. phospholine
Eckardt
  E. Heme-Stopper instrument
  E. temporary keratoprosthesis
eclamptic retinopathy
eclipse
  e. amblyopia
  e. blindness
  e. retinopathy
  e. scotoma
ECM
  extracellular matrix
Econochlor
Econopred
  E. Ophthalmic
  E. Plus
ectasia, ectasis
  corneal e.
  iris e.
  e. of sclera
  scleral e.
  stromal e.
ectatic
  e. cornea
  e. corneal dystrophy
  e. dilation
  e. marginal degeneration
ecthyma
  e. contagiosum
  e. gangrenosum
ectiris

E

ectochoroidea
ectocornea
ectopia
    cilia e.
    e. iridis
    e. lentis
    e. maculae
    macular e.
    posterior pituitary e.
    e. pupillae congenita
ectopic
    e. eyelash
    e. tissue
ectropion, ectropium
    Adams e.
    Adams operation for e.
    atonic e.
    Cibis e.
    e. cicatriceum
    cicatricial e.
    complex e.
    congenital e.
    e. of eyelid
    eyelid e.
    flaccid e.
    inflammatory e.
    involutional senile e.
    lid e.
    e. luxurians
    mechanical e.
    medial e.
    paralytic e.
    e. paralyticum
    pigment layer e.
    punctal e.
    e. sarcomatosum
    senescent e.
    senile e.
    e. senilis
    spastic e.
    e. spasticum
    tarsal e.
    e. uveae
ectropionize
eczematoid blepharitis
eczematosus
    pannus e.
eczematous
    e. conjunctivitis
    e. pannus
edema
    aphakic cystoid macular e.
    Berlin e.

boggy e.
brawny e.
central e.
cerebral e.
choroidal e.
conjunctival e.
e. of cornea
corneal e.
cystoid macular e. (CME)
diabetic macular e. (DME)
disk e.
endothelial cell e.
epithelial e.
eyelid e.
e. of eyelid
focal vasogenic e.
foveal e.
graft e.
hereditary corneal e.
Iwanoff retinal e.
lid e.
macular e.
microcystic e.
mucinous e.
e. of optic disk
optic disk e.
periorbital e.
periretinal e.
phakic cystoid macular e.
retinal e.
Stellwag brawny e.
stromal e.
subconjunctival e.
edge
    e. coating
    e. contour
    epithelial rolled e.
    fimbriated e.
    E. III hydrogel contact lens
    e. stand-off
EdgeAhead
    E. crescent knife
    E. microsurgical knives
    E. phaco slit knife
edge-light pupil cycle time
edging of spectacle lens
Edinger fiber
Edinger-Westphal nucleus
edipism
edrophonium
    e. chloride
    e. chloride test
Edwards syndrome

effect
    Abney e.
    autokinetic e.
    Bracken e.
    Braid e.
    cat's eye e.
    copper-wire e.
    Cotton e.
    Faden e.
    lens flexure e.
    Lythgoe e.
    Mizuo-Nakamura e.
    muscarinic cholinergic side e.
    myotonic dystrophy e.
    neuromuscular e.
    ocular motility e.
    pantoscopic e.
    prismatic e.
    pupillary e.
    Purkinje e.
    radiation e.
    Raman e.
    Stiles-Crawford e.
    sunburst e.
    telephoto e.
    threshold e.
    Tyndall e.
    venturi e.
    Zeeman e.
effective diameter
efferent
    e. fiber
    e. nerve
efficiency
    visual e.
effusion
    choroidal e.
    ciliochoroidal e.
    uveal e.
Efricel
Egger line
egilops
egocentric fixation distance
Egyptian
    E. conjunctivitis
    E. ophthalmia
Ehlers-Danlos syndrome

Ehrhardt lid forceps
Ehrlich-Türck line
Ehrmann test
eiconometer (*var. of* eikonometer)
eidoptometry
eight-ball
    e.-b. hemorrhage
    e.-b. hyphema
eighth cranial nerve
eikonometer, eiconometer
EKC
    epidemic keratoconjunctivitis
EKV
    erythrokeratodermia variabilis
elaioides
    degeneratio spherularis e.
elastic pseudoxanthoma
elasticum
    pseudoxanthoma e. (PXE)
    xanthoma e.
elastodysplasia
elastodystrophy
elastoid degeneration
Elastoplast
    E. bandage
    E. dressing
    E. eye occlusor
elastorrhexis
elastosis
    e. dystrophica
    senescent e.
    senile e.
elastotic band keratopathy
Eldridge-Green lamp
electric
    e. light blindness
    e. ophthalmia
    e. retinopathy
    e. shock cataract
electrica
    cataracta e.
    ophthalmia e.
electrocauterizer
electrocautery
    Fine micropoint e.
    Geiger e.
    Hildreth e.

E

NOTES

electrocautery *(continued)*
   Mentor wet-field e.
   Mira e.
   Mueller e.
   ophthalmic e.
   Op-Temp disposable e.
   Parker-Heath e.
   Prince e.
   Rommel e.
   Rommel-Hildreth e.
   Scheie e.
   Todd e.
   Valilab e.
   von Graefe e.
   Wadsworth-Todd e.
   wet-field e.
   Ziegler e.
electrocoagulation
electrode
   Berens e.
   Burian-Allen contact lens e.
   Cibis e.
   coagulating e.
   cyclodiathermy e.
   diathermy e.
   Gradle e.
   Guyton e.
   Kronfeld e.
   Pischel e.
   Schepens e.
   Walker e.
   Weve e.
electrodiaphake
electroencephalogram
electroepilation
electrokeratotome
   Castroviejo e.
electromagnetic
   e. energy
   e. radiation
   e. removal of foreign body
   e. scleral search coil
   e. spectrum
electromucotome
   Steinhauser e.
electron
   e. interferometer
   e. interferometry
   e. microscope
electronic tonometer
electronystagmogram (ENG)

electronystagmograph
electronystagmography (ENG)
electro-oculogram (EOG)
   monocular e.-o.
electro-oculograph
electro-oculography (EOG)
electroparacentesis
electroperimeter
electroretinogram (ERG)
   cone e.
   cone b-wave implicit time e.
   flash e.
   flicker e.
   focal e.
   full-field e.
   multifocal e.
   pattern e.
   pattern-evoked e. (PERG)
   peak latencies of pattern e.
   rod e.
   topographical e.
electroretinograph
   Ganzfeld e.
electroretinography (ERG)
   foveal cone e.
   topographic e.
electrostatic interaction
elegans
   Caenorhabditis e.
element
   encircling e.
   Kollmorgen e.
   Mira encircling e.
   retinal e.
elephantiasis oculi
elevation
   e. angle
   disk e.
   sensory e.
   e. topography
   e. topography map
elevator
   Desmarres lid e.
   Freer periosteal e.
   Joseph periosteal e.
   e. muscle
   e. palsy
   Tenzel e.
Eliasoph lid retractor
ELISA
   enzyme-linked immunosorbent assay
   ELISA antibody
Ellingson syndrome

Elliot
   E. corneal trephine
   E. operation
   E. sign
   E. trephine handle
ellipsoidal back surface
ellipsometer
   retinal e.
elliptic
   e. nystagmus
   e. pupil
elliptical
   e. nystagmus
   e. trephination
Ellis
   E. foreign body needle
   E. foreign body spud
   E. foreign body spud needle
   probe
   E. needle holder
Elrex
Elschnig
   E. blepharorrhaphy
   E. body
   E. canthorrhaphy
   E. canthorrhaphy operation
   E. capsule forceps
   E. cataract knife
   E. central iridectomy
   E. conjunctivitis
   E. corneal knife
   E. cyclodialysis spatula
   E. extrusion needle
   E. fixation forceps
   E. keratoplasty
   E. pearl
   E. pterygium knife
   E. refractor
   E. retractor
   E. spoon
   E. spot
   E. syndrome
   E. trephine
Elschnig-O'Brien forceps
Elschnig-O'Connor fixation forceps
Elschnig-Weber loupe
Ely operation

Emadine
embolism
   retinal e.
embryonal
   e. carcinoma
   e. epithelial cyst of iris
   e. medulloepithelioma
   e. medulloepithelioma of
   ciliary body
   e. nuclear cataract
   e. tumor of ciliary body
embryonic
   e. cataract
   e. fixation syndrome
   e. plate
embryopathic cataract
embryotoxon
   anterior e.
   posterior e.
Emcee lens
emedastine difurmarate ophthalmic
   solution
emergence
   angle of e.
emergency light reflex
emergent
   e. ray
   e. ray of light
Emerson one-piece segment bifocal
Emery lens
emissarial canal
emittance
   radiant e.
emmetrope
emmetropia
emmetropic
emmetropization
EMP
   epiretinal membrane proliferation
Empac-Cavitron irrigation/aspiration
   unit
emphysema
   e. of conjunctiva
   e. of orbit
   orbital e.
   subconjunctival e.
Empire needle

E

NOTES

empty
optically e.
e. sella
e. sella syndrome
encanthis
encapsulated bleb
encephalitis
e. periaxialis concentrica
e. periaxialis diffusa
encephalocele
basal e.
orbital e.
transsphenoidal e.
encephalofacial angiomatosis
encephalomyelitis
encephalomyelopathy
subacute necrotizing e.
encephalomyopathy
encephalo-ophthalmic dysplasia
encephalopathy
hypertensive e.
lead e.
Leigh e.
Wernicke e.
encephalotrigeminal angiomatosis
encircling
e. band
e. band for scleral buckle
e. element
e. explant
e. of globe operation
e. implant
e. polyethylene tube
e. of scleral buckle operation
e. silicone buckle
endarteritis
e. obliterans
end-gaze nystagmus
endocapsular
e. balloon
e. phacoemulsification
endocrine
e. exophthalmos
e. lid retraction
e. myopathy
e. ophthalmopathy
endocrine-inactive adenoma
endocryopexy
endocryophotocoagulation
endocryoretinopexy
endodiathermy
endogenous
e. dyslexia

e. endophthalmitis
e. uveitis
endoillumination
endoilluminator
Grieshaber e.
endolaser
diode e.
e. probe tip
endonasal laser
dacryocystorhinostomy (ENL-DCR)
endoneural cell
endonucleus
Endo Optics Microprobe
endophlebitis of retinal vein
endophotocoagulation
argon laser e.
diode e.
endophthalmitis
Acanthamoeba e.
bacterial e.
bleb-associated e.
candidal e.
chronic e.
endogenous e.
exogenous e.
fungal e.
granulomatous e.
infectious e.
Klebsiella e.
latent e.
metastatic e.
nocardial e.
e. ophthalmia nodosa
e. phacoallergica
phacoanaphylactic e.
e. phacoanaphylactica
phacoantigenic e.
e. phacogenetica
pneumococcal e.
postoperative e.
sterile e.
systemic bacterial e.
toxocariasis e.
endophthalmodonesis
endophthamitis
Ovadendron sulphureo-ochraceum e.
endophytum
glioma e.
endoplasmic reticulum
EndoProbe
endoretinal

endoscope
>Microprobe integrated laser e.
>ophthalmic e.

endoscopic raking

Endosol
>E. Extra

endothelial
>e. bleb
>e. cell
>e. cell analysis
>e. cell basement membrane
>e. cell count
>e. cell density
>e. cell dystrophy
>e. cell edema
>e. cell side down
>e. cell surface of cornea
>e. decompensation
>e. exudate
>iridocorneal e. (ICE)
>e. plaque
>e. rejection line
>vesiculosus linear e.

endothelialitis

endotheliitis
>diffuse e.
>disciform e.
>HSV e.
>linear e.
>peripheral e.

endothelioma
>Sidler-Huguenin e.

endotheliopathy
>autoimmune corneal e.
>idiopathic corneal e.
>progressive herpetic corneal e.

endothelitis

endothelium
>e. camerae anterioris bulbi
>corneal e.
>monolayered e.
>e. oculi

endotracheal
>e. anesthesia
>e. tube

end-point
>e.-p. color
>e.-p. nystagmus

end-position nystagmus

endrysone

energy
>electromagnetic e.
>facture e.
>radiant e.

enflurane

enfoldings

ENG
>electronystagmogram
>electronystagmography

engorgement
>conjunctival vascular e.
>episcleral vascular e.
>venous e.

enhancement
>astigmatic keratotomy e.

Enhydrina schistosa

enlargement
>blind spot e.
>corneal e.
>orbital e.

ENL-DCR
>endonasal laser
>dacryocystorhinostomy

enophthalmia

enophthalmos

enophthalmus
>senescent e.

enoxacin

Enroth sign

Enterobacter aerogenes

entero-Behçet disease

entochoroidea

entocornea

entophthalmia

entoptic
>e. phenomenon

entoptoscope

entoptoscopy

entoretina

entrance pupil

entrapment
>pupillary e.

E

NOTES

entropion, entropium
    acquired e.
    acute spastic e.
    atonic e.
    Celsus-Hotz e.
    Cibis e.
    e. cicatriceum
    cicatricial e.
    congenital e.
    eyelid e.
    e. forceps
    Hotz e.
    involutional senile e.
    marginal e.
    noncicatricial e.
    Poulard e.
    senescent e.
    senile e.
    spastic e.
    e. spasticum
    e. uveae
    uveal e.
entropionize
entry
    implant e.
enucleate
enucleation
    e. of eyeball operation
    Foix e.
    e. scissors
    e. scoop
    e. spoon
    whole-globe e.
    e. wire snare
enucleator
    Banner snare e.
    Botvin-Bradford e.
    Bradford snare e.
    Castroviejo snare e.
    Foster snare e.
    snare e.
Enuclene
enzymatic
    e. cleaner
    e. cleaner for extended wear
    e. galactosemia
    e. glaucoma
    e. sclerostomy
    e. zonulolysis
enzyme
    antioxidant e.
    e. cleaner
    e. defect

    e. glaucoma
    proteolytic e.
enzyme-linked immunosorbent assay (ELISA)
EOG
    electro-oculogram
    electro-oculography
EOM
    extraocular muscle
EOMI
    extraocular movement intact
eosinophilic
    e. globule
    e. granuloma
    e. intranuclear inclusion body
    e. reaction
    e. response
ependymoma tumor
epiblepharon
epibulbar
    e. dermoid cyst
    e. Fordyce nodule
    e. lesion
    e. limbal dermoid choristoma
    e. tissue
epicanthal
    e. correction
    e. inversus
    e. skin fold
epicanthic
epicanthine fold
epicanthus
    e. blepharophimosis
    e. caruncle
    e. inversus
    e. palpebralis
    e. supraciliaris
    e. tarsalis
epicapsular lens star
Epicar
epicauma
epicenter
Epic laser
epicorneascleritis
epidemic
    e. blindness
    e. conjunctivitis
    e. keratoconjunctivitis (EKC)
    e. typhus
epidermal inclusion cyst
epidermidis
    Staphylococcus e.

epidermoid
    e. carcinoma
    e. cyst
epidermolysis
    e. bullosa
    e. bullosa acquisita
epidiascope
Epifrin
epikeratophakia
epikeratophakic keratoplasty
epikeratoplasty
    e. lenticule
    tectonic e.
epikeratoprosthesis
epilation
epilator
epilens
epileptic nystagmus
E-Pilo
E-Pilo-x Ophthalmic
epimacular
    e. membrane
    e. proliferation
epimysium
Epinal
epinephrine
    e. bitartrate
    e. borate
    dipivalyl e.
    Duranest HCl with e.
    e. HCl
    lidocaine with e.
    Lidoject-1 with e.
    Marcaine HCl with e.
    Nervocaine with e.
    e. and pilocarpine
    pilocarpine and e.
    Sensorcaine with e.
    Xylocaine with e.
epinephryl borate
epinucleus
epipapillaris
    membrana e.
epipapillary membrane
epiphora
    atonic e.

epiretinal
    e. membrane (ERM)
    e. membrane proliferation (EMP)
episclera
episcleral
    e. angioma
    e. arterial circle
    e. artery
    e. blood vessel
    e. circulation
    e. explant
    e. eye plaque
    e. fibrosis
    e. hemangioma
    e. injection
    e. lamina
    e. nevus
    e. osteocartilaginous choristoma
    e. rheumatic nodule
    e. scarring
    e. space
    e. tissue
    e. vascular engorgement
    e. vein
    e. venous pressure (EVP)
episclerale
    spatium e.
    venae e.
episcleritis, episclerotitis
    circumscribed e.
    gouty e.
    e. multinodularis
    nodular e.
    e. partialis fugax
    e. periodica fugax
    simple e.
    syphilitic e.
episode
    ischemic e.
    stroke-like e.
episodic unilateral mydriasis
episphaeria
    Fusarium e.
epitarsus
    e. pterygium
epithelia (*pl. of* epithelium)

E

NOTES

epithelial
  e. adrenochrome deposition
  e. barrier
  e. basement layer
  e. basement membrane
  e. basement membrane disease
  e. basement membrane
    dystrophy
  e. bedewing
  e. bleb
  e. bleb disorder
  e. bulla
  e. cell
  e. debridement
  e. debris
  e. defect
  e. dendrite
  e. derma
  e. diffuse keratitis
  e. downgrowth
  e. dystrophy of Fuchs
  e. edema
  e. erosion
  e. herpetic disease
  e. hyperplasia
  e. hypertrophy
  e. implantation cyst
  e. inclusion
  e. inclusion cyst
  e. ingrowth
  e. invasion
  e. iron line
  e. keratopathy
  e. microcyst
  e. migration
  e. mitosis
  e. nerve plexus
  e. nevus
  e. orientation
  e. plug
  e. punctate haze
  e. punctate keratitis
  e. rolled edge
  e. scraper
  e. scraping
  e. slide
  e. transplantation
  e. tumor
  e. turnover
epithelialization
epitheliitis
  e. focal retinal pigment

  pigment e.
  retinal pigment e.
epitheliocapsularis
  fibrillopathia e.
epithelioid cell
epithelioma, pl. epitheliomata
  e. adenoides cysticum
  Contino e.
  intraepithelial e.
  Malherbe calcifying e.
  malignant ciliary e.
epitheliopathy
  acute multifocal placoid
    pigment e. (AMPPE)
  acute multifocal posterior
    placoid pigment e.
  acute posterior multifocal
    placoid pigment e.
    (APMPPE)
  advancing wave-like e. (AWE)
  dendritic e.
  multifocal posterior pigment e.
  pigment e.
  placoid pigment e.
  posterior pigment e.
  retinal pigment e.
epithelioplasty
epitheliosis desquamativa
  conjunctivae
epithelium, pl. epithelia
  e. anterius corneae
  ciliary e.
  corneal e.
  devitalized e.
  graft e.
  iris pigment e. (IPE)
  lens e.
  e. lentis
  migrating e.
  nonpigmented ciliary e.
  pigment e. (PE)
  e. pigmentosum iridis
  placoid pigmentation of e.
  e. posterius corneae
  retinal pigment e. (RPE)
  serous pigment e.
  stratified squamous e.
  subcapsular e.
Epitrate
epizootic keratoconjunctivitis
Eppendorf tube
Eppy/N

EPS
 exophthalmos-producing substance
EPSA
 early postoperative suture
 adjustment
Epstein
 E. collar stud acrylic implant
 E. collar stud acrylic lens
 E. symptom
Epstein-Barr virus (EBV)
equal
 pupils round, regular, and e.
 (PRRE)
equation
 Baker e. (corneal aspheric
 measurement)
equator
 anatomic e.
 e. bulbi oculi
 crystalline lens e.
 e. of crystalline lens
 eyeball e.
 geometric e.
 lens e.
 e. lentis
equatorial
 e. degeneration
 e. drusen
 e. lentis
 e. meridian
 e. ring scotoma
 e. staphyloma
equilateral hemianopsia
equilibrating operation
equilibrium disturbance
equipment
 laser e.
 Volk Plus non-contact adapter
 cap and e.
equivalent
 e. distance
 mean spherical e. (MSE)
 migraine e.
 e. oxygen percentage value
 e. power
 e. refracting plane
 spherical e.

ER
 erbium
eraser
 E. cautery
 Mentor curved e.
 Mentor wet-field e.
 Tano e.
Erbakan inferior fornix operation
erbium (ER)
 e. laser
Erdheim-Chester disease
erect illumination
ERG
 electroretinogram
 electroretinography
ERG-Jet disposable contact lens
ergograph
ergonovine
ergot
 e. alkaloid
**ErgoTec vitreoretinal instrument
 system**
Erhardt
 E. clamp
 E. lid forceps
erisophake, erisiphake
ERM
 epiretinal membrane
**Ernest-McDonald soft intraocular
 lens-folding forceps**
Ernest nucleus cracker
erosion
 coast e.
 corneal e.
 epithelial e.
 punctate epithelial e.
 recurrent corneal e.
 recurrent epithelial e.
 sphincter e.
erosive vitreoretinopathy
erroneous projection
error
 astigmagraphic e.
 astigmatic refractive e.
 asymmetric refractive e.
 field of view e.
 inborn e.

E

NOTES

error *(continued)*
  myopic e.
  position e.
  refractive e.
  retinal e.
  sampling e.
  spherical refractive e.
  velocity e.
eruptio
  zoster sine e.
eruptive keratoacanthoma
erysipelas
  coastal e.
erysiphake
  Barraquer e.
  Bell e.
  Castroviejo e.
  corneal e.
  Dimitry e.
  Dimitry-Bell e.
  Dimitry-Thomas e.
  Draeger high vacuum e.
  Esposito e.
  Floyd-Grant e.
  Harrington e.
  Johnson e.
  Johnson-Bell e.
  Kara e.
  L'Esperance e.
  Maumenee e.
  New York e.
  Nugent-Green-Dimitry e.
  oval cup e.
  Post-Harrington e.
  Sakler e.
  Searcy oval cup e.
  Simcoe nucleus e.
  Storz-Bell e.
  e. technique
  Viers e.
  Welch rubber bulb e.
  Welsh silastic e.
erythema
  e. chronicum migrans
  e. multiforme
  e. multiforme bullosum
  e. multiforme conjunctivitis
  e. multiforme exudativum
  e. multiforme major
Erythrocin
erythroclastic glaucoma

erythrocyte
  ghost e.
erythrokeratodermia variabilis (EKV)
erythrolabe
erythrometer
erythrometry
erythromycin
erythrophagocytosis
erythropsia, erythropia
escape
  e. phenomenon
  pupillary e.
Escapini cataract operation
Eschenbach low vision rehabilitation guide
Eschenback Optik lens
Escherichia coli
eserine
  Isopto E.
  e. sulfate
esocataphoria
esodeviation
  e. accommodation
  accommodative e.
  nonaccommodative e.
esophoria (E)
  accommodative e.
  classical congenital e.
  congenital e.
  nearpoint e.
  nonaccommodative e.
esophoric
esotropia (ET)
  A-e.
  e. accommodation
  accommodative e.
  acquired e.
  alternate day e.
  alternating e.
  A-pattern e.
  basic e.
  clock-mechanism e.
  congenital e.
  consecutive e.
  constant e.
  convergence excess e.
  cyclic e.
  essential infantile e.
  idiopathic congenital e.
  infantile e.
  intermittent e. (E(T))
  late-onset e.

left e.
mixed e.
near e. (ET')
nonaccommodative e.
nonrefractive accommodative e.
periodic e.
refractive accommodative e.
right e.
sensory e.
V-e.
V-pattern e.
X-e.
esotropic amblyopia
Esposito erysiphake
essential
e. anisocoria
e. blepharospasm
e. hypertension
e. hypotony
e. infantile esotropia
e. iris atrophy
e. phthisis
e. phthisis bulbi
e. progressive atrophy of iris
e. telangiectasia
Esser inlay operation
Esterman scale
esthesiometer, aesthesiometer
Cochet-Bonnet e.
Estivin
E. II Ophthalmic
estropia
ET
esotropia
ET'
near esotropia
E(T)
intermittent esotropia
etabonate
loteprednol e.
etafilcon A lenses
ETDRS
Early Treatment Diabetic
Retinopathy Study
ether
e. guard
e. theory of light

Ethicon
E. BV-75-3 needle
E. micropoint suture
E. Sabreloc suture
Ethicon-Atraloc suture
ethmoid
e. bone
e. bulla
e. canal
e. exenteration
e. sinus
ethmoidal
e. artery
e. incisure
e. lacrimal fistula
e. region
e. sinus
ethmoidalis
lamina orbitalis ossis e.
ethmoiditis
ethmoidolacrimalis
sutura e.
ethmoidomaxillaris
sutura e.
ethoxyzolamide
ethyl
e. alcohol amblyopia
e. cyanoacrylate
e. cyanoacrylate glue
ethylene glycol
etidocaine
EUA
exam under anesthesia
eucatropine
euchromatopsy
Euro Precision Technology
submicron lathe machine
euryopia
euthyphoria
evagination
optic e.
evaluation
visual function e.
evasion
macular e.

E

NOTES

event
   dark e.
   independent e.
Evergreen
   E. Lasertek coagulator
   E. Lasertek laser
Eversbusch operation
eversion
   double lid e.
   e. of eyelid
   lid e.
   e. of punctum
   single lid e.
everted
   e. eyelid
   e. punctum
everter
   Berens lid e.
   Berke lid e.
   lid e.
   Roveda lid e.
   Schachne-Desmarres lid e.
   Struble lid e.
   Walker lid e.
evisceration
   e. of eyeball
   e. operation
   e. spoon
evisceroneurotomy
E-Vista
evoked
   e. nystagmus gaze
   e. potential
evolutional cataract
EVP
   episcleral venous pressure
evulsion
evulsio nervi optici
Ewald law
EWCL
   extended-wear contact lens
Ewing
   E. capsule forceps
   E. operation
   E. sarcoma
ex
   e. amblyopia
   e. anopsia
examination
   anterior segment e.
   cytologic e.
   dark-field e.
   dilated retinal e.

dilated stereoscopic fundus e.
   e. of eye
   flashlight e.
   fundus e.
   funduscopic e.
   neurologic e.
   neuro-ophthalmologic e.
   ophthalmic e.
   ophthalmoscopic e.
   slit-lamp e. (SLE)
   Woods light e.
exam under anesthesia (EUA)
exanthematous conjunctivitis
excavated optic disk anomaly
excavatio
   e. disci
   e. papillae nervi optici
excavation
   atrophic e.
   glaucomatous e.
   e. of optic disk
   physiologic e.
   retinal e.
excess
   convergence e.
   divergence e.
   e. divergence
   e. esotropia convergence
excessive
   e. accommodation
   e. cyclodialysis cleft
   e. lacrimation
   e. rebound uveitis
exchange
   air-fluid e.
   fluid-air e.
   fluid-gas e.
   gas-fluid e.
   lens e.
ExciMed
   E. UV200 excimer laser
   E. UV200LA laser
excimer
   e. laser
   e. laser ablation
   e. laser, 193193-nm
   e. laser photoreactive
      keratectomy
   e. laser photorefractive
      keratectomy
   e. laser phototherapeutic
      keratectomy

e. laser transepithelial photoablation
e. laser trephination
excision
Arlt-Jaesche e.
bare-sclera e.
conjunctiva-Mueller muscle e.
e. of lacrimal gland operation
e. of lacrimal sac operation
pentagonal block e.
excitation
L cone e.
M cone e.
paradoxic levator e.
S cone e.
exciting eye
exclusion of pupil
excretory duct
excycloduction
excyclophoria
excyclotorsion
excyclotropia
excyclovergence
executive
e. bifocal
e. spectacle lens
e. trifocal
exenteration
ethmoid e.
eyelid-splitting orbital e.
Iliff e.
orbital e.
e. of orbital contents operation
exenteratio orbitae
exercise
antisuppression e.
blur and clear e.
convergent e.
pleoptic e.
exertional amblyopia
Exeter ophthalmoscope
exfoliation
e. glaucoma
e. of lens
e. of lens capsule
e. syndrome
true e.

exfoliative
e. glaucoma
e. keratitis
exit pupil
exocataphoria
exodeviation
comitant e.
exogenous
e. disease
e. endophthalmitis
e. ochronosis
exophoria (X, XP)
alternating e.
comitant e.
concomitant e.
constant e.
nearpoint e.
exophoric
exophthalmic
e. goiter
e. ophthalmoplegia
exophthalmogenic
exophthalmometer
Hertel e.
LICO Hertel e.
Luedde e.
Marco prism e.
exophthalmometric
exophthalmometry
Krahn e.
exophthalmos, exophthalmus
e. due to pressure
e. due to tower skull
endocrine e.
malignant e.
ophthalmoplegic e.
postural e.
pulsatile e.
pulsating e.
recurrent e.
substance e.
thyroid e.
thyrotoxic e.
thyrotropic e.
transient early e.
exophthalmos-producing substance (EPS)

E

NOTES

exoplant
scleral e.
exorbitism
exotropia (XT)
A-e.
alternating e.
A-pattern e.
basic e.
comitant e.
consecutive e.
convergence insufficiency e.
divergence excess e.
divergence insufficiency e.
flick e.
intermittent e. (X(T))
left e.
paralytic pontine e.
periodic e.
right e.
secondary e.
sensory e.
V-e.
V-pattern e.
X-e.
exotropic
expander
field e.
Graether pupil e.
scleral e.
Expeditions
Surgical Eye E. (SEE)
experiment
Mariotte e.
Scheiner e.
experimental diabetes
explant
encircling e.
episcleral e.
Molteno episcleral e.
posterior e.
scleral e.
segmental e.
silicone sponge e.
sponge e.
trypsin-digested e.
exploration
sclerotomy with e.
Expo
E. Bubble dressing
E. Bubble eye cover
E. Bubble eye shield

exposure
e. keratitis
e. keratopathy
expression
nuclear e.
expressor
Arroyo e.
Arruga e.
Bagley-Wilmer e.
Berens e.
Heath e.
Heyner e.
e. hook
hook e.
Hosford e.
Kirby hook e.
Kirby intracapsular lens e.
lens e.
e. loop
McDonald e.
meibomian gland e.
nucleus e.
ring lens e.
Rizzuti lens e.
Smith e.
Stahl nucleus e.
Verhoeff lens e.
Wilmer-Bagley e.
expulsive hemorrhage
EXT-DCR
external dacryocystorhinostomy
extended-range keratometry
extended round needle
extended-wear contact lens (EWCL)
extension
finger-like e.
orbital e.
Extenzyme
externa
axis oculi e.
folliculitis e.
membrana granulosa e.
membrana limitans e.
ophthalmoplegia e.
external
e. ankyloblepharon
e. axis of eye
e. beam radiation therapy
e. beam radiation treatment
e. canthotomy
e. dacryocystorhinostomy (EXT-DCR)
e. exudative retinopathy

e. geniculate body
e. hordeolum
e. limiting membrane
e. ophthalmopathy
e. ophthalmoplegia
e. orbital fracture
e. palsy
e. pterygoid levator synkinesis
e. route
e. squint
e. strabismus

externi
insufficiency of e.

externum
hordeolum e.

externus
axis bulbi e.

extinction
e. phenomenon
visual e.

extirpation
extorsion
Extra
AMO Endosol E.
Endosol E.

extracanthic
extracapsular
e. aphakia
e. cataract extraction (ECCE)
e. cataract extraction operation
e. extraction of cataract

extracellular matrix (ECM)
extraciliary fiber
extraconal fat reticulum
extracranial optic nerve decompression
extractable nuclear antigen
extraction
Arroyo cataract e.
Arruga cataract e.
cataract e. (CE)
Chandler-Verhoeff lens e.
e. of extracapsular cataract
extracapsular cataract e. (ECCE)
e. flap
foreign body e.

intracapsular cataract e. (ICCE)
e. of intracapsular cataract
intraocular cataract e.
magnetic e.
planned extracapsular cataract e.

extractor
Krwawicz cataract e.
Look cortex e.
Smirmaul nucleus e.
Visitec cortex e.
Welsh cortex e.

extrafoveal
e. retinal detachment

extramacular binocular vision
extramedullary
e. course
e. segment

extraocular
e. movement
e. movement intact (EOMI)
e. muscle (EOM)
e. muscle disorder
e. muscles of Tillaux
e. muscle testing

extraorbital disease
extrapyramidal
e. syndrome
e. system

extrarectus
extraretinal
e. neovascularization

extrascleral
e. outgrowth

Extra-Strength
MiraFlow E.-S.

extrastriate cortex lesion
extravisual zone
extrinsic muscle
extrusion
implant e.
e. needle
pellet e.

exudate
circinate e.
conjunctival e.
cotton-wool e.

E

NOTES

exudate *(continued)*
    endothelial e.
    fatty e.
    fibrin e.
    fibrinous e.
    foaming e.
    hard e.
    lipid e.
    retinal e.
    soft e.
    waxy e.
exudation
    proteinaceous aqueous e.
exudative
    e. choroiditis
    e. eye
    e. retinitis
    e. retinopathy
    e. senile maculopathy
    e. serous retinal detachment
    e. vitreoretinopathy
exudativum
    erythema multiforme e.
eye
    accessory organs of e.
    alkali burn to e.
    amaurotic cat's e.
    anterior segment of e.
    aphakic e.
    appendage of e.
    aqueous humor e.
    artificial e.
    axial length of e.
    e. bank
    E. Bank Association of
      America (EBAA)
    black e.
    both e.'s (OU)
    Bright e.
    bulb of e.
    bull's e.
    cat's e.
    centrally-fixing e.
    e. chamber
    e. chart
    cinema e.
    Clear E.'s
    closed surgery on e.
    e. color
    compound e.
    conjugate movement of e.'s
    e. contact

contact lens-induced acute
  red e. (CLARE)
contralateral e.
contusion of e.
crossed e.'s
e. cup
cyclopean e.
cystic e.
dancing e.
dark-adapted e.
deviating e.
disjugate movement of e.'s
disorder of e.
doll's e.
dominant e.
donor e.
e. dropper
e. drops
Dry E.'s
Easy E.'s
examination of e.
exciting e.
external axis of e.
exudative e.
fellow e.
fibrous coat of e.
fixating e.
fixing e.
following e.
Fox e.
fundus of e.
Gullstrand reduced e.
Gullstrand schematic e.
hare's e.
heavy e.
Helmholtz schematic e.
e. holder
hop e.
hot e.
e. implant conformer
e. infarction
inflammatory target site of e.
e. injury
internal axis of e.
iris e.
e. irrigating solution
Klieg e.
e. knife guard
lazy e.
left e. (LE, OS)
e. lens
light-adapted e.
Listing reduced e.

Listing schematic e.
e. magnet
master e.
master-dominant e.
medial angle of e.
micromovement of e.
monochromatic e.
e. movement
e. movement disorder
muscle of e.
e. muscle surgery
Nairobi e.
e. occluder
old e.
orbicular muscle of e.
oval e.
e. pad
e. pad dressing
parietal e.
patch e.
phakic e.
photopic e.
phthisical e.
pineal e.
e. plaque
e. plaque surgery
e. point
Pontocaine E.
posterior pole of e.
Preflex for Sensitive E.'s
e. pressing
primary e.
e. protector
protruding e.'s
pseudophakic e.
raccoon e.'s
red e.
reduced e.
e. reflex
e. removed in toto
e. restored to normotensive
  pressure
right e. (OD)
rolling of e.'s
e. rotated inferiorly
e. rotation
rudimentary e.

saccadic movements of e.
sagittal axis of e.
schematic e.
scotopic e.
secondary e.
Sensitive E.'s
e. shield
shipyard e.
e. size
Snellen reform e.
Soft Mate Comfort Drops for
  Sensitive E.'s
Soft Mate Saline for
  Sensitive E.'s
Soothe e.
e. speculum
e. spot
e. spud
squinting e.
stony-hard e.
e. strain
E. Stream solution
suspensory ligament of e.
e. suture scissors
e. sweep
sympathizing e.
tension of e.
tumor of interior of e.
vertical axis of e.
e. wall
e. wash
E. Wash solution
e. was quiet
watery e.
web e.
wet e.
white of e.

eyeball
e. compression reflex
dimpling of e.
e. equator
evisceration of e.
fibrous tunic of e.
luxation of e.
meridian of e.
pigmented layer of e.
posterior pole of e.

E

NOTES

eyeball *(continued)*
   e. sheath
   vascular coat of e.
eyeball-heart reflex
eyebrow
   e. fixation
   e. laceration
EyeClose
   E. Adhesive strip
   E. external eyelid weight
eye-closure reflex
Eye Con 5
Eye-Cool
Eyecor camera
Eye-Cort
eyecup
Eye Drops
   Optique 1 E.
eye/ear plane
eyeFix speculum system
Eye-Gene
eyeglasses
eyegrounds
eye-head
   e.-h. movement
   e.-h. shift
eyeing
eyelash
   ectopic e.
   piebald e.
eyelash-induced leak
eyelid
   angular junction of e.
   e. apraxia
   avulsion of e.
   baggy e.
   basal cell carcinoma of e.
   capillary hemangioma of e.
   carcinoma of e.
   e. coloboma
   e. contour
   e. crease
   e. crusting
   e. dermatochalasis
   e. disorder
   drooping of e.
   ecchymosis of e.
   e. ectropion
   ectropion of e.
   edema of e.
   e. edema
   e. entropion
   eversion of e.

everted e.
e. fissure
floppy e.
e. flutter
flutter of e.
e. fold
e. forceps
free margin of e.
e. fusion
gland of e.
incision into e.
inflammation of e.
insufficiency of e.
e. keratosis
lateral commissure of e.
levator muscle of upper e.
e. lichenification
lower e.
e. lymphangioma
e. margin
medial commissure of e.
melanoma of e.
e. milia
e. molluscum contagiosum
   infection
e. muscle
e. myokymia
e. neurilemoma
e. neurofibroma
e. nevus
e. nystagmus
one-stage reconstruction of eye
   socket and e.'s
orbital portion of e.
e. papilloma
e. plaque
plastic repair of e.
pseudobaggy e.
ptosis of e.
e. ptosis
reconstruction of e.
e. retraction
e. retractor
e. rhytids
sign of edema of lower e.
sluggish movements of eyes
   and e.'s
e. spacer
e. speculum
squamous cell carcinoma of e.
e. strawberry hemangioma
e. surgery
e.'s sutured closed

suturing of e.
e. syringoma
e. taping
tarsal portion of e.
e. tumor
tumor of e.
unilateral ptosis of e.
upper e.
e. vesiculation
xanthelasma around e.
eyelid-closure reflex
eyelid-splitting orbital exenteration
Eye-Lube-A Solution
EyeMap EH-290 corneal
   tomography system
Eye-Mo
Eye-Pak
   E.-P. II cover
   E.-P. II drape
   E.-P. II sheet
eyepatch
eyepiece
   comparison e.
   compensating e.
   demonstration e.
   huygenian e.
   negative e.
   position e.
   positive e.
   Ramsden e.
   wide-field e.

eye-popping reflex
eye-referenced stimulus
eye-refractometer
Eye-Sed solution
eyeshot
eyesight
Eyesine
   E. Ophthalmic
   E. solution
eyes-open coma
EyeSys
   E. charting
   E. corneal analysis system
   E. 2000 corneal topographic
      mapping system
   E. corneal topography system
   E. surface topography system
   E. System 2000
   E. Technologies corneal
      topography
   E. videokeratoscope
eyewash
eyewear
eyewire
Eye-Zine
EZE-FIT IOL system
EZVUE violet haptic intraocular
   lens

E

NOTES

165

F
    filial generation
    focus
    visual field
F2 Color Vision test
FA
    fluorescein angiography
Faber disease
Fab fragment
Fabry syndrome
face
    hyaloid f.
    f. line
    f. shield
    vitreous f.
face-down position
facet, facette
    corneal f.
facetted
    f. avascular disciform opacity
    f. corneal scar
faci
    no f.
facial
    f. anomaly
    f. block
    f. cleft
    f. hemangioma
    f. movement
    f. movement abnormality
    f. myokymia
    f. nerve
    f. nerve avulsion
    f. nerve lesion
    f. nerve misdirection
    f. nerve palsy
    f. nerve trunk
    f. neuroma
    f. pain
    f. paralysis
    f. perception
    f. spasm
    f. synkinesis
    f. vein
    f. vision
facialis
    vena f.
facies, pl. facies
    f. anterior corneae
    f. anterior iridis

    f. anterior lentis
    f. anterior palpebrarum
    f. antonina
    f. bovina
    Hutchinson f.
    mask-like f.
    f. orbitalis alae magnae
    f. orbitalis alae majoris
    f. orbitalis ossis frontalis
    f. orbitalis ossis zygomatici
    f. posterior corneae
    f. posterior iridis
    f. posterior lentis
    f. posterior palpebrarum
facility
    f. of outflow
    vergence f.
facio-auriculovertebral spectrum
FACT
    Functional Acuity Contrast Test
factitious
    f. blindness
    f. conjunctivitis
    f. mydriasis
facture energy
facultative
    f. hyperopia
    f. suppression
faculty
    fusion f.
    f. fusion
Faden
    F. effect
    F. operation
    F. procedure
    F. suture
fading time
faecalis
    Streptococcus f.
failed graft
failure
    lacrimal pump f.
    primary graft f.
faint flare
falciform
    f. fold of retina
    f. retinal fold
Falcon lens
Falls-Kertesz syndrome

F

false
   f. blepharoptosis
   f. image
   f. macula
   f. orientation
   f. projection
   f. ptosis
   f. vision
false-negative result
false-positive result
familial
   f. arteriolar tortuosity
   f. autonomic dysautonomia
   f. autonomic dysfunction
   f. colloid degeneration
   f. drusen
   f. episodic ataxia
   f. exudative vitreoretinopathy
   (FEVR)
   f. fibrosis
   f. foveal retinoschisis
   f. lecithin:cholesterol
   acyltransferase deficiency
   f. lipoprotein deficiency
   f. paroxysmal ataxia
   f. periodic paralysis
   f. pseudoinflammatory macular
   degeneration
   f. pseudoinflammatory
   maculopathy
   f. retinoblastoma
familiares
   cornea plana congenita f.
Fanconi syndrome
Fanta
   F. cataract operation
   F. speculum
fantascope
far
   f. phoria
   f. point
   f. point of accommodation
   (FPA)
   f. point of convergence
   f. sight
farinaceous epithelial keratitis
farinata
   cornea f.
Farnsworth
   F. D-15 panel
   F. Panel D-15 test
Farnsworth-Munsell 100-hue color
  vision test

far-point convergence
farsighted
farsightedness
Fary anterior chamber maintainer
Fas
   F. interaction
   F. receptor density
Fasanella
   F. lacrimal cannula
   F. operation
   F. retractor
Fasanella-Servat
   F.-S. procedure
   F.-S. ptosis operation
fascia, pl. **fasciae**
   f. band
   bulbar f.
   f. bulbi
   Crawford f.
   f. lata frontalis
   f. lata frontalis sling
   f. lata musculares bulbi
   f. lata musculares oculi
   f. lata sling for ptosis
   operation
   f. lata stripper
   muscular f.
   f. musculares bulbi
   f. musculares oculi
   orbital f.
   fasciae orbitales
   palpebral f.
fascicle
   abducens nerve f.
   oculomotor nerve f.
fascicular
   f. keratitis
   f. ophthalmoplegia
   f. ulcer
fasciculus
   inferior longitudinal f.
   longitudinal f.
   maculary f.
   medial longitudinal f. (MLF)
   rostral interstitial medial
   longitudinal f.
fasciitis
   nodular f.
   orbital f.
fashion
   in-tumbling f.
   McLean f.

stepwise f.
X-linked f.
FasL interaction
Fastpac
    F. 24-2 test
FASTPAC algorithm
fat
    f. cell
    f. embolism of retina
    f. graft
    mutton f.
    orbital f.
    f. pad
    f. reticulum
fatigue nystagmus
fatty
    f. change
    f. exudate
Faulkner folder
Favre dystrophy
FAZ
    foveal avascular zone
FB
    foreign body
fc
    footcandle
Fc fragment
FCT
    fluorescein clearance test
FDACL
    first definite apical clearance lens
Feaster
    F. Dualens lens
    F. K7-5460 hydrodissecting
      cannula
    F. radial keratotomy knife
Feather Touch CO₂ laser
feathery
    f. appearance
    f. clouding
Fechner
    F. intraocular lens
    F. ring forceps
Federov
    F. four-loop iris clip
    F. four-loop iris clip lens
      implant

F. type II intraocular lens
F. type II lens implant
F. type I intraocular lens
F. type I lens implant
feeder-frond technique
feeder vessel
Fehr macular dystrophy
Feldman
    F. adaptometer
    F. buffer solution
    F. RK optical center marker
fellow eye
felt
    f. disk polisher
    f. pad
fenestra, pl. **fenestrae**
fenestrated
    f. chain
    f. sheen macular dystrophy
fenestration
    optic nerve sheath f. (ONSF)
Fenhoff external and anterior
    segment
fenretinide
fentanyl
Fenzel
    F. angled manipulating hook
    F. insertion hook
    F. lens-manipulating hook
    F. manipulating hook
Féréol-Graux palsy
Ferguson implant
Fergus operation
ferning
    tear mucus f.
Ferree-Rand perimeter
Ferrein canal
ferric
    f. ferrocyanide
    f. hyaluronate gel
Ferris chart
Ferris-Smith
    F.-S. refractor
    F.-S. retractor
Ferris-Smith-Sewall
    F.-S.-S. refractor
    F.-S.-S. retractor

F

NOTES

ferrocholinate
ferrocyanide
  ferric f.
ferrous sulfate
Ferry line
Ferry-Porter law
fetal
  f. fibrovascular sheath
  f. hydantoin syndrome
  f. trimethadione syndrome
  f. warfarin syndrome
  f. Y suture
FEVR
  familial exudative vitreoretinopathy
FHC
  Fuchs heterochromic cyclitis
fiber
  accessory f.
  auxiliary f.
  Bernheimer f.'s
  Brücke f.
  f. cell
  chief f.
  cilioequatorial f.
  cilioposterocapsular f.
  circular ciliary muscle f.
  collagen f.
  cone f.
  congenital medullated optic
    nerve f.
  contiguous f.'s
  continuous f.
  corticonuclear f.
  Edinger f.
  efferent f.
  extraciliary f.
  fibrillenstruktur f.
  Gratiolet radiating f.
  f.'s of Henle
  interciliary f.
  intraocular myelination of
    retinal nerve f.
  f. layer of axon
  f. layer of Chievitz
  lens f.
  longitudinal f.
  main f.
  medullated nerve f.
  meridional ciliary muscle f.
  Müller f.
  myelinated retinal nerve f.
  myoclonic epilepsy with
    ragged-red f.

  nerve f.
  oblique f.
  optic nerve f.
  f. orbicularis oculi
  orbiculoanterocapsular f.
  orbiculociliary f.
  orbiculoposterocapsular f.
  parasympathetic f.
  peripapillary retinal nerve f.
  postganglionic f.
  principal f.
  pupilloconstrictor f.
  pupillomotor f.
  radial f.
  ragged-red f.
  Ritter f.
  rod f.
  Sappey f.
  sensory f.
  sphincter f.
  sustentacular f.
  trabecular f.
  vitreous f.
  zonular f.
Fiberlite microscope
fiberoptic
  f. diagnostic lens
  f. light projector
  f. pick
  f. videoendoscope
fiberscope
fibrae
  f. circulares musculi ciliaris
  f. lentis
  f. longitudinales musculi
    ciliaris
  f. meridionales musculi ciliaris
  f. radiales musculi ciliaris
  f. zonulares
Fibra Sonics phaco aspirator
fibril
  collagen f.
fibrillar material
fibrillenstruktur fiber
fibrillogranular deposit
fibrillogranuloma
fibrillopathia epitheliocapsularis
fibrin
  f. dusting
  f. exudate
  intravitreal f.
  f. layer
  postvitrectomy f.

f. pupillary block glaucoma
f. strand
f. thrombus
fibrinitis
iritis f.
fibrinogen glue
fibrinoid necrosis
fibrinolysis
local intra-arterial f. (LIF)
fibrinous
f. aqueous
f. cataract
f. exudate
f. iritis
f. rhinitis
fibroblastic
f. ingrowth
f. meningioma
fibroglial membrane
fibroid cataract
fibroma
orbital f.
fibromatosis
orbital f.
fibro-osseous tumor
fibroplasia
cicatricial retrolental f.
retrolental f. (RLF)
fibroproliferative membrane
fibrosa
cataracta f.
pseudophakia f.
fibrosarcoma
orbital f.
fibrosclerosis
multifocal f.
fibrosis
f. choroideae corrugans
congenital f.
cyst f.
cystic f.
episcleral f.
familial f.
preretinal macular f.
subepithelial f.
f. syndrome

fibrous
f. coat of eye
f. dysplasia
f. frond
f. proliferans
f. tissue cuff
f. tunic
f. tunic of eyeball
fibrovascular
f. frond
f. pannus
f. proliferation
f. sheath
f. tunic
Fick
anteroposterior axis of F.
F. axis
axis of F.
F. halo
longitudinal axis of F.
sagittal axis of F.
transverse axis of F.
vertical axis of F.
Z axis of F.
field
altitudinal f.
automated visual f.
binasal quadrant f.
binocular f.
bright empty f.
central f.
checkerboard visual f.
confrontation visual f.
cribriform f.
f. cut
dark empty f.
f. defect
depth of f.
f. diaphragm setting
f. expander
f. of fixation
fixation f.
Forel f.
frontal eye f.
f. of gaze
hysteric f.
hysterical constricted f.

NOTES

F

171

field *(continued)*
  keyhole f.
  f. lens
  f. loss
  paracentral visual f.
  peripheral visual f.
  receptive f.
  spiral f.
  star-shaped f.
  superonasal paracentral
   visual f.
  surplus f.
  Swiss-cheese visual f.
  temporal island of visual f.
  tubular visual f.
  f. of view
  f. of view error
  f. of vision
  visual f. (F, VF)
  wide f. (WF)
Fiessinger-Leroy-Reiter syndrome
fifth cranial nerve
figure
  Allen f.
  fortification f.
  Rey-Osterreith Complex F.
  Stifel f.
  Zöllner f.
figure-of-eight suture
filament
  branching f.
  corneal f.
  f. keratitis
  myosin f.
filamentary
  f. keratitis
  f. keratome
  f. keratopathy
filamentosa
  keratitis f.
filariasis
Filatov
  F. keratoplasty
  F. operation
Filatov-Marzinkowsky operation
fil d'Arion silicone tube
filial generation (F)
filiform dystrophy
filling
  choroidal f.
  retinal arterial f.
film
  absorbable gelatin f.

  aqueous layer of tear f.
  conditioning f.
  debris-laden tear f.
  gelatin f.
  precorneal tear f.
  preocular tear f. (POTF)
  proteinolipidic f.
  tear f.
filmtab
  Rondec F.
filter
  cobalt blue f.
  interference f.
  Millex f.
  Millipore f.
  neutral density f.
  Polaroid f.
  red f.
  red-free f.
  ultraviolet f.
  UV blocking f.
  Whatman f.
  Wrattan f.
filtering
  f. bleb
  f. cicatrix
  f. operation
  f. procedure
  f. wick
filtration
  f. angle
  f. surgery
  Van Herick f.
fimbriated
  f. edge
  f. margin
Finalite 1.6
final threshold
fine
  F. corneal carrying case
  f. fibrillar vitreal degeneration
  F. Finesse Triamond
  F. folding block
  f. iris process
  F. magnetic implant
  F. micropoint cautery
  F. micropoint electrocautery
  f. punctate keratopathy
  F. suture scissors
  F. suture-tying forceps
Fine-Castroviejo suturing forceps
fine-dissecting forceps
fine-needle aspiration

Fine-Thornton scleral fixation ring
fine-toothed forceps
fine-wire speculum
finger
   f. count
   counting f.'s (CF)
   f. counting
   f. mimicking
   f. tension
   f. vision
finger-counting
   down to f.-c.
finger-like extension
fingerprint
   f. body myopathy
   f. corneal dystrophy
   f. line
finished
   f. contact lens
   f. glass
   f. lens
Fink
   F. biprong marker
   F. cataract aspirator
   F. cul-de-sac irrigator
   F. curette
   F. irrigating/aspirating unit
   F. lacrimal retractor
   F. muscle marker
   F. oblique muscle hook
   F. operation
   F. refractor
   F. tendon tucker
Fink-Jameson muscle forceps
Fink-Weinstein two-way syringe
Finnoff transilluminator
first definite apical clearance lens
   (FDACL)
first-degree relative
first-grade fusion
Fisher
   F. eye needle
   F. lid retractor
   F. spoon
   F. spud
   F. syndrome
   F. test

Fisher-Arlt iris forceps
Fisher-Smith spatula
fishmouthing
fishmouth tear
Fison indirect binocular
   ophthalmoscope
fissura
   f. orbitalis inferior
   f. orbitalis superior
fissuratum
   acanthoma f.
fissure
   basin of inferior orbital f.
   calcarine f.
   choroid f.
   f. coloboma
   corneal f.
   eyelid f.
   inferior orbital f.
   interpalpebral f.
   lid f.
   orbital superior f.
   palpebral f.
   pterygomaxillary f.
   sphenoccipital f.
   sphenoidal f.
   sphenomaxillary f.
   superior orbital f. (SOF)
   water f.
   f. zone
fistula, pl. fistulae, fistulas
   carotid cavernous sinus f.
   cavernous sinus f.
   f. of cornea
   corneal f.
   dural cavernous sinus f.
   ethmoidal lacrimal f.
   internal lacrimal f.
   intraocular f.
   lacrimal f.
   f. lacrimalis
   scleral f.
   f. test
fistulizing surgery
fitting triangle
Fitz-Hugh-Curtis syndrome
Fitzpatrick sun-sensitivity scale

F

NOTES

fixate
fixating eye
fixation
  anomalous f.
  axis f.
  bifocal f.
  bifoveal f.
  binocular f.
  f. binocular forceps
  brow f.
  capsular f.
  central f.
  central, steady and
    maintained f. (CSM)
  cross f.
  crossed f.
  f. disparity
  eccentric f.
  eyebrow f.
  field of f.
  f. field
  f. forceps
  four-point f.
  graft f.
  Guyton-Noyes f.
  f. hook
  f. instrument
  f. light
  line of f.
  locus of f.
  f. mechanism
  microplate f.
  monocular f.
  near f.
  f. nystagmus
  f. object
  f. pick
  pigtail f.
  f. point
  point of f.
  f. reflex
  f. ring
  split f.
  sulcus f.
  f. suture
  f. target
  transscleral suture f.
fixational ocular movement
fixation/anchor
  f. forceps
  f. pick
  f. ring

fixed
  f. dilated pupil
  f. fold
  f. forceps
  f. mydriasis
  f. point
fix and follow
fixing eye
fixus
  strabismus f.
  vertical strabismus f.
Fizeau-Tolansky interferometer
flaccid
  f. canaliculus syndrome
  f. ectropion
Flajani
  F. disease
  F. operation
flame
  f. photometer
  f. spot
flame-shaped hemorrhage
flap
  advancement f.
  bicoronal scalp f.
  Blaskovics f.
  bridge pedicle f.
  cheek f.
  conjunctival f.
  conjunctivo-Tenon f.
  Cutler-Beard bridge f.
  donut-cut f.
  donut-shaped f.
  extraction f.
  fornix-based f.
  galeal f.
  Gunderson conjunctival f.
  hinged corneal f.
  Hughes tarsoconjunctival f.
  Imre sliding f.
  f. irregularity
  limbal-based f.
  Mustarde rotational cheek f.
  f. operation cataract
  partial conjunctival f. (PCF)
  pedicle f.
  pediculated f.
  retinal f.
  f. retraction
  scalp f.
  scleral f.
  skin f.
  sliding f.

swinging lid f.
tarsoconjunctival f.
f. tear
Tenon f.
Tenzel rotational cheek f.
total conjunctival f. (TCF)
Truc f.
Van Lint f.
FlapMaker
F. disposable microkeratome
F. microkeratome system
flare
aqueous f.
cell and f. (C&F)
f. and cell
faint f.
f. response
Flarex
flash
f. blindness
f. electroretinogram
f. keratoconjunctivitis
f.'s of light
f. ophthalmia
f. picture card
f. stimulus
f. visual evoked potential
flashlamp-pumped microsecond
pulse-dye laser
flashlight
f. examination
f. test
flat
f. anterior chamber
f. chorioretinal atrophy
f. contact lens
f. cornea
f. cup
f. demarcation line
f. eye spud
f. hook
f. top bifocal
Flatau-Schilder disease
flat-edge lens
flattening
keratometric f.

flavimaculatus
fundus f.
Flavobacterium meningosepticum
flavus
Aspergillus f.
fleck
intraretinal f.
flecked
f. corneal dystrophy
f. retina
f. retina disease
f. retina of Kandori
f. retina syndrome
flecken glaucoma
Fleischer
F. cataract
F. dystrophy
F. keratoconus ring
F. vortex
Fleischer-Strumpell ring
Flex-Care
flexible
f. loop
5139 f. retinal brush
f. translimbal iris retractor
flexible-wear
f.-w. contact lens
f.-w. lens
Flexlens lens
flexneri
Shigella f.
Flexner-Wintersteiner rosette
Flexner-Worst iris claw lens
Flexsol
flicher-fusion frequency technique
flick
f. exotropia
f. hypertropia
f. movement
flicker
f. amplitude
f. electroretinogram
f. fusion
f. fusion stimulus
f. perimetry
f. perimetry test

NOTES

flicker *(continued)*
    f. phenomenon
    f. photometer
Flieringa
    curved scleral-limbal incision
      of F.
    F. fixation ring
    F. scleral ring
Flieringa-Kayser
    F.-K. copper ring
    F.-K. fixation ring
Flieringa-LeGrand fixation ring
flight blindness
flint glass
flint-glass lens
flittering scotoma
floater
    meniscus f.
    pigment f.
    pupillary f.
    vitreous f.
flocculus
    cerebellar f.
    f. syndrome
flomoxef sodium
floor
    depression of orbital f.
    f. fracture
    orbital f.
floppy
    f. eyelid
    f. eyelid syndrome
flora
    ocular f.
Florentine iris
Floresoft
florid xanthelasma
floriform cataract
Floropryl
    F. Ophthalmic
Flouren law
Flouress
floury cornea
flow
    aqueous f.
    axoplasmic f.
    choroidal blood f. (ChBFlow)
    laminar f.
    reversed ophthalmic artery f.
      (ROAF)
    tear f.
flower petal pattern

flowmeter
    Heidelberg retinal f.
    laser Doppler f.
flowmetry
    confocal scanning laser
      Doppler f.
floxuridine
Floyd-Barraquer wire speculum
Floyd-Grant erysiphake
Flucaine
fluctuation
    diurnal f.
fluff
    f. dressing
    vitreous f.
fluffed gauze dressing
fluffy appearance
FLUFTEX gauze roll
fluid
    f. cataract
    cerebrospinal f. (CSF)
    f. contact lens
    intraocular f.
    f. mechanics
    perioptic cerebrospinal f.
    subarachnoid f.
    submembrane f.
    subretinal f.
    viscous ochre f.
    viscous xanthochromic f.
    Vitreon sterile intraocular f.
    xanthochromic f.
fluid-air exchange
fluid-attenuated inversion recovery
fluid-gas exchange
Fluidics
    Concentrix F.
fluidless contact lens
Fluoracaine
fluorescein
    f. angiogram
    f. angiogram test
    f. angiography (FA)
    f. clearance test (FCT)
    f. dilution test
    f. dye
    f. dye disappearance test
    f. dye and stain solution
    f. fundus angioscopy
    f. instillation test
    intravenous f.
    f. isothiocyanate
    parafoveal f.

sodium f. (NaFl)
f. sodium
f. staining
f. stick
f. strip test
fluorescence
f. microscopy
f. retinal photography
fluorescent
f. antibody test
f. lamp
f. treponemal antibody
absorption
Fluorescite
Fluoresoft
Fluorets
fluorexon
Fluor-I-Strip
Fluor-I-Strip-A.T.
fluorite
fluorobiprofen
fluorocarbon
f. in contact lens
fluorometer
CytoFluor II f.
fluorometholone
f. acetate
f. 0.1% ophthalmic suspension
(FML)
sulfacetamide sodium and f.
fluorometry
noninvasive corneal redox f.
Fluor-Op
fluorophosphate
diisopropyl f. (DFP)
fluorophotometer
Fluorotron Master f.
slit-lamp f.
fluorophotometry
vitreous f.
Fluoroplex
fluoroquinolone
f. antibiotic
Fluorotron
Coherent radiation F.
F. Master fluorophotometer
flurbiprofen sodium

Fluress
flush
choroidal f.
ciliary f.
circumciliary f.
hemifacial f.
flute needle
flutter
eyelid f.
f. of eyelid
ocular f.
flux
f. incident
luminous f.
oxygen f.
radiant f.
radiant and luminous f.
unit of luminous f.
fly
f. test
Titmus stereo f.
Flynn lens loop
FM-500
Kowa F.
FM-100 test
F/M base curve contact lens
FML
fluorometholone 0.1% ophthalmic
suspension
FML Forte
FML S.O.P.
FML-S
F.-S. Ophthalmic Suspension
foam cell
foaming exudate
focal
f. attenuation
f. choroiditis
f. constriction
f. depth
f. distance
f. dystonia
f. electroretinogram
f. granuloma
f. illumination
f. image point
f. interval

F

NOTES

177

focal *(continued)*
  f. laser photocoagulation
  f. length
  f. myasthenia
  f. scotoma
  f. staining
  f. vasogenic edema
foci *(pl. of* focus*)*
focimeter
focofilcon A
focus, pl. **foci (F)**
  aplanatic f.
  conjugate f.
  depth of f.
  detectable f.
  image-space f.
  object-space f.
  principal f.
  real f.
  virtual f.
fogging
  f. retinoscopy
  f. system of refraction
foil sheet
Foix
  F. enucleation
  F. syndrome
fold
  arcuate retinal f.
  choroidal f.
  ciliary f.
  concentric f.
  congenital retinal f.
  conjunctival semilunar f.
  Dennie-Morgan f.
  Descemet f.
  double lower lid f.
  dry f.
  epicanthal skin f.
  epicanthine f.
  eyelid f.
  falciform retinal f.
  fixed f.
  f. forceps
  glabellar f.
  Hasner f.
  iridial f.
  lacrimal f.
  Lange f.
  meridional f.
  mongolian f.
  nasojugal f.
  nasolabial f.

  palpebral f.
  palpebronasal f.
  primary retinal f.
  retinal fixed f.
  retrotarsal f.
  semilunar f.
  star f.
  stiff retinal f.
foldable
  f. intraocular lens
  f. intraocular lens surgery
folder
  Faulkner f.
folding spectacles
folic
  f. acid antagonist
  f. acid deficiency
follicle
  cilia f.
  conjunctival f.
  limbal f.
  lymphoid f.
  necrotic f.
follicular
  f. conjunctivitis
  f. hypertrophy
  f. iritis
  f. plugging
  f. trachoma
follicularis
  blepharitis f.
  keratosis f.
folliculitis
  f. externa
  f. interna
folliculorum
  Demodex f.
folliculosis
follow
  fix and f.
following
  f. eye
  f. movement
Foltz valve
fomivirsen
  f. sodium
Fontana
  F. canal
  space of F.
  F. space
footcandle (fc)
  f. meter

footplate
Müller cell f.
footprints of HSV
foramen, pl. **foramina**
Bozzi f.
cranial f.
inferior zygomatic f.
infraorbital f.
f. infraorbitale
lacerate anterior f.
lacerate middle f.
lacerate posterior f.
f. lacerum anterius
optic f.
f. opticum
orbitomalar f.
rotundum f.
f. of sclera
Soemmering f.
f. sphenoidalis
f. of sphenoid bone
supraorbital f.
f. supraorbitale
zygomatic f.
zygomaticofacial f.
zygomatico-orbital f.
f. zygomatico-orbitale
zygomaticotemporal f.
force
muscle f.
shear f.
forced
f. choice preferential looking
f. downward deviation
f. duction
f. generation
f. generation test
forced-duction
f.-d. test
f.-d. testing
forced-eye closure
forceps
0.12 f.
Adson f.
Alabama tying f.
Alabama University utility f.
Allen-Barkan f.

Allen-Barker f.
Allen-Braley f.
Allis f.
Alvis fixation f.
Ambrose suture f.
Amenabar capsule f.
angled capsule f.
Anis f.
Arroyo f.
Arruga capsule f.
Arruga-McCool capsule f.
Asch septal f.
ASSI IOL inserter f.
ASSI universal lens folding f.
Ayers chalazion f.
Azar lens-holding f.
Bailey chalazion f.
Baird chalazion f.
Ballen-Alexander f.
Bangerter muscle f.
Banner f.
Bard-Parker f.
Barkan iris f.
Barraquer cilia f.
Barraquer conjunctival f.
Barraquer corneal utility f.
Barraquer hemostatic
mosquito f.
Barraquer-von Mandach
capsule f.
bayonet f.
BB shot f.
beaked f.
Beaupre cilia f.
Bechert-McPherson angled
tying f.
Bennett cilia f.
Berens corneal transplant f.
Berens muscle f.
Berens ptosis f.
Berens suturing f.
Berkeley Bioengineering
ptosis f.
Berke ptosis f.
Bettman-Noyes fixation f.
binocular fixation f.
bipolar f.

F

NOTES

forceps *(continued)*

Birks Mark II Colibri f.
Birks Mark II grooved f.
Birks Mark II microneedle-
holder f.
Birks Mark II straight f.
Birks Mark II suture-tying f.
Birks Mark II toothed f.
Bishop-Harman foreign body f.
Bishop-Harman tissue f.
Blaydes corneal f.
Blaydes lens-holding f.
blepharochalasis f.
Bonaccolto fragment f.
Bonaccolto jeweler f.
Bonaccolto magnet tip f.
Bonaccolto utility f.
bone-biting f.
Bonn iris f.
Bonn suturing f.
Boruchoff f.
Botvin iris f.
Bracken fixation f.
Bracken iris f.
Bronson-Magnion f.
Bruening f.
Buratto ophthalmic f.
Calibri f.
Callahan fixation f.
capsule fragment f.
capsulorrhexis f.
Cardona corneal prosthesis f.
Cardona threading f.
Cartman lens insertion f.
Castroviejo-Arruga f.
Castroviejo capsule f.
Castroviejo clip-applying f.
Castroviejo-Colibri f.
Castroviejo corneal-holding f.
Castroviejo corneoscleral f.
Castroviejo fixation f.
Castroviejo lid f.
Castroviejo scleral fold f.
Castroviejo suture f.
Castroviejo suturing f.
Castroviejo tying f.
Castroviejo wide grip handle f.
Catalano corneoscleral f.
Catalano tying f.
chalazion f.
Chandler iris f.
Choyce lens-inserting f.
Cilco lens f.

cilia f.
Clark capsule fragment f.
Clark-Verhoeff capsule f.
Clayman lens-holding f.
Clayman lens implant f.
Clayman lens-inserting f.
clip-applying f.
coaptation bipolar f.
Cohen corneal f.
Coleman-Taylor IOL f.
Colibri f.
conjunctiva f.
cornea-holding f.
corneal fixation f.
corneal prosthesis f.
corneal splinter f.
corneoscleral f.
Cozean-McPherson tying f.
Crawford f.
cross-action capsule f.
Culler fixation f.
curved iris f.
curved tying f.
Dallas lens-inserting f.
Danberg iris f.
Dan chalazion f.
Dan-Gradle cilia f.
Davis f.
delicate serrated straight
dressing f.
Desmarres chalazion f.
disk f.
Dixon-Thorpe vitreous foreign
body f.
Dodick lens-holding f.
double-pronged f.
Douglas cilia f.
Draeger f.
dressing f.
Drews cilia f.
Drews-Sato tying f.
Eber needle-holder f.
Ehrhardt lid f.
Elschnig capsule f.
Elschnig fixation f.
Elschnig-O'Brien f.
Elschnig-O'Connor fixation f.
entropion f.
Erhardt lid f.
Ernest-McDonald soft
intraocular lens-folding f.
Ewing capsule f.
eyelid f.

Fechner ring f.
Fine-Castroviejo suturing f.
fine-dissecting f.
Fine suture-tying f.
fine-toothed f.
Fink-Jameson muscle f.
Fisher-Arlt iris f.
fixation f.
fixation/anchor f.
fixation binocular f.
fixed f.
fold f.
foreign body f.
Förster iris f.
Francis chalazion f.
Francis spud chalazion f.
Fuchs capsule f.
Fuchs extracapsular f.
Fuchs iris f.
Furniss cornea-holding f.
Gaskin fragment f.
25-gauge intraocular f.
Gelfilm f.
Gifford fixation f.
Gifford iris f.
Gill-Arruga capsular f.
Gill-Hess iris f.
Gill iris f.
Gills-Welsh capsule f.
Girard corneoscleral f.
Goldmann capsulorrhexis f.
Grabow f.
Gradle cilia f.
Graefe eye dressing f.
Graefe fixation f.
Graefe iris f.
Graefe tissue f.
Grayson corneal f.
Grayton corneal f.
Grazer blepharoplasty f.
Green capsule f.
Green chalazion f.
Green fixation f.
Grieshaber diamond coated f.
Grieshaber internal limiting
  membrane f.
Grieshaber iris f.

f. guard
Guist fixation f.
Gunderson muscle f.
Guyton-Clark fragment f.
Guyton-Noyes fixation f.
Halberg contact lens f.
Halsted curved mosquito
  hemostatic f.
Harman fixation f.
Harms corneal f.
Harms-Tubingen tying f.
Harms tying f.
Hartmann hemostatic f.
Hartmann mosquito
  hemostatic f.
Hasner lid f.
Heath chalazion f.
hemostatic f.
Hersh LASIK retreatment f.
Hertel stone f.
Hess f.
Hess-Barraquer f.
Hessburg lens f.
Hessburg lens-inserting f.
Hess-Horwitz f.
Heyner f.
Hirschman lens f.
Hirschman lens-inserting f.
Holth f.
Hoskins beaked Colibri f.
Hoskins-Dallas intraocular lens-
  inserting f.
Hoskins fine straight f.
Hoskins fixation f.
Hoskins-Luntz f.
Hoskins microstraight f.
Hoskins miniaturized micro
  straight f.
Hoskins-Skeleton fine f.
Hoskins-Skeleton micro-grooved
  broad-tipped f.
Hoskins straight microiris f.
Hoskins suture f.
host tissue f.
House miniature f.
Hubbard corneoscleral f.
Hunt chalazion f.

F

NOTES

forceps *(continued)*
Hyde corneal f.
Hyde double-curved f.
Ilg capsule f.
Ilg curved microtying f.
Ilg insertion f.
Inamura small incision
capsulorrhexis f.
intraocular f.
Iowa State fixation f.
iris f.
I-tech intraocular foreign
body f.
I-tech splinter f.
I-tech tying f.
Jacob capsule fragment f.
Jaffe capsulorrhexis f.
Jaffe suturing f.
Jameson muscle f.
Jansen-Middleton septotomy f.
Jensen intraocular lens f.
Jensen lens-inserting f.
Jervey capsule fragment f.
Jervey iris f.
jeweler f.
John Weiss f.
Jones f.
Judd f.
Kalt f.
Katena f.
Katzin-Barraquer f.
Keeler extended round tip f.
Keeler intraocular foreign body
grasping f.
Kelman-McPherson corneal f.
Kelman-McPherson tying f.
Kerrison f.
Kevorkian-Younge f.
King-Prince muscle f.
Kirby capsule f.
Kirby corneoscleral f.
Kirby iris f.
Kirby tissue f.
Knapp f.
Koby cataract f.
Kraff intraocular utility f.
Kraff lens-inserting f.
Kraff suturing f.
Kraff tying f.
Kraff-Utrata capsulorrhexis f.
Kraff-Utrata intraocular
utility f.
Kraft f.

Kratz lens-inserting f.
Kremer two-point fixation f.
Kronfeld suturing f.
Krukenberg pigment spindle f.
Kuhnt fixation f.
Kulvin-Kalt f.
Lambert chalazion f.
large-angled f.
Leahey chalazion f.
Leigh capsule f.
lens-holding f.
lens-threading f.
Lester fixation f.
lid f.
Lieberman-Pollock double
corneal f.
Lindstrom lens-insertion f.
Linn-Graefe iris f.
Lister f.
Littauer cilia f.
Livernois lens-holding f.
Livernois pickup and
folding f.
Llobera fixation f.
Lordan chalazion f.
Lucae dressing f.
Machemer diamond-dust-coated
foreign body f.
Malis f.
Manhattan Eye & Ear
suturing f.
marginal chalazion f.
matte black f.
Maumenee capsule f.
Maumenee-Colibri corneal f.
Maumenee corneal f.
Maumenee Suregrip f.
Max Fine f.
McCollough tying f.
McCullough suturing f.
McDonald lens folding f.
McGregor conjunctival f.
McGuire marginal chalazion f.
McLean capsule f.
McLean muscle recession f.
McPherson angled f.
McPherson bent f.
McPherson corneal f.
McPherson irrigating f.
McPherson microiris f.
McPherson microsuture f.
McPherson tying iris f.
McQueen vitreous f.

Mendez multi-purpose LASIK f.
Mentor-Maumenee Suregrip f.
Metico f.
micro Colibri f.
miniature f.
Moehle corneal f.
Moody fixation f.
Moore lens f.
Moore lens-inserting f.
mosquito hemostatic f.
muscle f.
Neubauer f.
Nevyas lens f.
New Orleans Eye & Ear fixation f.
New York Eye & Ear Hospital fixation f.
Noble f.
Noyes f.
Nugent fixation f.
Nugent rectus f.
Nugent superior rectus f.
O'Brien-Elschnig fixation f.
O'Brien fixation f.
Ochsner cartilage f.
Ochsner tissue f.
Ochsner tissue/cartilage f.
O'Connor-Elschnig fixation f.
O'Connor iris f.
O'Connor lid f.
O'Connor sponge f.
O'Gawa suture-fixation f.
Ogura cartilage f.
Ogura tissue f.
Ogura tissue/cartilage f.
Osher foreign body f.
Passarelli one-pass capsulorrhexis f.
Paton anterior chamber lens implant f.
Paton capsule f.
Paton corneal transplant f.
Paton suturing f.
Paton tying/stitch removal f.
Paufique suturing f.
Pavlo-Colibri corneal f.

Penn-Anderson scleral fixation f.
Perritt double-fixation f.
Peyman-Green vitreous f.
Phillips fixation f.
Pierse corneal Colibri-type f.
Pierse fixation f.
Pierse-Hoskins f.
Pierse-type Colibri f.
Pley extracapsular f.
Pollock f.
Primbs suturing f.
Prince muscle f.
ptosis f.
Puntenney f.
pupil spreader/retractor f.
Quevedo fixation f.
Quevedo suturing f.
Quire mechanical finger f.
recession f.
Reese muscle f.
Reisinger lens-extracting f.
Rhein capsulorrhexis cystotome f.
Rhein fine foldable lens-insertion f.
ring f.
ring-tip f.
Ritch-Krupin-Denver eye valve-insertion f.
Rizzuti fixation f.
Rizzuti-Furniss cornea-holding f.
Rizzuti rectus f.
Rizzuti scleral fixation f.
Rolf f.
roller f.
Russian f.
Rycroft tying f.
Sachs tissue f.
Sanders-Castroviejo suturing f.
Sandt f.
Sauer suture f.
Schaaf foreign body f.
Schaefer fixation f.
Scheie-Graefe fixation f.
Schepens f.

F

NOTES

forceps *(continued)*
Schweigger capsule f.
Schweigger extracapsular f.
scleral twist-grip f.
Scott lens-insertion f.
series five f.
serrated conjunctival f.
Sewall f.
Sheets lens-inserting f.
Sheets-McPherson tying f.
Shepard intraocular lens f.
Shepard intraocular utility f.
Shepard lens-inserting f.
Shepard-Reinstein f.
Shepard tying f.
Shields f.
Shoemaker intraocular lens f.
S5-1804-HUMER lens-
folding f.
silicone rod and sleeve f.
silicone sponge f.
Simcoe lens implant f.
Simcoe lens-inserting f.
Simcoe nucleus f.
Simcoe posterior chamber
lens f.
Sinskey micro-tying f.
Sinskey-Wilson foreign body f.
Skeleton fine f.
sleeve spreading f.
Smart f.
Smart-Leiske cross-action
intraocular lens f.
Smith-Leiske cross-action
intraocular lens f.
Snellen entropion f.
Snyder corneal spring f.
Sourdille f.
Spaleck f.
Spencer chalazion f.
Spero f.
splaytooth f.
Starr fixation f.
Stephens soft IOL-inserting f.
Stern-Castroviejo locking f.
Stern-Castroviejo suturing f.
Stevens iris f.
stitch-removal f.
Stolte capsulorrhexis f.
Storz-Bonn suturing f.
Storz capsule f.
Storz cilia f.
Storz corneal f.

Storz-Utrata f.
strabismus f.
straight-tip bipolar f.
straight tying f.
Strow corneal f.
superior rectus f.
suturing f.
Takahashi iris retractor f.
Tennant-Colibri corneal f.
Tennant lens-inserting f.
Tennant titanium suturing f.
Tennant-Troutman superior
rectus f.
Tennant tying f.
Tenner titanium suturing f.
Tenzel f.
Terson capsule f.
Terson extracapsular f.
Thomas fixation f.
Thornton fixation f.
Thorpe-Castroviejo corneal f.
Thorpe-Castroviejo fixation f.
Thorpe-Castroviejo vitreous
foreign body f.
Thorpe conjunctival f.
Thorpe corneal f.
Thorpe foreign body f.
Thrasher lens implant f.
three-toothed f.
tissue f.
titanium suturing f.
Troutman f.
Troutman-Barraquer corneal
fixation f.
Troutman-Barraquer corneal
utility f.
Troutman-Castroviejo corneal
fixation f.
Troutman-Llobera fixation f.
Troutman rectus f.
Troutman tying f.
tubing introducer f.
tying f.
tying/stitch removal f.
Universal II f.
Utrata capsulorrhexis f.
Utrata-Kershner capsulorrhexis
cystitome f.
Verhoeff capsule f.
vertical f.
Vickerall round ringed f.
Vickers f.
vitreous foreign body f.

von Graefe fixation f.
von Graefe iris f.
von Graefe tissue f.
von Mondak capsule fragment-clot f.
Wadsworth lid f.
Wainstock suturing f.
Waldeau fixation f.
Watzke f.
Weaver chalazion f.
Welsh pupil-spreader f.
Whitney superior rectus f.
Wies chalazion f.
Wilde f.
Wilkerson intraocular lens-insertion f.
Wills Hospital utility f.
Wills utility eye f.
Wolfe f.
Worth strabismus f.
Wullstein-House cup f.
Ziegler cilia f.

Fordyce nodule
forebrain dysplasia
foreign
   f. body (FB)
   f. body bur
   f. body cell
   f. body extraction
   f. body forceps
   f. body locator
   f. body needle
   f. body sclerotomy
   f. body spud
foreign-body sensation
Forel field
foreshortening
   fornical f.
Forker retractor
form
   f. perception
   f. sense
   f. vision
form-deprivation myopia
forme fruste

FormFlex
   F. lens
   F. lens loupe
formula
   Cellufresh F.
   Hoffer-Colenbrander f.
   Holladay f.
   lens-maker f.
   Lepper-Trier f.
   Sanders-Retzlaff-Kraff f. (SRK)
   SRK f.
fornical foreshortening
fornix, pl. fornices
   f. approach
   inferior conjunctival f.
   lacrimal f.
   f. reformation
   f. sacci lacrimalis
   superior conjunctival f.
fornix-based flap
Forsius-Eriksson syndrome
forskolin
Forssman carotid syndrome
Förster
   F. choroiditis
   F. conjunctiva
   F. disease
   F. enucleation snare
   F. iris forceps
   F. lacrimal sac
   F. operation
   F. photometer
   F. photoptometer
   F. sacci lacrimalis
   F. uveitis
Förster-Fuchs
   F.-F. black spot
   F.-F. spot
Forte
   AK-Sulf F.
   FML F.
   Inflamase F.
   Lipo-Tears F.
   Liquifilm F.
   Naphcon F.
   Ocu-Pred F.
   Pred F.

F

NOTES

Forte *(continued)*
Predair F.
Prednefrin F.
Sulfair F.
fortification
f. figure
f. spectrum
fortified antibiotic
fortuitum
Mycobacterium f.
forward
f. light scatter
f. traction test
foscarnet sodium
fossa, pl. **fossae**
f. glandulae lacrimalis
hyaloid f.
f. hyaloidea
interpeduncular f.
lacrimal gland f.
lacrimal sac f.
lenticular f.
optical f.
f. sacci lacrimalis
trochlear f.
f. trochlearis
f. tumor
fossette
Foster
F. enucleation snare
F. Kennedy syndrome
F. snare enucleator
F. suture
Fould entropion operation
four base-out prism testing
four-dot test
Fourier harmonic analysis
four-loop
f.-l. iris clip implant
f.-l. iris fixated implant
f.-l. lens
four-mirror
f.-m. goniolens
f.-m. goniolens lens
four-point fixation
four-sided cutting needle
fourth
f. cranial nerve
f. nerve palsy
fovea, pl. **foveae**
central f.
f. centralis
obscured f.

trochlear f.
f. trochlearis
foveal
f. avascular zone (FAZ)
f. burn
f. center
f. cone electroretinography
f. cyst
f. depression
f. dystopia
f. edema
f. flicker fusion frequency
f. image
f. ischemia
f. outer retinal dysfunction
f. outer retinal function
f. reflex
f. retinal detachment
f. sparing
f. splitting
f. traction
f. vision
foveola, pl. **foveolae**
f. ocularis
retinal f.
foveolar
f. choroidal circulation
f. reflex
f. retinal detachment
foveomacular
f. cone dysfunction syndrome
f. retinitis
f. retinopathy
f. vitelliform dystrophy
Foville syndrome
Foville-Wilson syndrome
fowleri
Naegleria f.
Fox
F. aluminum shield
F. conformer
F. eye
F. eye shield
F. irrigating/aspirating unit
F. operation
F. speculum
F. sphere implant
FOZR
front optic zone radius
FP
fundus photo
FPA
far point of accommodation

FR3
third framework region
fraction
Snellen f.
fracture
apex f.
blow-out f.
combined f.
comminuted orbital f.
depressed f.
external orbital f.
floor f.
midfacial f.
naso-orbital f.
f. of orbit
orbital blow-out f.
orbital floor f.
orbital rim f.
orbital wall f.
roof f.
zygomatic f.
fragilis
Bacillus f.
fragilitas ossium
Fragmatome
CooperVision F.
F. flute syringe
Gill-Hess F.
Girard F.
fragment
Cooper blade f.
Fab f.
Fc f.
Hoskins razor blade f.
fragmentation/aspiration handpiece
fragmented dendrite
fragmentor
Lieberman f.
frame
celluloid f.
cellulose acetate f.
cellulose nitrate f.
Lucite f.
molded f.
MTL trial f.
nylon f.
Oculus trial f.

optical f.
Optyl f.
Perspex f.
plastic f.
Plexiglas f.
polymethyl methacrylate f.
rimless f.
f. scotoma
spectacle f.
Stryker f.
trial f.
framework
scleral f.
uveal f.
Franceschetti
F. coreoplasty operation
F. corepraxy operation
F. deviation operation
F. disease
F. dystrophy
F. keratoplasty operation
F. pupil deviation operation
F. syndrome
Franceschetti-Klein syndrome
Franchesseti
oculodigital sign of F.
Francis
F. chalazion forceps
F. spud
F. spud chalazion forceps
Francisella tularensis
François
central cloudy dystrophy of F.
dermochondral corneal
dystrophy of F.
dyscephalic syndrome of F.
F. dystrophy
F. syndrome
frank corneal ulceration
Frankfort horizontal plane
Franklin
F. bifocal
F. glasses
F. spectacles
Franklin-style bifocal lenses
Fraser syndrome
Fraunfelder "no touch" technique

F

NOTES

187

Fraunhofer
F. diffraction
F. line
Frazier suction tube
freckle
iris f.
free
f. conjunctival autograft
f. margin of eyelid
f. operculum
f. running mode
f. skin autograft
f. tenotomy
Freeman
F. punctum plug
F. solution
Freeman-Sheldon syndrome
Freer
F. chisel
F. periosteal elevator
freeze
Keeler-Amoils f.
freeze-thaw cryotherapy
Frelex lens
French
F. catheter
F. hook spatula
F. lacrimal dilator
F. lacrimal probe
F. lacrimal spatula
F. needle holder
F. pattern spatula
Frenkel anterior ocular traumatic syndrome
Frenzel
F. goggles
F. lens
frequency
critical corresponding f. (CCF)
critical flicker fusion f.
F. Doubling Perimeter test
f. doubling perimetry
foveal flicker fusion f.
fusion f.
FreshLook ColorBlends lens
Fresnel
F. lens
F. membrane
F. optics
F. press-on prism
F. principle

Frey
F. syndrome
F. tunneled implant
Fricke operation
Fridenberg stigmatometric card
Friedenwald
F. funduscope
F. operation
F. ophthalmoscope
F. syndrome
Friedenwald-Guyton operation
Friede operation
Friedlander incision marker
Friedman
F. hand-held Hruby lens
F. Phaco/IOL manipulator
F. tantalum clip
F. test
Friedman-Hruby lens
Friedmann visual field analyzer
Friedreich
F. ataxia
F. syndrome
Frigitronics
Cilco F.
F. cryosurgical unit
F. freeze-thaw cryopexy probe
F. nitrous oxide cryosurgery apparatus
F. vitrector
frill
iris f.
plaited f.
Frin
Isopto F.
fringe
interference f.
Moiré f.
Fritz vitreous transplant needle
frog cortex remover
frond
fibrous f.
fibrovascular f.
sea f.
vascular f.
f. of vessel
front
f. build-up implant
f. optic zone radius (FOZR)
f. surface toric contact lens
f. vertex
frontal
f. axis

f. bone
f. craniotomy
f. diploic vein
f. eye field
f. incisure
f. lobe
f. lobe unilateral cerebral
  hemisphere lesion
f. nerve
f. sinus
f. sinusitis
f. triangle
f. tuber
frontalis
  facies orbitalis ossis f.
  fascia lata f.
  f. fascia lata suspension
  incisura f.
  incisura ethmoidalis ossis f.
  margo supraorbitalis ossis f.
  f. muscle
  f. muscle sling
  pars orbitalis ossis f.
  f. sling technique
  sulcus orbitales lobi f.
  vena diploica f.
frontolacrimalis
  sutura f.
frontolacrimal suture
**frontoparietal bilateral cerebral
  hemisphere lesion**
frontosphenoid suture
Frost
  F. scissors
  F. suture
Frost-Lang operation
frozen
  f. globe
  f. tissue
fruste
  forme f.
  keratoconus f.
Fuchs
  F. adenoma
  angle of F.
  F. aphakic keratopathy
  F. atrophy

F. black spot
F. canthorrhaphy operation
F. capsule forceps
F. combined corneal dystrophy
combined dystrophy of F.
F. crypt
dellen of F.
F. dimple
F. endothelial corneal
  dystrophy
F. endothelial-epithelial
  dystrophy
F. epithelial corneal dystrophy
epithelial dystrophy of F.
F. epithelial-endothelial
  dystrophy
F. extracapsular forceps
F. heterochromia
F. heterochromic cyclitis
  (FHC)
F. heterochromic iridocyclitis
F. inferior coloboma
F. iris bombe transfixation
  operation
F. iris forceps
F. keratitis
lamella of F.
F. lancet type keratome
F. retinal detachment syringe
F. spot coloboma
F. spur
F. syndrome
F. two-way syringe
F. uveitis
Fuchs-Kraupa syndrome
fucidic acid gel
fucidin gel
fugax
  amaurosis f.
  amaurosis partialis f.
  episcleritis partialis f.
  episcleritis periodica f.
  keratitis periodica f.
  saburral amaurosis f.
Fukala operation
Fukasaku pupil snapper hook
Fukasaku spatula

F

NOTES

full-dimpled Lucite implant
Fuller silicone sponge
Fullerview iris retractor
full-field
  f.-f. electroretinogram
  f.-f. system
full-thickness
  f.-t. autograft
  f.-t. corneal graft
  f.-t. corneal laceration
  f.-t. keratoplasty
full versions and ductions
fulminans
  glaucoma f.
fulminant
  f. abscess
  f. glaucoma
  f. myasthenia gravis
  f. ocular toxoplasmosis
Ful-Vue
  F.-V. bifocal
  F.-V. ophthalmoscope
  F.-V. spot retinoscope
  F.-V. streak retinoscope
fumagillin
Fumidil B
fumigatus
  Aspergillus f.
function
  bandpass f.
  binocular f.
  cone f.
  corneal epithelial barrier f.
  Easterman visual f.
  foveal outer retinal f.
  medial rectus f.
  modulation transfer f.
  motor f.
  peripheral rod f.
  rod f.
  spread f.
  transfer f.
  visual f.
functional
  F. Acuity Contrast Test
  (FACT)
  f. amblyopia
  f. blindness
  f. defect
  f. visual loss
fundal reflex
fundectomy
fundus, pl. **fundi**

albinotic f.
f. albipunctalis
albipunctate f.
f. albipunctatus
blond f.
f. camera
coloboma of f.
f. contact lens
f. diabeticus
f. examination
f. of eye
f. flavimaculatus
f. focalizing lens
Kowa f.
f. laser lens
leopard f.
f. microscopy
mottling of f.
normal f.
f. oculi
pepper-and-salt f.
f. photo (FP)
f. photograph
f. polycythemicus
prismatic f.
f. reflex
salt-and-pepper f.
tessellated f.
f. tigré
tigroid f.
tomato-ketchup f.
f. xerophthalmicus
Funduscein
Funduscein-10
Funduscein-25
funduscope
  Friedenwald f.
funduscopic examination
funduscopy
fundusectomy
fungal
  f. blepharitis
  f. corneal ulcer
  f. endophthalmitis
  f. infection
  f. keratitis
  f. uveitis
fungus, pl. **fungi**
  hyaline f.
  moniliaceous filamentous f.
funnel
  muscular f.
  vascular f.

funnel-shaped retinal detachment
furnacemen's cataract
Furniss cornea-holding forceps
furrow
    corneal marginal f.
    f. degeneration
    f. dystrophy
    f. keratitis
    marginal f.
    palpebral f.
    scleral f.
    superior palpebral f.
furrowing
Fusarium
    F. episphaeria
    F. moniliforme
    F. oxysporum
    F. solani
fusca
    lamina f.
    membrana f.
fuscin
fused
    f. bifocal lens
    f. multifocal lens
fusiform
    f. aneurysm
    f. cataract
fusion
    amplitude of f.
    f. area
    binocular f.
    f. breakpoint

    central f.
    color f.
    eyelid f.
    faculty f.
    f. faculty
    first-grade f.
    flicker f.
    f. frequency
    f. grade
    motor f.
    peripheral f.
    f. reflex
    second-grade f.
    sensory f.
    tenacious distance f.
    tenacious proximal f.
    third-grade f.
    f. tube
    f. with accommodation
    f. with amplitude
    Worth concept of f.
fusional
    f. convergence
    f. convergence amplitude
    f. divergence
    f. divergence amplitude
    f. movement
    f. reserve
    f. vergence
fusion-free
    f.-f. position
Fusobacterium

NOTES

F

191

Gaffee speculum
Gaillard-Arlt suture
galactose cataract
galactosemia
    g. cataract
    enzymatic g.
Galassi pupillary phenomenon
galeal flap
Galen vein
galeropia
galeropsia
Galezowski lacrimal dilator
Galilean
    G. magnification changer
    G. microscope
    G. telescope
Galin
    G. bleb cup
    G. intraocular implant lens
Gallie cryoenucleator
gallium
    g. citrate contrast
    g. citrate contrast material
    g. scan
    g. scanning
Galt aspirating cannula
galvanic nystagmus
Gamboscope
game
    E g.
gamma
    g. angle
    g. crystallin
    g. irradiation
ganciclovir
    g. cyclic phosphate
    g. sodium
    g. therapy
ganglia (pl. of ganglion)
ganglioglioma
ganglioma
ganglion, pl. ganglia
    basal g.
    g. cell
    g. cell layer
    cervical g.
    ciliary g.
    gasserian g.
    geniculate g.
    g. layer of optic nerve

    g. layer of retina
    lenticular g.
    long root of ciliary g.
    motor root of ciliary g.
    oculomotor root of ciliary g.
    ophthalmic g.
    optic g.
    orbital g.
    pterygopalatine g.
    retinal g.
    Schacher g.
    sensory root of ciliary g.
    short root of ciliary g.
    sphenopalatine g.
    g. stratum of optic nerve
    superior cervical g.
    trigeminal sensory g.
ganglioneuroma
ganglionic
    g. layer of optic nerve
    g. layer of retina
    g. stratum of optic nerve
    g. stratum of retina
ganglionitis
gangliosus ciliaris
gangraenescens
    granuloma g.
gangrenosa
    vaccinia g.
gangrenosum
    ecthyma g.
gangrenous rhinitis
Gans cyclodialysis cannula
Ganzfeld electroretinograph
Ganzfield bowl
gape
    wound g.
GAPO
    growth retardation, alopecia,
    pseudoanodontia, and optic atrophy
    GAPO syndrome
Garcia-Ibanez camera
Garcia-Novito eye implant
Gardner syndrome
garter
    Goffman eye g.
gas
    g. bubble
    C3F8 g.
    g. discharge lamp

G

gas *(continued)*
 hexafluoride g.
 inspired g.
 intraocular g.
 ISPAN intraocular g.
 laughing g.
 long-acting g.
 mustard g.
 octofluoropropane g.
 perfluorocarbon g.
 perfluoropropane g. (C3F8)
 SF6 g.
 sulfur g.
 sulfurhexafluoride g.
 g. tamponade
 tear g.
gas-exchange descemetopexy
gas-fluid exchange
Gaskin fragment forceps
gas-permeable
 g.-p. contact lens
 g.-p. daily cleaner
Gass
 G. cataract aspirating cannula
 G. corneoscleral punch
 G. dye applicator
 G. irrigating/aspirating unit
 G. macular hole classification
 G. muscle hook
 G. retinal detachment hook
 G. scleral marker
 G. scleral punch
 G. sclerotomy punch
 G. vitreous aspirating cannula
gasserian ganglion
gauge
 blade g.
 coin g.
 depth g.
 25-g. intraocular forceps
 Marco radius g.
 30-g. needle
 radius g.
 Reichert radius g.
 Shepard incision depth g.
 Stahl lens g.
 Steinert-Deacon incision g.
 20-g. straight bipolar pencil
 V-groove g.
Gaule
 G. pit
 G. spot
Gault reflex

gaussian
 g. distribution
 g. optical system
 g. optics
Gayet operation
gaze
 apraxia of g.
 cardinal direction of g.
 cardinal position of g.
 g. center
 conjugate g.
 diagnostic positions of g.
 disconjugate g.
 distant g.
 downward g.
 dysconjugate g.
 eccentric g.
 evoked nystagmus g.
 field of g.
 horizontal g.
 lateral g.
 left g.
 midline position of g.
 g. movement
 near g.
 near fixation position of g.
 g. nystagmus
 g. palsy
 parallelism of g.
 paralysis of g.
 ping-pong g.
 primary position of g.
 right g.
 spasticity of conjugate g.
 superior g.
 supranuclear paresis of
  vertical g.
 upward g.
 vertical g.
gaze-evoked
 g.-e. nystagmus
 g.-e. tinnitus
gaze-holding
 eccentric g.-h.
gaze-paretic nystagmus
G-banding
GC
 goniocurettage
GCA
 giant cell arteritis
GD
 glare disability

GDD
glaucoma drainage device
GDx nerve fiber analyzer
Geiger
G. cautery
G. electrocautery
gel
Aquasonic 100 g.
ferric hyaluronate g.
fucidic acid g.
fucidin g.
Gonio G.
H.P. Acthar G.
Pilopine g. 4%
Pilopine HS g.
silica g.
vitreous g.
gelatin
g. disk
g. film
gelatinous
g. dystrophy
g. mass
g. material
g. scleritis
gelatinous-appearing limbal
hypertrophy
Gel-Clean
Gel Clean
Gelfilm
G. cap
G. forceps
G. plate
G. retinal implant
Schepens G.
Gelfoam
gene
CYP1B1 g.
dominant g.
LMX1B g.
g. locus
myoclin g.
nonpenetrant g.
penetrant g.
peripherin/RDS g.
retinal degeneration slow
(RDS) g.

retinitis pigmentosa GTPase
regulator g. (RPGR)
syntenic g.
TIGR g.
general
g. anesthesia
g. anesthetic
g. cataract
generalized vaccinia
generating spectacle lens
generation
filial g. (F)
forced g.
Genesis
G. diamond blade
G. lens
Geneva lens measure
Geneye Ophthalmic
geniculate
g. body
g. ganglion
g. hemianopsia
g. nucleus
geniculocalcarine
g. radiation
g. tract
Genoptic
G. S.O.P.
G. S.O.P. Ophthalmic
Gentacidin
G. Ophthalmic
Gentafair
Gentak
G. Ophthalmic
gentamicin
prednisolone and g.
g. sulfate
GenTeal
G. lubricant eye drops
Gentex PDQ polycarbonate lens
gentian violet marking pen
GentleLASE laser
Gentrasul
geographic
g. atrophy
g. helicoid peripapillary
choroidopathy

G

NOTES

geographic *(continued)*
g. herpes simplex corneal ulcer
g. keratitis
g. lesion
g. peripapillary choroiditis
g. ulceration
geometric
g. axis
g. center
g. equator
g. optics
Geopen
Georgariou cyclodialysis operation
geotropic nystagmus
German Hefner candle
gerontopia
gerontoxon lentis
Gerstmann-Straussler-Scheinker disease
Gerstmann syndrome
gestational
g. diabetes
g. diabetes mellitus
g. injury
Geuder
G. implanter
G. keratoplasty needle
Ghormley double cannula
ghost
Bidwell g.
g. cell
g. cell glaucoma
dendritic g.
g. erythrocyte
g. image
g. ophthalmoscope
g. scarring
g. vessel
Gianelli sign
giant
g. aneurysm
g. axonal neuropathy
g. cell arteritis (GCA)
g. cyst of retina
g. drusen
g. epithelial cell
g. papilla
g. papillary conjunctivitis (GPC)
g. papillary hypertrophy (GPH)
g. retinal break
g. retinal tear (GRT)

Giardet corneal transplant scissors
Gibralter headrest
Gibson irrigating/aspirating unit
Gierke disease
Gifford
G. applicator
G. corneal curette
G. delimiting keratotomy operation
G. fixation forceps
G. iris forceps
G. needle holder
G. operation
G. reflex
G. sign
Gifford-Galassi reflex
Gill
G. blade
G. corneal knife
G. counterpressor
G. incision spreader
G. intraocular implant lens
G. iris forceps
G. scissors
Gill-Arruga capsular forceps
Gill-Fine corneal knife
Gill-Hess
G.-H. blade
G.-H. Fragmatome
G.-H. iris forceps
G.-H. knife
G.-H. scissors
Gillies scar correction operation
Gills
G. double irrigating-aspirating cannula
G. double Luer-Lok cannula
G. irrigating-aspirating cannula
G. pop-up arcuate diamond knife
Gills-Welsh
G.-W. aspirating cannula
G.-W. capsule forceps
G.-W. capsule polisher
G.-W. curette
G.-W. double-barreled irrigating-aspirating cannula
G.-W. guillotine port
G.-W. irrigating-aspirating cannula
G.-W. knife
G.-W. olive-tip cannula

G.-W. scissors
G.-W. spatula
Gills-Welsh-Vannas angled micro scissors
Gilmore
  G. intraocular implant lens
  G. lens
Girard
  G. anterior chamber needle
  G. cataract-aspirating needle
  G. corneoscleral forceps
  G. corneoscleral scissors
  G. Fragmatome
  G. irrigating cannula
  G. irrigating tip
  G. keratoprosthesis operation
  G. phacofragmatome needle
  G. phakofragmatome
  G. procedure
  G. scleral-expander ring
  G. ultrasonic unit
Girard-Swan knife needle
Giraud-Teulon law
girdle
  limbal g.
  limbus g.
  Vogt white limbal g.
Gish micro YAG laser
Givner lid retractor
glabella
glabellar fold
glabellum
glabrata
  Candida g.
  Torulopsis g.
Gladstone-Putterman
  G.-P. entropion clamp
  G.-P. transmarginal rotation entropion clamp
gland
  accessory lacrimal g.
  acinar lacrimal g.
  apocrine g.
  Baumgarten g.
  Bruch g.
  Ciaccio g.
  ciliary g.

conjunctival g.
drainage of lacrimal g.
g. of eyelid
Harder g.
harderian g.
Henle g.
inferior lacrimal g.
Krabbe disease g.
Krause lacrimal g.
lacrimal g.
Manz g.
meibomian g.
Moll g.
Mueller g.
nasolacrimal g.
palpebral g.
pineal g.
pituitary g.
Rosenmüller g.
salivary g.
sebaceous glands of conjunctiva g.
superior lacrimal g.
tarsal g.
tarsoconjunctival g.
trachoma g.
g. trachoma
Waldeyer g.
g. of Wolfring
Wolfring lacrimal g.
Zeis g.
g. of Zeis
zeisian g.
glandula
  g. lacrimalis
  g. lacrimalis inferior
  g. lacrimalis superior
glandulae
  g. ciliares conjunctivales
  g. conjunctivales
  g. lacrimales accessoriae
  g. mucosae conjunctivae
  g. sebaceae conjunctivales
  g. tarsales
glandular fossa of frontal bone
glare
  blinding g.

NOTES

G

glare *(continued)*
    dazzling g.
    direct g.
    g. disability (GD)
    g. disability measurement
    peripheral g.
    specular g.
    g. test
    veiling g.
    g. vision
glarometer
glass
    g. bead
    Chavasse g.
    Crookes g.
    crown g.
    finished g.
    flint g.
    High-Lite g.
    g. lens
    optical g.
    semifinished g.
    g. sphere implant
glassblower's cataract
Glasscock scissors
glasses
    bifocal g.
    cataract g.
    contact g.
    crutch g.
    Difei g.
    Franklin g.
    Grafco magnifying g.
    Hallauer g.
    hemianopic g.
    hyperbolic g.
    magnifying g.
    Masselon g.
    presbyopia g.
    reading g.
    red-green g.
    safety g.
    snow g.
    striated g.
    trifocal g.
glassine strand
glass-rod
    g.-r. negative phenomenon
    g.-r. positive phenomenon
glassworker's cataract
glassy
    g. membrane
    g. sheet

glaucoma
    absolute g.
    g. absolutum
    acute angle-closure g. (AACG)
    acute chronic g.
    acute congestive g.
    acute intermittent primary
      angle-closure g. (A/I-PACG)
    acute primary angle-closure g.
      (APACG)
    air-block g.
    alpha-chymotrypsin-induced g.
    angle-closure g. (ACG)
    angle-recession g.
    aphakic g.
    apoplectic g.
    aqueous misdirected g.
    auricular g.
    capsular g.
    chamber-deepening g.
    chronic angle-closure g.
    chronic narrow-angle g.
    chronic open-angle g. (COAG)
    chronic primary angle-
      closure g. (C-PACG)
    chronic simple g.
    ciliary block g.
    closed-angle g.
    combined-mechanism g.
    compensated g.
    congenital g.
    congestive g.
    g. consummatum
    Contino g.
    contusion angle g.
    corticosteroid-induced g.
    cyclocongestive g.
    90-day g.
    Donders g.
    g. drainage device (GDD)
    drug-induced g.
    enzymatic g.
    enzyme g.
    erythroclastic g.
    exfoliation g.
    exfoliative g.
    fibrin pupillary block g.
    g. field defect
    g. filtering surgery
    g. filtration surgery
    flecken g.
    g. fulminans
    fulminant g.

ghost cell g.
g. hemifield test
hemolytic g.
hemorrhagic g.
herpes zoster g.
high-tension g. (HTG)
hypersecretion g.
g. imminens
infantile g.
inflammatory g.
intermittent angle-closure g.
juvenile open-angle g. (JOAG)
laser-induced g.
latent angle-closure g.
lens exfoliation g.
lens-induced g.
lens-induced secondary open-angle g.
lens particle g.
lens protein g.
lenticular g.
low-pressure g.
low-tension g.
malignant g.
melanomalytic g.
monocular g.
mydriatic test for angle-closure g.
narrow-angle g. (NAG)
neovascular angle-closure g.
noncongestive g.
normal-pressure g.
normal-tension g. (NTG)
obstructive g.
ocular hypertension g.
ocular hypertensive g.
open-angle g. (OAG)
g. pencil
penetrating keratoplasty and g. (PKPG)
phacogenic g.
phacolytic g.
phacomorphic g.
phakic g.
pigmentary dispersion g.
primary angle-closure g.
primary infantile g.

primary open-angle g. (PAOG, POAG)
prodromal g.
pseudoexfoliative g. (PEXG)
pseudoexfoliative capsular g.
pupil block g.
pupillary block g.
recessed-angle g.
recession-angle g.
retrobulbar hemorrhage g.
rubeotic g.
scleral shell g.
secondary neovascular g.
simple g.
g. simplex
simplex g.
steroid g.
steroid-induced g.
g. suspect
trabeculitis g.
transscleral neodymium:yttrium-aluminum-garnet cyclophotocoagulation for g.
traumatic g.
uveitic g.
vitreociliary g.
vitreous block g.
wide-angle g.
Glaucoma-Scope
glaucomatocyclitic crisis
glaucomatologist
glaucomatosa
  iritis g.
glaucomatous
  g. atrophy
  g. cataract
  g. cul-de-sac
  g. cup
  g. cupping
  g. damage detection by retinal thickness mapping
  g. excavation
  g. habit
  g. halo
  g. nerve-fiber bundle scotoma
  g. optic nerve damage (GOND)

G

NOTES

glaucomatous *(continued)*
  g. optic neuropathy
  g. pannus
  g. ring
  g. visual field loss
Glaucon
glaucosis
Glaucotest
GlaucTabs
glaukomflecken of Vogt
GLCIA **locus**
glia
glial
  g. fibrillary acidic protein
    antibody
  g. proliferation
  g. ring
glial-neural hamartoma
glide
  Hessburg intraocular lens g.
  intraocular lens g.
  lens g.
  Sheets lens g.
glioblastoma multiforme
gliocyte
  retinal g.
glioma
  astrocytic g.
  chiasmal g.
  g. endophytum
  hypothalamic g.
  intracranial g.
  g. of optic chiasm
  optic nerve g.
  orbital g.
  peripheral g.
  g. of retina
  retinal g.
  g. sarcomatosum
  telangiectatic g.
gliomatosis
gliomatous
glioneuroma
gliosarcoma
  retinal g.
gliosis
  neonatal g.
  premacular g.
  preretinal g.
  retinal g.
  traumatic g.

gliotic
  g. membrane
  g. strip
glissade
glissadic
global
  g. cataract
globe
  contact burns of g.
  contusion of g.
  disorganized g.
  frozen g.
  luxation of g.
  g. perforation
  ruptured g.
globosa
  cornea g.
globule, pl. globuli, globules
  eosinophilic g.
  Morgagni g.
  morgagnian g.
  ora g.
globus pallidus (GP)
glove
  Biogel Sensor surgical g.
glower
  Nernst g.
GLP
  grid laser photocoagulation
glucocorticoid
  ophthalmic g.
  systemic g.
  topical g.
glucose 6-phosphate dehydrogenase
glue
  butyl cyanoacrylate g.
  ethyl cyanoacrylate g.
  fibrinogen g.
  Histoacryl g.
  methyl cyanoacrylate g.
  g. patch
  g. patch leak
glued-on hard contact lens
glutamyltransferase
  β-g.
glycerin
glyceringlycerol
glycerin-preserved graft
glycerol
  anhydrase g.
glyceryl monostearate
glycogen granule

glycol
    ethylene g.
    polyethylene g.
    propylene g.
Glyrol
GMS
    Grocott-Gomori methenamine silver
    nitrate
goblet
    g. cell
    g. cell hyperplasia
Goffman eye garter
goggles
    Frenzel g.
    night-vision g.
    pinhole g.
    plethysmographic g.
    swimmer's g.
goiter
    exophthalmic g.
gold
    g. dust retinopathy
    G. eyelid load implant
    g. eye plaque
    g. sphere implant
    g. tattoo pigment
    g. weight
Goldberg
    G. side port splitter
    G. syndrome
Goldenhar-Gorlin syndrome
Goldenhar syndrome
Goldmann
    G. applanation tonometer
    G. capsulorrhexis forceps
    G. Coherent radiation
    G. contact lens prism
    G. diagnostic contact lens
    G. fundus contact lens
    G. goniolens
    G. kinetic perimetry
    G. kinetic technique
    G. macular contact lens
    G. manual projection perimeter
    G. multi-mirror lens
    G. perimeter
    G. serrated knife

    G. static technique
    G. three-mirror implant
    G. three-mirror lens
    G. three-mirror prism
Goldmann-Favre
    G.-F. disease
    G.-F. dystrophy
    G.-F. syndrome
Goldmann-Larson
    G.-L. foreign body
    G.-L. foreign body operation
Goldmann-Weekers dark
    adaptometer
Gold-Mules implant
Goldstein
    G. anterior chamber syringe
    G. cannula
    G. golf-club spud
    G. lacrimal sac retractor
    G. lacrimal syringe
    G. refractor
golf-club eye spud
Golgi
    G. apparatus
    G. complex
    G. II neuron
    G. I neuron
Goltz-Gorlin syndrome
Goltz syndrome
Gomez-Marquez lacrimal operation
Gonak
GOND
    glaucomatous optic nerve damage
gondii
    Toxoplasma g.
Gonin
    G. cautery
    G. cautery operation
    G. marker
    G. operation
Gonin-Amsler marker
goniocurettage (GC)
goniodysgenesis
goniofocalizing lens
Gonio Gel
goniogram
    Becker g.

G

NOTES

201

goniolaser
  Thorpe four-mirror g.
goniolens
  Allen-Thorpe g.
  Barkan g.
  four-mirror g.
  Goldmann g.
  Koeppe g.
  g. lens
  P.F. Lee pediatric g.
  single-mirror g.
  Thorpe-Castroviejo g.
  Thorpe four-mirror g.
  Zeiss g.
goniometer
  Bailliart g.
goniophotocoagulation
goniophotography
gonioplasty
gonioprism
  Posner diagnostic g.
  Posner surgical g.
  Swan-Jacob g.
goniopuncture knife
gonioscope
  Jacob-Swann g.
  Lovac g.
  Sussman four-mirror g.
  Thorpe surgical g.
  Troncoso g.
  Zeiss g.
gonioscopic
  g. implant
  g. lens
  g. prism
gonioscopy
  compression g.
  indentation g.
  Koeppe g.
gonioseton implantation
Goniosol
goniostasis
goniosynechia
goniosynechiae
goniosynechialysis (GSL)
goniotomy
  g. knife
  g. knife cannula
  g. needle holder
  g. operation
  photoablative laser g. (PLG)
gonoblennorrhea

gonococcal
  g. bacillus
  g. conjunctivitis
  g. ophthalmia
gonorrheal
  g. conjunctivitis
  g. ophthalmia
gonorrhoeae
  Neisseria g.
Good retractor
Goppert sign
gossamer scarring
gouge
  lacrimal sac g.
  spud g.
  g. spud
  Todd g.
  West g.
Gould intraocular implant lens
gout conjunctivitis
gouty
  g. diabetes
  g. episcleritis
  g. iritis
Gower sign
GP
  globus pallidus
GPC
  giant papillary conjunctivitis
GPH
  giant papillary hypertrophy
Grabow forceps
graceful swirling rod
grade
  fusion g.
Gradenigo syndrome
gradient
  hydrostatic g.
  g. method
grading
  Broders g.
  g. of retinal nerve fiber layer
Gradle
  G. cilia forceps
  G. corneal trephine
  G. electrode
  G. keratoplasty operation
  G. refractor
  G. retractor
graduated tenotomy
Graefe
  G. cataract knife
  G. cystitome

G. cystitome knife
G. disease
G. eye dressing forceps
G. fixation forceps
G. iris forceps
G. needle
G. operation
G. sign
G. strabismus hook
G. syndrome
G. tissue forceps
Graether
G. button hook
G. collar button
G. collar-button micro-iris
retractor
G. mushroom hook
G. pupil expander
G. refractor
Grafco
G. eye shield
G. magnifying glasses
graft
Amsler corneal g.
annular corneal g.
autogenous dermis fat g.
bone g.
g. carrier spoon
conjunctival patch g.
corneal g.
corneolimbal ring g.
crescent corneal g.
dermis fat g.
dermis patch g.
donor g.
g. edema
g. epithelium
failed g.
fat g.
g. fixation
full-thickness corneal g.
glycerin-preserved g.
g. infection
lamellar corneal g.
Marquez-Gomez conjunctival g.
mucous membrane g.
mushroom corneal g.

Mustarde g.
patch g.
pattern-cut corneal g.
penetrating corneal g.
penetrating full-thickness
corneal g.
g. preservation solution
retroauricular complex g.
scleral patch g.
skin g.
split-calvarial bone g.
tarsoconjunctival composite g.
tectonic corneal g.
Tenon patch g.
Tudor-Thomas g.
Wolfe g.
graft-host interface
grafting
surgical patch g.
graft-versus-host disease
gramicidin
neomycin, polymyxin B,
and g.
gram-negative
g.-n. bacteria
g.-n. medium
gram-positive
g.-p. bacteria
g.-p. bacterial keratitis
g.-p. cocci
granular
g. appearance
g. conjunctivitis
g. corneal dystrophy
g. lid
g. ophthalmia
g. trachoma
granularity
granule
Birbeck g.
cone g.
dense core g.
glycogen g.
keratohyaline g.
Langerhans g.
pigment g.

G

NOTES

granule *(continued)*
  rod g.
  scintillating g.
granuliformis
  degeneratio hyaloidea g.
granulocytic sarcoma
granuloma
  caseating orbital g.
  cholesterol g.
  chorioretinal g.
  choroidal g.
  conjunctival g.
  diffuse g.
  discrete g.
  eosinophilic g.
  focal g.
  g. gangraenescens
  intracranial g.
  g. iridis
  lethal midline g.
  midline g.
  noncaseating conjunctival g.
  orbital g.
  palisading orbital g.
  peripheral g.
  pyogenic g.
  reparative giant cell g.
  sclerosing orbital g.
  zonal g.
granulomatous
  g. anterior uveitis
  g. endophthalmitis
  g. inflammatory cell
  g. iridocyclitis
  g. panuveitis
  g. vasculitis
granulosus
  Echinococcus g.
graph
  shadow g.
grating
  g. acuity
  Arden g.
  Cambridge low-contrast g.
  sinusoidal g.
Gratiolet radiating fiber
Graves
  G. disease
  G. hyperthyroidism
  G. ophthalmopathy
  G. orbitography
  G. orbitopathy
  G. strabismus

gravidarum
  retinitis g.
gravidic
  g. retinitis
  g. retinopathy
gravid retinitis
gravis
  fulminant myasthenia g.
  myasthenia g.
Grawitz tumor
gray
  g. atrophy
  g. cataract
  g. line
  g. plaque
graying
  g. of macula
  macular g.
grayline incision
gray-scale ultrasonogram
Grayson corneal forceps
Grayson-Wilbrandt anterior corneal dystrophy
Gray Standardized Oral Reading Paragraphs
Grayton corneal forceps
gray-white corneal scar
Grazer blepharoplasty forceps
greater
  g. ring of iris
  g. superficial petrosal nerve
  g. superficial temporal artery biopsy
  g. wing of sphenoid
Greaves operation
green
  g. blindness
  G. calipers
  G. capsule forceps
  g. cataract
  G. cataract
  G. cataract knife
  G. chalazion forceps
  G. corneal dissector
  G. corneal knife
  G. corneal marker
  G. curette
  G. double spatula
  G. eye shield
  G. fixation forceps
  indocyanine g. (ICG)
  G. iris replacer
  g. laser

G. lens spatula
G. muscle hook
G. muscle tucker
G. needle holder
G. refractor
G. replacer spatula
G. strabismus hook
G. strabismus tucker
Topographic Scanning System/indocyanine g. (TopSS/ICG)
G. trephine
g. vision
Green-Kenyon corneal marker
Greig syndrome
Grey-Hess screen
grid
    Amsler g.
    Bernell g.
    g. laser photocoagulation (GLP)
    g. method
Gridley intraocular lens
Grieshaber
    G. blade
    G. calibrated trephine
    G. corneal trephine
    G. diamond coated forceps
    G. endoilluminator
    G. flexible iris retractor
    G. internal limiting membrane forceps
    G. iris forceps
    G. keratome
    G. micro-bipolar coagulator
    G. needle holder
    G. opthalmic needle
    G. power injector system
    G. ruby knife
    G. three-function manipulator
    G. two-function manipulator
    G. ultrasharp knife
    G. ultrasharp microsurgery instrument
    G. vertical cutting scissors
    G. vitreous scissors

Griffith sign
Grimsdale operation
grinding
    bicentric g.
    slab-off g.
grip
    scleral g.
grittiness
Grocco sign
Grocott-Gomori methenamine silver nitrate (GMS)
Groenholm
    G. refractor
    G. retractor
Groenouw
    G. corneal dystrophy
    G. type I dystrophy
    G. type II dystrophy
    G. type II maculopathy
Grolman photographic system
Grönblad-Strandberg syndrome
groove
    Blessig g.
    corneal lamellar g.
    corneoscleral g.
    infraorbital g.
    lacrimal g.
    lamellar g.
    limbal g.
    nasolacrimal g.
    optic g.
    g. suture
    Verga lacrimal g.
grooved
    g. director
    g. incision
    g. silicone implant
    g. silicone sponge
Gross
    G. retractor
    G. stercopsis
Grossmann operation
ground glass sheet
group
    nonocular muscle g.
growth-onset diabetes

G

NOTES

growth retardation, alopecia,
  pseudoanodontia, and optic
  atrophy (GAPO)
GRT
  giant retinal tear
Gruber syndrome
Gruening magnet
Grunert spur
GS
  Optisol GS
GS-9
  G. blade
  G. needle
GSA-9 blade
GSL
  goniosynechialysis
gt
  gutta (drop)
gtt
  guttae (drops)
guard
  cataract knife g.
  ether g.
  eye knife g.
  forceps g.
  Hansen keratome g.
  keratome g.
  knife g.
  scalpel g.
Guardian scalpel with myoguard
  depth resistor
Guarnieri inclusion body
Gudden
  commissure of G.
  G. commissure
Gueder keratoplasty needle
Guibor
  G. chart
  G. duct tube
  G. shield
  G. Silastic tube
guide
  Clayman g.
  Eschenbach low vision
    rehabilitation g.
  vacuum-centering g.
guillotine
  g. cutting tip
  g. vitrectomy instrument
guillotine-type cutter
Guimaraes ophthalmic spatula
Guist
  G. enucleation hemostat

G. enucleation scissors
G. fixation forceps
G. speculum
G. sphere implant
Guist-Bloch speculum
Gullstrand
  G. law
  G. lens
  G. loupe
  G. ophthalmoscope
  G. reduced eye
  G. schematic eye
  G. six-surface eye model
  G. slit lamp
gun-barrel field defect
Gunderson
  G. conjunctival flap
  G. muscle forceps
Gunn
  G. dot
  G. jaw-winking phenomenon
  G. pupil
  G. pupillary reflex
  G. sign
  G. syndrome
gustatolacrimal reflex
gustatory lacrimation
Guthrie fixation hook
gutta, pl. guttae
  g. amaurosis
  g. serena
gutta (drop) (gt)
guttae (drops) (gtt)
guttat.
  guttatim (drop by drop)
guttata
  absent g.
  g. of cornea
  cornea g.
  corneal g.
guttate choroidopathy
guttatim (drop by drop) (guttat.)
gutter dystrophy
guttering
  corneal g.
  limbal g.
  limbus g.
Gutzeit dacryostomy operation
guy suture
Guyton
  G. corneal transplant trephine
  G. electrode
  G. ptosis operation

Guyton-Clark fragment forceps
Guyton-Friedenwald suture
Guyton-Lundsgaard
    G.-L. cataract knife
    G.-L. keratome
    G.-L. scalpel
    G.-L. sclerotome
Guyton-Maumenee speculum
Guyton-Minkowski potential acuity meter
Guyton-Noyes
    G.-N. fixation
    G.-N. fixation forceps
Guyton-Park
    G.-P. eye speculum
    G.-P. lid speculum

GV
    Healon GV
gymnastics
    ocular g.
gyrata
    atrophia g.
gyrate
    g. atrophy
    g. atrophy of choroid and retina
gyrus
    angular g.

NOTES

G

H
 hyperopia
 hyperopic
 hyperphoria
 H band
HA
 headache
 hydroxyapatite
Haab
 H. knife needle
 H. magnet
 H. reflex
 H. scleral resection knife
 H. stria
Haag-Streit
 H.-S. distometer
 H.-S. fluorescein dye
 H.-S. keratometer
 H.-S. ophthalmometer
 H.-S. slit lamp
habit
 glaucomatous h.
Hadeco intraoperative Doppler
Haefliger cleaver
haemolyticus
 Staphylococcus h.
Haemophilus
 H. aegypticus
 H. influenzae
haemorrhagica
 retinitis h.
Haenel symptom
Haenig irrigating scissors
Hagberg-Santavuori syndrome
Hague cataract lamp
Haidinger brush test
Haik implant
hair
 h. bulb incubation test
 h. follicle tumor
halation
Halberg
 H. contact lens forceps
 H. indirect ophthalmoscope
 H. trial clip
 H. trial clip occluder
**Halberstaedter-Prowazek inclusion
 body**
Haldrone
half-glass spectacles

half-moon syndrome
half vision
HALK
 hyperopic automated lamellar
 keratoplasty
Hallauer
 H. glasses
 H. spectacles
Hall dermatome
Haller
 circle of H.
 H. layer
 H. membrane
halleri
 circulus arteriosus h.
**Hallermann-Streiff-Francois
 syndrome**
Hallermann-Streiff syndrome
Hallervorden-Spatz syndrome
Hallgren syndrome
Hallpike maneuver
hallucination
 hypnagogic h.
 hypnopompic h.
 irritative h.
 migrainous h.
 peduncular h.
 release h.
 visual h.
 h. with eye closure
hallucinogenic
halo
 h. demonstrator
 Fick h.
 glaucomatous h.
 parafoveal h.
 h. phenomenon
 pigmentary h.
 h. saturninus
 senescent h.
 senile h.
 h. sheathing
 h. symptom
 h. vision
 visual h.
halogen
 h. Finhoff transilluminator
 h. ophthalmoscope
halogenated hydroxyquinoline
halogram

H

halometer
halometry
haloscope
    phase difference h.
halothane
Halpin operation
Halsey needle holder
Halsted
    H. curved mosquito clamp
    H. curved mosquito hemostatic
    forceps
    H. hemostat
    H. strabismus scissors
    H. straight mosquito clamp
Haltia-Santavuori type of Batten
    syndrome
hamartoblastoma
hamartoma
    astrocytic h.
    glial-neural h.
    melanocytic h.
    orbit h.
    orbital h.
    uveal tract h.
    vascular h.
hamartomatosis
hamartomatous lesion
hammock pupil
hamular procedure
hamulus
    h. lacrimalis
    trochlear h.
hand
    h. motion (HM)
    h. movement
hand-held
    h.-h. eye magnet
    h.-h. fundus camera
    h.-h. Hruby lens
    h.-h. magnifying reticle
    h.-h. rotary prism
    h.-h. trephine
handle
    Beaver h.
    DORC h.
    Elliot trephine h.
    Storz h.
hand motion at 3 feet (HM/3ft)
hand-motion visual acuity test
hand-movement visual acuity test
handpiece
    Avit h.
    B-mode h.

    Cavitron I/A h.
    fragmentation/aspiration h.
    Kelman irrigating h.
    Lightning high-speed
    vitrectomy h.
    MicroSeal ophthalmic h.
    Packer Wick extrusion h.
    phacoemulsification h.
    ProFinesse II ultrasonic h.
    SITE Phaco II h.
    soft-tipped extrusion h.
    Storz h.
    Vit Commander h.
Handy non-mydriatic video fundus
    camera
Hanna trephine
Hannover canal
hansatome
    Chiron h.
Hansen
    H. keratome
    H. keratome guard
haplopia
haploscope
    mirror h.
haploscopic
    h. test
    h. vision
haptic
    h. angulation
    h. contact
    lamellar h.
    h. loop
    h. plate lens
    Slant h.
    violet h.
Harada
    H. disease
    H. syndrome
Harada-Ito procedure
hard
    h. cataract
    h. contact lens (HCL)
    h. drusen
    h. exudate
hardened spectacle lens
hardening of lens
Harder gland
harderian gland
Hardesty
    H. tendon hook
    H. tenotomy hook
hard-finger tension

Hardy
   H. lensometer
   H. punch
Hardy-Rand-Ritter
   H.-R.-R. pseudoisochromatic
     plate
   H.-R.-R. screening plate
   H.-R.-R. test
hare's eye
Harman
   H. eye dressing
   H. fixation forceps
   H. operation
harmonious
   h. abnormal retinal
     correspondence
   h. retinal correspondence
Harms
   H. corneal forceps
   H. trabeculotome
   H. trabeculotomy probe
   H. tying forceps
Harms-Dannheim trabeculotomy
operation
Harms-Tubingen tying forceps
Harrington
   H. erysiphake
   H. retractor
   H. tonometer
Harrington-Flocks
   H.-F. multiple pattern
   H.-F. test
Harrison
   H. retractor
   H. scissors
Harrison-Stein nomogram
Hartinger Coincidence
refractionometer
Hartmann
   H. clamp
   H. hemostatic forceps
   H. mosquito hemostatic forceps
Hart pediatric three-mirror lens
Hartstein
   H. irrigating/aspirating unit
   H. irrigating iris retractor

   H. irrigator
   H. refractor
Hashimoto thyroiditis
Hasner
   H. fold
   H. lid forceps
   H. operation
   valve of H.
   H. valve
Hassall body
Hassall-Henle
   H.-H. body
   H.-H. wart
hay fever conjunctivitis
Hay-Wells syndrome
haze
   aerial h.
   corneal h.
   epithelial punctate h.
   interface h.
   late-onset corneal h.
   reticular h.
   stromal h.
   subepithelial corneal h.
   vitreous h.
HBO
   hyperbaric oxygen therapy
HCL
   hard contact lens
HCl
   hydrochloride
   antazoline phosphate and
     naphazoline HCl
   apraclonidine HCl
   betaxolol HCl
   carteolol HCl
   dapiprazole HCl
   dipivefrin HCl
   Duranest HCl
   epinephrine HCl
   levobunolol HCl
   levocabastine HCl
   Marcaine HCl
   mepivacaine HCl
   naphazoline HCl
   pheniramine maleate and
     naphazoline HCl

NOTES

H

HCl *(continued)*
    pilocarpine HCl
    proparacaine HCl
head
    h. mirror
    h. nystagmus
    optic nerve h. (ONH)
    h. tremor
headache (HA)
    brain tumor h.
    cluster h.
    cough h.
    migraine h.
    muscle contraction h.
    postherpetic h.
    posttraumatic h.
    retroorbital h.
    sinus h.
head-nodding
headrest
    Gibralter h.
head-tilt test
head-turning reflex
Healon
    H. cannula
    H. GV
    H. solution
hearing loss
heater
    broad-spectrum h. (BSH)
    infrared h.
heat-generated cataract
Heath
    H. chalazion curette
    H. chalazion forceps
    H. dilator
    H. expressor
heat-ray cataract
heavy
    h. eye
    h. ion irradiation
    h. ion radiation
Hebra
    H. blade
    H. curette
    H. hook
hedger cataract
Hedges Corneal Wetting Pak
Heerfordt syndrome
hefilcon A
Heidelberg
    H. laser tomographic scanner
    H. retinal angiography

    H. retinal flowmeter
    H. retinal tomography
    H. retina tomograph (HRT)
Heidenhain syndrome
height
    buckle h.
    contact lens h.
    orbital h.
    peripapillary retinal h.
    sagittal h.
Heine
    H. cyclodialysis
    H. Lambda 100 retinometer
    H. operation
    H. penlight
Heisrath operation
helcoma
helicoid
    h. choroidopathy
    h. peripapillary atrophy
helium-ion aiming laser
helium-neon
    h.-n. aiming laser
    h.-n. neon beam
Helmholtz
    H. keratometer
    H. line
    H. ophthalmoscope
    H. schematic eye
    H. theory of accommodation
    H. theory of color vision
helminthic disease
helper/inducer T cell
Helveston
    H. Great Big Barbie retractor
    H. scleral marking ruler
Helvestoon hook
hemangioblastoma
    optic nerve h.
hemangioendothelioma
    orbital h.
hemangioma
    capillary h.
    cavernous h.
    choroidal h.
    conjunctival h.
    episcleral h.
    eyelid strawberry h.
    facial h.
    orbital h.
    periorbital h.
    racemose h.
    strawberry h.

uveal tract h.
venous h.
hemangiomatosis
racemose h.
hemangiopericytoma
lacrimal sac h.
meningeal h.
orbital h.
hematic cyst
hematogenous
h. metastasis
h. pigmentation
hematoma
orbital h.
subdural h.
hematopoietic metastasis
hematopsia
hemeralopia
hemeranopia
hemiachromatopsia
hemiakinetopsia
hemi-alexia
hemiamblyopia
hemianopia
altitudinal h.
bilateral h.
checkerboard h.
homonymous h.
nasal h.
postgeniculate congenital
homonymous h.
hemianopic
h. dyslexia
h. glasses
h. scotoma
h. spectacles
hemianopsia, hemianopia
absolute h.
altitudinal h.
bilateral homonymous h.
binasal h.
binocular h.
bitemporal fugax h.
complete h.
congenital h.
congruous h.
crossed h.

double homonymous h.
equilateral h.
geniculate h.
heteronymous h.
homonymous h.
horizontal h.
incomplete h.
incongruous h.
lateral h.
lower h.
nasal h.
quadrant h.
quadrantic h.
relative h.
temporal h.
true h.
unilateral h.
uniocular h.
upper h.
vertical h.
hemianoptic
hemianosmia
hemiastigmatism
hemichiasma
hemichromatopsia
hemicrania
hemicraniosis
hemi-CRVO
hemifacial
h. atrophy
h. blepharospasm
h. flush
h. spasm
hemifield
H. glaucoma test
h. slide phenomenon
hemimicropsia
hemiopalgia
hemiopia
hemiopic
h. hypoplasia
h. pupillary reaction
hemiplegia
alternating oculomotor h.
hemiplegic migraine
hemiscotosis
hemi-seesaw nystagmus

NOTES

H

213

hemisensory
  h. deficit
  h. loss
hemisphere
  cerebellar h.
  h. eye implant
  h. projection perimetry
  silicone h.
hemispherical
hemocytic mesenchyme
hemolytic glaucoma
hemophthalmia
hemophthalmos
hemophthalmus
hemorrhage
  arachnoid h.
  blot h.
  blot-and-dot h.
  caudate h.
  cerebellar h.
  choroidal h.
  conjunctival h.
  delayed massive
    suprachoroidal h.
  disk drusen h.
  dot h.
  dot-and-blot h.
  eight-ball h.
  expulsive h.
  flame-shaped h.
  intralenticular h.
  intraocular h.
  intraretinal h.
  intraventricular h. (IVH)
  intravitreal h.
  kissing suprachoroidal h.
  nerve fiber layer h.
  ochre h.
  orbital h.
  peripheral intraretinal h.
  premacular subhyaloid h.
  prepapillary h.
  preretinal h.
  punctate h.
  retinal h.
  retinopathy h.
  retrobulbar h.
  retrohyaloid premacular h.
  round h.
  salmon-patch h.
  splinter disk h.
  subarachnoid h.

  subconjunctival h.
  subhyaloid h.
  subinternal limiting
    membrane h.
  subjunctival h.
  subretinal h.
  suprachoroidal h. (SCH, SH)
  vitreal h.
  vitreous h. (VH)
  vitreous break-through h.
  white-centered h.
  yellow-ochre h.
hemorrhagic
  h. conjunctivitis
  h. disciform lesion
  h. disorder
  h. glaucoma
  h. iritis
  h. retinopathy
  h. RPE
  h. sarcoma
hemorrhagica
  Leber lymphangiectasia h.
hemosiderosis bulbi
hemostat
  Corboy h.
  Guist enucleation h.
  Halsted h.
  Kelly h.
hemostatic forceps
Henderson-Patterson inclusion body
HeNe beam
Henle
  H. body
  H. fiber layer
  fibers of H.
  H. gland
  H. layer of the macula
  H. membrane
  H. wart
henselae
  Bartonella h.
Hensen body
Henson CFS 2000 perimeter
heparan sulfate
heparin
  h. surface-modified intraocular
    lens (HSM)
  h. surface-modified polymethyl
    methacrylate
hepatolenticular degeneration
herapathite

Herbert
  H. operation
  H. peripheral pit
Herbit pit
hereditaria
  atrophia bulborum h.
  degeneratio hyaloideoretinae h.
hereditary
  h. anterior membrane
    dystrophy
  h. benign intraepithelial
    dyskeratosis
  h. benign intraepithelial
    dyskeratosis syndrome
  h. cerebellar ataxia
  h. corneal edema
  h. degeneration
  h. epithelial corneal dystrophy
  h. hemorrhagic macular
    dystrophy
  h. macular dystrophy
  h. optic atrophy
  h. optic atrophy syndrome
  h. optic neuropathy
  h. progressive arthro-
    ophthalmopathy
  h. renal-retinal dysplasia
  h. vitelliform dystrophy
heredity maculopathy
heredodegeneration
  macular h.
heredodegenerative
  h. atrophy
  h. neurologic syndrome
heredofamilial optic atrophy
heredomacular degeneration
Hering
  H. after-image mechanism
  H. law
  H. law of equal innervation
  H. law of equivalent
    innervation
  H. law of motor
    correspondence
  H. test
  H. theory of color vision
Hering-Bielschowsky after-image test

Hering-Hellebrand deviation
Hermann grid illusion
Hermansky-Pudlak syndrome
hernia
  h. of iris
  orbital h.
  vitreous h.
herniation
  hippocampal gyrus h.
  vitreous h.
Herpchek
herpes
  h. corneae
  h. epithelial tropic ulceration
  h. follicular keratoconjunctivitis
  h. iridis
  ocular h.
  h. ophthalmicus
  h. panuveitis
  h. simplex blepharitis
  h. simplex
    blepharoconjunctivitis
  h. simplex cellulitis
  h. simplex conjunctivitis
  h. simplex corneal ulcer
  h. simplex iridocyclitis
  h. simplex keratitis
  h. simplex keratoconjunctivitis
  h. simplex keratouveitis
  h. simplex retinitis
  h. simplex scar
  h. simplex scleritis
  h. simplex uveitis
  h. simplex virus (HSV)
  h. simplex virus type I
  h. zoster conjunctivitis
  h. zoster glaucoma
  h. zoster iridocyclitis
  h. zoster keratitis
  h. zoster keratoconjunctivitis
  h. zoster ophthalmicus
  h. zoster oticus
  h. zoster virus
herpesvirus
herpetic
  H. Eye Disease Study
  h. keratoconjunctivitis

NOTES

H

215

herpetic *(continued)*
  h. metakeratitis
  h. necrotizing retinopathy
  h. ocular disease
  h. ocular infection
  h. stromal keratitis
  h. ulcer
herpetic-fungal keratitis
herpetoid lesion
Herplex
  H. Liquifilm
  H. Qphthalmic
Herrick
  H. lacrimal plug
  H. silicone lacrimal implant
Hersh
  H. LASIK retreatment forceps
  H. LASIK retreatment spatula
Hertel
  H. exophthalmometer
  H. stone forceps
Hertwig-Magendie
  H.-M. phenomenon
  H.-M. syndrome
Hertzog
  H. lens spatula
  H. pliable probe
Hess
  H. diplopia screen
  H. eyelid operation
  H. forceps
  H. ptosis operation
  H. screen test
  H. spoon
Hess-Barraquer forceps
Hessburg
  H. corneal shield
  H. eye shield
  H. intraocular lens glide
  H. lacrimal needle
  H. lens
  H. lens forceps
  H. lens-inserting forceps
  H. subpalpebral lavage system
Hessburg-Barron
  H.-B. suction trephine
  H.-B. vacuum trephine
Hess-Horwitz forceps
Hess-Lee screen
heterochromia
  atrophic h.
  binocular h.
  congenital h.

Fuchs h.
  h. iridis
  h. of iris
monocular h.
simple h.
sympathetic h.
heterochromic
  h. cataract
  h. Fuchs cyclitis
  h. iridocyclitis
  h. uveitis
heterogeneity
  optical h.
heterogeneous
  h. cell
  h. donor material
heterogenous keratoplasty
heterokeratoplasty
heterometropia
heteronymous
  h. diplopia
  h. hemianopsia
  h. image
  h. parallax
heterophoralgia
heterophoria
  h. method
heterophoric position
heterophthalmia, heterophthalmos,
  heterophthalmus
heteropsia
heteroptics
heteroscope
heteroscopy
heterotopia
  cerebral h.
  diabetic macular h.
heterotropia, heterotropy
  circadian h.
  comitant h.
  concomitant h.
  h. maculae
  noncomitant h.
  paralytic h.
heterotropic deviation
Hexadrol
  H. Phosphate
hexafluoride
  h. gas
  sulfur h.
hexagonal keratotomy
hexahydrate
  trisodium phosphonoformate h.

hexametaphosphate
  sodium h.
hexamethonium chloride
hexamidine
Hexon illumination system
hex procedure
hexylcaine
Heyer-Schulte microscope
Heyner
  H. curette
  H. dilator
  H. double cannula
  H. double needle
  H. expressor
  H. forceps
HGM
  H. argon green laser
  H. intravitreal laser
  H. ophthalmic laser
HHH
  hyperornithinemia,
  hyperammonemia, and
  homocitrullinuria
HHH syndrome
Hidex glass lens
Hiff
  H. operation
  H. ptosis
high
  h. convex
  h. hyperopia
  h. intensity illuminator
  h. myopia
high-add bifocals
higher visual function test
high-frequency ultrasound
  biomicroscope
high-gain
  h.-g. artifact
  h.-g. digital ultrasound
Highlight spectral indirect
  ophthalmoscope
High-Lite glass
high-magnification (HM)
high-pass resolution perimetry

high-tension
  h.-t. glaucoma (HTG)
  h.-t. suturing technique
high-vacuum phacoemulsification
Hildreth
  H. cautery
  H. electrocautery
Hill
  H. operation
  H. procedure
  H. retractor
Hillis
  H. refractor
  H. retractor
Hilton
  H. self-retaining infusion
  cannula
  H. sutureless infusion cannula
hinged corneal flap
Hippel
  H. disease
  H. operation
Hippel-Lindau syndrome
hippocampal gyrus herniation
hippocampus
Hirschberg
  H. magnet
  H. method
  H. reflex
  H. reflex assessment
  H. test
Hirschman
  H. iris hook
  H. lens forceps
  H. lens-inserting forceps
  H. microiris hook
  H. spatula
  H. speculum
Hismanal
histiocytic
  h. disorder
  h. lymphoma
  h. tumor
Histoacryl
  H. glue
  H. glue patch

NOTES

H

histolyticum
   Clostridium h.
Histoplasma
   H. capsulatum
   H. duboisii
histoplasmic choroiditis
histoplasmosis
   h. maculopathy
   ocular h.
   presumed ocular h.
   h. syndrome
history
   neuro-ophthalmologic case h.
   past ocular h. (POH)
histo spot
HIV-specific antibody
Hl
   latent hyperopia
HLA-A29 antigen
HLA-B15 antigen
HLA-B27 antigen
HLA-B5 antigen
HLA-B7 antigen
HLA-DR4 antigen
HM
   hand motion
   high-magnification
Hm
   manifest hyperopia
HM/3ft
   hand motion at 3 feet
HMS Liquifilm
Hoaglund sign
hockey-end temple
Hoffer
   H. forward-cutting knife
   cannula
   H. optical center marker
Hoffer-Colenbrander formula
Hoffer-Laseridge intraocular lens
Hogan operation
holder
   Alabama-Green needle h.
   Arruga needle h.
   baby Barraquer needle h.
   Barraquer curved h.
   Barraquer needle h.
   Belin double-ended needle h.
   Birks Mark II micro cross-action h.
   Birks Mark II micro lock-type needle h.
   Birks Mark II needle h.

   Bodkin thread h.
   Boyce needle h.
   Boynton needle h.
   Castroviejo-Barraquer needle h.
   Castroviejo blade h.
   Castroviejo-Kalt needle h.
   Castroviejo needle h.
   Clerf needle h.
   Cohen needle h.
   Corboy needle h.
   Crile needle h.
   Dean knife h.
   Derf needle h.
   Ellis needle h.
   eye h.
   French needle h.
   Gifford needle h.
   goniotomy needle h.
   Green needle h.
   Grieshaber needle h.
   Halsey needle h.
   Ilg microneedle h.
   Ilg needle h.
   I-tech cannula h.
   I-tech needle h.
   Jaffe needle h.
   Kalt needle h.
   Keeler-Catford microjaws needle h.
   McIntyre fish-hook needle h.
   McPherson needle h.
   needle h.
   Neumann razor blade fragment h.
   Paton needle h.
   Schaefer sponge h.
   Stangel modified Barraquer microsurgical needle h.
   Stephenson needle h.
   Stevens needle h.
   Tilderquist needle h.
   Troutman needle h.
   Vickers needle h.
   Webster needle h.
holding clip
hole
   atrophic h.
   cystoid macular h.
   iatrogenic retinal h.
   idiopathic macular cyst and h.
   impending macular h.
   lamellar h.
   macular h. (MH)

operculated h.
retinal h.
senescent macular h.
Holladay
H. contrast acuity test
H. formula
H. posterior capsule polisher
Hollenhorst plaque
hollowing and shadowing
hollow-sphere implant
Holmes-Adie
H.-A. pupil
H.-A. tonic pupil syndrome
Holmgren
H. color test
H. method
H. skein
H. wool skein test
holmium
h. laser
h. laser sclerostomy
h. YAG laser sclerectomy
Holofax Oxford retroillumination cataract camera
Holth
H. forceps
H. iridencleisis
H. operation
H. scleral punch
H. sclerectomy
Holthouse-Batten superficial choroiditis
Holt-Oram syndrome
Holzknecht unit
Homatrocel
homatropine
h. hydrobromide
Isopto H.
h. refraction
Homén syndrome
Homer-Wright rosette
hominis
Staphylococcus h.
homocitrullinuria
hyperornithinemia, hyperammonemia, and h. (HHH)

homogeneous donor material
homogenous keratoplasty
homokeratoplasty
homonymous
h. crescent
h. diplopia
h. field defect
h. hemianopia
h. hemianopic scotoma
h. hemianopsia
h. hemiopic hypoplasia
h. hemioptic hypoplasia
h. image
h. parallax
h. quadrantanopsia
homoplastic keratomileusis
homotropic antibody
Honan
H. balloon
H. cuff
H. manometer
honey bee lens
honeycomb
h. dystrophy
h. macula
hook
Amenabar discission h.
anchor h.
angled discission h.
Azar lens-manipulating h.
Berens scleral h.
Birks Mark II h.
boat h.
Bonn microiris h.
Catalano muscle h.
corneal h.
Crawford h.
Culler muscle h.
discission h.
Drews-Sato suture-pickup h.
expressor h.
h. expressor
Fenzel angled manipulating h.
Fenzel insertion h.
Fenzel lens-manipulating h.
Fenzel manipulating h.
Fink oblique muscle h.

NOTES

H

hook *(continued)*
  fixation h.
  flat h.
  Fukasaku pupil snapper h.
  Gass muscle h.
  Gass retinal detachment h.
  Graefe strabismus h.
  Graether button h.
  Graether mushroom h.
  Green muscle h.
  Green strabismus h.
  Guthrie fixation h.
  Hardesty tendon h.
  Hardesty tenotomy h.
  Hebra h.
  Helvestoon h.
  Hirschman iris h.
  Hirschman microiris h.
  Hunkeler ball-point h.
  iris h.
  Jaeger h.
  Jaffe lens-manipulating h.
  Jaffe microiris h.
  Jameson muscle h.
  Katena boat h.
  Kennerdell muscle h.
  Kennerdell nerve h.
  Kirby muscle h.
  Knapp iris h.
  Kratz K push-pull iris h.
  Kuglen manipulating h.
  Laqua black line retinal h.
  Maidera-Stern suture h.
  Manson double-ended
    strabismus h.
  Maumenee iris h.
  McIntyre irrigating h.
  McReynolds lid-retracting h.
  muscle h.
  Nugent h.
  oblique muscle h.
  Ochsner h.
  O'Connor flat h.
  O'Connor muscle h.
  O'Connor sharp h.
  O'Connor tenotomy h.
  ophthalmic h.
  Osher h.
  Praeger iris h.
  retinal detachment h.
  Russian four-pronged
    fixation h.
  scleral h.

  Scobee oblique muscle h.
  sharp h.
  Sheets microiris h.
  Shepard microiris h.
  Shepard reversed iris h.
  Sinskey lens h.
  Sinskey lens-manipulating h.
  Sinskey microiris h.
  Sinskey microlens h.
  skin h.
  Smith expressor h.
  Smith lid h.
  h. spatula
  spatula h.
  squint h.
  Stamler side-port fixation h.
  Stevens tenotomy h.
  St. Martin-Franceschetti
    cataract h.
  strabismus h.
  suture-pickup h.
  Tennant anchor lens-
    insertion h.
  Tennant lens-manipulating h.
  tenotomy h.
  Tomas iris h.
  Tomas suture h.
  twist fixation h.
  Tyrell iris h.
  Visitec angled lens h.
  Visitec corneal suture
    manipulating h.
  Visitec micro double-iris h.
  Visitec microiris h.
  Visitec straight lens h.
  von Graefe muscle h.
  von Graefe strabismus h.
  Wiener corneal h.
  Wiener scleral h.
  Y h.
hook-shaped cataract
hook-type implant
**Hooper Visual Organization Test
  (HVOT)**
Hoopes corneal marker
hop eye
Hopkins rod lens telescope
Horay operation
hordeolum
  external h.
  h. externum
  internal h.

h. internum
h. meibomianum
horizontal
  h. band pallor
  h. cells
  h. deviation
  h. diplopia
  h. gaze
  h. gaze center
  h. hemianopsia
  h. mattress suture
  h. meridian
  h. nystagmus
  h. plane
  h. prism bar
  h. raphe
  h. retinal disparity
horn
  cutaneous h.
  lateral h.
  medial h.
Horner
  H. law
  H. muscle
  H. ptosis
  H. pupil
  H. syndrome
Horner-Bernard syndrome
Horner-Trantas
  H.-T. dot
  H.-T. spot
horopter
  Vieth-Mueller h.
horopteric
horror fusionis
horseshoe tear
Horton syndrome
Horvath operation
Hosford
  H. expressor
  H. lacrimal dilator
  H. spud
Hoskins
  H. beaked Colibri forceps
  H. fine straight forceps
  H. fixation forceps
  H. lens

H. microstraight forceps
H. miniaturized micro straight
  forceps
H. razor blade fragment
H. razor fragment blade
H. straight microiris forceps
H. suture forceps
Hoskins-Barkan goniotomy infant
  lens
Hoskins-Castroviejo corneal scissors
Hoskins-Dallas intraocular lens-
  inserting forceps
Hoskins-Drake implant
Hoskins-Luntz forceps
Hoskins-Skeleton
  H.-S. fine forceps
  H.-S. micro-grooved broad-
    tipped forceps
Hoskins-Westcott tenotomy scissors
hospital
  King Khaled Eye Specialist H.
  (KKESH)
  Wills Eye H.
host
  h. incision
  h. tissue forceps
  h. trephination
host-graft junction
hot eye
Hotz
  H. entropion
  H. entropion operation
Hotz-Anagnostakis operation
Hough drape
House
  H. lacrimal dilator
  H. miniature forceps
  H. myringotomy knife
House-Bellucci alligator scissors
House-Dieter nipper
Houser
  H. cul-de-sac irrigator T-tube
  H. cul-de-sac irrigator tube
House-Urban-Pentax camera
Hovius
  H. canal
  H. circle

NOTES

H

Hovius *(continued)*
  H. membrane
  H. plexus
Howard abrader
Hoya
  H. AR-570 autorefractor
  H. HDR objective
    refractometer
  H. MRM objective
    refractometer
Ho:YAG laser
Hoyt-Spencer triad
H.P. Acthar Gel
HPMC
  hydroxypropyl methylcellulose
HR
  hypertensive retinopathy
HRT
  Heidelberg retina tomograph
Hruby
  H. contact lens
  H. implant
HS
  Pilopine HS
HSM
  heparin surface-modified intraocular
  lens
HSV
  herpes simplex virus
  HSV endotheliitis
  HSV epithelial keratitis
  footprints of HSV
  HSV ocular disease
  HSV stromal disease
  HSV trophic keratopathy
HT
  hypertropia
Ht
  total hyperopia
HTG
  high-tension glaucoma
Hubbard corneoscleral forceps
Huco diamond knife
Hudson line
Hudson-Stähli
  H.-S. line
  H.-S. line of corneal
    pigmentation
hue
  salmon patch h.
  100 h. test
Hueck ligament
28 Hue de Roth test

Huey scissors
Hughes
  H. classification of chemical
  injury
  H. implant
  H. modification of Burch
  technique
  H. operation
  H. tarsoconjunctival flap
human
  h. immunodeficiency virus
  h. leukocyte antigen
  h. T-lymphotropic virus
Hummelsheim
  H. operation
  H. procedure
humor, gen. humoris
  aqueous h.
  h. aquosus
  h. cristallinus
  crystalline h.
  ocular h.
  plasmoid aqueous h.
  vitreous h.
humoral immunity
Humorsol
  H. Ophthalmic
Humphrey
  H. ATLAS Eclipse corneal
  topography system
  H. automatic refractor
  H. B-scan
  H. field analyzer
  H. glaucoma hemifield test
  H. Instruments vision analyzer
  H. Instruments vision analyzer
    overrefraction system
  H. lens analyzer
  H. Mastervue corneal
    topography system
  H. perimeter
  H. retina imager
  H. ultrasonic pachometer
  H. visual field analyzer
Humphriss binocular balance
Hunkeler
  H. ball-point hook
  H. frown incision marker
  H. lens
Hunt
  H. chalazion forceps
  H. chalazion scissors
Hunter-Hurler syndrome

Hunter syndrome
Hunt-Transley operation
Hurler
   H. disease
   H. syndrome
Hurler-Scheie
   H.-S. compound
   H.-S. syndrome
hurricane keratopathy
Huschke valve
Hutchinson
   H. facies
   H. patch
   H. pupil
   H. sign
   H. syndrome
   H. triad
Hutchinson-Tays central guttate
   choroiditis
huygenian eyepiece
HVOT
   Hooper Visual Organization Test
hyaline
   h. artery
   h. body
   h. degeneration
   h. fungus
   h. mass
   h. material
   h. membrane
   h. plaque
hyalinosis cutis et mucosae
hyalitis
   h. of anterior membrane
   asteroid h.
   h. punctata
   punctate h.
   h. suppurativa
   suppurative h.
Hyall
hyaloid
   h. artery
   h. asteroid
   h. body
   h. canal
   h. clouding
   h. corpuscle

   h. face
   h. fossa
   h. membrane detachment
   h. posterior membrane
   h. system
hyaloidal fibrovascular proliferation
hyaloidea
   fossa h.
   membrana h.
   stella lentis h.
hyaloideocapsular ligament
hyaloideoretinal degeneration
hyaloideus
   canalis h.
hyaloiditis
hyaloidotomy
hyalomucoid
hyalonyxis
hyalosis
   asteroid h.
   punctate h.
hyaluronate
   h. sodium
   h. sodium with chondroitin
Hyde
   H. astigmatism ruler
   H. corneal forceps
   H. double-curved forceps
   H. irrigating/aspirating unit
   H. irrigator/aspirator unit
Hydeltrasol
Hyde-Osher keratometric ruler
Hydracon contact lens
Hydrasoft contact lens
Hydrate Injection
hydration
   stromal h.
hydraulic retinal reattachment
hydroa vacciniforme
hydroblepharon
hydrobromide
   homatropine h.
   hydroxyamphetamine h.
HydroBrush keratome
Hydrocare preserved saline
hydrochloride (HCl)
   apraclonidine h.

NOTES

H

223

hydrochloride *(continued)*
  benoxinate h.
  betaxolol h.
  carteolol h.
  ciprofloxacin h.
  cocaine h.
  cyclopentolate h.
  dapiprazole h.
  diphenhydramine h.
  dorzolamide h.
  hydromorphone h.
  levobunolol h.
  levocabastine h.
  lidocaine h.
  lignocaine h.
  meperidine h.
  naloxone h.
  Neo-Synephrine H.
  oxymorphone h.
  papaverine h.
  phenacaine h.
  phencyclidine h.
  phenmetrazine h.
  phenoxybenzamine h.
  phenylephrine h.
  phenylpropanolamine h.
  piperocaine h.
  procaine h.
  proparacaine h.
  protriptyline h.
  quinacrine h.
  tetracaine h.
  tetrahydrozoline h.
  thioridazine h.
  thymoxamine h.
  trifluoperazine h.
  trifluperidol h.
  tyramine h.
hydrocortisone
  h. acetate
  bacitracin, neomycin, polymyxin
    B, and h.
  chloramphenicol, polymyxin B,
    and h.
  Chloromycetin/H.
  neomycin and h.
  neomycin, polymyxin B,
    and h.
  oxytetracycline and h.
  h. suspension
Hydrocorton Acetate
Hydrocortone
  H. Phosphate

Hydrocurve II lens
hydrodelamination
hydrodelineation
hydrodiascope
hydrodissection
  cortical cleaving h.
  Kellan h.
hydrodissector
  cortical cleaving h.
  Pearce nucleus h.
hydrodissector/rotator
  5195 nucleus h.
hydrogel
  h. contact lens
Hydrokeratome Mark I
hydrolysis
  Koch nucleus h.
  h. of solution
hydrometric chamber
hydromorphone hydrochloride
Hydron
  American H.
  H. lens
Hydronol
hydrophila
  Aeromonas h.
hydrophilic
  h. contact lens
hydrophobic contact lens
hydrophthalmia, hydrophthalmos,
  hydrophthalmus
  anterior h.
  posterior h.
  total h.
hydropic degeneration
hydrops of iris
hydroquinone
Hydrosight lens
hydrostatic gradient
Hydroview lens
hydroxide
  calcium h.
  potassium h. (KOH)
  sodium h.
hydroxocobalamin
hydroxyamphetamine
  h. hydrobromide
  h. and tropicamide
hydroxyapatite (HA)
  h. ocular implant
  h. orbital implant
hydroxychloroquine sulfate
hydroxyethyl cellulose

hydroxyethylmethacrylate
hydroxymethylprogesterone
hydroxypropyl methylcellulose
(HPMC)
hydroxyquinoline
    halogenated h.
hydroxystilbamidine isethionate
hydroxyzine pamoate
Hy-Flow
hyfrecator
hygroblepharic
hygroma
    perioptic h.
Hygroton
hyicus
    Staphylococcus h.
Hylashield
Hymenolepis nana
hyoscine
    Isopto H.
    scopolamine h.
hyoscyamine
hyperactivity
    sympathetic h.
hyperacuity
hyperacute conjunctivitis
hyperbaric oxygen therapy (HBO)
hyperbolic glasses
hypercalcemic
hyperdeviation
    alternate h.
    dissociated h.
hyperemia
    ciliary h.
    conjunctival h.
hyperemic
hyperesophoria
hyperesthesia
    optic h.
    h. optica
hypereuryopia
hyperexophoria
hyperfluorescence
    choroidal h.
    stippled h.
hyperfluorescent window defect
hypergranulation tissue

hyperintense foci image
hyperkalemic periodic paralysis
hyperkeratotic
    h. disorder
    h. plaque
hypermaturation
hypermature
    h. cataract
    h. lens
hypermetrope
hypermetropia
    index h.
hypermetropia (*var. of* hyperopia)
hypermetropic astigmatism
hyperope
hyperophthalmopathic syndrome
hyperopia, hypermetropia (H)
    absolute h.
    axial h.
    curvature h.
    facultative h.
    high h.
    index h.
    h. index
    latent h. (Hl)
    manifest h. (Hm)
    refractive h.
    relative h.
    total h. (Ht)
hyperopic (H)
    h. ablation
    h. astigmatism
    h. automated lamellar
      keratoplasty (HALK)
    h. LASIK
    h. shift
hyperornithinemia
    h., hyperammonemia, and
      homocitrullinuria (HHH)
hyperphoria (H)
    circumduction h.
    left h.
    right h.
hyperplasia
    epithelial h.
    goblet cell h.
    iris epithelial h.

NOTES

H

hyperplasia *(continued)*
    lymphoid h.
    pseudoepitheliomatous h.
    pseudosarcomatous
        endothelial h.
    retinal epithelial pigment h.
hyperplastic
    h. primary vitreous
    h. vitreous
hyperpresbyopia
hyperreflective tissue
Hypersal
hypersecretion
    h. glaucoma
hypersensitivity reaction
hyperteloric
hypertelorism
    canthal h.
    ocular h.
    orbital h.
hypertension
    adrenal h.
    arterial h.
    essential h.
    idiopathic intracranial h. (IIH)
    intracranial h.
    malignant h.
    ocular h. (OHT)
hypertensive
    h. encephalopathy
    h. iridocyclitis
    h. neuroretinopathy
    h. oculopathy
    h. retinitis
    h. retinopathy (HR)
hyperthermia
    malignant h.
    microwave h.
hyperthyroidism
    Graves h.
    ophthalmic h.
hyperthyroid stare
hypertonia oculi
hypertonic
    h. drops
    h. osmotherapy
    h. saline
    h. solution
hypertrophic
    h. dendriform epithelial lesion
    h. interstitial neuropathy
    h. rhinitis

hypertrophy
    epithelial h.
    follicular h.
    gelatinous-appearing limbal h.
    giant papillary h. (GPH)
    papillary conjunctival h.
    pigment epithelial h.
    retinal pigment epithelial h.
    RP h.
hypertropia (HT)
    alternating h.
    constant h.
    dissociated double h. (DDHT)
    double dissociated h.
    flick h.
    left h. (LHT)
    right h.
hyperviscosity
    h. syndrome
hyphema
    black-ball h.
    eight-ball h.
    layered h.
    microscopic h.
    postsurgical h.
    spontaneous h.
    total h.
    traumatic h.
    uveitis glaucoma h. (UGH)
hyphemia
hypnagogic hallucination
hypnopompic hallucination
hypocalcemic cataract
Hypoclear
hypocyclosis
hypoesophoria
hypoesthesia
    corneal h.
hypoexophoria
hypoglobus
hypoglycemic cataract
hypointense foci image
hypointensity
hypokalemic periodic paralysis
hypometric saccade
hypoorbitism
hypophoria
hypophyseal artery
hypopigmentation
    oculocutaneous h.
hypoplasia
    bow-tie h.
    hemiopic h.

homonymous hemiopic h.
homonymous hemioptic h.
macular h.
optic nerve h.
segmental h.
thymic h.
hypoplastic disk
hypopyon
h. keratitis
keratoiritis h.
recurrent h.
sterile h.
h. ulcer
hyposcleral
HypoTears
H. PF Solution
H. Solution
hypotelorism
ocular h.
orbital h.
hypotension
intracranial h.
spontaneous intracranial h.
hypotensive retinopathy
hypothalami
pars optica h.
hypothalamic glioma
hypothalamic-pituitary-thyroid axis
hypothalamus
hypothesis
Knudson h.
Lyon h.
h. testing

hypothyroidism
hypotonia, hypotony
h. oculi
hypotonic solution
hypotonus
hypotony (*var. of* hypotonia)
bilateral h.
essential h.
ocular h.
persistent postdrainage h.
(PPH)
hypotropia
alternating h.
constant h.
hypoxia
orbital h.
retinal h.
hypoxic eyeball syndrome
hypsiconchous
Hyrexin-50 Injection
hysteric
h. amaurosis
h. amblyopia
h. field
hysterical
h. amblyopia
h. blindness
h. constricted field
h. nystagmus
hysteropia
Hyzine-50

NOTES

H

I
  luminous intensity
I&A
  irrigating-aspirating
  irrigation-aspiration
  irrigation and aspiration
  Simcoe I&A system
I/A
  irrigation/aspiration
  I/A machine
Ialo photocoagulator
ianthinopsia
iatrogenic
  i. keratoconus
  i. limbal stem cell deficiency
  i. retinal break
  i. retinal hole
  i. retinal tear
ICAM-1 antigen
ICaps
  I. ocular vitamins
  I. Plus
  I. TR dietary supplement
ICCE
  intracapsular cataract extraction
ICD
  intercanthal distance
ICE
  iridocorneal endothelial
  iridocorneal endothelial syndrome
  ICE syndrome
ice
  i. ball
  i. test
ICG
  indocyanine green
  ICG angiography
ICGA
  indocyanine green angiography
I-Chlor
ichthyosis
  congenital i.
  i. cornea
ICK
  infectious crystalline keratopathy
ICL
  implantable contact lens
ICP
  intracranial pressure

ICSC
  idiopathic central serous
  chorioretinopathy
icteric
icterus
  scleral i.
IDDM
  insulin-dependent diabetes mellitus
identical point
identification acuity
IDI corneoscope
idiocy
  amaurotic i.
  amaurotic familial i.
idiopathic
  i. acquired retinal telangiectasia
  i. arteritis of Takayasu
  i. central serous
  chorioretinopathy (ICSC)
  i. congenital esotropia
  i. corneal endotheliopathy
  i. demyelinating optic neuritis
  i. epiretinal membrane (IERM)
  i. facial palsy
  i. inflammatory pseudotumor
  i. intracranial hypertension
  (IIH)
  i. juxtafoveal retinal
  telangiectasis
  i. lipid keratopathy
  i. macular cyst and hole
  i. myositis
  i. nongranulomatous optic
  neuritis
  i. orbital inflammatory
  syndrome (IOIS)
  i. perioptic neuritis
  i. polypoidal choroidal
  vasculopathy (IPCV)
  i. preretinal membrane
  i. retinal vasculitis
  i. scleritis
  i. sclerosing inflammation of
  the orbit
  i. vitreitis
  i. vitritis
idioretinal light
idoxuridine (IDU)
I-Drops

IDU
idoxuridine
IERM
idiopathic epiretinal membrane
I-Gent
ignipuncture
I-Homatrine
II
ALGERBRUSH II
Jones test II
Lens Opacities Classification
System II (LOCS II)
LOCS II
Lens Opacities Classification
System II
membranoproliferative
glomerulonephritis type II
Microputor II (MR2)
Schirmer test II
Thomas subretinal instrument
set II
Vaper Vac II
IIH
idiopathic intracranial hypertension
III
Clear Image III
IK
interstitial keratitis
I-knife
Alcon I.-k.
ILC
Integrated Light Control
Ilg
I. capsule forceps
I. curved microtying forceps
I. insertion forceps
I. lens loupe
I. microneedle holder
I. needle
I. needle holder
I. probe
I. push/pull
Iliff
I. approach
I. exenteration
I. lacrimal probe
I. lacrimal trephine
I. operation
Iliff-Haus operation
Iliff-House sclerectomy
Iliff-Park speculum
Iliff-Wright fascia needle
I-Liqui Tears

illacrimation
illaqueation
Illiterate
I. E chart
I. eye chart
illuminance
illuminated
i. near card (INC)
i. suction needle
illumination
axial i.
background i.
central i.
coaxial i.
contact i.
critical i.
dark-field i.
dark-ground i.
direct i.
erect i.
focal i.
Köhler i.
lateral i.
Macbeth i.
narrow-slit i.
oblique i.
photopic i.
slit i.
vertical i.
illuminator
high intensity i.
Luxo surgical i.
illusion
Hermann grid i.
Kuhnt i.
i. of movement
oculogravic i.
oculogyral i.
optical i.
passive i.
illusory visual spread
ILM
internal limiting membrane
Ilotycin
I. Ophthalmic
I-Lube
image
accidental i.
i. analysis
astigmatic i.
catatropic i.
i. degradation
direct i.

i. displacement
false i.
foveal i.
ghost i.
heteronymous i.
homonymous i.
hyperintense foci i.
hypointense foci i.
incidental i.
inversion of i.
inverted i.
i. jump
i. of mires
mirror i.
negative i.
ocular i.
optical i.
Placido disk i.
i. point
pseudostereo i.
Purkinje i.
Purkinje-Sanson mirror i.
real i.
retinal i.
Sanson i.
Scheimpflug slit i.
spectacular i.
specular i.
stigmatic i.
true i.
unequal retinal i.
virtual i.
visual i.
ImageNet image digitizing system
imager
Digital fundus i.
Digital slit-lamp i.
Humphrey retina i.
image-space
i.-s. focus
imaging
cine-magnetic resonance i.
color Doppler i.
magnetic resonance i. (MRI)
off-axis i.
on-axis i.
posterior visual pathway i.

stereoscopic i.
i. technology
imbalance
binocular i.
central vestibular i.
Imbert-Fick principle
imbrication
retinal i.
immature cataract
immersion
i. lens
i. method
imminens
glaucoma i.
immitis
Coccidioides i.
coccidioidomycosis i.
immune
i. complex
i. mechanism
i. reaction
i. response
i. stromal keratitis (ISK)
i. system
i. Wessely ring
immunity
adaptive i.
cell-mediated i.
humoral i.
immunoadsorption therapy
immunodiagnostic method
immunofluorescent
i. assay
i. staining
immunohistochemical technique
immunologic
i. memory
i. reaction
immunological conjunctivitis
immunology
ocular i.
immunoperoxidase staining
immunosuppressive drug
impact resistance
impaired vergence eye movement
impairment
adduction i.

NOTES

impairment *(continued)*
cortical visual i.
sensation i.
visual i. (VI)
impatency
congenital i.
impending macular hole
impetigo contagiosa
IMPEX diamond radial keratotomy
knife
impingement
implant
acorn-shaped eye i.
acrylic i.
Ahmed valve i.
Allen-Braley i.
Allen-ePTFE ocular i.
Allen orbital i.
Alpar i.
Arroyo i.
Arruga i.
Arruga-Moura-Brazil i.
Baerveldt glaucoma i.
Baerveldt seton i.
Barkan infant i.
Barraquer i.
Berens conical i.
Berens pyramidal i.
Berens-Rosa scleral i.
Binkhorst collar stud lens i.
Binkhorst four-loop iris-
fixated i.
Binkhorst two-loop intraocular
lens i.
Bio-Eye ocular i.
Biomatrix ocular i.
Boberg-Ans lens i.
Bonaccolto monoplex orbital i.
Boyd orbital i.
Brawner orbital i.
Brown-Dohlman Silastic
corneal i.
build-up i.
Bunker i.
Cardona focalizing fundus
lens i.
Cardona goniofocalizing i.
Castroviejo acrylic i.
Choyce i.
Choyce Mark VIII i.
Cogan-Boberg-Ans lens i.
conical i.
conus shell type eye i.

conventional shell i.
Cooper i.
Copeland i.
corneal i.
cosmetic contact shell i.
Cryo-Barrages vitreous i.
curlback shell i.
Cutler i.
Dannheim eye i.
45-degree bent reform i.
Dermostat i.
Doherty sphere i.
encircling i.
i. entry
Epstein collar stud acrylic i.
i. extrusion
Federov four-loop iris clip
lens i.
Federov type I lens i.
Federov type II lens i.
Ferguson i.
Fine magnetic i.
four-loop iris clip i.
four-loop iris fixated i.
Fox sphere i.
Frey tunneled i.
front build-up i.
full-dimpled Lucite i.
Garcia-Novito eye i.
Gelfilm retinal i.
glass sphere i.
Gold eyelid load i.
Goldmann three-mirror i.
Gold-Mules i.
gold sphere i.
gonioscopic i.
grooved silicone i.
Guist sphere i.
Haik i.
hemisphere eye i.
Herrick silicone lacrimal i.
hollow-sphere i.
hook-type i.
Hoskins-Drake i.
Hruby i.
Hughes i.
hydroxyapatite ocular i.
hydroxyapatite orbital i.
intracanalicular collagen i.
intraocular lens i.
intravitreal ganciclovir i.
Iovision i.
Iowa orbital i.

Ivalon sponge i.
Jordan i.
keratolens i.
King orbital i.
Koeppe gonioscopic i.
Krupin-Denver long-valve i.
Kryptok i.
Landegger orbital i.
Lemoine orbital i.
lens i.
i. lens
Levitt i.
Lincoff scleral sponge i.
Lovac fundus contact lens i.
Lovac six-mirror gonioscopic
  lens i.
Lucite i.
Lucite sphere i.
Lyda-Ivalon-Lucite i.
i. magnet
magnetic i.
McCannel i.
McGhan i.
MedDev i.
Medical Optics PC11NB
  intraocular lens i.
Medical Workshop intraocular
  lens i.
Medicornea Kratz intraocular
  lens i.
Medpor i.
Melauskas acrylic i.
Melauskas orbital i.
meridional i.
methyl methacrylate i.
i. migration
Molteno i.
motility i.
Mueller i.
Muhlberger orbital i.
Mules i.
Nocito eye i.
Oculo-Plastik ePTFE ocular i.
O'Malley self-adhering lens i.
Ophtec occlusion i.
optic i.
orbital floor i.

peanut i.
piggyback i.
i. placement
plastic sphere i.
Platina intraocular lens i.
Plexiglas i.
polyethylene i.
porous orbital i.
posterior chamber lens i.
  (PCLI)
posterior tube shunt i.
Precision Cosmet intraocular
  lens i.
primary lens i.
pseudophake i.
Radin-Rosenthal eye i.
Rayner-Choyce i.
retinal Gelfilm i.
reverse-shape i.
Ridley anterior chamber lens i.
Ridley Mark II lens i.
Rodin orbital i.
Rosa-Berens orbital i.
Ruedemann eye i.
Ruiz plano fundus lens i.
Schepens hollow hemisphere i.
Schocket tube i.
scleral i.
secondary lens i.
segmental i.
semishell i.
Severin i.
Shearing posterior chamber
  intraocular lens i.
shelf-type i.
shell i.
Sichi orbital i.
Silastic scleral buckler i.
silicone mesh i.
i. sleeve
sleeve i.
sling for i.
Smith orbital floor i.
Snellen conventional reform i.
solid silicone with Supramid
  mesh i.
sphere i.

NOTES

implant *(continued)*
  spherical i.
  i. sponge
  sponge i.
  Stone i.
  Stone-Jordan i.
  Strampelli lens i.
  subperiosteal i.
  Supramid-Allen i.
  Supramid lens i.
  surface i.
  tantalum mesh i.
  Teflon i.
  temporary intracanalicular
    collagen i.
  Tennant i.
  Tensilon i.
  i. tire
  tire i.
  Troncoso gonioscopic lens i.
  Troutman i.
  tunneled i.
  Ultex lens i.
  Universal i.
  Uribe orbital i.
  VA magnetic orbital i.
  Varigray i.
  Varilux lens i.
  Vitallium i.
  Vitrasert intravitreal i.
  Volk conoid lens i.
  Walter Reed i.
  Wheeler eye sphere i.
  wire mesh i.
implantable contact lens (ICL)
implantation
  Ahmed glaucoma valve i.
  gonioseton i.
  in-the-bag i.
  intraocular lens i.
  i. of lens
  PHEMA KPro i.
  radon seed i.
implanter
  Geuder i.
implantoptic
Implens intraocular lens
impletion
implicit time
impression
  basilar i.
  i. cytology

  i. debridement
  i. tonometer
imprint
improvement
  no i.
  pinhole no i. (PHNI)
Imre
  I. keratoplasty
  I. lateral canthoplasty
  I. lateral canthoplasty operation
  I. sliding flap
  I. treatment
inactive trachoma
INAD
  infantile neuroaxonal dystrophy
inadequacy
  blink i.
Inamura small incision
  capsulorrhexis forceps
I-Naphline
  I.-N. Ophthalmic
inattention
  visual i.
inborn error
INC
  illuminated near card
Inc.
  Akorn, I.
  Integrated Orbital Implants, I.
incandescent lamp
incarceration
  iris i.
incidence
  plane of i.
incident
  i. angle
  flux i.
  i. point
  ray i.
  i. ray of light
incidental
  i. color
  i. image
incipient cataract
incision
  Abex-Turner i.
  Agnew-Verhoeff i.
  arcuate i.
  buttonhole i.
  centrifugal i.
  centripetal i.
  chevron i.
  chord i.

clear corneal step i.
clear corneal tunnel i.
conjunctival i.
corneal i.
corneoscleral i.
corridor i.
cutdown i.
grayline i.
grooved i.
host i.
i. into eyelid
lateral canthal i.
limbal i.
Lynch medial canthal i.
nasal buttonhole i.
posterior i.
relaxing i.
scleral-limbal-corneal i.
scleral tunnel i.
i. spreader
sub-2 i.
subciliary i.
Swan i.
T-i.
temporal self-sealing clear
  corneal i.
i. terminus
trap i.
trapezoid single-plane clear
  corneal i.
von Noorden i.
incisura
i. ethmoidalis ossis frontalis
i. frontalis
i. lacrimalis
i. maxillae
i. supraorbitalis
incisure
ethmoidal i.
frontal i.
lacrimal i.
supraorbital i.
inclinometer
inclusion
i. blennorrhea
i. body
i. conjunctivitis

i. cyst
epithelial i.
intranuclear i.
mascara particle i.
incomitance
incomitant
i. vertical deviation
i. vertical strabismus
incomplete
i. achromatopsia
i. hemianopsia
i. pupil-sparing oculomotor
  nerve paresis
incongruent nystagmus
incongruous
i. field defect
i. hemianopsia
incontinentia pigmenti
increment
i. threshold spectral sensitivity
incrementally
incycloduction
incyclophoria
incyclotropia
incyclovergence
indentation
i. gonioscopy
i. operation
prominent i.
scleral i.
i. tonometer
i. tonometry
independent event
index, gen. **indicis,** pl. **indices,**
  indexes
i. amblyopia
i. ametropia
i. case
i. hypermetropia
i. hyperopia
hyperopia i.
i. myopia
myopia i.
Ophthalmic Confidence I.
  (OCI)
i. of refraction (n)
resistive i.

NOTES

i. nasal artery
i. nasal vein
i. oblique
i. oblique extraocular muscle
i. oblique overaction
i. olivary nucleus
i. ophthalmic vein
i. orbital fissure
i. orbital rim
i. palpebral vein
i. pole
i. punctum
i. rectus (IR)
i. rectus extraocular muscle
i. retinal arcade
i. salivary nucleus
i. steepening
i. tarsal muscle
i. tarsus
i. tarsus palpebra
i. temporal arcade
i. temporal artery
i. temporal vein
vena ophthalmica i.
venula macularis i.
venula nasalis retinae i.
venula temporalis retinae i.
i. zone of retina
i. zygomatic foramen

inferiores
venae palpebrales i.

inferioris
pars orbitalis gyri frontalis i.

inferiorly
eye rotated i.

inferonasal artery
inferonasally
inferotemporal
i. arcade
i. artery

inferotemporally
infiltrate
annular i.
bacterial infectious corneal i.
central stromal i.
i. in cornea
corneal punctate i.

crystalline i.
inflammatory cellular i.
leukemic i.
patchy anterior stromal i.
peripheral ring i.
plasmacytoid i.
ring i.
ring-shaped stromal i.
stromal annular i.
stromal ring i.
subepithelial punctate corneal i.
white stromal i.
wreath pattern stromal i.

infiltration
branching i.
choroidal i.
dermal amyloid i.
inflammatory cell i.
linear i.
lymphocytic i.
lymphoid i.
mononuclear cell i.
perivascular neutrophil i.
radial i.
sarcoidosis i.

infiltrative optic neuropathy
infinite distance
Infirmary
Massachusetts Eye & Ear I.

Inflamase
I. Forte
I. Forte Ophthalmic
I. Mild
I. Mild Ophthalmic

inflammation
anterior chamber i.
anterior segment i.
ciliary body i.
corneal nerve i.
i. of eyelid
ocular i.

inflammatory
i. cell
i. cell infiltration
i. cellular infiltrate
i. changes of retina
i. ectropion

NOTES

inflammatory *(continued)*
  i. glaucoma
  i. mediator
  i. meibomian gland disease
  i. myopathy
  i. optic neuritis
  i. optic neuropathy
  i. retinopathy
  i. target site of eye
inflow
  aqueous i.
influenzae
  Haemophilus i.
influenza virus
infraciliary
infraduct
infraduction
infraepitrochlear nerve
infranasal
infranuclear
  i. disorder
  i. ophthalmoplegia
  i. pathway
infraorbital
  i. anesthesia
  i. artery
  i. canal
  i. foramen
  i. groove
  i. margin
  i. margin of maxilla
  i. nerve
  i. region
  i. sulcus of maxilla
  i. suture
infraorbitale
  foramen i.
infraorbitalis
  nervus i.
  sutura i.
infrapalpebralis
  sulcus i.
infrapalpebral sulcus
infrared
  i. cataract
  i. heater
  i. oculography
  i. optometer
  i. pupillometry
  i. radiation
  i. slit lamp
infratentorial arteriovenous
  malformation

infratrochlear nerve
infravergence
infraversion
infundibular cyst
infusion
  i. cannula
  i. suction cutter vitreous cutter
ingrowth
  epithelial i.
  fibroblastic i.
  stromal i.
inhalation anesthetic
inhibition
  lateral i.
  paradoxic levator i.
inhibitional
  i. palsy
  i. palsy of contralateral
    antagonist
injection
  botulinum i.
  ciliary i.
  circumcorneal i.
  conjunctival ciliary i.
  Cytoxan I.
  episcleral i.
  Hydrate I.
  Hyrexin-50 I.
  intraocular gas i.
  intravitreal i.
  i. molding
  Neosar I.
  Osmitrol I.
  peribulbar i.
  periocular i.
  posterior sub-Tenon i.
  Predcor-TBA I.
  retrobulbar alcohol i.
  silicone oil i.
  subconjunctival i.
  sub-Tenon corticosteroid i.
  Toradol I.
  Ureaphil I.
  Van Lint i.
injector
  automatic twin syringe i.
  Dyonics syringe i.
injury
  chemical i.
  concussion i.
  contrecoup i.
  coup i.
  eye i.

gestational i.
Hughes classification of
 chemical i.
levator i.
microwave radiation i.
ocular i.
optic nerve i.
penetrating i.
radiation i.
shearing i.
ultraviolet-induced i.

inlay
corneal i.

inner
i. canthus
i. limiting membrane
i. nuclear layer
i. plexiform layer
i. punctate choroidopathy
i. retina
i. segment

innervate
innervation
Hering law of equal i.
Hering law of equivalent i.
levator i.
reciprocal i.
regeneration of i.
Sherrington law of
 reciprocal i.

innocens
diabetes i.

Innovar
INNOVA System 920
Innovatome
INO
internuclear ophthalmoplegia

inoculum
inositus
diabetes i.

input
nerve i.
i. nerve
supranuclear i.

inserter
AMO-PhacoFlex lens and i.
Lens-Eze i.

insertion
tendinous i.
tensor i.

insipidus
diabetes i.

insonification
ultrasonic i.

inspired gas
instability
tear film i.

instillation
Institute
Dartmouth Eye I.
Wilmer Eye I.
Wilmer Ophthalmological I.

instrument
Alcon Surgical i.
American Hydron i.
AO Reichert I.'s
Argyll-Robertson i.
Ascon i.
Ayerst i.
Biophysic Ophthascan S i.
Birks Mark II i.
Carl Zeiss i.
Daisy irrigation-aspiration i.
DORC backflush i.
Eckardt Heme-Stopper i.
fixation i.
Grieshaber ultrasharp
 microsurgery i.
guillotine vitrectomy i.
IOLAB titanium i.
Karl Ilg i.
Kerato-Kontours i.
matte black i.
optical centering i.
Retinomax refractometry i.
Rizzuti-Bonaccolto i.
Rizzuti-Fleischer i.
Rizzuti-Kayser-Fleischer i.
Rizzuti-Lowe i.
Rizzuti-Maxwell i.
Rizzuti-Soemmering i.
Rumex titanium i.
Sutcliffe laser shield and
 retracting i.

NOTES

instrument *(continued)*
    Sutherland rotatable
      microsurgery i.
    Thomas Kapsule i.
    topographic
      scanning/indocyanine green
      angiography combination i.
    UTAS 2000
      electroretinography i.
    vitrectomy i.
instrument/apparatus
    Squid i./a.
instrumentation
insufficiency
    accommodation i.
    convergence i. (CI)
    cortical visual i.
    divergence i.
    dynamic accommodation i.
    i. of externi
    i. of eyelid
    i. of eyelid closure
    muscular i.
    static accommodation i.
insular scotoma
insulin-deficient diabetes
insulin-dependent diabetes mellitus (IDDM)
insulin resistance
Intacs ring
intact
    extraocular movement i. (EOMI)
Integrated
    I. Light Control (ILC)
    I. Orbital Implants, Inc.
integrity
    break in retinal i.
intensity
    luminous i. (I)
    radiant i.
    unit of luminous i.
interaction
    bipolar horizontal i.
    contour i.
    drug i.
    electrostatic i.
    Fas i.
    FasL i.
    spatial i.
intercalary staphyloma
intercanthal distance (ICD)
intercanthic

intercellular space
intercept
    corneal i.
interciliary fiber
intercilium
interface
    graft-host i.
    i. haze
    macular paramacular
      vitreoretinal i.
    i. opacity
    parallel i.
    i. phenomena
    vitreomacular i.
    vitreoretinal i.
interfasciale
    spatium i.
interfascial space
interference
    i. filter
    i. fringe
    i. visual acuity test
interferometer
    electron i.
    Fizeau-Tolansky i.
interferometry
    electron i.
    laser i.
interferon
    i. alfa-2a
    i. alfa-2b
interior eye tumor
interlacing of collagen lamellae
interlamellar space
intermediate
    i. posterior curve (IPC)
    i. uveitis
Intermedics
    I. intraocular tonometer
    I. lens
    I. Phaco I/A unit
    Pharmacia I.
intermedius
    i. nerve
    nervus i.
    Staphylococcus i.
intermittent
    i. angle-closure glaucoma
    i. deviation
    i. esotropia (E(T))
    i. exotropia (X(T))
    i. strabismus
    i. tropia

intermuscular
   i. membrane
   i. septum
interna
   axis oculi i.
   folliculitis i.
   membrana granulosa i.
   membrana limitans i.
   ophthalmoplegia i.
internal
   i. axis of eye
   i. capsule syndrome
   i. carotid artery
   i. hordeolum
   i. lacrimal fistula
   i. limiting membrane (ILM)
   i. nucleus hydrodelineation
     needle
   i. ophthalmopathy
   i. ophthalmoplegia
   i. ostium
   i. palsy
   i. reflectivity
   i. squint
   i. strabismus
internuclear
   i. ophthalmoparesis
   i. ophthalmoplegia (INO)
   i. paralysis
internuclearis
   ophthalmoplegia i.
internum
   hordeolum i.
internus
   axis bulbi i.
interosseous wiring
interpalpebral
   i. fissure
   i. zone
interpeduncular fossa
interplexiform cell
interpolation
interpupillary
   i. distance (IPD)
interrogans
   Leptospira i.
interrupted nylon suture

Intersol
Interspace YAG laser lens
interstitial
   i. keratitis (IK)
   i. neovascularization
   i. nucleus of Cajal
   i. pneumonitis
interthalamic commissure
intervaginale
   spatium i.
intervaginal space of optic nerve
interval
   focal i.
   Sturm i.
   i. of Sturm
interweaving
   collagen fibril i.
Interzeag bowl perimeter
in-the-bag
   i.-t.-b. implantation
   i.-t.-b. lens
intorsion
intortor muscle
intoxification amaurosis
intra-axonal
intracameral suture
intracanalicular
   i. anatomy
   i. collagen implant
   i. optic nerve
intracanicular
intracapsular
   i. cataract extraction (ICCE)
   i. extraction of cataract
intracavernous carotid artery
intracorneal
   i. cyst
   i. ring
intracranial
   i. anatomy
   i. aneurysm
   i. glioma
   i. granuloma
   i. hypertension
   i. hypotension
   i. mass
   i. optic nerve

NOTES

intracranial *(continued)*
  i. optic nerve decompression
  i. pressure (ICP)
intracytoplasmic inclusion body
intradermal nevus
intraepithelial
  i. cyst
  i. dyskeratosis
  i. epithelioma
  i. microcyst
  i. neoplasia
  i. plexus
intralacrimal papilloma
intralenticular hemorrhage
intraluminal suture
intraluminar pressure
intramarginal sulcus
intramedullary segment
intranuclear
  i. eosinophilic inclusion body
  i. inclusion
intraocular
  i. administration
  i. air
  i. anatomy
  i. cataract extraction
  i. cilia
  i. coccidioidomycosis
  i. cysticercus
  i. distance
  i. fistula
  i. fluid
  i. forceps
  i. foreign body
  i. gas
  i. gas bubble
  i. gas injection
  i. hemorrhage
  i. lens (IOL)
  i. lens dialer
  i. lens dislocation
  i. lens glide
  i. lens implant
  i. lens implantation
  i. lens power (IOLP)
  i. lymphoma
  i. melanoma
  Miostat I.
  i. muscle (IOM)
  i. myelination of retinal nerve
    fiber
  i. optic nerve
  i. optic neuritis

  i. pressure (IOP)
  i. pressure spike
  i. retinoblastoma
  i. silicone oil tamponade
  i. tension
  i. tuberculosis
intraoperative
  i. adjustable suture surgery
  i. blood loss
  i. suture adjustment (ISA)
IntraOptics lensometer
intraorbital
  i. anatomy
  i. anesthesia
  i. foreign body
  i. margin of orbit
  i. nerve dysfunction
intraosseous optic nerve
intrapapillary drusen
intraretinal
  i. bleeding
  i. fleck
  i. hemorrhage
  i. lipid deposit
  i. microvascular abnormality
    (IRMA)
intrascleral
  i. nerve loop
  i. plexus
intrasellar tumor
intrasheath tenotomy
intrastromal
  i. corneal ring
  i. laser
intratemporal segment
intravenous
  i. fluorescein
  i. fluorescein angiography
  i. thyrotropin-releasing hormone
    test
intraventricular hemorrhage (IVH)
intravitreal
  i. fibrin
  i. ganciclovir implant
  i. hemorrhage
  i. injection
  i. tPA
intrinsic
  i. light
  i. ocular muscle
introducer
  Carter sphere i.
  silicone i.

sphere i.
Weaver trocar i.
Intron A
intrusion
saccadic i.
intubation
monocanalicular i.
O'Donoghue silicone i.
Silastic i.
silicone i.
in-tumbling fashion
intumescent cataract
invasion
epithelial i.
invasive adenoma
Inventory
Color Screening I.
inversa
retinitis pigmentosa i.
inverse
i. astigmatism
i. ocular bobbing
inversion of image
inversus
blepharophimosis i.
epicanthal i.
epicanthus i.
inverted image
Inverter vitrectomy system
investigation
neuro-ophthalmological i.
invisible bifocal
involutional
i. blepharoptosis
i. senile ectropion
i. senile entropion
i. senile ptosis
i. stenosis
inward rectifier
Iocare
I. balanced salt solution
I. titanium needle
iodide
echothiophate i.
Metubine I.
Phospholine I.
potassium i.

iodochlorhydroxyquin
iodopsin
iodoquinol
IOIS
idiopathic orbital inflammatory
syndrome
IOL
intraocular lens
Kearney side-notch IOL
IOLAB
I. 108 B lens
I. I&A photocoagulator
I. intraocular lens
I. irrigating/aspirating
photocoagulator
I. irrigating/aspirating unit
I. irrigating needle
I. taper-cut needle
I. taper-point needle
I. titanium instrument
I. titanium needle
IOLP
intraocular lens power
IOM
intraocular muscle
ION
ischemic optic neuropathy
IONDT
Ischemic Optic Neuropathy
Decompression Trial
ionizing radiation
ion laser
IOP
intraocular pressure
Iopidine
Ioptex
I. laser intraocular lens
I. TabOptic lens
Iovision implant
Iowa
I. orbital implant
I. State fixation forceps
I/P
iris and pupil
I-Paracaine
I-Parescein

NOTES

IPC
    intermediate posterior curve
IPCV
    idiopathic polypoidal choroidal
    vasculopathy
IPD
    interpupillary distance
IPE
    iris pigment epithelium
I-Pentolate
I-Phrine
    I.-P. Ophthalmic Solution
I-Picamide
I-Pilocarpine
I-Pilopine
I-Pred
I-Prednicet
ipsilateral
    i. antagonist
    i. centrocecal scotoma
    i. iris
    i. proptosis
IR
    inferior rectus
Irene lens
I-Rescein
iridal
iridalgia
iridauxesis
iridectasis
iridectome
iridectomesodialysis
iridectomize
iridectomy
    argon laser i.
    basal i.
    Bethke i.
    buttonhole i.
    Castroviejo i.
    central i.
    Chandler i.
    complete i.
    Elschnig central i.
    laser i.
    i. operation
    optic i.
    optical i.
    patent i.
    peripheral i. (PI)
    preliminary i.
    preparatory i.
    pupil-to-root i.
    i. scissors

    sector i.
    stenopeic i.
    superior sector i.
    therapeutic i.
iridectopia
iridectropium
iridemia
iridencleisis
    Holth i.
    i. operation
iridentropium
irideremia
irides (*pl. of* iris)
iridescent
    i. spot
    i. vision
iridesis
iridiagnosis
iridial, iridian, iridic
    i. angle
    i. fold
    i. muscle
iridica
    stella lentis i.
iridis
    angulus i.
    atresia i.
    coloboma i.
    ectopia i.
    epithelium pigmentosum i.
    facies anterior i.
    facies posterior i.
    granuloma i.
    herpes i.
    heterochromia i.
    ligamentum pectinatum i.
    margo ciliaris i.
    margo pupillaris i.
    melanosis i.
    plicae i.
    i. rubeosis
    rubeosis i.
    sinus circularis i.
    spatia anguli i.
    sphincter i.
    vitiligo i.
    xanthelasmatosis i.
    xanthomatosis i.
iridization
iridoavulsion
iridocapsular intraocular lens
iridocapsulitis

iridocapsulotomy
    i. scissors
iridocele
iridochoroiditis
iridociliary
    i. process contact
    i. sulcus
iridocoloboma
iridoconstrictor
iridocorneal
    i. angle
    i. endothelial (ICE)
    i. endothelial syndrome (ICE)
    i. epithelial syndrome
    i. mesodermal dysgenesis
    i. synechia
    i. touch
iridocornealis
    angular i.
    angulus i.
    ligamentum anguli i.
    ligamentum pectinatum
      anguli i.
    spatia anguli i.
iridocorneosclerectomy
iridocyclectomy
iridocyclitis
    Fuchs heterochromic i.
    granulomatous i.
    herpes simplex i.
    herpes zoster i.
    heterochromic i.
    hypertensive i.
    i. masquerade syndrome
    nongranulomatous i.
    posttraumatic i.
    i. septica
    varicella i.
iridocyclochoroidectomy
    Peyman i.
iridocyclochoroiditis
iridocycloretraction
iridocystectomy
iridodesis
iridodiagnosis

iridodialysis
    i. operation
    i. spatula
iridodiastasis
iridodilator
iridodonesis
iridoendothelial syndrome
iridogoniocyclectomy
iridogoniodysgenesis
iridokeratitis
iridokinesis, iridokinesia
iridokinetic
iridolenticular contact
iridoleptynsis
iridology
iridolysis
iridomalacia
iridomesodialysis
iridomotor
iridoncosis
iridoncus
iridoparalysis
iridopathy
iridoperiphakitis
iridoplasty
    argon laser peripheral i.
      (ALPI)
    laser i.
iridoplegia
    i. accommodation
    complete i.
    i. reflex
    sympathetic i.
iridoptosis
iridopupillary
iridorrhexis
iridoschisis
iridoschisma
iridosclerotomy
iridosteresis
iridotasis operation
iridotomy
    Abraham i.
    Castroviejo radial i.
    laser i. (LPI)
    i. lens
    i. operation

NOTES

iridotomy *(continued)*
   radial i.
   i. scissors
iridovitreosynechiae
iridozonular contact
I-Rinse
IRIS
   I. LIO500
   I. OcuLight SLx indirect
      ophthalmoscope delivery
      system
iris, pl. irides
   angle of i.
   i. architecture
   arterial circle of greater i.
   arterial circle of lesser i.
   i. atrophy
   i. bombé
   i. capture
   i. chafing
   ciliary margin of i.
   circle of greater i.
   circle of lesser i.
   i. coloboma
   coloboma of i.
   i. concavity
   congenital cleft of i.
   i. contraction reflex
   cosmetic i.
   i. crypt
   i. cyst
   i. dehiscence
   detached i.
   i. diameter
   i. diastasis
   i. dilator
   i. ectasia
   embryonal epithelial cyst of i.
   i. epithelial hyperplasia
   i. eye
   Florentine i.
   i. forceps
   i. freckle
   i. frill
   greater ring of i.
   hernia of i.
   heterochromia of i.
   i. hook
   i. hook cannula
   hydrops of i.
   i. incarceration
   ipsilateral i.
   i. knife needle

leiomyoma of i.
lesser ring of i.
major arterial circle of i.
melanoma of i.
i. neovascularization
neovascularization of the i.
   (NVI)
i. neurofibroma
i. nodule
notch of i.
I. Oculight SLx MicroPulse
   laser
i. pearl
pectinate ligament of i.
i. pigment dusting
pigmented epithelium of i.
pigmented layer of i.
i. pigment epithelium (IPE)
i. pit
plateau i.
i. process
prolapse of i.
i. prolapse
i. and pupil (I/P)
pupillae muscle of i.
pupillary margin of i.
i. repositor
i. retraction syndrome of
   Campbell
retroflexion of i.
i. ring
ring of i.
i. roll
i. root
i. scissors
shredded i.
i. spatula
i. sphincter
i. sphincter muscle
i. sphincter tear
i. strand
stroma of i.
i. stroma
i. support
i. suture
i. sweep
i. synechia
torn i.
transfixion of i.
i. transillumination defect
tremulous i.
i. tuck
umbrella i.

I

Iriscorder
iris-fixated lens
iris-fixation technique
iris-lens diaphragm
iris-nevus syndrome
Iri-Sol
irisopsia
iris-supported lens
iritic
iritides
iritis
    i. blenorrhagique à rechutes
    i. catamenialis
    diabetic i.
    Doyne guttate i.
    i. fibrinitis
    fibrinous i.
    follicular i.
    i. glaucomatosa
    gouty i.
    hemorrhagic i.
    i. nodosa
    nodular i.
    i. obturans
    i. papulosa
    plastic i.
    postoperative i.
    purulent i.
    quiet i.
    i. recidivans staphylococcal
      allergica
    i. roseata
    serous i.
    spongy i.
    sympathetic i.
    syphilitic i.
    tuberculous i.
    uratic i.
iritoectomy
iritomy
IRMA
    intraretinal microvascular
      abnormality
iron
    i. deposit
    i. deposition

    i. Fleischer ring
    i. line
iron-ferry line
iron-Hudson-Stähli line
iron-leaking bleb
iron-Stocker line
irotomy
irradiation
    cataract i.
    i. cataract
    gamma i.
    heavy ion i.
    ^{90}Sr-plaque i.
irregular
    i. astigmatism
    i. nystagmus
    i. pupil
irregularity
    flap i.
    surface i.
irreversible amblyopia
Irrigate eye wash
irrigating
    i. anterior chamber vectis
    i. cannula
    i. cystitome
    i. solution
    i. vectis loop
irrigating-aspirating (*var. of*
    irrigation-aspiration) **(I&A)**
irrigating/aspirating
    i. cannula
    i. vectis
irrigation
    dilation and i. (D&I)
irrigation-aspiration, irrigating-
    aspirating (I&A)
    i.-a. system
    i.-a. unit
irrigation/aspiration (I/A)
irrigator
    anterior chamber i.
    Birch-Harman i.
    Bishop-Harman anterior
      chamber i.
    cul-de-sac i.
    Fink cul-de-sac i.

NOTES

irrigator *(continued)*
  Hartstein i.
  olive-tip i.
  Randolph i.
  Sylva anterior chamber i.
  Vidaurri i.
irritation
  ocular i.
irritative
  i. hallucination
  i. miosis
Irvine
  I. irrigating/aspirating unit
  I. operation
  I. probe-pointed scissors
Irvine-Gass syndrome
ISA
  intraoperative suture adjustment
I-scan
ischemia
  carotid i.
  choroidal i.
  foveal i.
  limbal i.
  i. of optic nerve
  i. retinae
  retinal i.
  transient i.
  transient vertebrobasilar i.
ischemic
  i. atherosclerosis
  i. chiasmal syndrome
  i. choroidal atrophy
  i. disk
  i. episode
  i. ocular syndrome
  i. oculomotor palsy
  i. optic atrophy
  i. optic neuropathy (ION)
  I. Optic Neuropathy
    Decompression Trial (IONDT)
  i. papillitis
  i. papillopathy
  i. retina
  i. retinal whitening
  i. retinopathy
I-Scrub
iseikonia
iseikonic lens
isethionate
  dibromopropamidine i.
  hydroxystilbamidine i.

  pentamidine i.
  propamidine i.
Ishihara
  I. I-Temp cautery
  I. IV slit lamp
  I. pseudoisochromatic plate
  I. test for color blindness
ISK
  immune stromal keratitis
island
  central i.
  isolated i.
  Traquair i.
Ismotic
isobutyl 2-cyanoacrylate
Isocaine
isochromatic plate
isocoria
isoflurophate
isoiconia
isoiconic
  i. lens
I-Sol
isolated
  i. fixed dilated pupil
  i. island
  i. oculomotor nerve
    dysfunction
isomerase
  retinal i.
  retinene i.
isomerization
isometropia
isophoria
isopia
isopter
  nasal i.
  sloping i.'s
Isopto
  I. Atropine
  I. Carbachol
  I. Carbachol Ophthalmic
  I. Carpine
  I. Carpine Ophthalmic
  I. Cetamide
  I. Cetamide Ophthalmic
  I. Cetapred
  I. Cetapred ophthalmic
  I. Eserine
  I. Frin
  I. Homatropine
  I. Homatropine Ophthalmic
  I. Hyoscine

I. Hyoscine Ophthalmic
I. P-ES
I. Plain
I. Plain Solution
I. Prednisolone
I. Sterofrin
I. Tears
I. Tears Solution
isoscope
isosorbide
isothiocyanate
fluorescein i.
isotonic solution
isotope scan
isotretinoin
ISPAN intraocular gas
I-Sulfacet
I-Sulfalone
I-tech
I.-t. cannula
I.-t. cannula holder
I.-t. cannula tray
I.-t. Castroviejo bladebreaker

I.-t. intraocular foreign body
forceps
I.-t. needle holder
I.-t. splinter forceps
I.-t. tying forceps
I-Temp cautery
Ito procedure
I-Trol
I-Tropine
IV
I. retinal fluorescein
angiography
I. slit lamp
Ivalon sponge implant
IVEX system
IVH
intraventricular hemorrhage
Iwanoff
I. cysts
I. retinal edema
I-Wash
I-White
Ixodes dammini

NOTES

J
joule
J loop
jack-in-the-box phenomenon
Jackson
   J. cross cylinder
   J. lacrimal intubation set
Jacob
   J. capsule fragment forceps
   J. membrane
   J. ulcer
Jacobson retinitis
Jacob-Swann
   J.-S. gonioscope
   J.-S. gonioscopic prism
Jacoby
   border tissue of J.
Jacod syndrome
Jacquart angle
Jadassohn
   nevus sebaceus of J.
Jadassohn-type anetoderma
Jaeger
   J. acuity card
   J. grading system
   J. hook
   J. keratome
   J. lid plate
   J. notation
   J. retractor
   J. system
   J. test type
   J. visual test
Jaesche-Arlt operation
Jaesche operation
Jaffe
   J. capsulorrhexis forceps
   J. Cilco lens
   J. intraocular spatula
   J. laser blepharoplasty and facial resurfacing set
   J. lens-manipulating hook
   J. lens spatula
   J. lid retractor
   J. lid retractor set
   J. lid speculum
   J. microiris hook
   J. needle holder
   J. suturing forceps
Jaffe-Bechert nucleus rotator

Jaffe-Givner lid retractor
Jahnke syndrome
Jaime lacrimal operation
Jamaican optic neuropathy
jamb
   sphenoid door j.
Jameson
   J. calipers
   J. muscle forceps
   J. muscle hook
   J. operation
Janelli clip
Jannetta procedure
Jansen-Middleton septotomy forceps
Jansky-Bielschowsky
   J.-B. disease
   J.-B. syndrome
Jardon eye shield
Jarisch-Herxheimer reaction
Javal
   J. keratometer
   J. ophthalmometer
Javal-Schiotz ophthalmometer
jaw
   j. muscle pain
   j. winking
jaw-winking
   j.-w. phenomenon
   j.-w. syndrome
JCAHPO
   Joint Commission on Allied Health Personnel in Ophthalmology
JC virus
Jedmed A-scan
Jedmed/DGH A-scan
Jellinek sign
Jendrassik sign
Jenning test
Jensen
   J. capsule scratcher
   J. choroiditis juxtapapillaris
   J. disease
   J. intraocular lens forceps
   J. jerk nystagmus
   J. juxtapapillary choroiditis
   J. lens-inserting forceps
   J. operation
   J. polisher/scratcher
   J. retinitis
   J. transposition procedure

J

**Jensen-Thomas irrigating-aspirating
cannula**
jequirity ophthalmia
jerk
  macro square-wave j.'s
  j. nystagmus
  square-wave j.'s
Jervey
  J. capsule fragment forceps
  J. iris forceps
Jeune syndrome
jeweler
  j. forceps
  j. tweezers
J-loop
  J.-l. PC lens
  J.-l. posterior chamber
    intraocular lens
JOAG
  juvenile open-angle glaucoma
Joal lens
Joffroy sign
John
  J. Green calipers
  J. Weiss forceps
Johnson
  J. double cannula
  J. erysiphake
  J. evisceration knife
  J. operation
  J. syndrome
Johnson-Bell erysiphake
Johnson-Tooke corneal knife
Joint
  J. Commission on Allied
    Health Personnel in
    Ophthalmology (JCAHPO)
  J. Review Committee for
    Ophthalmic Medical Personnel
    (JRCOMP)
Jones
  J. dye test
  J. forceps
  J. II test
  J. I test
  J. keratome
  J. operation
  J. punctum dilator
  J. Pyrex tube
  J. repair
  J. tear duct tube
  J. test I
  J. test II

  J. towel clamp
  J. tube procedure
Jordan implant
Joseph
  J. device
  J. periosteal elevator
Josephberg probe
Joubert syndrome
joule (J)
Jr.
  Optelec Spectrum J.
JRCOMP
  Joint Review Committee for
  Ophthalmic Medical Personnel
J-shaped
  J.-s. irrigating/aspirating cannula
  J.-s. sella
Judd forceps
Judson-Smith manipulator
jump
  image j.
junction
  basal j.
  corneoscleral j.
  craniocervical j.
  host-graft j.
  mucocutaneous j.
  myoneural j.
  parieto-occipital-temporal j.
  sclerocorneal j.
  scotoma j.
  j. scotoma
junctional
  j. bay
  j. nevus
  j. scotoma
  j. scotoma of Traquair
  j. zone
Jung-Schaffer intraocular lens
Just
  J. Tears
  J. Tears Solution
juvenile
  j. arcus
  j. corneal epithelial dystrophy
  j. developmental cataract
  j. diabetes
  j. diabetes mellitus
  j. epithelial dystrophy
  j. iris xanthogranuloma
  j. macular degeneration
  j. melanoma
  j. nevoxanthoendothelioma

j. open-angle glaucoma
(JOAG)
j. optic atrophy
j. pilocytic astrocytoma
j. reflex
j. retinoschisis
j. xanthogranuloma (JXG)
juvenilis
angiopathia retinae j.
arcus j.
juxtacanicular
juxtafoveal
j. choroidal neovascularization
j. microaneurysm

juxtalimbal suture
juxtapapillaris
Jensen choroiditis j.
retinochoroiditis j.
juxtapapillary
j. leakage
j. nerve fiber layer
j. perfusion
j. retina
juxtaposition
juxtapupillary choroiditis
JXG
juvenile xanthogranuloma

J

NOTES

K
cornea curvature
kelvin
keratometric power
phylloquinone
K readings
K Sol preservation solution
K1
Canon Autokeratometer K.
Kainair
Kaiser speculum
Kalt
K. corneal needle
K. forceps
K. needle holder
K. needle holder clamp
K. spoon
Kamdar microscissors
Kamerling Capsular 90 lens
Kamppeter anomaloscope
kanamycin
Kandori
flecked retina of K.
Kaposi
K. sarcoma
xeroderma of K.
kappa angle
Kara
K. cataract-aspirating cannula
K. cataract needle
K. erysiphake
Karakashian-Barraquer scissors
Karickhoff
K. double cannula
K. laser lens
Karl Ilg instrument
Kasabach-Merritt syndrome
Katena
K. boat hook
K. double-edged sapphire blade
K. forceps
K. iris spatula
K. product
K. quick switch I/A system
K. speculum
K. trephine
katophoria
katotropia
Katzin
K. operation

K. scissors
K. trephine
Katzin-Barraquer forceps
Kaufman
K. medium
K. type II retractor
K. type II vitrector
K. vitreophage
Kayser-Fleischer cornea ring
KCS
keratoconjunctivitis sicca
Kearney
K. side-notch IOL
K. side-notch lens
Kearns-Sayre syndrome (KSS)
Keeler
K. cryoextractor
K. cryophake
K. cryophake unit
K. cryosurgical unit
K. extended round tip forceps
K. intraocular foreign body
grasping forceps
K. intravitreal scissors
K. lancet tip
K. micro round tip
K. microscissors
K. micro spear tip
K. ophthalmoscope
K. panoramic lens
K. panoramic loupe
K. pantoscope
K. prism
K. Pulsair tonometer
K. puncture tip
K. razor tip
K. retinoscope
K. retractable blade
K. ruby knife
K. specular microscope
K. Tearscope
K. triple facet tip
K. ultrasonic cataract removal
lancet
Keeler-Amoils
K.-A. curved cataract probe
K.-A. freeze
K.-A. glaucoma probe
K.-A. long-shank retinal probe

Keeler-Amoils *(continued)*
- K.-A. microcurved cataract probe
- K.-A. Ophthalmic Cryosystem
- K.-A. ophthalmic curved cataract probe
- K.-A. ophthalmic long-shank probe
- K.-A. ophthalmic Machemer retinal probe
- K.-A. ophthalmic microcurved cataract probe
- K.-A. ophthalmic retinal probe
- K.-A. ophthalmic straight cataract probe
- K.-A. ophthalmic vitreous probe
- K.-A. straight cataract probe
- K.-A. vitreous probe

Keeler-Catford
- K.-C. microjaws needle holder
- K.-C. needle holder with microjaws

Keeler-Fison tissue retractor
Keeler-Keislar lacrimal cannula
Keeler-Konan Specular microscope
Keeler-Meyer diamond knife
Keeler-Pierse
- K.-P. eye speculum
- K.-P. speculum

Keeler-Rodger iris retractor
Keith-Wagener
- K.-W. change (KW)
- K.-W. retinopathy

Keith-Wagener-Barker classification
Keizer-Lancaster
- K.-L. eye speculum
- K.-L. lid retractor
- K.-L. speculum

Kellan
- K. capsular sparing system
- K. hydrodissection
- K. sutureless incision blade

Kelly-Descemet membrane punch
Kelly hemostat
Kelman
- K. air cystitome
- K. aspirator
- K. cryoextractor
- K. cryophake
- K. cryosurgical unit
- K. cyclodialysis cannula
- K. flexible tripod lens

- K. iris retractor
- K. irrigating/aspirating unit
- K. irrigating handpiece
- K. knife
- K. Multiflex II lens
- K. Omnifit II intraocular lens
- K. operation
- K. PC 27LB CapSul lens
- K. phacoemulsification unit
- K. Quadriflex anterior chamber intraocular lens
- K. tip

Kelman-Cavitron
- K.-C. I/A unit
- K.-C. irrigating/aspirating unit

Kelman-McPherson
- K.-M. corneal forceps
- K.-M. tying forceps

kelvin (K)
Kenacort
Kenaject-40
Kenalog
Kenalog-10
Kenalog-40
Kennedy syndrome
Kennerdell
- K. muscle hook
- K. nerve hook

Keracor laser
KeraCorneoScope
Keradiscs
Kerascan
keratalgia
keratan sulfate
keratectasia
keratectomy
- automated lamellar k.
- Castroviejo k.
- excimer laser photoreactive k.
- excimer laser photorefractive k.
- excimer laser phototherapeutic k.
- laser-scrape photorefractive k.
- no-touch transepithelial photorefractive k.
- k. operation
- photoastigmatic refractive k. (PARK)
- photorefractive k.
- photorefractive astigmatic k.
- phototherapeutic k. (PTK)
- k. scissors
- superficial k.

surface photorefractive k.
tracker-assisted
   photorefractive k. (T-PRK)
keratic precipitate (KP)
keratinization
   canthal k.
keratin layer
keratinoid degeneration
keratitic precipitate
keratitis
   Acanthamoeba k.
   acne rosacea k.
   actinic k.
   aerosol k.
   alphabet k.
   amebic k.
   ameboid k.
   annular k.
   arborescent k.
   artificial silk k.
   avascular k.
   bacterial k.
   band k.
   k. band
   k. bandelette
   band-shaped k.
   bank k.
   k. bullosa
   candidal k.
   catarrhal ulcerative k.
   chronic superficial k.
   classic dendritic k.
   Cogan interstitial k.
   confocal microscopy
      identification of
      Acanthamoeba k.
   contact lens-related
      microbial k.
   corneal k.
   Corynebacterium k.
   Cryptococcus laurentii k.
   deep punctate k.
   deep pustular k.
   dendriform k., dendritic k.
   dendritic herpes zoster k.
   desiccation k.
   diffuse deep k.

   diffuse lamellar k.
   Dimmer nummular k.
   disciform herpes simplex k.
   k. disciformis
   epithelial diffuse k.
   epithelial punctate k.
   exfoliative k.
   exposure k.
   farinaceous epithelial k.
   fascicular k.
   filament k.
   filamentary k.
   k. filamentosa
   Fuchs k.
   fungal k.
   furrow k.
   geographic k.
   gram-positive bacterial k.
   herpes simplex k.
   herpes zoster k.
   herpetic-fungal k.
   herpetic stromal k.
   HSV epithelial k.
   hypopyon k.
   immune stromal k. (ISK)
   infectious epithelial k.
   interstitial k. (IK)
   lagophthalmic k.
   lamellar keratectomy for
      nontuberculous
      mycobacterial k.
   lattice k.
   k. lesion
   letter-shaped k.
   k. linearis migrans
   luetic interstitial k.
   Lyme disease k.
   lymphogranuloma venereum k.
   marginal k.
   metaherpetic k.
   microbial k.
   mixed bacterial-fungal k.
   mixed fungal k.
   k. molluscum contagiosum
   Moraxella k.
   mumps k.
   Mycobacterium k.

K

NOTES

keratitis *(continued)*
mycotic k.
necrogranulomatous k.
necrotizing interstitial k.
necrotizing stromal k.
necrotizing ulcerative k.
neuroparalytic k.
neurotrophic k.
Nocardia k.
non-*Acanthamoeba* amebic k.
nonulcerative interstitial k.
nummular k.
k. nummularis
onchocercal sclerosing k.
oyster shuckers' k.
paddy k.
parenchymatous k.
k. periodica fugax
peripheral ulcerative k. (PUK)
k. petrificans
phlyctenular k.
polymorphic superficial k.
k. post vaccinulosa
k. profunda
pseudodendritic k.
k. punctata
k. punctata leprosa
k. punctata profunda
k. punctata subepithelialis
punctate epithelial k.
purulent k.
k. pustuliformis profunda
pyknotic k.
radiation k.
k. ramificata superficialis
reaper's k.
reticular k.
ribbon-like k.
ring k.
k. rosacea
rosacea k.
rubeola k.
Schmidt k.
sclerosing k.
scrofulous k.
secondary k.
serpiginous k.
k. sicca
striate k.
stromal k.
subepithelial k.
superficial linear k.
superficial punctate k. (SPK)

suppurative k.
syphilitic k.
Thygeson superficial
punctate k.
trachomatous k.
trophic k.
tuberculous k.
ulcerative k.
k. urica
k. vaccinia
vaccinial k.
varicella k.
vascular k.
vasculonebulous k.
vesicular k.
xerotic k.
zonular k.
keratoacanthoma
eruptive k.
keratocele
keratocentesis operation
keratoconjunctivitis
adenoviral k.
allergic k.
atopic eczema k.
bilateral k.
epidemic k. (EKC)
epizootic k.
flash k.
herpes follicular k.
herpes simplex k.
herpes zoster k.
herpetic k.
limbic vernal k.
phlyctenular k.
shipyard k.
k. sicca (KCS)
staphylococcal allergic k.
superior limbic k. (SLK)
Theodore k.
ultraviolet k.
vernal k. (VKC)
viral k.
welder's k.
keratoconus
anterior k.
Collaborative Longitudinal
Evaluation of K. (CLEK)
k. cornea
k. dystrophy
k. fruste
iatrogenic k.

posterior k.
Sato k.
keratocyte
keratoderma
k. blennorrhagica
keratodermatocele
keratoectasia
keratoepitheliomileusis
keratoepithelioplasty
keratoglobus
k. cornea
keratographer
Keravue k.
keratography
keratohelcosis
keratohemia
keratohyaline granule
keratoid
keratoiridocyclitis
keratoiridoscope
keratoiritis hypopyon
Kerato-Kontours instrument
keratokyphosis
keratolens implant
keratolenticuloplasty
keratoleptynsis
keratoleukoma
keratolimbal allograft (KLA)
Keratolux fixation device
keratolysis
keratoma, pl. **keratomas, keratomata**
solar k.
keratomalacia
keratome
Agnew k.
Bard-Parker k.
Beaver k.
Berens partial k.
Castroviejo angled k.
Czermak k.
Draeger modified k.
K. excimer laser system
filamentary k.
Fuchs lancet type k.
Grieshaber k.
k. guard
Guyton-Lundsgaard k.

Hansen k.
HydroBrush k.
Jaeger k.
Jones k.
Kirby k.
Lancaster k.
Martinez k.
McReynolds k.
Rowland k.
Storz k.
Tri-Beeled trapezoidal k.
Wiener k.
keratometer
Bausch & Lomb manual k.
Canon auto refraction k.
Haag-Streit k.
Helmholtz k.
Javal k.
manual k.
Marco manual k.
k. mires
Osher surgical k.
10 SL/O Zeiss k.
Storz k.
Terry k.
Topcon k.
keratometric
k. astigmatism
k. flattening
k. power (K)
k. reading (K readings)
keratometry
extended-range k.
surgical k.
keratomileusis (KM)
automated laser k. (ALK)
homoplastic k.
laser-assisted intrastromal k. (LASIK)
laser-assisted in situ k.
laser intrastromal k.
laser in situ k.
myopic k. (MKM)
k. operation
keratomycosis
keratoneuritis
pathognomonic radial k.

NOTES

keratonosis
keratonyxis
keratopathy
  aphakic bullous k. (ABK)
  band k.
  band-shaped k.
  Bietti k.
  bullous k.
  calcific band k.
  central striate k.
  chloroquine k.
  chronic actinic k.
  climatic droplet k.
  climatic proteoglycan
    stromal k.
  climatic stromal k.
  contact lens-induced k.
  crystalline k.
  dendritic k.
  elastotic band k.
  epithelial k.
  exposure k.
  filamentary k.
  fine punctate k.
  Fuchs aphakic k.
  HSV trophic k.
  hurricane k.
  idiopathic lipid k.
  indomethacin toxicity k.
  infectious crystalline k. (ICK)
  Labrador k.
  lamellar k.
  linear k.
  lipid k.
  Nama k.
  neuroparalytic k.
  neurotrophic k.
  pearl diver's k.
  phenothiazine k.
  plaque k.
  postinfectious epithelial k.
  pseudophakic bullous k. (PBK)
  punctate epithelial k. (PEK)
  striate k.
  superficial punctate k.
  Thygeson superficial
    punctate k.
  trigeminal neuropathic k.
  trophic k.
  urate band k.
  uveitic band k.
  vesicular k.
  vortex k.

keratophakia
keratophakic keratoplasty
keratoplasty
  allopathic k.
  Arroyo k.
  Arruga k.
  autogenous k.
  automated lamellar k. (ALK)
  deep lamellar k. (DLK)
  Elschnig k.
  epikeratophakic k.
  Filatov k.
  full-thickness k.
  heterogenous k.
  homogenous k.
  hyperopic automated
    lamellar k. (HALK)
  Imre k.
  keratophakic k.
  lamellar k. (LKP)
  lamellar refractive k.
  laser thermal k. (LTK)
  layered k.
  manual lamellar k.
  Morax k.
  nonpenetrating k.
  k. operation
  optic k.
  optical k.
  partial k.
  Paufique k.
  penetrating k. (PK, PKP)
  perforating k.
  photorefractive k. (PRK)
  punctate epithelial k.
  refractive k.
  k. scissors
  Sourdille k.
  superficial lamellar k.
  surface lamellar k.
  tectonic k.
  thermal k. (TKP)
  total k.
keratoplasty-Excimer
  automated lamellar k.-E.
    (ALK-E)
keratoprosthesis
  Eckardt temporary k.
  Lander wide-field temporary k.
  PHEMA core-and-skirt k.
keratorefractive
  k. procedure
keratorrhexis

keratorus
keratoscleritis
keratoscope
    Klein k.
    Polack k.
    wire-loop k.
keratoscopy
keratosis
    actinic k.
    eyelid k.
    k. follicularis
    k. follicularis spinulosa
      decalvans
    seborrheic k.
    senescent k.
    senile k.
    solar k.
keratostomy
keratotome
keratotomy
    Analysis of Radial K. (ARK)
    arcuate transverse k.
    astigmatic k. (AK)
    delimiting k.
    hexagonal k.
    laser k.
    k. operation
    prospective evaluation of
      radial k. (PERK)
    radial k. (RK)
    refractive k.
    Ruiz trapezoidal k.
    trapezoidal k.
keratotorus
keratouveitis
    herpes simplex k.
    stromal k.
Keratron corneal topographer
KeraVision ring
Keravue keratographer
kerectasis
kerectomy
Kerlone Oral
Kermix antibody
keroid

Kerrison
    K. forceps
    K. mastoid rongeur
Kestenbaum
    K. capillary count
    K. procedure
    K. rule
ketorolac
    k. tromethamine
    k. tromethamine ophthalmic
      solution, 0.5%
ketosis-prone diabetes
ketosis-resistant diabetes
Kevorkian-Younge forceps
keyhole
    k. bridge
    k. field
    lacrimal k.
    k. pupil
    k. vision
Key operation
Keystone view stereopsis test
Khodadoust line
Khosia cautery
kibisitome
    k. cystitome
killer cell
Kiloh-Nevin syndrome
Kilp lens
Kimmelstiel-Wilson
    K.-W. disease
    K.-W. syndrome
Kimura platinum spatula
kindergarten eye chart
kinematogram
    random-dot k.
kinematography
    random-dot k.
kinescope
kinetic
    k. echography
    k. perimeter
    k. perimetry
    k. strabismus
    k. ultrasound
    k. visual field testing

K

NOTES

King
- K. clamp
- K. corneal trephine
- K. Khaled Eye Specialist Hospital (KKESH)
- K. operation
- K. orbital implant

King-Prince
- K.-P. knife
- K.-P. muscle forceps

Kirby
- K. angulated iris spatula
- K. capsule forceps
- K. cataract knife
- K. corneoscleral forceps
- K. cylindrical zonal separator
- K. flat zonal separator
- K. hook expressor
- K. intracapsular lens expressor
- K. intracapsular lens loupe
- K. intracapsular lens spoon
- K. intraocular lens loupe
- K. intraocular lens scoop
- K. iris forceps
- K. iris spatula
- K. keratome
- K. lens
- K. lens dislocator
- K. lid retractor
- K. muscle hook
- K. operation
- K. refractor
- K. scissors
- K. tissue forceps

Kirby-Bauer disk sensitivity test
Kirisawa uveitis
Kirschner wire
Kirsch test
Kishi lens
kissing suprachoroidal hemorrhage
kit
- Bergland-Warshawski phaco/cortex k.
- Lacrimedics occlusion starter k.
- Massachusetts Vision K. (MVK)
- OPTIMUM rigid gas permeable starter k.
- Shearing suction k.
- Tearscope Plus tear film k.

Kjer
- K. disease
- K. dominant optic atrophy

KKESH
- King Khaled Eye Specialist Hospital

KLA
- keratolimbal allograft

Klebsiella
- *K. oxytoca*
- *K. pneumoniae*

Klebsiella **endophthalmitis**
Kleen
- Velva K.

Klein
- K. curved cannula
- K. keratoscope
- K. punch

Klein-Tolentino ring
Klieg eye
Klippel-Feil anomaly
Kloti vitreous cutter
Klumpke paralysis
Klyce/Wilson scale
KM
- keratomileusis

Knapp
- K. blade
- K. cataract knife
- K. eye speculum
- K. forceps
- K. iris hook
- K. iris probe
- K. iris repositor
- K. iris scissors
- K. iris spatula
- K. knife needle
- K. lacrimal sac retractor
- K. law
- K. lens loop
- K. lens spoon
- K. operation
- K. procedure
- K. refractor
- K. rule
- K. scoop
- K. streak
- K. stria

Knapp-Culler speculum
Knapp-Imre operation
Knapp-Wheeler-Reese operation
Knies sign
knife, pl. **knives**
- Agnew canaliculus k.
- Alcon A-OK crescent k.
- Alcon A-OK ShortCut k.
- Alcon A-OK slit k.

ASICO multi-angled diamond k.
Bard-Parker k.
Barkan goniotomy k.
Barraquer keratoplasty k.
Beard k.
Beaver goniotomy needle k.
Beaver Xstar k.
Beer canaliculus k.
Beer cataract k.
Berens cataract k.
Berens glaucoma k.
Berens keratoplasty k.
Berens ptosis k.
Bishop-Harman k.
blade k.
bladebreaker k.
Castroviejo discission k.
Castroviejo twin k.
cataract k.
Celita elite k.
Celita sapphire k.
corneal k.
Cusick goniotomy k.
Dean iris k.
Desmarres k.
Deutschman cataract k.
Diamatrix trapezoidal diamond k.
diamond blade k.
diamond-dusted k.
diamond phaco k.
Diamontek k.
discission k.
dissector k.
Duredge k.
EdgeAhead crescent k.
EdgeAhead microsurgical knives
EdgeAhead phaco slit k.
Elschnig cataract k.
Elschnig corneal k.
Elschnig pterygium k.
Feaster radial keratotomy k.
Gill corneal k.
Gill-Fine corneal k.
Gill-Hess k.

Gills pop-up arcuate diamond k.
Gills-Welsh k.
Goldmann serrated k.
goniopuncture k.
goniotomy k.
Graefe cataract k.
Graefe cystitome k.
Green cataract k.
Green corneal k.
Grieshaber ruby k.
Grieshaber ultrasharp k.
k. guard
Guyton-Lundsgaard cataract k.
Haab scleral resection k.
House myringotomy k.
Huco diamond k.
IMPEX diamond radial keratotomy k.
Johnson evisceration k.
Johnson-Tooke corneal k.
Keeler-Meyer diamond k.
Keeler ruby k.
Kelman k.
King-Prince k.
Kirby cataract k.
Knapp cataract k.
KOI diamond k.
Lancaster k.
Laseredge microsurgical k.
Lowell glaucoma k.
Lundsgaard k.
Martinez k.
Maumenee goniotomy k.
McPherson-Wheeler k.
McPherson-Ziegler k.
McReynolds pterygium k.
Meyer Swiss diamond lancet k.
Meyer Swiss diamond mini-angled k.
Meyer Swiss diamond wedge k.
Microknife k.
micrometer k.
microsurgical k.
Myocure k.

NOTES

263

knife *(continued)*
k.-needle
Optima diamond k.
Parker discission k.
Paton corneal k.
Paufique graft k.
Paufique keratoplasty k.
Phaco-4 diamond step k.
ptosis k.
Quantum enhancement k.
radial keratotomy k.
razor blade k.
Reese ptosis k.
Rhein Advantage diamond k.
Rhein clear corneal
  diamond k.
Rizzuti-Spizziri k.
Rizzuti-Spizziri cannula k.
ruby diamond k.
sapphire k.
SatinCrescent implant k.
SatinShortCut implant k.
SatinSlit implant k.
Sato corneal k.
scarifier k.
Scheie goniopuncture k.
Scheie goniotomy k.
scleral resection k.
Sharpoint microsurgical k.
Sharpoint slit k.
ShortCut A-OK small-
  incision k.
Sichel k.
slit blade k.
Smith k.
Smith-Fisher k.
Smith-Green cataract k.
Spizziri cannula k.
Stealth DBO free-hand
  diamond k.
Step-Knife diamond blade k.
stiletto k.
stitch-removing k.
Storz cataract k.
Storz-Duredge steel cataract k.
Swan discission k.
swift-cut phaco incision k.
Tooke corneal k.
Tooke cornea-splitting k.
Tooke-Johnson corneal k.
Troutman corneal k.
Troutman-Tooke corneal k.
Unicat k.

Universal Pathfinder k.
V-lancet k.
von Graefe cataract k.
Wallace-Maloney fixation
  diamond k.
wave-edge k.
Weber k.
Weck k.
Wheeler discission k.
Wilder cystitome k.
Zaldivar k.
Ziegler k.
knife-edged lens
Knolle
  K. capsule polisher
  K. capsule scraper
  K. capsule scratcher
  K. lens cortex spatula
  K. lens nucleus spatula
  K. lens speculum
Knolle-Kelman cannulated
  cystihtome
Knolle-Pearce irrigating lens loop
Knoll refraction technique
knot
  bow-tie k.
  partial throw surgeon's k.
  Tripier operation throw
    square k.
knuckle
  k. of choroid
  k. of loose vitreous
Knudson hypothesis
Koby
  K. cataract
  K. cataract forceps
  superficial reticular degeneration
    of K.
Koch
  K. chopper
  K. nucleus hydrolysis
  K. phaco manipulator
Kocher sign
Koch-Salz nucleus splitter
Koch-Weeks
  K.-W. bacillus
  K.-W. conjunctivitis
Kodak Surecell Chlamydia test
Koeller illumination system
Koenen tumor
Koeppe
  K. diagnostic lens
  K. disease

K. goniolens
K. gonioscopic implant
K. gonioscopy
K. nodule
K. syndrome
Koerber-Salus-Elschnig syndrome
Koffler operation
KOH
    potassium hydroxide
Köhler illumination
KOI diamond knife
Kollmorgen element
Kollner
K. law
K. rule
Kolmer crystalloid structure
Kolmogorov-Smirnov test
Konan
K. fixed-frame method
K. SP8000 image analysis
    system
K. SP8000 noncontact specular
    microscope
Konig bar chart
Konoto tetrad
Kooijman eye model
Korb
K. contact lens
K. lens
koroscope
koroscopy
Kowa
K. fluorescein system
K. FM-500
K. FM-500 laser flare meter
K. fundus
K. hand-held slit lamp
K. laser flare-cell photometer
K. laser flare photometer
K. Optimed slit lamp
K. PRO II retinal camera
K. RC-XV fundus camera
Koyter muscle
Kozlowski degeneration
KP
    keratic precipitate
KR-7000P auto-kerato-refractometer

Krabbe disease gland
Kraff
K. capsule polisher
K. capsule polisher curette
K. cortex cannula
K. intraocular utility forceps
K. lens-inserting forceps
K. nucleus lens loupe
K. nucleus splitter
K. suturing forceps
K. tying forceps
Kraff-Utrata
K.-U. capsulorrhexis
K.-U. capsulorrhexis forceps
K.-U. intraocular utility forceps
Kraft forceps
Krahn exophthalmometry
Krakau tonometer
Kramp scissors
Krasnov lens
Kratz
K. angled cystitome
K. capsule scraper
K. capsule scratcher
K. diamond-dusted needle
K. elliptical-style lens
K. K push-pull iris hook
K. lens-inserting forceps
K. lens needle
K. polisher
K. polisher/scratcher
K. posterior chamber
    intraocular lens
K. "soft" J-loop intraocular
    lens
K. speculum
Kratz-Barraquer wire eye speculum
Kratz-Jensen
K.-J. polisher/scratcher
K.-J. scratcher
Kratz-Johnson lens
Kratz-Sinskey
K.-S. intraocular lens
K.-S. loop configuration
Kraupa operation
Krause
K. lacrimal gland

K

NOTES

Krause *(continued)*
K. syndrome
transverse suture of K.
K. valve
Kreiger-Spitznas vibrating scissors
Kreiker
K. blepharochalasis
K. operation
Kremer
K. excimer laser
K. two-point fixation forceps
Krieberg operation
Krieger wide-field fundus lens
Krill
K. disease
K. disk
Krimsky
K. method
K. prism test
Krimsky-Prince accommodation rule
Kronfeld
K. electrode
K. refractor
K. retractor
K. suturing forceps
Krönlein
K. operation
K. procedure
Krönlein-Berke operation
Krukenberg
K. corneal spindle
K. pigment spindle
K. pigment spindle forceps
K. sponge
Krumeich-Baraquer lasitome
Krumeich-Barraquer microkeratome
Krupin
K. device
K. eye disk
K. valve
Krupin-Denver
K.-D. long-valve implant
K.-D. valve
krusei
Candida k.
Kruskal-Wallis test
Krwawicz cataract extractor
Krymed Cryopexy unit
Kryptok
K. bifocal
K. implant
K. lens

krypton
k. photocoagulation
k. red laser
K-Sol medium
KSS
Kearns-Sayre syndrome
Kufs syndrome
Kuglein
K. irrigating lens manipulator
K. push/pull
K. refractor
K. retractor
Kuglen manipulating hook
Kugler lens manipulator
Kuhnt
K. corneal scarifier
K. dacryostomy
K. eyelid operation
K. fixation forceps
K. illusion
K. meniscus
K. postcentral vein
K. space
K. tarsectomy
Kuhnt-Helmbold operation
Kuhnt-Junius
K.-J. disease
K.-J. macular degeneration
K.-J. maculopathy
K.-J. repair
Kuhnt-Szymanowski
K.-S. operation
K.-S. procedure
Kuhnt-Thorpe operation
Kuler panoramic lens
Kulvin-Kalt forceps
Kurova Shursite lens series
Kurz syndrome
Kveim
K. antigen
K. test
KW
Keith-Wagener change
KW change
Kwitko
K. conjunctival spreader
K. operation
Kynex
Kyrle disease

LA
 Dexone L.
L.A.
 Dexasone L.
 Solurex L.
labeling
 in situ DNA nick end l.
 (TUNEL)
Labrador keratopathy
labyrinthine nystagmus
LaCarrere operation
lacerate
 l. anterior foramen
 l. middle foramen
 l. posterior foramen
laceration
 canalicular l.
 central stellate l.
 conjunctival l.
 corneal l.
 corneoscleral l.
 eyebrow l.
 full-thickness corneal l.
 lid margin l.
 partial-thickness corneal l.
 tarsal l.
lacertus musculi recti lateralis bulbi
lachrymal (*var. of* lacrimal)
Lacramore
Lacricath lacrimal duct catheter
Lacril
 L. Ophthalmic Solution
Lacri-Lube NP
Lacri-Lube S.O.P.
lacrimal, lachrymal
 l. abscess
 l. acinar lobule
 l. angle duct anomaly
 l. anterior crest
 l. apparatus
 l. artery
 l. awl
 l. balloon catheter
 l. bay
 l. bone
 l. calculus
 l. canal
 l. canaliculus
 l. caruncle
 l. caruncula

 l. conjunctivitis
 l. dilator
 l. drainage
 l. duct
 l. ductal cyst
 l. duct anlage
 duct T-tube l.
 l. duct T-tube
 l. fistula
 l. fold
 l. fornix
 l. gland
 l. gland acinus
 l. gland epithelial tumor
 l. gland fossa
 l. gland gallium uptake
 l. gland repair
 l. groove
 l. incisure
 l. intubation probe
 l. irrigating cannula
 l. irrigation test
 l. keyhole
 l. lake
 l. lens
 l. nerve
 l. notch
 l. nucleus aplasia
 l. osteotome
 l. outflow
 l. papilla
 l. point
 l. posterior crest
 l. power
 l. process
 l. pump failure
 l. punctal stenosis
 l. punctum
 l. reflex
 l. sac
 l. sac bur
 l. sac chisel
 l. sac fossa
 l. sac gouge
 l. sac hemangiopericytoma
 l. sac retractor
 l. sac rongeur
 l. scintillography
 l. sound
 l. stent

L

267

lacrimal *(continued)*
l. sulcus
l. sulcus of lacrimal bone
l. sulcus of maxilla
l. surgery
l. syringe
l. system
l. testing
l. transit time
l. trephine
l. tubercle
l. vein
lacrimale
os l.
punctum l.
lacrimales
ductus l.
lacrimalin
lacrimalis
ampulla canaliculi l.
ampulla ductus l.
apparatus l.
avulsion of caruncula l.
canaliculus l.
caruncula l.
fistula l.
fornix sacci l.
Förster sacci l.
fossa glandulae l.
fossa sacci l.
glandula l.
hamulus l.
incisura l.
lacus l.
nervus l.
pars orbitalis glandulae l.
pars palpebralis glandulae l.
plica l.
rivus l.
sacculus l.
saccus l.
vena l.
lacrimarum
stillicidium l.
lacrimase
lacrimation
l. disorder
excessive l.
gustatory l.
l. reflex
lacrimator
lacrimatory
Lacrimedics occlusion starter kit

lacrimo-auriculo-dento-digital
syndrome
lacrimoconchalis
sutura l.
lacrimoconchal suture
lacrimoethmoidal suture
lacrimomaxillaris
sutura l.
lacrimomaxillary suture
lacrimonasal duct
lacrimotome
lacrimotomy
lacrimoturbinal suture
Lacrisert
Lacrivial
Lacrivisc
L. unit dose
lactate
ammonium l.
l. dehydrogenase
lacteal cataract
Lactoplate
lacuna, pl. **lacunae**
Blessig l.
vitreous l.
lacunata
Moraxella l.
lacus lacrimalis
LADARVision
L. excimer laser system
Ladarvision Platform
Ladd-Franklin theory
LaForce knife spud
lag
adduction l.
l. dilation
dilation l.
lid l.
Lagleyze
L. needle
L. operation
Lagleyze-Trantas operation
lagophthalmia, lagophthalmos,
lagophthalmus
l. conjunctivitis
spastic l.
lagophthalmic keratitis
Lagrange
L. operation
L. sclerectomy scissors
Laird spatula
laissez-faire lid operation

lake
    lacrimal l.
    tear l.
lambda
    l. angle
    L. Physik EMG 103 laser
Lambert chalazion forceps
Lambert-Eaton myasthenic
    syndrome
Lambert-Heiman scissors
lamella, gen. and pl. **lamellae**
    collagen l.
    corneal l.
    corneoscleral l.
    l. of Fuchs
    interlacing of collagen lamellae
    Rabl l.
lamellar
    l. calcification
    l. channel
    l. corneal graft
    l. corneal transplant
    l. developmental cataract
    l. groove
    l. haptic
    l. hole
    l. keratectomy for
    nontuberculous mycobacterial
    keratitis
    l. keratopathy
    l. keratoplasty (LKP)
    l. refractive keratoplasty
    l. separation of lens
    l. zonular perinuclear cataract
lamellation
lamina
    anterior limiting l.
    basal l.
    basalis choroideae l.
    basalis corporis ciliaris l.
    Bowman l.
    l. choriocapillaris
    l. choroidocapillaris
    l. cribrosa
    l. cribrosa sclerae
    l. densa
    l. dot

    l. elastica anterior
    l. elastica posterior
    episcleral l.
    l. fusca
    l. fusca sclerae
    l. limitans anterior corneae
    l. limitans posterior corneae
    limiting l.
    l. lucida
    orbital l.
    l. orbitalis ossis ethmoidalis
    l. papyracea
    posterior limiting l.
    l. superficialis musculi
    suprachoroid l.
    l. suprachoroidea
    l. vasculosa choroideae
    l. vitrea
    vitreal l.
    vitreous l.
laminar flow
laminated
    l. acellular mass
    l. spectacle lens
laminin
lamp
    Bausch-Lomb-Thorpe slit l.
    biomicroscope slit l.
    Birch l.
    Birch-Hirschfeld l.
    Burton l.
    Campbell slit l.
    carbon arc l.
    Coburn-Rodenstock slit l.
    Coherent LaserLink slit l.
    Duke-Elder l.
    Eldridge-Green l.
    fluorescent l.
    gas discharge l.
    Gullstrand slit l.
    Haag-Streit slit l.
    Hague cataract l.
    incandescent l.
    infrared slit l.
    Ishihara IV slit l.
    IV slit l.
    Kowa hand-held slit l.

L

NOTES

lamp *(continued)*
    Kowa Optimed slit l.
    Marco slit l.
    Nikon zoom photo slit l.
    Nitra l.
    Posner slit l.
    Reichert slit l.
    Rodenstock slit l.
    Specular reflex slit l.
    Thorpe slit l.
    Topcon SL-7E photo slip l.
    Topcon SL-E Series slit l.
    Topcon SL-1E slit l.
    tungsten-halogen l.
    Universal slit l.
    VG slit l.
    V-slit l.
    Wood l.
    Zeiss carbon arc slit l.
    Zeiss-Comberg slit l.
    Zeiss slit l.
Lancaster
    L. Cross
    L. eye magnet
    L. eye speculum
    L. keratome
    L. knife
    L. lid speculum
    L. operation
    L. red-green projector
    L. red/green test
    L. screen test
Lancaster-O'Connor speculum
Lancaster-Regan
    L.-R. dial 1 chart
    L.-R. dial 2 chart
    L.-R. test
lance
    Rolf l.
Lancereaux diabetes
lancet
    Keeler ultrasonic cataract
      removal l.
    Meyer Swiss diamond knife l.
    suture l.
    l. suture
    Swan l.
    ultrasonic cataract-removal l.
Lanchner operation
lancing pain
Landegger orbital implant
Landers
    L. biconcave lens

    L. contact lens
    L. irrigating vitrectomy ring
    L. vitrectomy ring
Landers-Foulks temporary
    keratoprosthesis lens
Lander wide-field temporary
    keratoprosthesis
Landolt
    L. body
    L. broken ring
    L. broken-ring chart
    L. broken-ring test
    L. C acuity chart
    L. C ring
    L. operation
Landry ascending paralysis
Landström muscle
Lane needle
Lang
    L. speculum
    L. stereo test
    L. stereotest
Lange
    L. blade
    L. fold
    L. speculum
Langenbeck operation
Langer-Giedion
    trichorhinophalangeal syndrome
Langerhans granule
Langerman diamond knife system
lantern test
Laqua black line retinal hook
Larcher sign
Largactil
large
    l. kappa angle
    l. physiologic cup
large-angled forceps
large-cell lymphoma
Larsen syndrome
larva
    ocular l.
larval conjunctivitis
Lasag
    L. Micropter II laser
LASAG microruptor
Laschal precision suture tome
lase
laser
    l. activity
    Aesculap argon ophthalmic l.
    Aesculap excimer l.

Aesculap-Meditec excimer l.
Allergan Humphrey l.
AMO YAG 100 l.
Apex Plus excimer l.
ArF excimer l.
argon blue l.
argon-fluoride excimer l.
argon green l.
argon-pumped tunable dye l.
Atlas-Elite l.
Atlas ophthalmic l.
Autonomous Technologies l.
l. biomicroscopy
Biophysic Medical YAG l.
blue-green argon l.
Britt argon/krypton l.
Britt argon pulsed l.
Britt BL-12 l.
Britt krypton l.
Britt pulsed argon l.
l. burn
l. burst
candela l.
carbon dioxide l.
Cardona l.
Carl Zeiss YAG l.
l. cavity
l. cell and flare meter
  (LCFM)
Cilco argon l.
Cilco Frigitronics l.
Cilco Hoffer Laseridge l.
Cilco krypton l.
Cilco/Lasertek A/K l.
Cilco/Lasertek argon l.
Cilco/Lasertek krypton l.
Cilco YAG l.
CO₂ l.
Coherent 7910 l.
Coherent 900 argon l.
Coherent 920 argon l.
Coherent 920 argon/dye l.
Coherent dye l.
Coherent EPIC l.
Coherent krypton l.
Coherent Medical YAG l.

Coherent Novus Omni
  multiwavelength l.
Coherent radiation
  argon/krypton l.
Coherent radiation argon model
  800 l.
Coherent Selecta 7000 l.
continuous l.
continuous-wave argon l.
continuous-wave diode l.
Cool Touch l.
Cooper 2000 l.
Cooper 2500 l.
Cooper Laser Sonics l.
CooperVision argon l.
CooperVision YAG l.
CO₂ Sharplan l.
l. cyclotherapy
Derma-K l.
diode l.
l. Doppler flowmeter
l. Doppler velocimeter
l. Doppler velocimetry
dye yellow l.
EC-5000 excimer l.
Epic l.
l. equipment
erbium l.
Evergreen Lasertek l.
ExciMed UV200 excimer l.
ExciMed UV200LA l.
excimer l.
Feather Touch CO₂ l.
l. flare-cell meter
l. flare-cell photometry
l. flare meter (LFM)
l. flare photometry
flashlamp-pumped microsecond
  pulse-dye l.
GentleLASE l.
Gish micro YAG l.
green l.
helium-ion aiming l.
helium-neon aiming l.
HGM argon green l.
HGM intravitreal l.
HGM ophthalmic l.

L

NOTES

laser *(continued)*
holmium l.
Ho:YAG l.
l. interferometry
intrastromal l.
l. intrastromal keratomileusis
ion l.
l. iridectomy
l. iridoplasty
l. iridotomy (LPI)
Iris Oculight SLx
MicroPulse l.
Keracor l.
l. keratotomy
Kremer excimer l.
krypton red l.
Lambda Physik EMG 103 l.
Lasag Micropter II l.
laser l.
Laserex Era 4106 YAG l.
LaserHarmonic l.
Lasertek l.
l. lens
liquid organic dye l.
LPK-80 II argon l.
Lumonics l.
l. manipulation
MC-7000 multi-wavelength l.
MC-7000 ophthalmic l.
Meditec l.
MEL 60 excimer l.
MEL 70 flying spot l.
MEL 60 scanning l.
Merrimac l.
Microlase transpupillary
diode l.
Microprobe ophthalmic l.
mode-locked Nd:YAG l.
molectron l.
Nanolas Nd:YAG l.
Nd:YAG l.
Nd:YLF l.
neodymium:YAG l. (Nd:YAG)
neodymium:yttrium aluminum
garnet l.
neodymium:yttrium lithium
fluoride l. (Nd:YLF)
neodymium:yttrium-lithium-
fluoride photodisruptive l.
Nidek EC-1000 excimer l.
Nidek Laser System l.
193-nm excimer l.
OcuLight SL diode l.

OcuLight SLx ophthalmic l.
oculocutaneous l.
OmniMed argon-fluoride
excimer l.
Ophthalas argon l.
Ophthalas argon/krypton l.
Ophthalas krypton l.
Opmilas 144 surgical l.
l. optometer
orange dye l.
l. panretinal photocoagulation
PC EDO ophthalmic office l.
l. photocoagulator
photodisrupting l.
PhotoPoint l.
photovaporation l.
photovaporizing l.
Prima KTP/532 l.
Q-switched Er:YAG l.
Q-switched neodymium:YAG l.
Q-switched ruby l.
l. refractometry
l. ridge
ruby l.
scanning excimer l.
Sharplan argon l.
l. in situ keratomileusis
Summit Apex l.
Summit excimer l.
Summit OmniMed excimer l.
Summit SVS Apex l.
Summit UV 200 Excimed l.
l. surgery
Takata l.
TE MOO mode beam l.
THC:YAG l.
l. therapy
l. thermal keratoplasty (LTK)
l. thermokeratoplasty
l. tomography scanner (LST)
T-PRK l.
tracker-assisted PRK laser
l. trabeculoplasty
tracker-assisted PRK l. (T-PRK
laser)
transpupillary l.
l. transscleral
cyclophotocoagulation
l. tube
tunable\ dye l.
twenty/twenty argon-fluoride
excimer l.
UltraPulse l.

URAM E2 compact
MicroProbe l.
Veinlaser Captured-Pulse l.
Visulas argon C l.
Visulas argon/YAG l.
Visulas Nd:YAG l.
Visulas YAG C l.
Visulas YAG E l.
Visulas YAG S l.
VisuMed MEL60 l.
VISX 2020 excimer l.
VISX Star S2 l.
VISX Twenty/Twenty
excimer l.
VitaLase Er:YAG l.
white l.
YAG l.
    yttrium-aluminum-garnet laser
yellow dye l.
yttrium-aluminum-garnet l.
(YAG laser)
Zeiss VISULAS 532 l.
Zeiss VISULAS YAG II l.
laser-argon device
laser-assisted
l.-a. intrastromal keratomileusis
(LASIK)
l.-a. in situ keratomileusis
lasered
Laseredge microsurgical knife
Laserex Era 4106 YAG laser
laser-filtering surgery
Laserflex
L. coagulator
L. lens
LaserHarmonic laser
Laseridge
Cilco Hoffer L.
L. Optics lens
laser-induced glaucoma
laser-ruby device
laser-scrape
l.-s. photorefractive keratectomy
l.-s. technique
Lasertek
L. laser

lash
l. abrasion of cornea
l. margin
misdirected l.
LASIK
laser-assisted intrastromal
keratomileusis
hyperopic LASIK
lasing
Lasiodiplodia theobromae
lasitome
Krumeich-Baraquer l.
lasso
lens l.
LAT
limbal autograft transplantation
lata
Tenon fascia l.
latanoprost
l. ophthalmic solution
l. solution 0.005%
late
l. phase detachment
l. postoperative suture
adjustment (LPSA)
latent
l. angle-closure glaucoma
l. deviation
l. diabetes
l. endophthalmitis
l. hyperopia (Hl)
l. nystagmus
l. squint
l. strabismus
late-onset
l.-o. corneal haze
l.-o. esotropia
l.-o. myope
l.-o. myopia
lateral
l. aberration
l. angle
l. canthal incision
l. canthal tendon
l. canthotomy
l. canthus
l. commissure of eyelid

L

NOTES

lateral *(continued)*
  l. gaze
  l. geniculate body (LGB)
  l. geniculate body lesion
  l. geniculate nucleus (LGN)
  l. hemianopsia
  l. horn
  l. illumination
  l. inhibition
  l. margin of orbit
  l. medullary infarction
  l. medullary syndrome
  l. nystagmus
  l. oblique conus
  l. orbital decompression
  l. orbital tubercle
  l. orbitotomy
  l. orbit tubercle
  l. palpebral ligament
  l. palpebral raphe
  l. palpebral tubercle
  l. phoria
  l. rectus (LR)
  l. rectus extraocular muscle
  l. rectus palsy
  l. rectus recession
lateralis
  angulus oculi l.
  commissura palpebrarum l.
  raphe palpebralis l.
lateroduction
lateropulsion
laterotorsion
lathe-cut contact lens
lathe lens
lathing procedure
lattice
  l. corneal dystrophy
  l. degeneration of retina
  l. dystrophy of cornea
  l. keratitis
  l. retinal degeneration
Lauber disease
laughing gas
Laurence-Biedl syndrome
Laurence-Moon-Bardet-Biedl
  syndrome
Laurence-Moon-Biedl syndrome
Laurence-Moon syndrome
laurentii
  Cryptococcus l.
Lauth canal
lavage

Lavoptik eye wash
law
  Alexander l.
  Ångström l.
  Beer l.
  Bunsen-Roscoe l.
  Descartes l.
  Desmarres l.
  Donders l.
  Ewald l.
  Ferry-Porter l.
  Flouren l.
  Giraud-Teulon l.
  Gullstrand l.
  Hering l.
  Horner l.
  Knapp l.
  Kollner l.
  Listing l.
  Plateau-Talbot l.
  Poiseuille l.
  reciprocity l.
  l. of refraction
  Riccò l.
  Roscoe-Bunsen l.
  Sherrington l.
  Snell l.
  Stefan l.
  Talbot l.
  Weber l.
  Wundt-Lamansky l.
Lawford syndrome
Lawton corneal scissors
laxity
  lid l.
  lower lid l.
Layden infant lens
layer
  aqueous tear l.
  bacillary l.
  basal l.
  Bowman l.
  Bruch l.
  Chievitz fiber l.
  choriocapillary l.
  columnar l.
  cuticular l.
  epithelial basement l.
  fibrin l.
  ganglion cell l.
  grading of retinal nerve
    fiber l.
  Haller l.

Henle fiber l.
inner nuclear l.
inner plexiform l.
juxtapapillary nerve fiber l.
keratin l.
limiting l.
lipid tear l.
molecular external l.
molecular inner l.
molecular internal l.
molecular outer l.
mucin l.
mucous tear l.
nerve fiber l. (NFL)
nerve fiber bundle l.
nuclear external l.
nuclear inner l.
nuclear internal l.
nuclear outer l.
oil l.
outer nuclear l.
outer plexiform l. (OPL)
peripapillary nerve fiber l.
pigment l.
plexiform external l.
plexiform inner l.
plexiform internal l.
plexiform outer l.
posterior collagenous l. (PCL)
retinal ganglion cell l.
retinal nerve fiber l. (RNFL)
retinochoroidal l.
l. of rods and cones
Sattler l.
suprachoroid l.
tear l.
layered
    l. hyphema
    l. keratoplasty
lazy eye
LC-65
L-Caine
LCFM
    laser cell and flare meter
l-cone
L cone excitation
LD+2

L/D ratio
LE
    left eye
Le
    L. Grand-Geblewics
    phenomenon
    L. Grand-Gullstrand eye model
lead
    l. encephalopathy
    l. incrustation of cornea
lead-filled mallet
Leahey
    L. chalazion forceps
    L. operation
leak
    eyelash-induced l.
    glue patch l.
    macular l.
leakage
    corneal l.
    juxtapapillary l.
    microaneurysmal l.
    parafoveal microvascular l.
    progressive fluorescein l.
leaking filtering bleb
least diffusion circle
Lea Symbol chart
leaves of capsule
Lebensohn
    L. reading chart
    L. visual acuity chart
Leber
    L. cell
    L. congenital amaurosis
    L. disease
    L. hereditary optic atrophy
    L. hereditary optic atrophy
    reverse dot-blot assay
    L. hereditary optic neuropathy
    (LHON)
    L. idiopathic stellate
    retinopathy
    L. lymphangiectasia
    hemorrhagica
    L. miliary aneurysm
    L. plus syndrome
    L. syndrome

L

NOTES

275

LED
light-emitting diode
LED-illuminated ring
Lefler-Wadsworth-Sidbury foveal dystrophy
left
l. deorsumvergence
l. esotropia
l. exotropia
l. eye (LE, OS)
l. gaze
l. hyperphoria
l. hypertropia (LHT)
l. inferior oblique recession
l. inferior rectus muscle
l. superior oblique tuck
l. superior rectus muscle
l. sursumvergence
left-beating nystagmus
left-handed cornea scissors
left-to-right shunting
Legacy Series 2000
Cavitron/Kelman phaco-emulsifier aspirator
legal blindness
legally blind
Leigh
L. capsule forceps
L. disease
L. encephalopathy
leiomyoma
l. of iris
l. of uveal tract
Leishman classification
Leishman-Donovan body
leishmaniasis
American l.
Leishmania tropica
Leiske lens
Leitz microscope
Leland refractor
lema
lemniscus, pl. **lemnisci**
optic l.
Lemoine
L. orbital implant
L. serrefine
Lemoine-Searcy fixation anchor loupe
lemon-drop nodule
Lempert rongeur

Lempert-Storz
L.-S. lens
L.-S. loupe
Lems lens
length
axial l. (AL)
chord l.
focal l.
primary focal l.
secondary focal l.
temple l.
lens, pl. **lenses**
l. aberration
Abraham iridectomy laser l.
Abraham peripheral button iridotomy l.
Abraham YAG laser l.
accommodation of crystalline l.
Accugel l.
achromatic spectacle l.
acrylic l.
AcrySof foldable intraocular l.
Acrysof MA60 l.
Acuvue disposable contact l.
adherent l.
Airy cylindric l.
Alcon MA30BA optic Acrysof l.
Alges bifocal contact l.
Allen-Thorpe l.
Allergan AMO Array S155 l.
all-Perspex CQ l.
all-Perspex Kelman Omnifit l.
all-PMMA intraocular l.
Amenabar l.
American Medical Optics Baron l.
amnifocal l.
AMO Array foldable intraocular l.
AMO Array multifocal ultraviolet-absorbing silicone posterior chamber intraocular l.
AMO intraocular l.
AMO IOPTEX Model ACR 360 foldable acrylic l.
AMO Phacoflex II foldable intraocular l.
amorphic l.
Amsoft l.
anastigmatic l.
angle-fixated l.

angle-supported l.
aniseikonic l.
Anis staple l.
annular bifocal contact l.
anterior chamber intraocular l.
(ACIOL)
AO l.
AO-XT 166 l.
aphakic l.
aplanatic l.
apochromatic l.
Appolionio l.
Aquaflex contact l.
Aquasight l.
Arlt l.
Arruga l.
artificial l.
Artisan l.
Arysoft foldable acrylic l.
aspherical ophthalmoscopic l.
aspheric cataract l.
aspheric contact l.
aspheric spectacle l.
aspheric-viewing l.
aspiration of l.
astigmatic l.
auxiliary l.
l. axis
axis of cylindric l. (x)
Azar l.
back surface toric contact l.
Bagolini l.
Baikoff l.
ballasted contact l.
bandage soft contact l.
Barkan gonioscopic l.
Barkan goniotomy l.
Baron l.
Barraquer l.
baseball l.
Bausch & Lomb Optima l.
Bausch & Lomb Surgical
L161U l.
Bayadi l.
8.4 BC disposable l.
Bechert 7-mm l.
Beebe l.

beveled-edge l.
bicentric spectacle l.
biconcave contact l.
biconvex l.
bicurve contact l.
bicylindrical l.
Bietti l.
bifocal contact l.
bifocal intracorneal l.
bifocal spectacle l.
Binkhorst four-loop iris-
fixated l.
Binkhorst-Fyodorov l.
Binkhorst intraocular l.
Binkhorst iridocapsular l.
Binkhorst two-loop l.
biomicroscopic indirect l.
Bi-Soft l.
bispherical l.
bitoric contact l.
blooming of l.
blooming spectacle l.
Boberg-Ans l.
Boston contact l.
Boston Envision l.
Bowling l.
Boys-Smith laser l.
Brücke l.
Burian-Allen contact l.
Byrne expulsive hemorrhage l.
Calendar monthly disposable
contact l.
l. capsule
capsule of l.
Cardona fiberoptic diagnostic l.
Carl Zeiss l.
cast resin l.
cataract l.
CeeOn foldable l.
CeeOn intraocular l.
cellulose acetate butyrate
contact l.
Centra-Flex l.
central posterior curve of
contact l.
central retinal l.
central thickness of contact l.

L

NOTES

lens *(continued)*
Charles intraocular l.
Charles irrigating contact l.
chemically treated spectacle l.
Chiroflex C11UB l.
Choyce intraocular l.
Choyce Mark VIII l.
Cibasoft contact l.
Cibathin l.
Cilco intraocular l.
Cilco MonoFlex multi-piece
 PMMA intraocular l.
Cilco-Simcoe II l.
Cilco-Sonometrics l.
CIMA*flex* 411 foldable
 silicone l.
Clayman intraocular l.
Clayman posterior chamber l.
L. Clear
clear crystalline l.
l. clip
C-loop intraocular l.
C-loop posterior chamber l.
coating of l.
coating for spectacle l.
Coburn intraocular l.
collagen bandage l.
coloboma of l.
Comberg contact l.
ComfortKone l.
composition of spectacle l.
compound l.
concave spectacle l.
concavoconcave l.
concavoconvex l.
condensing l.
conoid l.
constructional ability contact l.
contact l. (CL)
contact bandage l.
contact low-vacuum l.
contour l.
converging meniscus l.
convex l.
convexoconcave l.
convexoconvex l.
convex plano l.
convex spectacle l.
CooperVision PMMA-ACL
 Flex l.
Copeland panchamber l.
Copeland radial panchamber
 intraocular l.

Copeland radial panchamber
 UV l.
coquille plano l.
corneal contact l.
corrected spectacle l.
cortical substance of l.
cosmetic shell contact l.
CR-39 l.
crocodile l.
Crookes l.
crossed l.
crown glass l.
l. crystallina
crystalline l.
CSI l.
curvature of l.
curves of spectacle l.
cylinder spectacle l.
cylindrical l. (C, cyl.)
Dailies contact l.
daily-wear contact l. (DWCL)
Darin l.
decentered l.
l. decentration
decentration of l.
diagnostic contact l.
diagnostic fiberoptic l.
66-diopter iridectomy laser l.
direct gonioscopic l.
dislocated l.
l. dislocation
dislocation of l.
dispersing l.
disposable contact l.
distortion of l.
diverging meniscus l.
dot-like l.
double concave l.
double convex l.
Doubra l.
l. dressing
Drews l.
dual l.
Dulaney l.
Durasoft 2 contact l.
Dura-T l.
Edge III hydrogel contact l.
edging of spectacle l.
Emcee l.
Emery l.
l. epithelium
Epstein collar stud acrylic l.
l. equator

equator of crystalline l.
ERG-Jet disposable contact l.
Eschenback Optik l.
etafilcon A lenses
l. exchange
executive spectacle l.
exfoliation of l.
l. exfoliation glaucoma
l. expressor
extended-wear contact l.
(EWCL)
eye l.
EZVUE violet haptic
intraocular l.
Falcon l.
Feaster Dualens l.
Fechner intraocular l.
Federov type II intraocular l.
Federov type I intraocular l.
l. fiber
fiberoptic diagnostic l.
field l.
finished l.
first definite apical clearance l.
(FDACL)
flat contact l.
flat-edge l.
flexible-wear l.
Flexlens l.
Flexner-Worst iris claw l.
l. flexure effect
flint-glass l.
fluid contact l.
fluidless contact l.
F/M base curve contact l.
foldable intraocular l.
FormFlex l.
four-loop l.
four-mirror goniolens l.
Franklin-style bifocal lenses
Frelex l.
Frenzel l.
FreshLook ColorBlends l.
Fresnel l.
Friedman hand-held Hruby l.
Friedman-Hruby l.
front surface toric contact l.

fundus contact l.
fundus focalizing l.
fundus laser l.
fused bifocal l.
fused multifocal l.
Galin intraocular implant l.
gas-permeable contact l.
generating spectacle l.
Genesis l.
Gentex PDQ polycarbonate l.
Gill intraocular implant l.
Gilmore l.
Gilmore intraocular implant l.
glass l.
l. glide
glued-on hard contact l.
Goldmann diagnostic contact l.
Goldmann fundus contact l.
Goldmann macular contact l.
Goldmann multi-mirror l.
Goldmann three-mirror l.
goniofocalizing l.
goniolens l.
gonioscopic l.
Gould intraocular implant l.
Gridley intraocular l.
Gullstrand l.
hand-held Hruby l.
haptic plate l.
hard contact l. (HCL)
hardened spectacle l.
hardening of l.
Hart pediatric three-mirror l.
heparin surface-modified
intraocular l. (HSM)
Hessburg l.
Hidex glass l.
Hoffer-Laseridge intraocular l.
honey bee l.
Hoskins l.
Hoskins-Barkan goniotomy
infant l.
Hruby contact l.
Hunkeler l.
Hydracon contact l.
Hydrasoft contact l.
Hydrocurve II l.

NOTES

lens *(continued)*
hydrogel contact l.
Hydron l.
hydrophilic contact l.
hydrophobic contact l.
Hydrosight l.
Hydroview l.
hypermature l.
immersion l.
l. implant
implant l.
implantable contact l. (ICL)
implantation of l.
Implens intraocular l.
inert material for intraocular l.
infant Karickhoff laser l.
infant three-mirror laser l.
Intermedics l.
Interspace YAG laser l.
in-the-bag l.
intraocular l. (IOL)
IOLAB 108 B l.
IOLAB intraocular l.
Ioptex laser intraocular l.
Ioptex TabOptic l.
Irene l.
iridocapsular intraocular l.
iridotomy l.
iris-fixated l.
iris-supported l.
iseikonic l.
isoiconic l.
Jaffe Cilco l.
J-loop PC l.
J-loop posterior chamber
intraocular l.
Joal l.
Jung-Schaffer intraocular l.
Kamerling Capsular 90 l.
Karickhoff laser l.
Kearney side-notch l.
Keeler panoramic l.
Kelman flexible tripod l.
Kelman Multiflex II l.
Kelman Omnifit II
intraocular l.
Kelman PC 27LB CapSul l.
Kelman Quadriflex anterior
chamber intraocular l.
Kilp l.
Kirby l.
Kishi l.
knife-edged l.

Koeppe diagnostic l.
Korb l.
Krasnov l.
Kratz elliptical-style l.
Kratz-Johnson l.
Kratz posterior chamber
intraocular l.
Kratz-Sinskey intraocular l.
Kratz "soft" J-loop
intraocular l.
Krieger wide-field fundus l.
Kryptok l.
Kuler panoramic l.
lacrimal l.
lamellar separation of l.
laminated spectacle l.
Landers biconcave l.
Landers contact l.
Landers-Foulks temporary
keratoprosthesis l.
laser l.
Laserflex l.
Laseridge Optics l.
l. lasso
lathe l.
lathe-cut contact l.
Layden infant l.
Leiske l.
Lempert-Storz l.
Lems l.
lenticular-cut contact l.
lenticular spectacle l.
Lewis l.
Lieb-Guerry l.
Lindstrom Centrex l.
Liteflex l.
l. localizer
long-wearing contact l.
l. loop
loose l.
lotrafilcon A l.
l. loupe
Lovac gonioscopic l.
L. Lubricant
luxated l.
luxation of l.
Lynell intraocular l.
Machemer flat l.
Machemer infusion contact l.
Machemer magnifying
vitrectomy l.
macular contact l.
magnifying l.

Mainster-HM retinal laser l.
Mainster retinal laser l.
Mainster-S retinal laser l.
Mainster Ultra Field PRP laser l.
Mainster-WF retinal laser l.
Mainster wide field l.
Mandelkorn suture laser lysis l.
l. manipulator
March laser l.
Mark II Magni-Focuser l.
Mark IX l.
L. Mate
mature l.
McCannel l.
McGhan 3M intraocular l.
McLean prismatic fundus laser l.
Medallion l.
Medical Optics PC11NB intraocular l.
Medical Workshop intraocular l.
Meditec bandage contact l.
meniscus concave l.
Meso contact l.
meter l.
microbevel edge l.
microthin l.
mid-coquille l.
MiniQuad XL l.
minus spectacle l.
4-Mirror Gonio l.
modified C-loop intraocular l.
modified C-loop UV l.
modified J-loop intraocular l.
modified J-loop UV l.
mold-injected l.
Momose l.
multicurve contact l.
Multiflex anterior chamber l.
multifocal spectacle l.
Multi-Optics l.
negative meniscus l.
Neolens l.
New Orleans l.

NewVues l.
Nikon aspheric l.
Nokrome bifocal l.
Nova Aid l.
Nova Curve broad C-loop posterior chamber l.
Nova Curve Omnicurve l.
Nova Soft II l.
nuclear sclerosis of l.
nucleus of l.
Nuvita l.
occupational l.
Oculaid l.
ocular l.
Ocular oamboscope l.
O'Malley-Pearce-Luma l.
Omnifit intraocular l.
one-piece multifocal l.
one-piece plate haptic silicone intraocular l.
one-plane l.
L. Opacification Classification System (LOCS)
L. Opacities Case-Control Study
L. Opacities Classification System II (LOCS II)
open l.
Ophtec Co. l.
optical center of spectacle l.
optical contact l.
Optical Radiation l.
optical zone of contact l.
optics of intraocular l.
Optiflex l.
Optima contact l.
Opti-Vu l.
Opt-Visor l.
Optycryl 60 contact l.
Opus III contact l.
orbital l.
ORC intraocular l.
Orthogon l.
orthoscopic l.
O'Shea l.
Osher gonio/posterior pole l.
Osher pan-fundus l.

L

NOTES

lens *(continued)*
Osher surgical gonio/posterior pole l.
overall diameter of contact l. (OAD)
panchamber UV l.
Pannu intraocular l.
Pannu type II l.
PanoView Optics l.
Paraperm O2 contact l.
l. particle glaucoma
PBII blue loop l.
Pearce posterior chamber intraocular l.
pediatric Karickhoff laser l.
pediatric three-mirror laser l.
Percepta progressive l.
peripheral curve on contact l.
periscopic concave l.
periscopic convex l.
Permaflex l.
Permalens l.
Perspex CQ-Shearing-Simcoe-Sinskey l.
Petrus single-mirror laser l.
Peyman-Green vitrectomy l.
Peyman-Tennant-Green l.
Peyman wide-field l.
PhacoFlex II SI30NB intraocular l.
Phakic 6 l.
Pharmacia intraocular l.
Pharmacia Visco J-loop l.
photobrown lenses
photochromic l.
photogray l.
photosensitive l.
photosun l.
piggyback contact l.
pigmentary deposits on l.
l. pit
l. placode
placode l.
l. plane
plano l.
planoconcave l.
planoconvex nonridge l.
Plano T l.
plastic l.
plate-haptic silicone l.
Platina clip l.
L. Plus
L. Plus daily cleaner

L. Plus Oxysept
L. Plus Oxysept System
L. Plus rewetting drops
L. Plus saline
plus spectacle l.
polarizing l.
polycarbonate l.
Polycon I contact l.
Polycon II contact l.
Polymacon l.
polymethyl methacrylate contact l.
positive meniscus l.
Posner diagnostic l.
posterior chamber intraocular l. (PCIOL)
posterior pole of l.
l. power
l. power calculation
Precision Cosmet l.
press-on Fresnel l.
primary l.
prismatic contact l.
prismatic effect by l.
prismatic gonioscopic l.
prismatic gonioscopy l.
prismatic goniotomy l.
prismatic spectacle l.
progressive addition l.
progressive multifocal l.
prolonged-wear contact l.
prosthetic l.
protective l.
l. protein glaucoma
punctal l.
pupillary l.
QuadPediatric fundus l.
radius of l.
Rayner l.
Red Reflex Lens Systems l.
refractive contact l.
l. removal
retroscopic l.
Revolution l.
ridge l.
Ridley l.
rigid contact l.
Ritch contact l.
Ritch nylon suture laser l.
Ritch trabeculoplasty laser l.
RLX l.
Rodenstock panfundus l.
rudiment l.

Ruiz fundus contact l.
Ruiz fundus laser l.
safety l.
SaturEyes contact l.
Saturn II contact lenses
Sauflon l.
Sauflon PW l.
Schachar l.
Scharf l.
Schlegel l.
scleral contact l.
scratch-resistant spectacle l.
secondary l.
secondary curve on contact l.
segmental l.
self-stabilizing vitrectomy l.
semifinished l.
semiscleral contact l.
Severin l.
Shearing intraocular l.
Shearing planar posterior
  chamber intraocular l.
Sheets l.
short C-loop l.
Signet Optical l.
silicone acrylate contact l.
silicone elastomer l.
Silsoft contact l.
Simcoe II PC l.
simple plus l.
single-cut contact l.
Sinskey intraocular l.
l. size
slab-off l.
Slant haptic single-piece
  intraocular l.
SlimFit ovoid intraocular l.
SlimFit small-incision ovoid l.
Snellen soft contact l.
Soflens 66 l.
Soflens contact l.
SoFlex series lenses
soft contact l. (SCL)
soft intraocular l.
SoftSITE high add aspheric
  multifocal contact l.

Sola Optical USA Spectralite
  high index l.
Soper cone l.
Sovereign bifocal l.
special spectacle l.
spectacle l.
Spectralite Transitions l.
spherical l. (S, sph.)
spherical equivalent l.
spherocylindric l.
spherocylindrical l.
spin-cast l.
l. sponge
spontaneous extrusion of l.
l. spoon
Staar AA 4207 l.
Staar implantable contact l.
Staar intraocular l.
Staar toric l.
Staar 4203VF l.
Staar 4207VF l.
Stableflex anterior chamber l.
l. star
star l.
steep contact l.
stigmatic l.
Stokes l.
Storz CAPSULORBLUE
  intraocular l.
Strampelli l.
Style S2 clear-loop l.
styrene contact l.
subluxated l.
subluxation of l.
subluxed l.
substance of l.
Super Field NC slit lamp l.
Surefit AC 85J l.
Surevue contact l.
Surgidev intraocular l.
Surgidev PC BUV 20-24
  intraocular l.
Sussman l.
Sutherland l.
suture of l.
T l.

L

NOTES

283

lens *(continued)*
Tano double mirror peripheral
  vitrectomy l.
telescopic l.
Tennant Anchorflex AC l.
therapeutic contact l.
thick l.
thin l.
Thorpe four-mirror
  goniolaser l.
Thorpe four-mirror vitreous
  fundus laser l.
three-mirror contact l.
three-piece acrylic intraocular l.
three-piece silicone
  intraocular l.
tight contact l.
Tillyer bifocal l.
tilting l.
tinted contact l.
tinting of spectacle l.
Tolentino prism l.
Tolentino vitrectomy l.
Topcon aspheric l.
toric contact l.
Toric intraocular l.
Toric-Optima series l.
toric spectacle l.
toroidal contact l.
Touchlite zoom l.
transsclerally sutured posterior
  chamber l. (TS-SPCL)
trial case and l.
tricurve contact lenses
trifocal l.
Trokel l.
Trokel-Peyman laser l.
truncated contact l.
Trupower aspherical l.
TruVision l.
two-plane l.
Ultex l.
Ultra mag l.
Ultra view SP slit lamp l.
Ultravue l.
uncut spectacle l.
Uniplanar style PC II l.
Univis l.
Univision low-vision
  microscopic l.
Urrets-Zavalia retinal
  surgical l.
Uvex l.

UV Nova Curve l.
Varigray l.
Varilux l.
vaulting of contact l.
vergence of l.
l. vesicle
Viscolens l.
Vision Tech l.
VISITEC Company l.
Volk aspheric l.
Volk coronoid l.
Volk High Resolution
  aspherical l.
Volk 3 Mirror ANF+ l.
Volk 3 Mirror gonio fundus
  laser l.
Volk Quadraspheric l.
Volk SuperField aspherical l.
Volk SuperField NC l.
Volk SuperQuad 160 contact l.
Volk SuperQuad 160
  panretinal l.
Volk Transequator l.
Wang l.
Weber-Elschnig l.
Wesley-Jessen l.
L. Wet
whorl l.
Wild l.
WildEyes costume contact l.
Wise iridotomy laser l.
Wise iridotomy-sphincterotomy
  laser l.
with contact lenses (c̄cl)
Wood l.
Woods Concept l.
Worst Claw l.
Worst goniotomy l.
Worst Medallion l.
Worst Platina iris-fixated l.
X chrom l.
Yannuzzi fundus laser l.
Youens l.
Zeiss l.
Zeiss-Gullstrand l.
zero power lenses
l. zonule
lens blank
LensCheck Advanced Logic
  lensometer
lensectomy
Charles l.

clear l.
coal-mining l.
Lensept
lenses (*pl. of* lens)
Lens-Eze inserter
Lens Fresh
lens-holding forceps
lens-induced
    l.-i. glaucoma
    l.-i. secondary open-angle
      glaucoma
    l.-i. UGH syndrome
    l.-i. uveitis
lens-iris diaphragm
lens-maker formula
Lensmeter
    L. 701
    Badal L.
    Nagel L.
    Zeiss LA 110 projection L.
lensometer
    Allergan l.
    Allergan Humphrey l.
    AO l.
    AO Reichert Instruments l.
    Carl Zeiss l.
    Coburn l.
    Hardy l.
    IntraOptics l.
    LensCheck Advanced Logic l.
    Marco l.
    Reichert Lenschek advanced
      logic l.
    Topcon LM P5 digital l.
lensopathy
Lensrins
lens-sparing vitrectomy
lens-threading forceps
Lens-Wet
lenta
    ophthalmia l.
lentectomize
lentectomy
lenticonus
    anterior l.
    posterior l.
lenticula

lenticular
    l. astigmatism
    l. body
    l. bowl
    l. cataract
    l. contact lens
    l. degeneration
    l. fossa
    l. fossa of vitreous body
    l. ganglion
    l. glaucoma
    l. myopia
    l. nucleus
    l. opacity
    l. ring
    l. spectacle lens
    l. vesicle
lenticular-cut
    l.-c. contact lens
lenticule
    epikeratoplasty l.
lenticuli (*pl. of* lenticulus)
lenticulocapsular
lenticulo-optic
lenticulostriate
lenticulothalamic
lenticulus, pl. **lenticuli**
lentiform
    l. nodule
    nucleus l.
lentigines
    l., electrocardiogram
      abnormalities, ocular
      hypertelorism, pulmonary
      stenosis, abnormal genitalia,
      retardation of growth, and
      deafness (LEOPARD)
lentiglobus
lentis
    apparatus suspensorius l.
    l. articularis
    axis l.
    caligo l.
    capsula l.
    cellulae l.
    chalcosis l.
    coloboma l.

L

NOTES

lentis *(continued)*
    cortex l.
    ectopia l.
    epithelium l.
    equator l.
    equatorial l.
    facies anterior l.
    facies posterior l.
    fibrae l.
    gerontoxon l.
    nucleus l.
    polus anterior l.
    polus posterior l.
    radius of l.
    siderosis l.
    spontaneous ectopia l.
    substantia corticalis l.
    Topia l.
    tunica vasculosa l.
    vortex l.
Lenz syndrome
leonine appearance
LEOPARD
    lentigines, electrocardiogram
    abnormalities, ocular
    hypertelorism, pulmonary stenosis,
    abnormal genitalia, retardation of
    growth, and deafness
    LEOPARD syndrome
leopard
    l. fundus
    l. retina
Lepper-Trier formula
leprae
    Mycobacterium l.
leprosa
    keratitis punctata l.
leptomeningeal metastasis
Leptospira
    L. interrogans
leptotrichosis conjunctivae
lesion
    acquired abducens nerve l.
    Archer l.
    basal ganglia l.
    bilateral occipital lobe l.
    boomerang-shaped l.
    brainstem l.
    branching l.
    bull's eye macular l.
    cerebellar l.
    cerebellopontine angle l.
    cerebral hemisphere l.

    cervical l.
    chiasm l.
    chiasmal l.
    chorioretinal l.
    choroidal l.
    concentric l.
    congenital abducens nerve l.
    conjunctival melanotic l.
    cornea guttate l.
    corneal punctate l.
    corpus callosum l.
    CPA l.
    cracked windshield stromal l.
    dendriform corneal l.
    dendriform epithelial l.
    dendritic epithelial l.
    diencephalic l.
    epibulbar l.
    extrastriate cortex l.
    facial nerve l.
    frontal lobe unilateral cerebral
      hemisphere l.
    frontoparietal bilateral cerebral
      hemisphere l.
    geographic l.
    hamartomatous l.
    hemorrhagic disciform l.
    herpetoid l.
    hypertrophic dendriform
      epithelial l.
    keratitis l.
    lateral geniculate body l.
    LGB l.
    linear streak l.
    lipocytic l.
    lymphoepithelial l.
    lytic l.
    malignant pituitary l.
    medulla l.
    melanocytic conjunctival l.
    melanotic l.
    mesencephalic l.
    mesencephalon l.
    neural l.
    occipital lobe unilateral
      cerebral hemisphere l.
    oculomotor nerve l.
    optic chiasmal l.
    optic nerve l.
    optic radiation l.
    optic tract l.
    l. of orbit
    orbital l.

osseous l.
parasellar l.
parietal lobe bilateral cerebral
  hemisphere l.
parietal lobe unilateral cerebral
  hemisphere l.
periventricular l.
phototoxic l.
pigmented l.
pons l.
pontine l.
precancerous l.
preganglionic l.
pseudocancerous l.
punched-out l.
recurrent corneal l. (RCL)
retinal l.
retrobulbar compressive l.
retrogeniculate l.
satellite l.
sonolucent l.
space-occupying l.
subarachnoid oculomotor
  nerve l.
sunburst-type l.
supranuclear l.
suprasellar l.
temporal lobe unilateral
  cerebral hemisphere l.
trochlear nerve l.
unifocal optic nerve l.
unilateral l.
VZV disciform l.
waxy l.
weeping eczematous l.
white laser l.
L'Esperance erysiphake
lesser
  l. ring of iris
  l. wing of sphenoid
Lester
  L. fixation forceps
  L. Jones operation
  L. Jones tube
  L. lens dialer
  L. lens manipulator
Lester-Burch speculum

lethal midline granuloma
letter
  l. blindness
  Sloan l.'s
  Snellen l.'s
  test l.
  l. test
letterbox technique
Letterer-Siwe syndrome
letter-shaped keratitis
leucitis
leukemic
  l. cell
  l. infiltrate
  l. infiltration of the optic disk
  l. retinitis
  l. retinopathy
leukocoria, leukokoria
leukoderma
  periorbital l.
leukokoria, leukocoria
leukoma, pl. **leukomata**
  l. adherens
  adherent l.
  l. corneae
  corneal l.
leukomatous corneal opacity
leukopathia, leukopathy
  congenital l.
leukopsin
leukoscope
leukotomy
  transorbital l.
levator
  l. aponeurosis defect
  l. aponeurosis disinsertion
  l. aponeurosis repair
  l. function testing
  l. injury
  l. innervation
  l. muscle of upper eyelid
  l. palpebrae superioris
  l. palpebrae superioris muscle
  l. resection
  l. trochlear muscle
Levine spud
Levitt implant

L

NOTES

levobunolol
  l. HCl
  l. hydrochloride
levocabastine
  l. HCl
  l. hydrochloride
levoclination
levocycloduction
levocycloversion
levoduction
levo-epinephrine
levotorsion
levoversion
Lewicky
  L. formed cystitome
  L. needle
  L. self-retaining chamber
    maintainer
  L. threaded infusion cannula
Lewis
  L. lens
  L. lens loupe
  L. scoop
Lewy body
Lexan
Lexer operation
LFM
  laser flare meter
LGB
  lateral geniculate body
  LGB lesion
LGN
  lateral geniculate nucleus
LHA-B27-associated uveitis
LHON
  Leber hereditary optic neuropathy
LHT
  left hypertropia
library temple
lichenification
  eyelid l.
lichenified lid
Lichtenberg corneal trephine
LICO
  L. disposable penlight
  L. Hertel exophthalmometer
lid
  l. agglutination
  l. block
  Celsus l.
  l. closure reaction
  l. closure reflex
  l. crease

  l. crusting
  crusting l.
  l. droop
  droopy l.
  l. ectropion
  l. edema
  l. eversion
  l. everter
  l. fissure
  l. forceps
  granular l.
  l. imbrication syndrome
  l. lag
  l. laxity
  lichenified l.
  l. loading
  lower l. (LL)
  l. margin
  l. margin laceration
  l. notching
  l. nystagmus
  l. plate
  l. retraction
  l. scrub
  l. scurf
  l. speculum
  l. thrush
  tonic l.
  l. trephine
  upper l. (UL)
  l. vesicle
LidFix speculum
lidocaine
  l. hydrochloride
  l. with epinephrine
Lidoject
Lidoject-1 with epinephrine
lids, lashes, lacrimals, lymphatics
  (LLLL)
lid-triggered synkinesia
Lid Wipes-SPF
Lieberman
  L. fragmentor
  L. K-Wire speculum
  L. MicroFinger manipulator
  L. phaco crusher
Lieberman-Pollock double corneal
  forceps
Lieb-Guerry lens
Liebreich symptom
Lieppman cystitome
LIF
  local intra-arterial fibrinolysis

life-belt cataract
ligament
    canthal l.
    check l.
    ciliary l.
    cribriform l.
    Hueck l.
    hyaloideocapsular l.
    lateral palpebral l.
    Lockwood l.
    medial canthal l.
    medial palpebral l.
    palpebral l.
    pectinate l.
    pectineal l.
    suspensory l.
    Weigert l.
    Whitnall l.
    Wieger l.
    Zinn l.
ligamentum
    l. anguli iridocornealis
    l. circulare corneae
    l. pectinatum anguli
      iridocornealis
    l. pectinatum iridis
light
    l. adaptation
    l. argon laser burn
    autokinesis visible l.
    axial ray of l.
    Barkan l.
    L. Blade laser workstation
    central l.
    l. coagulation
    cobalt blue l.
    convergent l.
    dichromatic l.
    l. difference
    l. differential threshold
    l. discrimination
    divergent l.
    emergent ray of l.
    ether theory of l.
    fixation l.
    flashes of l.
    idioretinal l.

    incident ray of l.
    intrinsic l.
    Lumiwand l.
    marginal ray of l.
    l. microscope
    l. microscopy
    minimum l.
    monochromatic l.
    near reaction to l.
    oblique ray of l.
    ophthalmoscopy with
      reflected l.
    l. optometer reflex
    paraxial ray of l.
    l. perception (LP)
    peripheral ray of l.
    pipe l.
    l. pipe pick
    polarized l.
    polychromatic l.
    l. projection
    l. projection test
    l. reaction
    reflected l.
    l. reflex ring
    refracted l.
    l. response of pupil
    l. scatter
    l. scattering
    l. sensation
    l. sense
    l. sensitivity
    Serdarevic Circle of L.
    l. stimulus
    l. toxicity
    l. transmission
    transmitted l.
    ultraviolet l.
    unit of l.
    white l.
    Young theory of l.
light-adapted eye
LightBlade
    Novatec L.
light/dark amplitude ratio (L/D ratio)
light-emitting diode (LED)

L

NOTES

Lighthouse
   L. Distance Visual Acuity Test
   L. ET-DRS acuity chart
   L. Low Vision Service
lighting
   paraxial l.
light-near dissociation
lightning
   l. cataract
   l. eye movement
   L. high-speed vitrectomy
      handpiece
   l. streak
light-optometer
light-peak to dark-trough ratio
light-stress test
ligneous
   conjunctivitis l.
   l. conjunctivitis
lignocaine
   l. hydrochloride
lilacinus
   Paecilomyces l.
limbal
   l. allograft
   l. approach
   l. arcade
   l. autografting
   l. autograft transplantation
      (LAT)
   l. bleeding
   l. choristoma
   l. compression
   l. dermoid
   l. follicle
   l. girdle
   l. girdle of Vogt
   l. groove
   l. guttering
   l. incision
   l. ischemia
   l. luteus retinae
   l. neurofibroma
   l. palisades of Vogt
   l. papillae
   l. parallel orientation
   l. stem cell
   l. stem-cell deficiency
   l. stem-cell transplantation
   l. stroma
   l. tissue
   l. vasculitis
   l. zone

limbal-based flap
limbi (*pl. of* limbus)
limbic
   l. vernal keratoconjunctivitis
limbitis
Limbitrol
limbus, pl. **limbi**
   balding the l.
   blue l.
   circumferential vascular plexus
      of the l.
   congenital dermoid of l.
   conjunctival l.
   l. of cornea
   corneal inferior l.
   corneoscleral l.
   cystoid cicatrix of l.
   l. girdle
   l. guttering
   l. mass
   l. palpebrales anteriores
   l. palpebrales posteriores
   l. parallel orientation straddling
      tattoo mark
   l. of perception
   l. of sclera
limit
   Rayleigh l.
limitation
   eccentric l.
limited gallium scan
limiting
   l. angle
   l. lamina
   l. lamina anterior
   l. layer
   l. membrane
Lincoff
   L. balloon
   L. balloon catheter
   L. lens sponge
   L. operation
   L. scleral sponge implant
Lindau disease
Lindau-von Hippel disease
Linde cryogenic probe
Lindner
   L. operation
   L. sclerotomy
   L. spatula
Lindsay operation
Lindstrom
   L. arcuate incision marker

L. astigmatic marker
L. Centrex lens
L. lens-insertion forceps
L. Star
L. Star nucleus manipulator
Lindstrom-Casebeer algorithm
Lindstrom-Chu aspirating speculum
line
 absorption l.
 A Maddox l.
 angular l.
 Arlt l.
 atopic l.
 blue l.
 corneal iron l.
 l. of direction
 distance between nasal l.'s
  (DBL)
 Donders l.
 Egger l.
 Ehrlich-Türck l.
 endothelial rejection l.
 epithelial iron l.
 face l.
 Ferry l.
 fingerprint l.
 l. of fixation
 flat demarcation l.
 Fraunhofer l.
 gray l.
 Helmholtz l.
 Hudson l.
 Hudson-Stähli l.
 iron l.
 iron-ferry l.
 iron-Hudson-Stähli l.
 iron-Stocker l.
 Khodadoust l.
 mare's hair l.
 mare's tail l.
 Morgan l.
 Paton l.
 pigment demarcation l.
 principal l.
 pupillary l.
 rejection l.
 retinal stress l.

 Sampaoelesi l.
 Schwalbe l. (SL)
 l. of sight
 Snellen l.
 Stähli pigment l.
 Stocker l.
 stromal l.
 superficial corneal l.
 l. test
 triradiate l.
 Turk l.
 l. of vision
 visual l.
 Vogt l.
 Zöllner l.
linea, gen. and pl. **lineae**
 l. corneae senilis
 l. visus
linear
 l. endotheliitis
 l. infiltration
 l. keratopathy
 l. scar
 l. scarring
 l. sebaceous nevus sequence
 l. streak lesion
 l. subcutaneous atrophy
 l. vision
 l. visual acuity test
linkage analysis
Linn-Graefe iris forceps
lint-free sponge
LIO500
 IRIS L.
Lions
 L. Doheny Eye and Tissue
  Transplant Bank
 L. Low Vision Center
lip
 anterior l.
 scleral l.
lipemia
 l. retinalis
lipemic
 l. retina
 l. retinopathy

L

NOTES

lipid
> l. accumulation
> l. cell
> l. degeneration
> l. deposit
> l. exudate
> l. keratopathy
> l. tear layer

lipoatrophic diabetes
lipocytic lesion
lipodermoid
> conjunctival l.

lipoidosis
> l. corneae

lipoma
> orbital l.

lipomatosis
> ptosis l.

lipoplethoric diabetes
Lipo-Tears Forte
lippa
lippitude, lippitudo
Lipschütz inclusion body
lipuric diabetes
liquefaciens
> *Serratia l.*

liquefaction
> contraction and l.
> vitreal l.

liquid
> l. organic dye laser
> l. perfluorocarbon
> l. Pred
> l. vitreous-aspirating cannula

liquified vitreous
Liquifilm
> Albalon L.
> Betagan L.
> Bleph-10 L.
> L. Forte
> L. Forte Solution
> Herplex L.
> HMS L.
> Prefrin Z L.
> P.V. Carpine L.
> L. Tears
> L. Tears Solution
> L. Wetting

liquor
> l. corneae
> Morgagni l.

Lisch
> L. nodule
> L. spot

Lister
> L. forceps
> L. lens manipulator
> L. scissors

Listeria
Listing
> L. law
> L. plane
> L. reduced eye
> L. schematic eye

Liteflex lens
Lite-Pred
literal alexia
lithiasis
> l. conjunctivae
> conjunctival l.
> l. conjunctivitis

lithotriptor
> candela laser l.

Littauer
> L. cilia forceps
> L. dissecting scissors

Littler dissecting scissors
Littmann Galilean magnification
> **changer**

Livernois
> L. lens-holding forceps
> L. pickup and folding forceps

Livingston peribulbar wedge
Living Water Eye Lotion
Livostin
LKP
> lamellar keratoplasty

LL
> lower lid

LLLL
> lids, lashes, lacrimals, lymphatics

Llobera fixation forceps
Lloyd stereocampimeter
LMX1B **gene**
loa
> *Loa l.*

loading
> lid l.

loafer temple
Loa loa
lobe
> frontal l.
> occipital l.
> palpebral l.

parietal l.
temporal l.
temporoparietal l.
lobule
lacrimal acinar l.
lobuli
coloboma l.
local
l. anesthetic
l. intra-arterial fibrinolysis
(LIF)
l. outgrowth
l. tic
l. tonic pupil
localization
Comberg l.
spatial l.
localized
l. albinism
l. amyloidosis
localizer
Berman l.
lens l.
Roper-Hall l.
Wildgen-Reck l.
location anomaly
locator
Berman foreign body l.
Bronson-Turner foreign body l.
foreign body l.
Roper-Hall l.
Sweet l.
Wildgen-Reck l.
loci (*pl. of* locus)
lock
Luer cannula l.
Lockwood
L. ligament
L. light reflex
superior tendon of L.
L. tendon
LOCS
Lens Opacification Classification
System
LOCS II
Loctoplate
locus, pl. **loci**

l. of fixation
gene l.
GLCIA l.
preferred retinal l. (PRL)
retinoblastoma l.
trained retinal l.
lodoxamide
l. tromethamine
l. tromethamine ophthalmic
solution
Loewi
L. reaction
L. sign
Löfgren syndrome
**logarithmic Minimum Angle of
Resolution (logMAR)**
logistic discriminant analysis
logMAR
logarithmic Minimum Angle of
Resolution
logMAR chart
log unit
Löhlein operation
Lombart
L. radioscope
L. tonometer
lomustine
Londermann
L. corneal trephine
L. operation
long
l. ciliary artery
l. ciliary nerve
l. posterior ciliary artery
l. root of ciliary ganglion
l. sight
long-acting gas
longi
nervi ciliares l.
longitudinal
l. aberration
l. axis
l. axis of Fick
l. ciliary muscle
l. fasciculus
l. fiber
long-scale contrast

NOTES

long/short occluder
longsightedness
long-wearing contact lens
Look
L. capsule polisher
L. cortex extractor
L. cystitome
L. I/A coaxial cannula
L. irrigating lens loop
L. irrigating vectis
L. micropuncture device
L. retrobulbar needle
L. suture
looking
forced choice preferential l.
preferential l.
loop
Axenfeld nerve l.
C l.
Clayman-Knolle irrigating
lens l.
closed l.
expressor l.
flexible l.
Flynn lens l.
haptic l.
intrascleral nerve l.
irrigating vectis l.
J l.
Knapp lens l.
Knolle-Pearce irrigating lens l.
lens l.
Look irrigating lens l.
Meyer-Archambault l.
Meyer temporal l.
modified J l.
nerve l.
nylon l.
open l.
Pearce-Knolle irrigating lens l.
prepapillary arterial l.
prepapillary vascular l.
temporal l.
two-angled polypropylene l.
vascular l.
venous l.
loose
l. contact lens
l. lens
Lopez-Enriquez
L.-E. operation
L.-E. scleral trephine
loratadine

Lordan chalazion forceps
lorgnette
l. occluder
Loring ophthalmoscope
loss
axonal l.
blood l.
chiasmal visual field l.
field l.
functional visual l.
glaucomatous visual field l.
hearing l.
hemisensory l.
intraoperative blood l.
migrainous vision l.
nasal field l.
nonorganic visual l.
nonphysiologic visual field l.
progressive hearing l.
retrochiasmal visual field l.
scintillating vision l.
scotopic sensitivity l.
sudden visual l.
transient visual l.
unilateral hearing l.
vascular optical disk swelling
without visual l.
l. of vision
vitreous l.
l. of vitreous
Lotemax
L. ophthalmic suspension
loteprednol
l. etabonate
l. etabonate ophthalmic
suspension 0.5%
Lotion
Living Water Eye L.
Lotman Visometer
lotrafilcon A lens
Lo-Trau side-cutting needle
Lotze local sign
louchettes
loupe
Amenabar lens l.
angled lens l.
angled nucleus removal l.
Arlt lens l.
Atwood l.
Beebe l.
Berens lens l.
binocular l.
Callahan lens l.

Castroviejo lens l.
Elschnig-Weber l.
FormFlex lens l.
Gullstrand l.
Ilg lens l.
Keeler panoramic l.
Kirby intracapsular lens l.
Kirby intraocular lens l.
Kraff nucleus lens l.
Lemoine-Searcy fixation
  anchor l.
Lempert-Storz l.
lens l.
Lewis lens l.
magnifying l.
Mark II Magni-Focuser l.
New Orleans lens l.
nucleus delivery l.
nucleus removal l.
Ocular Gamboscope l.
operating l.
Opt-Visor l.
panoramic l.
Simcoe l.
Simcoe double-end lens l.
Simcoe II PC nucleus
  delivery l.
Simcoe nucleus delivery l.
Simcoe nucleus lens l.
Snellen lens l.
Troutman lens l.
Visitec nucleus removal l.
Weber-Elschnig lens l.
Wilder lens l.
Zeiss-Gullstrand l.
Zeiss operating field l.
Lovac
  L. fundus contact lens implant
  L. gonioscope
  L. gonioscopic lens
  L. six-mirror gonioscopic lens
    implant
low
  l. contrast
  l. convex
  l. profile R-K marker
  l. vision

Lowe
  L. oculocerebrorenal syndrome
  L. ring
Lowell glaucoma knife
Löwenstein-Jensen medium
Löwenstein operation
lower
  l. eyelid
  l. hemianopsia
  l. lid (LL)
  l. lid laxity
  l. lid retractor
  l. lid sling procedure
  l. punctum
  l. retina
Lowe-Terrey-MacLachlan syndrome
low-pressure glaucoma
Lowry assay
low-tension glaucoma
low-vision aid
loxophthalmus
LP
  light perception
LPI
  laser iridotomy
LPK-80 II argon laser
LPSA
  late postoperative suture adjustment
LR
  lateral rectus
LST
  laser tomography scanner
L.T. Jones tear duct tube
LTK
  laser thermal keratoplasty
lubricant
  Lens L.
  silicone l.
lubricating drops
lubrication
  surface l.
Lubricoat
Lubrifair
LubriTears Solution
Lucae dressing forceps
lucency, pl. **lucencies**

NOTES

lucida
 camera l.
 lamina l.
lucidum
 tapetum l.
Lucite
 L. frame
 L. implant
 L. sphere implant
Luedde
 L. exophthalmometer
 L. transparent rule
Luer
 L. cannula lock
 L. connection
 L. tube
Luer-Lok
 L.-L. syringe
 Yale L.-L.
luetic
 l. chorioretinitis
 l. interstitial keratitis
 l. neuropathy
lugdunensis
 Staphylococcus l.
lumbar puncture
lumbricoides
 Ascaris l.
lumen, pl. **lumina, lumens**
 capillary l.
luminance
 background l.
 l. setting
luminosity
 l. curve
luminous
 l. flux
 l. intensity (I)
 l. retinoscope
lumirhodopsin
Lumiwand light
Lumonics laser
lunata
 plica l.
Lundsgaard
 L. knife
 L. rasp
 L. sclerotome
Lundsgaard-Burch
 L.-B. corneal rasp
 L.-B. sclerotome
Luneau retinoscopy rack
Luntz-Dodick punch

lupus
 l. erythematosus cell test
 l. oculopathy
Lurocoat
luster
 binocular l.
 corneal l.
 polychromatic l.
lusterless
lustrous central yellow point
lutea
 macula l.
luteum
 punctum l.
lux
 l. setting
luxated lens
luxation
 l. of eyeball
 l. of globe
 l. of lens
 superior oblique muscle and
 trochlear l.
Luxo surgical illuminator
luxurians
 ectropion l.
luxury perfusion
LX needle
Lyda-Ivalon-Lucite implant
Lyle syndrome
Lyme disease keratitis
lymphangioma
 conjunctival l.
 eyelid l.
lymphatic drainage
lymphatics
 lids, lashes, lacrimals, l.
 (LLLL)
lymphaticus
 nodulus l.
lymphoblastic lymphoma
lymphocytic
 l. infiltration
 l. interstitial pneumonitis
lymphoepithelial lesion
lymphoepithelioma
Lymphogranuloma
 L. venereum conjunctivitis
lymphogranuloma venereum
 keratitis
lymphoid
 l. follicle
 l. hyperplasia

l. infiltration
l. pseudotumor
l. tumor
lymphoma
anterior chamber l.
histiocytic l.
intraocular l.
large-cell l.
lymphoblastic l.
MALT l.
non-Hodgkin l.
oculocerebral l.
orbital l.
porcupine l.
primary central nervous
system l. (PCNSL)
primary ocular l.
reticulum cell l.
signet-ring l.
T-cell l.
zone B-cell l.

lymphomatosis
ocular l.
lymphophagocytosis
lymphoproliferative tumor
Lynch
L. approach
L. medial canthal incision
Lynell intraocular lens
Lyon hypothesis
lysed
lysis
cell l.
l. of restricting strand
symblepharon l.
lysozyme
serum l.
Lythgoe effect
lytic lesion
Lytico-Bodig syndrome

NOTES

L

M
myopia
myopic
  M band
  M cell
  M cone excitation
3M
  3M small aperture Steri-Drape
  3M Steri-Drape drape
M4-400 freedom blade
Macbeth
  M. ColorChecker
  M. illumination
MacCallan classification
Macewen sign
Machado-Joseph disease
**Machat superior flap LASIK
  marker**
Mach band
Machek-Blaskovics operation
Machek-Brunswick operation
Machek-Gifford operation
Machek ptosis operation
Machemer
  M. calipers
  M. diamond-dust-coated foreign
  body forceps
  M. flat lens
  M. infusion contact lens
  M. magnifying vitrectomy lens
  M. vitreous cutter
machine
  Catalyst m.
  CooperVision I/A m.
  Euro Precision Technology
  submicron lathe m.
  I/A m.
  Stat m.
  Stat Scrub handwasher m.
  Visual-Tech m.
Mackay-Marg
  M.-M. electronic tonometer
  M.-M. principle
Mack-Brunswick operation
Mackool system
macroaneurysm
  arterial m.
  retinal m.
macroblepharia
macrocornea

macrocupping
  pseudoglaucomatous m.
macrocyst
macrocytic anemia
macrodisc
  congenital m.
macroerosion
macroperforation
macrophthalmia
macrophthalmic
macrophthalmous
macropsia
macroptic
macroreticular dystrophy
macrosaccadic oscillation
macro square-wave jerks
macrostereognosis
macrovessel
macula, pl. **maculae**
  m. adherens
  maculae ceruleae
  cherry-red spot in m.
  m. corneae
  dragged m.
  ectopia maculae
  false m.
  m. flava retinae
  graying of m.
  Henle layer of the m.
  heterotropia maculae
  honeycomb m.
  inferior m.
  m. lutea
  m. lutea retinae
  parafoveal m.
  m. retinae
  superonasal m.
  temporal m.
  vitelliform degeneration of m.
**macula-off rhegmatogenous retinal
  detachment**
macular, maculate
  m. aplasia
  m. area
  m. arteriole
  m. arteriole occlusion
  m. binocular vision
  m. branch retinal vein
  occlusion (MBRVO)
  m. choroiditis

M

macular *(continued)*
m. cluster
m. CMV
m. coloboma
m. contact lens
m. corneal dystrophy
m. cytomegalovirus
m. detachment
m. disciform degeneration
m. disease
m. displacement
m. dragging
m. drusen
m. dysplasia
m. ectopia
m. edema
m. epiretinal membrane
m. evasion
m. graying
m. heredodegeneration
m. hole (MH)
m. hole surgery
m. hypoplasia
m. leak
m. neuroretinopathy
m. ocular histoplasmosis
   syndrome
m. OHS
m. paramacular vitreoretinal
   interface
m. photocoagulation
M. Photocoagulation Study
   (MPS)
m. photostress
m. pucker
m. puckering
m. retinoblastoma
m. retinopathy
m. sparing
m. splitting
m. star
m. stereopsis
m. suppression
m. surface wrinkling
m. traction
m. translocation
m. venule
maculary
   m. fasciculus
macule
maculocerebral
maculopapillary bundle

maculopapular bundle
maculopathy
age-related m. (ARM)
atrophic degenerative m.
bull's eye m.
cellophane m.
cystoid m.
diabetic m.
dry senile degenerative m.
exudative senile m.
familial pseudoinflammatory m.
Groenouw type II m.
heredity m.
histoplasmosis m.
Kuhnt-Junius m.
myopic m.
niacin m.
nicotinic acid m.
operating microscope-induced
   phototoxic m.
photic m.
phototoxic m.
pigment epithelial
   detachment m.
serous detachment m.
solar m.
Sorsby m.
Stargardt m.
toxic m.
unilateral acute idiopathic m.
vitelliform m.
MaculoScope
maculovesicular
MacVicar double-end strabismus
   retractor
madarosis
Maddox
M. LASIK spatula
M. prism
M. rod
M. rod method
M. rod occluder
M. rod test
M. wing test
Madribon
madurae
   Actinomadura m.
Maeder-Danis dystrophy
mafilcon A
Magendie
M. sign
M. symptom

Magendie-Hertwig
  M.-H. sign
  M.-H. syndrome
Magitot keratoplasty operation
magnae
  facies orbitalis alae m.
magnet
  Bronson-Magnion eye m.
  eye m.
  Gruening m.
  Haab m.
  hand-held eye m.
  Hirschberg m.
  implant m.
  Lancaster eye m.
  m. operation
  original Sweet eye m.
  rare earth intraocular m.
  Schumann giant type eye m.
  Storz-Atlas hand eye m.
  Storz Microvit m.
  Sweet original m.
magnetic
  m. extraction
  m. field-search coil test
  m. implant
  m. operation
  m. resonance angiography
    (MRA)
  m. resonance imaging (MRI)
  m. resonance imaging scan
  m. resonance spectroscopy
    (MRS)
magnification
  relative spectacle m.
magnifier
  Circline m.
  Optelec Passport m.
  spectacle m.
magnifying
  m. glasses
  m. lens
  m. loupe
  m. power
magnocellular
  m. cell
  m. visual pathway

Magnus operation
Maguire-Harvey vitreous cutter
Maidera-Stern suture hook
Maier
  M. sinus
  sinus of M.
main fiber
Mainster
  M. retinal laser lens
  M. Ultra Field PRP laser lens
  M. wide field lens
Mainster-HM retinal laser lens
Mainster-S retinal laser lens
Mainster-WF retinal laser lens
maintainer
  Blumenthal anterior
    chamber m.
  Fary anterior chamber m.
  Lewicky self-retaining
    chamber m.
Majewsky operation
major
  m. amblyoscope
  m. amblyoscope test
  annulus iridis m.
  m. arcade
  m. arterial circle of iris
  circulus arteriosus iridis m.
  erythema multiforme m.
  m. histocompatibility antigen
  m. histocompatibility complex
  m. meridian
majoris
  facies orbitalis alae m.
Maklakoff tonometer
malalignment
Malbec operation
Malbran operation
maleate
  chlorpheniramine m.
  naphazoline and
    pheniramine m.
  pilocarpine and timolol m.
  timolol m.
malformation
  Arnold-Chiari m.
  arteriovenous m.

M

NOTES

301

malformation *(continued)*
Chiari m.
congenital brain m.
dural arteriovenous m.
infratentorial arteriovenous m.
orbital arteriovenous m.
retinal arteriovenous m.
supratentorial arteriovenous m.
Malherbe calcifying epithelioma
malignant
m. choroidal melanoma
m. ciliary epithelioma
m. dyskeratosis
m. epithelial tumor
m. exophthalmos
m. glaucoma
m. hypertension
m. hyperthermia
m. melanoma of the choroid
m. myopia
m. neurilemoma
m. pituitary lesion
m. schwannoma
m. scleritis
Malis
M. bipolar coagulating/cutting system
M. forceps
Mallazine Eye Drops
mallet
lead-filled m.
malprojection
MALT lymphoma
Manche LASIK speculum
Mandelkorn suture laser lysis lens
maneuver
Carlo Traverso m. (CTM)
doll's eye m.
doll's head m.
Hallpike m.
notch-and-roll m.
Nylen-Barany m.
oculocephalic m.
Valsalva m.
wall push m.
Manhattan
M. Eye & Ear probe
M. Eye & Ear spatula
M. Eye & Ear suturing forceps
manifest
m. deviation
m. hyperopia (Hm)

m. latent nystagmus
m. refraction (MR)
m. strabismus
manifestation
neuro-ophthalmic m.
neurovisual m.
manipulation
laser m.
pharmacologic m.
physical m.
manipulator
angled m.
button-tip m.
Drysdale nucleus m.
Friedman Phaco/IOL m.
Grieshaber three-function m.
Grieshaber two-function m.
Judson-Smith m.
Koch phaco m.
Kuglein irrigating lens m.
Kugler lens m.
lens m.
Lester lens m.
Lieberman MicroFinger m.
Lindstrom Star nucleus m.
Lister lens m.
McIntyre irrigating iris m.
Rappazzo intraocular m.
Visitec m.
manner
McLean m.
Mannis
M. probe
M. suture
mannitol
mannosidosis
Mann sign
Mann-Whitney U test
manometer
Honan m.
Tycos m.
manometry
manoptoscope
Manson-Aebli corneal section scissors
Manson double-ended strabismus hook
Mantel-Haenszel method
manual
m. keratometer
m. kinetic perimetry
m. lamellar keratoplasty
Manz gland

MAO
Montana Academy of
Ophthalmology
map
axial curvature m.
m. dystrophy
elevation topography m.
m. pattern
rastersteriography-based
elevation m.
map-dot corneal dystrophy
map-dot-fingerprint corneal
epithelial dystrophy
mapping
axial curvature m.
deletion m.
glaucomatous damage detection
by retinal thickness m.
placido-based axial
curvature m.
visually evoked potential m.
mapropsia
marbleization
Marcaine
M. HCl
M. HCl with epinephrine
marcescens
Serratia m.
March
M. laser lens
M. laser sclerostomy needle
Marco
M. chart projector
M. lensometer
M. manual keratometer
M. perimeter
M. prism exophthalmometer
M. radius gauge
M. refractor
M. slit lamp
M. SurgiScope
Marcus
M. Gunn dot
M. Gunn jaw-winking
phenomenon
M. Gunn jaw-winking
syndrome

M. Gunn pupil (MG)
M. Gunn pupillary sign
M. Gunn relative afferent
defect
M. Gunn test
mare's
m. hair line
m. tail line
margin
ciliary m.
eyelid m.
fimbriated m.
infraorbital m.
lash m.
lid m.
orbital m.
marginal
m. blepharitis
m. catarrhal ulcer
m. chalazion forceps
m. corneal degeneration
m. corneal ulcer
m. crystalline dystrophy
m. degeneration of cornea
m. entropion
m. furrow
m. furrow degeneration
m. keratitis
m. melt
m. myotomy
m. ray of light
m. reflex distance (MRD)
m. ring ulcer of cornea
m. tear strip
marginalis
blepharitis m.
marginoplasty
margo
m. ciliaris iridis
m. infraorbitalis orbitae
m. lacrimalis maxillae
m. lateralis orbitae
m. medialis orbitae
m. orbitalis
m. palpebra
m. pupillaris iridis

M

NOTES

margo *(continued)*
  m. supraorbitalis orbitae
  m. supraorbitalis ossis frontalis
Marie ataxia
Marinesco-Sjögren syndrome
Mariotte
  blind spot of M.
  M. blind spot
  M. experiment
  M. scotoma
Maritima
  succus cineraria M.
Mark
  M. II Magni-Focuser lens
  M. II Magni-Focuser loupe
  M. IX lens
mark
  limbus parallel orientation
    straddling tattoo m.
marker
  Amsler scleral m.
  Arrowsmith corneal m.
  astigmatic m.
  biprong muscle m.
  Bores axis m.
  Castroviejo corneal
    transplant m.
  Castroviejo scleral m.
  Chayet corneal m.
  corneal transplant m.
  Dell astigmatism m.
  Desmarres m.
  Feldman RK optical center m.
  Fink biprong m.
  Fink muscle m.
  Friedlander incision m.
  Gass scleral m.
  Gonin m.
  Gonin-Amsler m.
  Green corneal m.
  Green-Kenyon corneal m.
  Hoffer optical center m.
  Hoopes corneal m.
  Hunkeler frown incision m.
  Lindstrom arcuate incision m.
  Lindstrom astigmatic m.
  low profile R-K m.
  Machat superior flap
    LASIK m.
  McDonald optic zone m.
  Mendez corneal m.
  Neumann-Shepard corneal m.

  Neumann-Shepard oval optical
    center m.
  Nordin-Ruiz trapezoidal m.
  O'Brien m.
  O'Connor m.
  ocular m.
  optical zone m.
  Osher-Neumann corneal m.
  radial keratotomy m.
  RK m.
  Ruiz-Nordan trapezoidal m.
  scleral m.
  Shepard optical center m.
  Simcoe corneal m.
  Soll suture and incision m.
  Storz radial incision m.
  Thornton 360 degree
    arcuate m.
  Thornton K3-7991 360 degree
    arcuate m.
  Thornton optical center m.
  Visitec RK zone m.
  Zaldivar m.
markers for zone
marking pen
Markwell
  method of M.
Marlex mesh
Marlin Salt System II
Marlow test
Marmor
  pattern dystrophy of pigment
    epithelium of Byers and M.
Marquez-Gomez
  M.-G. conjunctival graft
  M.-G. operation
Marshall syndrome
Martegiani
  area M.
Martinez
  M. corneal transplant centering
    ring
  M. corneal trephine blade
  M. disposable corneal trephine
  M. dissector
  M. keratome
  M. knife
Martin Surefit lens pusher
mascara particle inclusion
Masciuli silicone sponge
masked diabetes
mask-like facies
masque biliaire

masquerade
    m. syndrome
    m. technique
mass
    choroidal m.
    cicatricial m.
    coalescent m.
    gelatinous m.
    hyaline m.
    intracranial m.
    laminated acellular m.
    limbus m.
    mulberry-shaped m.
    mycelial m.
    ochre m.
    ovoid m.
    yellow-white choroidal m.
Massachusetts
    M. Eye & Ear Infirmary
    M. Vision Kit (MVK)
    M. XII vitrectomy system
    (MVS)
massage
    ocular m.
Masselon
    M. glasses
    M. spectacles
massive
    m. granuloma of sclera
    m. periretinal proliferation
    (MPP)
mast
    m. cell
    m. cell stabilizer
Mastel
    M. compass-guided arcuate
    keratotomy system
    M. diamond compass
    M. trifaceted diamond blade
master-dominant eye
master eye
Masuda-Kitahara disease
Mate
    Lens M.
    Soft M.
material
    alloplastic donor m.

    autogenous donor m.
    coating m.
    contrast m.
    cyanographic contrast m.
    cyanographin contrast m.
    donor m.
    fibrillar m.
    gallium citrate contrast m.
    gelatinous m.
    heterogeneous donor m.
    homogeneous donor m.
    hyaline m.
    m.'s primary dye
    M.'s Testing System
matogenous retinal detachment
matrix
    acellular m.
    extracellular m. (ECM)
    stromal m.
matte
    m. black forceps
    m. black instrument
matter
    particulate m.
    periaqueductal gray m.
Mattis corneal scissors
mattress suture
maturation
    delayed visual m.
mature
    m. cataphoria
    m. cataract
    m. lens
maturity-onset diabetes
Mauksch-Maumenee-Goldberg
  operation
Mauksch operation
Maumenee
    M. capsule forceps
    M. corneal forceps
    M. erysiphake
    M. goniotomy knife
    M. goniotomy knife cannula
    M. iris hook
    M. knife goniotomy cannula
    M. Suregrip forceps

NOTES

305

Maumenee *(continued)*
M. vitreous-aspirating needle
M. vitreous sweep spatula
Maumenee-Colibri corneal forceps
Maumenee-Goldberg operation
Maumenee-Park eye speculum
Maunoir iris scissors
Maurice corneal depot technique
mauritaniensis
Acanthamoeba m.
Mauthner test
Max
M. Fine forceps
M. Fine scissors
Maxidex
maxilla, gen. **maxillae,** pl. **maxillae**
incisura maxillae
infraorbital margin of m.
infraorbital sulcus of m.
lacrimal sulcus of m.
margo lacrimalis maxillae
processus zygomaticus maxillae
sulcus infraorbitalis maxillae
zygomatico-orbital process of
the m.
maxillaris
nervus m.
maxillary
m. bone
m. nerve
m. osteomyelitis
m. sinusitis
maximum tolerated medical therapy
Maxitrol
MaxiVision dietary supplement
Maxwell
M. ring
M. spot
Maxwell-Lyons sign
Mayo
M. scissors
M. stand
May sign
Mazzotti reaction
MBRVO
macular branch retinal vein
occlusion
MC-7000
M. multi-wavelength laser
M. ophthalmic laser
McCannel
M. implant
M. lens

M. ocular pressure reducer
M. suture
M. suture technique
McCarey-Kaufman (M-K)
M.-K. medium
M.-K. transport medium
McCarthy reflex
McClure iris scissors
McCollough tying forceps
McCool capsule retractor
McCullough suturing forceps
McCune-Albright syndrome
McDonald
M. expressor
M. lens folding forceps
M. optic zone marker
McGannon
M. refractor
M. retractor
McGavic operation
McGhan
M. implant
M. 3M intraocular lens
McGregor conjunctival forceps
McGuire
M. conformer
M. corneal scissors
M. I/A system
M. marginal chalazion forceps
M. operation
McIntyre
M. coaxial cannula
M. coaxial irrigating-aspirating
system
M. fish-hook needle holder
M. I/A needle
M. I/A system
M. infusion set
M. irrigating/aspirating unit
M. irrigating hook
M. irrigating iris manipulator
M. irrigation/aspiration needle
M. irrigation/aspiration system
M. nylon cannula connector
M. reverse cystitome
M. spatula
M. truncated cone
McIntyre-Binkhorst irrigating
cannula
McKee speculum
McKinney
M. eye speculum
M. fixation ring

McLaughlin operation
McLean
  M. capsule forceps
  M. capsulotomy scissors
  M. classification of melanoma
  M. fashion
  M. manner
  M. muscle recession forceps
  M. operation
  M. prismatic fundus laser lens
  M. suture
  M. technique
  M. tonometer
McNeill-Goldmann
  M.-G. blepharostat
  M.-G. ring
McNemar test
McPherson
  M. angled forceps
  M. bent forceps
  M. corneal forceps
  M. corneal section scissors
  M. irrigating forceps
  M. microiris forceps
  M. microsuture forceps
  M. needle holder
  M. spatula
  M. speculum
  M. trabeculotome
  M. tying iris forceps
McPherson-Castroviejo corneal
section scissors
McPherson-Vannas microiris scissors
McPherson-Westcott
  M.-W. conjunctival scissors
  M.-W. stitch scissors
McPherson-Wheeler
  M.-W. blade
  M.-W. knife
McPherson-Ziegler knife
McQueen vitreous forceps
McReynolds
  M. keratome
  M. lid-retracting hook
  M. operation
  M. pterygium knife
  M. pterygium scissors

  M. pterygium transplant
  M. spatula
  M. technique
mean
  m. acuity
  m. corneal power
  m. episcleral heat dose
  m.'s sign
  m. spherical equivalent (MSE)
measure
  Geneva lens m.
measurement
  box m.
  color-contrast sensitivity m.
  criterion-free m.
  diurnal intraocular pressure m.
  glare disability m.
  post occlusion m.
  prism cover m.
  Rushton ocular m.
  Stenstrom ocular m.
mechanical
  m. acquired ptosis
  m. ectropion
  m. lid retraction
  m. strabismus
  m. vitrector
mechanics
  fluid m.
mechanism
  m. of action
  cAMP mediated m.
  cholinergic m.
  fixation m.
  Hering after-image m.
  immune m.
  oculogyric m.
  primary m.
  pursuit m.
  secondary m.
  trigger m.
mechanized scissors
Mecholyl test
MED
  minimal effective diameter
Medallion lens
MedDev implant

NOTES

media (*pl. of* medium)
medial
  m. angle
  m. angle of eye
  m. arteriole of retina
  m. canthal ligament
  m. canthal repair
  m. canthal tendon
  m. canthus
  m. commissure of eyelid
  m. ectropion
  m. horn
  m. longitudinal fasciculus
  (MLF)
  m. palpebral ligament
  m. rectus (MR)
  m. rectus extraocular muscle
  m. rectus function
  m. rectus muscle
  m. rectus palsy
  m. rectus transposition
  m. superior temporal (MST)
  m. superior temporal visual
  area
  m. temporal (MT)
  m. temporal visual area
  m. venulae of retina
  m. vestibular nucleus (MVN)
medialis
  angulus oculi m.
  commissura palpebrarum m.
  venula retinae m.
mediaometer
mediator
  inflammatory m.
medical
  m. adenomectomy
  m. ophthalmoscopy
  M. Optics PC11NB intraocular
  lens
  M. Optics PC11NB intraocular
  lens implant
  m. tattooing
  M. Workshop intraocular lens
  M. Workshop intraocular lens
  implant
medicamentosa
  conjunctivitis m.
Medicornea
  M. Kratz intraocular lens
  implant
Medi-Duct ocular fluid management
system

Meditec
  M. bandage contact lens
  M. laser
Mediterranean anemia
medium, pl. media
  anaerobic m.
  chondroitin sulfate m.
  media clearing
  contrast m.
  corneal storage m.
  culture m.
  dextran m.
  dioptric m.
  gram-negative m.
  Kaufman m.
  K-Sol m.
  Löwenstein-Jensen m.
  McCarey-Kaufman m.
  McCarey-Kaufman transport m.
  M-K m.
  ocular m.
  media opacity
  opaque m.
  Optisol m.
  Page m.
  refracting m.
  refractive m.
  Sabouraud m.
MedJet microkeratome
Medmont M600 perimeter
Medpor implant
medroxyprogesterone acetate
medrysone
medulla
  m. lesion
medullary
  m. cystic disease
  m. optic disease
  m. ray
medullated nerve fiber
medulloblastoma tumor
medulloepithelioma
  adult m.
  embryonal m.
  orbital m.
Meek operation
Meesman
  M. epithelial corneal dystrophy
  M. juvenile epithelial
  dystrophy
megalocornea
megalopapilla

megalophthalmus
 anterior m.
megalopsia, megalopia
megophthalmus
meibomian
 m. blepharitis
 m. conjunctivitis
 m. cyst
 m. disease
 m. duct
 m. gland
 m. gland carcinoma
 m. gland expressor
 m. gland obstruction
 m. gland orifice metaplasia
 m. secretion
 m. sty
meibomianitis
meibomianum
 hordeolum m.
meibomitis
Meige syndrome
MEL
 M. 60 excimer laser
 M. 70 flying spot laser
 M. 60 scanning laser
melanin
melaninogenicus
 Bacteroides m.
melanocyte
 uveal m.
melanocytic
 m. conjunctival lesion
 m. hamartoma
 m. iris tumor
 m. nevus
melanocytoma
melanocytosis
 congenital ocular m.
 congenital oculodermal m.
 ocular m.
 oculodermal m.
melanokeratosis
 striate m.
melanoma, pl. **melanomata**
 amelanotic choroidal m.
 cavitary uveal m.

 choroidal m.
 ciliochoroidal m.
 conjunctival m.
 cutaneous m.
 m. of eyelid
 intraocular m.
 m. of iris
 juvenile m.
 malignant choroidal m.
 McLean classification of m.
 nodular m.
 ocular m.
 orbital m.
 pagetoid m.
 posterior uveal m.
 spindle A m.
 spindle B m.
 spindle cell m.
 tapioca iris m.
 uveal m.
melanoma-associated retinopathy
melanomalytic glaucoma
melanomata (*pl. of* melanoma)
melanosis
 acquired m.
 m. bulbi
 diabetic m.
 m. iridis
 m. oculi
 oculodermal m.
 presenile m.
 primary acquired m.
 m. sclerae
melanotic
 m. lesion
 m. sarcoma
 m. schwannoma
Melauskas
 M. acrylic implant
 M. orbital implant
Melkersson-Rosenthal syndrome
Melkersson syndrome
Meller
 M. lacrimal sac retractor
 M. operation
 M. refractor
Mellinger speculum

M

NOTES

mellitus
    adult-onset diabetes m.
    (AODM)
    diabetes m. (DM)
    gestational diabetes m.
    insulin-dependent diabetes m.
    (IDDM)
    juvenile diabetes m.
    non-insulin-dependent
    diabetes m.
melt
    corneal m.
    corneoscleral m.
    marginal m.
    sterile m.
    stromal m.
membrana, gen. and pl. **membranae**
    ˉm. capsularis lentis posterior
    m. choriocapillaris
    m. epipapillaris
    m. fusca
    m. granulosa externa
    m. granulosa interna
    m. hyaloidea
    m. limitans externa
    m. limitans interna
    m. nictitans
    m. pupillaris
    m. ruyschiana
    m. vitrea
membranacea
    cataracta congenita m.
membrane
    amniotic m.
    anterior hyaloid m. (AHM)
    Barkan m.
    basement m. (BM)
    bilaminar m.
    Biopore m.
    Bowman m.
    Bruch m.
    choroidal neovascular m.
    (CNVM)
    conjunctival m.
    connective tissue m.
    contraction of cyclitic m.
    cyclitic m.
    Descemet m.
    diabetic m.
    Duddell m.
    endothelial cell basement m.
    epimacular m.
    epipapillary m.

epiretinal m. (ERM)
epithelial basement m.
external limiting m.
fibroglial m.
fibroproliferative m.
Fresnel m.
glassy m.
gliotic m.
Haller m.
Henle m.
Hovius m.
hyaline m.
hyalitis of anterior m.
hyaloid posterior m.
idiopathic epiretinal m. (IERM)
idiopathic preretinal m.
inner limiting m.
intermuscular m.
internal limiting m. (ILM)
Jacob m.
limiting m.
m. lipid cell
macular epiretinal m.
mucous m.
neovascular m.
nictitating m.
ochre m.
onion skin-like m.
outer limiting m.
panretinal m.
m. peeler-cutter
m. peeling
periorbital m.
pigmented preretinal m.
posterior hyaloid m. (PHM)
preretinal m.
pupillary m.
purpurogenous m.
reduplication of Descemet m.
Reichert m.
retrocorneal m.
Ruysch m.
ruyschian m.
secondary m.
serous m.
stripping m.
subfoveal neovascular m.
subretinal m. (SRM)
subretinal neovascular m.
(SRNVM)
tarsal m.
Tenon m.
trabecular m.

vitreal m.
vitreous m.
Wachendorf m.
wrinkling m.
Zinn m.
membranectomy
membranoproliferative
glomerulonephritis type II
membranotomy
membranous
m. cataract
m. conjunctivitis
m. rhinitis
memory
immunologic m.
visual m.
MemoryLens
Mentor ORC M.
Mendez
M. astigmatism dial
M. corneal marker
M. cystitome
M. multi-purpose LASIK
forceps
meningeal
m. carcinomatosis
m. cell
m. hemangiopericytoma
meningioma
angioblastic m.
fibroblastic m.
nerve sheath m.
ocular m.
optic nerve sheath m. (ONSM)
orbital m.
perioptic sheath m.
psammomatous m. (PM)
sphenoid wing m.
suprasellar m.
meningitidis
Neisseria m.
meningitis
carcinomatous m.
cryptococcal m.
meningocele
meningococcosis
meningococcus conjunctivitis

meningocutaneous angiomatosis
meningoencephalocele
meningosepticum
Flavobacterium m.
meniscus, pl. menisci
m. concave lens
converging m.
diverging m.
m. floater
Kuhnt m.
negative m.
periscopic m.
positive m.
tear of m.
Mentanium vitreoretinal instrument
set
Mentor
M. B-VAT II BVS contour
circles distance stereoacuity
test
M. B-VAT II BVS random
dot E distance stereoacuity
test
M. B-VAT II monitor
M. B-VAT II video acuity
tester
M. curved eraser
M. Exeter ophthalmoscope
M. fine-focus microscope
M. ORC MemoryLens
M. pre-cut drain
M. wet-field cautery
M. wet-field electrocautery
M. wet-field eraser
Mentor-Maumenee Suregrip forceps
meperidine hydrochloride
mepivacaine
m. HCl
mercurialentis
mercuric oxide
mercury
millimeters of m. (mmHg, mm
Hg)
m. pressure
meridian
m. of cornea
corneal m.

NOTES

311

meridian *(continued)*
   equatorial m.
   m. of eyeball
   horizontal m.
   major m.
   steepest m.
   vertical m.
meridiani bulbi oculi
meridianus
meridional
   m. aberration
   m. amblyopia
   m. balance
   m. ciliary muscle fiber
   m. fold
   m. implant
   m. refractometer
Merkel cell neoplasm
Merocel
   M. sponge
   M. surgical spear
meropia
Merrimac laser
Mersilene suture
mesencephalic
   m. lesion
   m. lid retraction
mesencephalon lesion
mesenchymal
   m. dysgenesis
   m. ridge
   m. tumor
mesenchyme
   hemocytic m.
   neurogenic m.
   orbital m.
mesenchymoma
mesh
   Marlex m.
   tantalum m.
meshwork
   trabecular m. (TM)
mesiris
mesoblastic tissue
mesochoroidea
Meso contact lens
mesocornea
mesoderm
   paraxial m.
mesodermal dysgenesis
mesodermalis
   primary dysgenesis m.
mesophryon

mesopia
mesopic perimetry
mesoretina
mesoridazine
mesoropter
mesylate
   nelfinavir m.
metabolic
   m. coma
   m. syndrome cataract
metacontrast
metaherpetic
   m. keratitis
   m. ulcer
   m. ulceration of the cornea
metakeratitis
   herpetic m.
metameric color
metamorphopsia
   cerebral m.
   m. varians
metaplasia
   conjunctival m.
   meibomian gland orifice m.
   squamous m.
metaplastic epithelial cell
metarhodopsin
metastasis, pl. metastases
   chiasmal m.
   choroidal m.
   hematogenous m.
   hematopoietic m.
   leptomeningeal m.
   orbital m.
   pyogenic m.
   m. of tumor
   tumor m.
   uveal m.
metastatic
   m. carcinoma
   m. choroidal tumor
   m. choroiditis
   m. endophthalmitis
   m. ophthalmia
   m. retinitis
Metcher speculum
Metenier sign
meter
   m. angle
   footcandle m.
   Guyton-Minkowski potential
     acuity m.
   Kowa FM-500 laser flare m.

laser cell and flare m.
(LCFM)
laser flare m. (LFM)
laser flare-cell m.
m. lens
potential acuity m. (PAM)
straylight m.
Vuero m.
meter-candle
methacholine chloride
methacrylate
heparin surface-modified
polymethyl m.
methyl m.
passivated polymethyl m.
polymethyl m. (PMMA)
MethaSite
methazolamide
methicillin-resistant *Staphylococcus*
aureus
method
Barraquer m.
Bio-Optics Bambi fixed-
frame m.
confrontation m.
Con-Lish polishing m.
contact m.
corners m.
Crawford m.
Credé m.
Cuignet m.
direct m.
divide-and-conquer m.
dot m.
gradient m.
grid m.
heterophoria m.
Hirschberg m.
Holmgren m.
immersion m.
immunodiagnostic m.
Konan fixed-frame m.
Krimsky m.
Maddox rod m.
Mantel-Haenszel m.
m. of Markwell
Mishima-Hedbys m.

modified band lid m.
Mueller m.
optical density m.
Pfeiffer-Komberg m.
push-up m.
rag-wheel m.
m. of the sphere
Sweet m.
twirling m.
von Graefe prism
dissociation m.
Westergren m.
Wheeler m.
Wolfe m.
Methopto
methosulfate
trimethidium m.
Methulose
methyl
m. cyanoacrylate glue
m. methacrylate
m. methacrylate implant
methylcellulose
hydroxypropyl m. (HPMC)
methylergonovine
methylmethacrylate
methylparaben
methylpentynol
methylphenidate
cocaine m.
methyl-phenyl-tetrahydropyridine
(MPTP)
methylprednisolone
methylsulfate
neostigmine m.
methysergide
Metico forceps
Meticorten
Metimyd
M. Ophthalmic
metipranolol
metoprolol
Metreton
metric
m. ophthalmoscope
m. ophthalmoscopy
metrizamide

M

NOTES

metronoscope
Metubine Iodide
Metycaine
Meyer
    M. Swiss diamond knife lancet
    M. Swiss diamond lancet knife
    M. Swiss diamond mini-angled
    knife
    M. Swiss diamond wedge
    knife
    M. temporal loop
Meyer-Archambault loop
Meyer-Schwickerath
    M.-S. coagulator
    M.-S. light coagulation
    M.-S. operation
Meyhoeffer
    M. chalazion
    M. chalazion curette
Meynert
    M. commissure
    superior commissura of M.
MG
    Marcus Gunn pupil
MH
    macular hole
mica spectacles
micelles in vitreous
Michaelson
    M. counter pressure
    M. operation
Michel
    M. pick
    M. spur
miconazole
Micra double-edged diamond blade
micro
    m. Colibri forceps
    m. eye movement
    M. One pneumatonometer
    M. punctum plug
    m. round-tip needle
    m. scissors
    m. Westcott scissors
microadenoma
microaneurysm
    juxtafoveal m.
microaneurysmal leakage
microangiography
microangiopathy
    circumpapillary telangiectatic m.
    occlusive m.
microanisocoria

microbevel edge lens
microbial keratitis
microbiallergic conjunctivitis
microblepharia, microblepharism,
    microblepharon, microblephary
Microcap scalpel
microcautery unit
microcirculation
    retinal m.
microcoria
microcornea
microcyst
    Blessig-Iwanoff m.
    epithelial m.
    intraepithelial m.
    punctate epithelial m.
microcystic
    m. corneal dystrophy
    m. edema
    m. epithelial dystrophy
micro-dots
microembolism, pl. microemboli
    retinal m.
microendoscope
    ophthalmic laser m. (OLM)
microendoscopic test card
microforceps
    Birks-Mathelone m.
    Colibri m.
    Sparta m.
Microfuge tube
Micro-Glide corneal suture
microgonioscope
microhemagglutination test
microhook
    Visitec m.
microhyphema
microinfarction
microjaw
    Keeler-Catford needle holder
    with m.'s
Microjet-based cutting and
    debriding device
microkeratome
    automated m.
    Barraquer m.
    Barraquer-Carriazo m.
    Chiron ACS m.
    Corneal Shaper m.
    FlapMaker disposable m.
    Krumeich-Barraquer m.
    MedJet m.
    Ruiz m.

Microknife
Microlase transpupillary diode laser
micromanipulator
    self-centering m.
Micromatic ophthalmometer
micromegalopsia
micromesh sheeting
micrometer
    diamond m.
    m. disk
    m. knife
    Tolman m.
    ultrasonic m.
micromovement of eye
micronystagmus
micropannus
microperforation
microperimeter
microperimetry
microphakia
microphotography
microphthalmia, microphthalmos,
    microphthalmus
    colobomatous m.
    cystic m.
microphthalmoscope
micropigmentation system
micropins
    Pischel m.
microplate fixation
micropoint
    m. needle
    m. suture
Microprobe
    Endo Optics M.
    M. integrated laser endoscope
    M. integrated laser and
      endoscope system
    M. ophthalmic laser
microproliferation
micropsia
    cerebral m.
    convergence-accommodative m.
    psychogenic m.
    retinal m.
microptic

micropuncture
    anterior stromal m.
Microputor II (MR2)
microruptor
    LASAG m.
microsaccades
microscalpel
    Oasis feather m.
microscissors
    DORC microforceps and m.
    Kamdar m.
    Keeler m.
    Twisk m.
microscope
    Beckerscope binocular m.
    Bio-Optics specular m.
    Bitumi monobjective m.
    Cohan-Barraquer m.
    confocal m.
    CooperVision m.
    corneal m.
    Czapski m.
    electron m.
    Fiberlite m.
    Galilean m.
    Heyer-Schulte m.
    Keeler-Konan Specular m.
    Keeler specular m.
    Konan SP8000 noncontact
      specular m.
    Leitz m.
    light m.
    Mentor fine-focus m.
    Moller m.
    OM 2000 operation m.
    operating m.
    OPMI PRO magis m.
    OPMI VISU 200 m.
    PRO CEM-4 m.
    Project Research Ophthalmic
      specular m.
    Pro-Koester wide-field
      SCM m.
    scanning slit confocal m.
    slit-lamp m.
    SMZ-10A zoom stereo m.
    specular m.

M

NOTES

microscope *(continued)*
   Storz m.
   tandem scanning confocal m.
   Topcon SP-1000 non-contact
     specular m.
   transmission electron m.
   video specular m.
   Weck m.
   white light tandem-scanning
     confocal m.
   Wild operating m.
   Zeiss-Barraquer cine m.
   Zeiss-Barraquer surgical m.
   Zeiss OM-3 operating m.
   Zeiss OpMi-6 FR m.
microscopic hyphema
microscopy
   confocal m.
   fluorescence m.
   fundus m.
   light m.
   specular m.
microscotometry
MicroSeal
   M. ophthalmic handpiece
   Storz M.
Micro-Sharp blade
microspatula
   Birks Mark II m.
microspectroscope
microspherometer
microspherophakia
microsponge
   Alcon m.
   M. Teardrop sponge
microstrabismic amblyopia
microstrabismus
microsurgery
microsurgical knife
microthin
   m. contact lens
   m. lens
MicroTip phaco tip
microtome
Microtonometer
   Computon M.
MicroTrac Direct Specimen Test
microtrauma
microtremor
   ocular m.
   superior oblique m.
   unilateral m.
microtropia

microtropic syndrome
microtubule
microvascular
   m. abnormality
   m. decompression
microvillus, pl. **microvilli**
Microvit
   M. probe
   M. probe system
   Storz Premiere M.
   M. vitrector
microvitrector
microvitreoretinal (MVR)
   m. blade
   m. spatula
microwave
   m. hyperthermia
   m. plaque thermotherapy
   m. radiation injury
midbrain
   m. corectopia
   m. disease
   m. ptosis
mid-coquille lens
middle
   m. cerebral artery
   m. temporal visual area
midfacial fracture
midget system
midline
   m. granuloma
   m. position
   m. position of gaze
midperiphery
midsightedness
midstromal
Mietens syndrome
migraine
   basilar m.
   m. equivalent
   m. headache
   hemiplegic m.
   ophthalmic m.
   m. ophthalmoplegia
   ophthalmoplegic m.
   retinal m.
   transformed m.
migrainous
   m. hallucination
   m. ophthalmoplegia
   m. vision loss
migrans
   erythema chronicum m.

keratitis linearis m.
ocular larva m.
visceral larva m. (VLM)
migrating epithelium
migration
bleb m.
epithelial m.
implant m.
pigmentary m.
m. theory
migratory ophthalmia
Mikamo double-eyelid operation
Mikulicz disease
mild
m. chromic suture
Inflamase M.
Pred M.
milia
eyelid m.
miliary aneurysm
milk-alkali syndrome
milky cataract
Millard-Gubler syndrome
Millennium
M. CX microsurgical system
M. LX microsurgical system
Miller-Fisher
M.-F. syndrome
M.-F. variant
Miller-Nadler glare tester
Miller syndrome
Milles syndrome
millet seed nodule
Millex filter
**millimeters of mercury (mmHg,
mm Hg)**
Millipore filter
Milroy Artificial Tears
mimicking
finger m.
mind blindness
miner's
m. blindness
m. disease
m. nystagmus

miniature
m. blade
m. forceps
minicircular capsulorrhexis
mini-excimer
Compak-200 m.-e.
miniflap
scleral m.
mini-keratoplasty
Castroviejo m.-k.
m.-k. stitch scissors
minimal
m. amplitude nystagmus
m. brain dysfunction
m. effective diameter (MED)
m. pigment oculocutaneous
albinism
minimum
m. deviation
m. light
m. light threshold
m. perceptible acuity
m. separable acuity
m. separable angle
m. visible angle
m. visual angle
miniophthalmic drape
miniplate
titanium m.
Vitallium m.
MiniQuad XL lens
Mini-tip culturette
minor
annulus iridis m.
circulus arteriosus iridis m.
Minsky
M. circle
M. intramarginal splitting
M. operation
minus
m. carrier
m. carrier contact lens
cyclophoria m.
m. cyclophoria
m. cyclotropia
cyclotropia m.

NOTES

minus *(continued)*
  m. cylinder
  m. spectacle lens
Miocel
Miochol
  M. solution
Miochol-E
miosis
  congenital m.
  irritative m.
  paralytic m.
  pupil m.
  pupillary m.
  senescent m.
  senile m.
  spastic m.
  spinal m.
  traumatic pupillary m.
Miostat
  M. Intraocular
miotic
  m. alkaloid
  m. pupil
  m. therapy
Mira
  M. AGL-400
  M. cautery
  M. diathermy
  M. diathermy unit
  M. electrocautery
  M. encircling element
  M. endovitreal cryopencil
  M. photocoagulator
  M. Pola test
  M. silicone rod
Miracon
MiraFlow
  M. Extra-Strength
MiraSept System
MiraSol
mire
  image of m.'s
  keratometer m.'s
  m.'s of ophthalmometer
mirror
  m. area
  m. coating
  concave m.
  contact lens training m.
  convex m.
  4-M. Gonio lens
  m. haploscope
  head m.

  m. image
  power of m.
  m. rocking test
misdirected lash
misdirection
  aqueous m.
  facial nerve m.
  oculomotor nerve m.
  m. phenomenon
Mishima-Hedbys method
misty vision
mitochondrial
  m. disease
  m. myopathy
mitosis
  epithelial m.
mitotic
Mittendorf dot
Mitzuo phenomenon
mivacurium
mixed
  m. astigmatism
  m. bacterial-fungal keratitis
  m. cataract
  m. esotropia
  m. fungal keratitis
  m. strabismus
  m. tumor
mixing
  color m.
mixture
  Neo-Synephrine cocaine m.
Miyake technique
Mizuo-Nakamura
  M.-N. effect
  M.-N. phenomenon
M-K
  McCarey-Kaufman
MK IV ophthalmoscope
MKM
  myopic keratomileusis
M-K medium
MLF
  medial longitudinal fasciculus
mmHg, mm Hg
  millimeters of mercury
Möbius
  M. disease
  M. sign
  M. syndrome
Möbius-von Graefe-Stellway sign
mode
  m. of action

free running m.
pulse m.
model
Bohr m.
Gullstrand six-surface eye m.
Kooijman eye m.
Le Grand-Gullstrand eye m.
reduced eye m.
von Helmholtz eye m.
mode-locked Nd:YAG laser
modification
Deller m.
Smith m.
Van Herick m.
modified
m. band lid method
M. Clinical Technique test
m. C-loop intraocular lens
m. C-loop UV lens
m. corncrib (inverted T)
procedure
m. J loop
m. J-loop intraocular lens
m. J-loop UV lens
m. monovision
m. Van Lint anesthesia
m. Van Lint block
m. Wies procedure
Modular One pneumatonometer
modulation transfer function
Moehle
M. cannula
M. corneal forceps
Mohs microsurgical resection
Moiré fringe
moistened fine mesh gauze dressing
moisture
m. chamber
M. Ophthalmic Drops
molded
m. frame
m. pressing
molding
cast m.
compression m.
injection m.
mold-injected lens

molectron laser
molecular
m. dissociation theory
m. external layer
m. inner layer
m. internal layer
m. outer layer
Moll
M. gland
M. gland cystadenoma
Moller microscope
molluscum
conjunctivitis m.
m. conjunctivitis
m. contagiosum
m. virus
Molteno
M. episcleral explant
M. implant
M. shunt tube
Momose lens
Monakow syndrome
Monarch IOL delivery system
Moncrieff
M. cannula
M. discission
M. operation
mongolian
m. fold
m. spot
mongoloid slant
moniliaceous filamentous fungus
moniliforme
Fusarium m.
monitor
Mentor B-VAT II m.
monoblepsia
monocanalicular intubation
monochroic
monochromacy
monochromasia
monochromasy
blue cone m.
rod m.
monochromat
cone m.
rod m.

M

NOTES

monochromatic
  m. aberration
  m. cone
  m. eye
  m. light
  m. ray
monochromatism
  blue cone m.
  cone m.
  rod m.
  X-linked blue cone m.
monocle
monoclonal antibody
monocular
  m. aphakia
  m. bandage
  m. bobbing movement
  m. confrontation visual field
    test
  m. depth perception
  m. diplopia
  m. dressing
  m. electro-oculogram
  m. field defect
  m. fixation
  m. glaucoma
  m. heterochromia
  m. indirect ophthalmoscope
  m. nystagmus
  m. occlusion
  m. oscillopsia
  m. patch
  m. strabismus
  m. telescope
  m. temporal crescent
  m. vision
monocular-estimate-method dynamic
retinoscopy
monoculus
monodiplopia
monofilament nylon suture
monofixational phoria
monofixation syndrome
monolateral strabismus
monolayered endothelium
mononuclear
  m. cell infiltration
  m. reaction
  m. response
monophosphate
  adenosine m. (AMP)
  cyclic adenosine m.

  cyclic guanidine m.
  cyclic guanosine m.
monophthalmica
  polyopia m.
monophthalmos
monopia
monostearate
  glyceryl m.
monovision
  modified m.
montage
  retinal m.
Montana Academy of
Ophthalmology (MAO)
Moody fixation forceps
moon blindness
Moore
  M. lens forceps
  M. lens-inserting forceps
  M. lightning streak
Mooren corneal ulcer
Moore-Troutman corneal scissors
Moran
  M. operation
  M. proptosis
Morax
  M. keratoplasty
  M. operation
Morax-Axenfeld conjunctivitis
Moraxella
  M. bovis
  M. catarrhalis
  M. keratitis
  M. lacunata
  M. nonliquefaciens
Morck
  M. cement
  M. cement bifocal
Morel-Fatio-Lalardie operation
Morgagni
  M. cataract
  M. globule
  M. liquor
  M. sphere
morgagnian
  m. cataract
  m. globule
Morgan
  M. dot
  M. line
Moria
  M. obturator

M. one-piece speculum
M. trephine
Moria-France dacryocystorhinostomy clamp
morning
  m. glory disk
  m. glory optic atrophy
  m. glory optic disk anomaly
  m. glory retinal detachment
  m. glory syndrome
  m. ptosis
morpheaform pattern
Morquio-Brailsford syndrome
Morquio syndrome
Morse code pattern
mosaic pattern
Mosher operation
Mosher-Toti operation
Mosler diabetes
mosquito
  m. clamp
  m. hemostatic forceps
Moss
  M. operation
  M. traction
Motais operation
motile scotoma
motility
  m. implant
  ocular m.
motion
  against m.
  m. automated perimetry
  m. and displacement perimetry
  hand m. (HM)
  m. parallax
  m. perception disorder
  scotoma for m.
  skew m.
  m. vision
  with m.
motoneuron
  ocular m.
motor
  m. function
  m. fusion
  m. nerve

m. oculi
m. root
m. root of ciliary ganglion
m. tic
Visuscope m.
motor-output disability
Mot-R-Pak vitrectomy system
mottled appearance
mottling
  early receptor potential m.
  m. of fundus
  pigment m.
  retinal pigment epithelium m.
Moulton lacrimal duct tube
mounds
  pearl white m.
mount
  unstained wet m.
  wet m.
movement
  cardinal ocular m.
  cogwheel ocular m.
  cogwheel pursuit m.
  conjugate horizontal eye m.
  conjugate ocular m.
  corrective m.
  Developmental Eye M. (DEM)
  disconjugate roving eye m.
  disjugate m.
  disjunctive m.
  drift m.
  extraocular m.
  eye m.
  eye-head m.
  facial m.
  fixational ocular m.
  flick m.
  following m.
  fusional m.
  gaze m.
  hand m.
  illusion of m.
  impaired vergence eye m.
  lightning eye m.
  micro eye m.
  monocular bobbing m.
  nonoptic reflex eye m.

M

NOTES

movement *(continued)*
    nonrapid eye m.
    nystagmoid m.
    ocular m.
    paradoxical m. of eyelids
    perverted ocular m.
    pursuit m.
    rapid eye m. (REM)
    reflex eye m.
    roving eye m.
    saccadic eye m.
    scissors m.
    slow conjugate roving eye m.
    slow eye m. (SEM)
    smooth-pursuit m.
    synkinetic m.
    torsional m.
    vergence eye m. (VEM)
    vermiform m.
    version m.
    vertical m.
    voluntary eye m.
    yoke m.
MPC automated intravitreal scissors
Mport lens insertion system
MPP
    massive periretinal proliferation
MPS
    Macular Photocoagulation Study
MPTP
    methyl-phenyl-tetrahydropyridine
MP video endoscopic lens attachment
MR
    manifest refraction
    medial rectus
MR2
    Microputor II
MRA
    magnetic resonance angiography
Mr. Color test
MRD
    marginal reflex distance
MRI
    magnetic resonance imaging
    MRI scan
M-Rinse
MRS
    magnetic resonance spectroscopy
MSE
    mean spherical equivalent

MST
    medial superior temporal
    MST visual area
MT
    medial temporal
    MT visual area
M-TEC 2000 Surgical System
MTL trial frame
mucin
    m. layer
    m. strand
    m. of tear
mucinous
    m. adenocarcinoma tumor
    m. edema
mucocele
    sinus m.
mucocutaneous junction
mucoid discharge
mucolipidosis, pl. **mucolipidoses**
    m. IV
mucomycosis
mucopurulent conjunctivitis
mucormycosis
    rhino-orbital m.
mucosae
    hyalinosis cutis et m.
mucosal
    m. associated lymphoid tissue
    m. neuroma
    m. pemphigoid
mucotome
    Castroviejo m.
mucous
    m. assay
    m. discharge
    m. membrane
    m. membrane graft
    m. ophthalmia
    m. tear layer
    m. thread
mucous-like strand
mucus
    ropy m.
    m. strand
    stringy m.
Mueller
    M. cautery
    cells of M.
    M. electric corneal trephine
    M. electrocautery
    M. electronic tonometer
    M. eye shield

M. gland
M. implant
M. lacrimal sac retractor
M. method
M. muscle
M. operation
radial cells of M.
M. refractor
M. speculum
M. trigone
Muhlberger orbital implant
mulberry-shaped mass
mulberry-type papilloma
Muldoon lacrimal dilator
Mules
M. implant
M. operation
M. scoop
M. vitreous sphere
Mulibrey nanism
Müller
M. cell
M. cell footplate
M. fiber
multicore disease
multicurve contact lens
multifactorial disease
Multiflex anterior chamber lens
multifocal
m. chorioretinal disease
m. choroiditis
m. electroretinogram
m. fibrosclerosis
m. hemorrhagic sarcoma
m. posterior pigment
epitheliopathy
m. spectacle lens
multiforme
erythema m.
glioblastoma m.
multilocular vesicle
Multilux
multinodularis
episcleritis m.
multinucleated
m. giant epithelial cell
Multi-Optics lens

multiple
m. evanescent white-dot
syndrome
m. lentigines syndrome
m. myeloma
m. ocular motor palsies
m. sclerosis
m. vision
Multi-Purpose
ReNu M.-P.
multiscope
roaming optical access m.
(ROAM)
multivesicular body
mumps keratitis
Munsell color
Munson sign
mural cell
Murdock eye speculum
Murdock-Wiener eye speculum
Murdoon eye speculum
murine
M. Plus
M. Plus Ophthalmic
m. retina
M. Solution
M. sterile saline
Muro
M. 128
M. Opcon
M. Opcon A
M. Tears
Murocel
M. Ophthalmic Solution
Murocoll-2 Ophthalmic
musca, pl. **muscae**
muscae volitantes
muscarinic cholinergic side effect
muscle
abductor m.
adductor m.
agonist m.
m. belly
belly of m.
bound-down m.
Bowman m.
Brücke m.

M

NOTES

muscle *(continued)*
ciliary m.
circular ciliary m.
m. clamp
m. cone
m. contraction headache
corrugator m.
cyclorotary m.
cyclovertical m.
m. depressor
m. dilator
dilator m.
disinserted m.
elevator m.
extraocular m. (EOM)
extrinsic m.
m. of eye
eyelid m.
m. force
m. forceps
frontalis m.
m. hook
Horner m.
inferior oblique extraocular m.
inferior rectus extraocular m.
inferior tarsal m.
intortor m.
intraocular m. (IOM)
intrinsic ocular m.
iridial m.
iris sphincter m.
Koyter m.
Landström m.
lateral rectus extraocular m.
left inferior rectus m.
left superior rectus m.
levator palpebrae superioris m.
levator trochlear m.
longitudinal ciliary m.
medial rectus m.
medial rectus extraocular m.
Mueller m.
oblique m.
ocular m.
oculorotatory m.
orbicularis oculi m.
orbicularis oris m.
orbital m.
palpebrae superioris m.
palsy of m.
m. paretic nystagmus
preseptal orbicularis m.
pupillary sphincter m.

radial dilator m.
recession of m.
rectus lateralis m.
rectus medialis m.
resection of m.
m. resection
Riolan m.
Rouget m.
m. sheath
sphincter m.
superciliary m.
superior oblique extraocular m.
superior rectus extraocular m.
superior tarsal m.
tarsal m.
temporalis m.
m. transposition
trochlear m.
trochlea of superior oblique m.
vertical m.
yoked m.
muscle-eye-brain disease
muscular
m. asthenopia
m. balance
m. dystrophy
m. fascia
m. funnel
m. insufficiency
m. strabismus
m. vein
musculus, gen. and pl. musculi
musculi bulbi
m. ciliaris
m. corrugator supercilii
m. depressor supercilii
m. dilator pupilla
lamina superficialis musculi
m. levator palpebrae superioris
m. obliquus inferior bulbi
m. obliquus inferior oculi
m. obliquus superior bulbi
m. obliquus superior oculi
musculi oculi
m. orbicularis
m. orbicularis oculi
m. orbitalis
m. procerus
m. rectus inferior bulbi
m. rectus inferior oculi
m. rectus lateralis bulbi
m. rectus lateralis oculi
m. rectus medialis bulbi

m. rectus medialis oculi
m. sphincter pupilla
m. tarsalis inferior
m. tarsalis superior
mushroom
corneal m.
m. corneal graft
mustache technique
Mustarde
M. awl
M. graft
M. operation
M. rotational cheek flap
mustard gas
mutton-fat
m.-f. deposit
m.-f. keratic precipitate
mutton fat
MVB blade
MVK
Massachusetts Vision Kit
MVN
medial vestibular nucleus
MVR
microvitreoretinal
MVR blade
MVS
Massachusetts XII vitrectomy
system
Myambutol
myasthenia
focal m.
m. gravis
neonatal m.
ocular m.
pediatric m.
m. syndrome
myasthenia-like syndrome
myasthenic
m. crisis
m. nystagmus
mycelial mass
Mycitracin
mycobacteria
atypical m.
Mycobacteriaceae
mycobacterial disease

Mycobacterium
M. *africanum*
M. *avium*
M. *bovis*
M. *chelonei*
M. *fortuitum*
M. *keratitis*
M. *leprae*
M. *smegmatis*
M. *tuberculosis*
Mycobutin
Mycostatin
mycotic
m. infection
m. keratitis
m. snowball opacity
mycotoxicity
Mydfrin
M. Ophthalmic Solution
Mydramide
Mydrapred
Mydriacyl
Mydriafair
mydriasis
accidental m.
alternating m.
amaurotic m.
bounding m.
congenital m.
episodic unilateral m.
factitious m.
fixed m.
paralytic m.
postoperative m.
spasmodic m.
spastic m.
spinal m.
springing m.
transient unilateral m.
traumatic m.
mydriatic
m. provocative test
m. rigidity
m. test for angle-closure
glaucoma
mydriatic-cycloplegic therapy
Mydrilate

M

NOTES

myectomy
    m. operation
    orbicularis m.
    selective facial m.
myelinated
    m. retinal nerve fiber
myelination
    optic nerve m.
    m. of retinal nerve
    retinal nerve fiber m.
myelin disorder
myelitis
myeloidin
myeloma
    multiple m.
    osteosclerotic m.
myelomatosis
    disseminated nonosteolytic m.
myelo-optic neuropathy
myiasis
    cutaneous m.
    ocular m.
MYOC
    myocilin
Myochrysine
myocilin (MYOC)
myoclin gene
myoclonal
myoclonic epilepsy with ragged-red fiber
myoclonus
    m. nystagmus
    ocular m.
    oculopalatal m.
    startle m.
    vertical m.
myoculator
Myocure
    M. blade
    M. blade scalpel
    M. knife
    M. phacoblade
myodesopsia
myodiopter
myoepithelial cell
myofibril
myogenic acquired ptosis
myoid visual cell
myokymia
    eyelid m.
    facial m.
    superior m.
    superior oblique m.

myoneural
    m. junction
myopathic
    m. disorder
    m. eyelid retraction
    m. ptosis
myopathy
    centronuclear m.
    congenital m.
    endocrine m.
    fingerprint body m.
    inflammatory m.
    mitochondrial m.
    nemaline m.
    ocular m.
    proximal myotonic m.
    reducing body m.
    rod m.
    systemic m.
    toxin-induced m.
    traumatic m.
    visceral m.
myope
    early-onset m.
    late-onset m.
myopia (M)
    abnormal nearwork-induced transient m.
    axial m.
    choroiditis m.
    chromic m.
    crescent m.
    curvature m.
    degenerative m.
    early-onset m.
    form-deprivation m.
    high m.
    index m.
    m. index
    late-onset m.
    lenticular m.
    malignant m.
    night m.
    nyctalopia with congenital m.
    pathologic m.
    pernicious m.
    physiologic m.
    prematurity m.
    primary m.
    prodromal m.
    progressive m.
    refractive m.
    school m.

senile lenticular m.
simple m.
space m.
transient m.
vision deprivation m.
myopic (M)
  m. anisometropia
  m. astigmatism (AsM)
  m. choroidal atrophy
  m. choroidopathy
  m. conus
  m. crescent
  m. error
  m. keratomileusis (MKM)
  m. maculopathy
  m. reflex
  m. regression
  m. retinal degeneration
myorhythmia
  oculomasticatory m.
myoscope
myosin filament

myosis
myositis
  idiopathic m.
  infective m.
  orbital m.
  systemic m.
myotomy
  marginal m.
  m. operation
  Z m.
myotonia
  chondrodystrophic m.
  m. congenita
  m. dystrophica
myotonic
  m. dystrophy
  m. dystrophy cataract
  m. dystrophy effect
  m. pupil
myringotomy blade
Mysoline
Mytrate

NOTES

M

N
  nasal
n
  index of refraction
NA
  numerical aperture
naboctate
  n. HCl
Nadbath
  N. akinesia
  N. block
  N. facial block
Nadler superior radial scissors
nadolol
Naegeli syndrome
Naegleria
  N. cyst
  N. fowleri
Nafazair
  N. Ophthalmic
Naffziger operation
NaFl
  sodium fluorescein
NAG
  narrow-angle glaucoma
Nagahara karate chopper
Nagel
  N. anomaloscope
  N. Lensmeter
  N. test
Nager syndrome
NAION
  nonarteritic anterior ischemic optic
  neuropathy
Nairobi eye
naked vision (Nv)
nalorphine
naloxone
  n. hydrochloride
Nama keratopathy
naming
  color n.
nana
  Hymenolepis n.
nanism
  Mulibrey n.
Nanolas Nd:YAG laser
nanophthalmia, nanophthalmos
naphazoline
  n. and antazoline

n. and antazoline phosphate
  n. HCl
  n. and pheniramine maleate
Naphcon
  N. Forte
  N. Forte Ophthalmic
  N. Ophthalmic
Naphcon-A
  N.-A. Ophthalmic
naphthalinic cataract
naproxen sodium
narrow-angle glaucoma (NAG)
narrowed arteriole
narrowing
  arteriolar n.
  n. of retinal arteriole
narrow-slit illumination
Nasahist B
nasal (N)
  n. architecture
  n. arteriole of retina
  n. border of optic disk
  n. buttonhole incision
  n. canal
  n. duct
  n. field loss
  n. hemianopia
  n. hemianopsia
  n. isopter
  n. periphery
  n. speculum
  n. step
  n. step defect
  n. venule of retina
nasalis
  commissura palpebrarum n.
nasalization
nasi
  cancrum n.
  inferior meatus n.
nasion
nasoantritis
nasociliaris
  nervus n.
nasociliary
  n. nerve
  n. neuralgia
nasofrontalis
  vena n.
nasofrontal vein

N

nasojugal fold
nasolabial fold
nasolacrimal
   n. blockade
   n. canal
   n. drainage system
   n. duct (NLD)
   n. duct obstruction
   n. duct probe
   n. gland
   n. groove
   n. reflex
   n. sac
nasolacrimalis
   ductus n.
naso-orbital fracture
Natacyn
natamycin
National Eye Institute Visual
  Function Questionnaire
natural
   N. Tears
   n. UV radiation
Naturale
   Duratears N.
   Tears N.
Nature's Tears Solution
NCT
   noncontact tonometer
ND-Stat
Nd:YAG
   neodymium:YAG laser
   Nd:YAG cyclophotocoagulation
   Nd:YAG laser
   Nd:YAG laser
     cyclophotocoagulation
Nd:YLF
   neodymium:yttrium lithium fluoride
   laser
   Nd:YLF laser
Neale Reading Analysis
near
   n. acuity testing
   n. add
   distance and n. (D&N)
   n. esotropia (ET')
   n. fixation
   n. fixation position of gaze
   n. gaze
   n. light reflex
   n. point absolute
   n. point of accommodation
     (NPA)

   n. point of convergence (NPC)
   n. reaction
   n. reaction to light
   n. reflex spasm
   n. response
   n. sight
   n. triad
   n. vision
   n. vision test
   n. vision testing
   n. visual acuity (NVA)
   n. visual point (NVP)
nearpoint
   n. esophoria
   n. exophoria
   n. phoria
near-point
   n.-p. accommodation
   n.-p. relative
near-reflex spasm
nearsighted
nearsightedness
nebula, pl. nebulae
   corneal n.
nebular stromal opacity
necrobiotic xanthogranuloma
necrogranulomatous keratitis
necrosis
   acute retinal n. (ARN)
   anterior segment n.
   caseous n.
   conjunctival n.
   fibrinoid n.
   perifascicular myofiber n.
   progressive outer retinal n.
     (PORN)
   retinal n.
   stromal n.
   white retinal n.
necrotic
   n. follicle
   n. infectious conjunctivitis
necroticans
   scleritis n.
necrotizing
   n. interstitial keratitis
   n. nodular scleritis
   n. papillitis
   n. retinitis
   n. retinopathy
   n. sclerocorneal ulceration
     (NSU)

n. stromal keratitis
n. ulcerative keratitis
needle
  ACS n.
  Agnew tattooing n.
  Agrikola tattooing n.
  Alcon CU-15 4-mil n.
  Alcon irrigating n.
  Alcon reverse cutting n.
  Alcon spatula n.
  Alcon taper cut n.
  Alcon taper point n.
  Amsler aqueous transplant n.
  aqueous transplant n.
  Atkinson retrobulbar n.
  Atkinson single-bevel blunt-
   tip n.
  Atkinson tip peribulbar n.
  Barraquer n.
  Barraquer-Vogt n.
  B-D n.
  bent blunt n.
  bent 22-gauge n.
  blunt n.
  Bowman cataract n.
  Bowman stop n.
  Burr butterfly n.
  butterfly n.
  BV100 n.
  Calhoun n.
  Calhoun-Hagler lens n.
  Calhoun-Merz n.
  Castroviejo vitreous
   aspirating n.
  cataract n.
  cataract-aspirating n.
  CD-5 n.
  Charles flute n.
  Charles vacuuming n.
  Chiba eye n.
  Cibis ski n.
  CIF4 n.
  Cleasby spatulated n.
  Colorado n.
  CooperVision irrigating n.
  CooperVision spatulated n.
  corneal n.

couching n.
Crawford n.
CU-8 n.
CUA n.
Curran knife n.
Daily cataract n.
Davis knife n.
Dean knife n.
discission n.
Drews cataract n.
DS-9 n.
Ellis foreign body n.
Elschnig extrusion n.
Empire n.
Ethicon BV-75-3 n.
extended round n.
extrusion n.
Fisher eye n.
flute n.
foreign body n.
four-sided cutting n.
Fritz vitreous transplant n.
30-gauge n.
Geuder keratoplasty n.
Girard anterior chamber n.
Girard cataract-aspirating n.
Girard phacofragmatome n.
Girard-Swan knife n.
Graefe n.
Grieshaber opthalmic n.
GS-9 n.
Gueder keratoplasty n.
Haab knife n.
Hessburg lacrimal n.
Heyner double n.
n. holder
n. holder clamp
Ilg n.
Iliff-Wright fascia n.
illuminated suction n.
internal nucleus
  hydrodelineation n.
Iocare titanium n.
IOLAB irrigating n.
IOLAB taper-cut n.
IOLAB taper-point n.
IOLAB titanium n.

N

NOTES

needle *(continued)*
iris knife n.
Kalt corneal n.
Kara cataract n.
Knapp knife n.
Kratz diamond-dusted n.
Kratz lens n.
Lagleyze n.
Lane n.
Lewicky n.
Look retrobulbar n.
Lo-Trau side-cutting n.
LX n.
March laser sclerostomy n.
Maumenee vitreous-aspirating n.
McIntyre I/A n.
McIntyre irrigation/aspiration n.
micropoint n.
micro round-tip n.
nucleus hydrolysis n.
Oaks double n.
peribulbar n.
probe n.
n. probe
puncture n.
puncture-tip n.
razor n.
razor-tip n.
retrobulbar n.
Reverdin suture n.
reverse-cutting n.
Riedel n.
Rycroft n.
Sabreloc n.
Sato cataract n.
Scheie cataract-aspirating n.
sclerostomy n.
Sharpoint Ultra-Guide
    ophthalmic n.
side-cutting spatulated n.
Simcoe aspirating n.
Simcoe II PC aspirating n.
Simcoe suture n.
SITE irrigating/aspirating n.
SITE macrobore plus n.
SITE Phaco I/A n.
ski n.
n. spatula
spatulated n.
n. spoon
spoon n.
n. spud
spud n.

n. stick
Stocker n.
Straus curved retrobulbar n.
Subco n.
subconjunctival n.
Surgicraft suture n.
suturing n.
Swan n.
taper-cut n.
taper-point n.
tattooing n.
tax double n.
TG-140 n.
Thornton n.
titanium n.
translocation n.
triple facet-tip n.
ultrasonic cataract-removal
    lancet n.
Ultrasonic lancet n.
Viers n.
vitreous aspirating n.
vitreous transplant n.
Vogt-Barraquer corneal n.
Vogt-Barraquer eye n.
von Graefe knife n.
Weeks n.
Wergeland double n.
Wooten n.
Worst n.
Wright fascia n.
Wright ophthalmic n.
Yale Luer-Lok n.
Ziegler iris knife-n.
Ziegler knife-n.

negative
n. accommodation
n. afterimage
n. convergence
n. eyepiece
n. image
n. meniscus
n. meniscus lens
n. scotoma
n. vertical divergence
n. vertical vergence
n. visual phenomenon

neglect dyslexia

Neher operation

Nehra-Mack operation

Neisseria
N. gonorrhoeae
N. meningitidis

neisserial conjunctivitis
Neitz
  N. CT-R cataract camera
  N. Instruments Company
nelfinavir mesylate
Nelson grading system
nemaline myopathy
Nembutal
Neocidin
Neo-Cobefrin
Neo-Cortef
NeoDecadron
  N. Ophthalmic
  N. Topical
Neo-Dexair
Neo-Dexameth Ophthalmic
neodymium:YAG laser (Nd:YAG)
neodymium:yttrium
  n. aluminum garnet laser
  n. lithium fluoride laser
    (Nd:YLF)
neodymium:yttrium-lithium-fluoride
  n.-l.-f. laser segmentation
  n.-l.-f. photodisruptive laser
Neo-Flow
neoformans
  Cryptococcus n.
Neo-Hydeltrasol
NeoKnife cautery
Neolens lens
Neolyte laser indirect
  ophthalmoscope
Neo-Medrol
Neomixin
neomycin
  n. and dexamethasone
  n. and hydrocortisone
  n., polymyxin B, and
    gramicidin
  n., polymyxin B, and
    hydrocortisone
  n., polymyxin B, and
    prednisolone
  n. sulfate
Neomycin-Dex
neonatal
  n. gliosis

n. inclusion blennorrhea
n. inclusion conjunctivitis
n. myasthenia
n. ophthalmia
neonatorum
  blennorrhea n.
  ophthalmia n.
neoplasia
  conjunctival intraepithelial n.
    (CIN)
  conjunctival squamous cell n.
  corneal conjunctival
    intraepithelial n.
  intraepithelial n.
neoplasm
  choroidal n.
  Merkel cell n.
  orbital n.
  secondary malignant n.
neoplastic angioendotheliomatosis
Neo-Polycin
Neosar Injection
Neosporin
  N. drops
  N. Ophthalmic Ointment
  N. Ophthalmic Solution
neostigmine
  n. methylsulfate
  n. test
Neo-Synephrine
  N.-S. cocaine mixture
  N.-S. Hydrochloride
  N.-S. Ophthalmic Solution
Neo-Tears
Neotricin
  N. HC Ophthalmic Ointment
neovascular
  n. angle-closure glaucoma
  n. membrane
  n. net
  n. tuft
neovascularization
  choroidal n. (CNV)
  choroidovitreal n.
  classic choroidal n.
  corneal n.
  disk n.

N

NOTES

neovascularization *(continued)*
n. of disk (NVD)
disseminated asymptomatic
  unilateral n.
extraretinal n.
interstitial n.
n. of the iris (NVI)
iris n.
juxtafoveal choroidal n.
n. of new vessels elsewhere
  (NVE)
occult choroidal n.
peripapillary subretinal n.
preretinal n.
n. of retina
retinal quadrant n.
secondary n.
stromal n.
subfoveal choroidal n.
subretinal n. (SRNV)
vitreous n.
nephritica
retinitis n.
nephropathic cystinosis
Neptazane
Nernst glower
nerve
abducens n.
abducent n. (N.VI)
aberrant regeneration of n.
aberrant reinnervation of the
  oculomotor n.
acoustic n.
afferent n.
aplasia of optic n.
atrophy of optic n.
basal epithelial n.
block n.
n. block
cavernous portion of the
  oculomotor n.
ciliary n.
coloboma of optic n.
n. core
corneal n.
cranial n. (CN)
n. cross section
cupping of optic n.
efferent n.
eighth cranial n.
facial n.
n. fiber

N. Fiber Analyzer laser
  ophthalmoscope
n. fiber axon
n. fiber bundle
n. fiber bundle defect
n. fiber bundle layer
n. fiber layer (NFL)
n. fiber layer analyzer
n. fiber layer dropout
n. fiber layer hemorrhage
n. fiber layer infarct
fifth cranial n.
fourth cranial n.
frontal n.
ganglionic layer of optic n.
ganglionic stratum of optic n.
ganglion layer of optic n.
ganglion stratum of optic n.
greater superficial petrosal n.
n. head angioma
n. head drusen
infraepitrochlear n.
infraorbital n.
infratrochlear n.
input n.
n. input
intermedius n.
intervaginal space of optic n.
intracanalicular optic n.
intracranial optic n.
intraocular optic n.
intraosseous optic n.
ischemia of optic n.
lacrimal n.
n. layer of retina
long ciliary n.
n. loop
maxillary n.
motor n.
myelination of retinal n.
nasociliary n.
oculomotor n. (N.III)
ophthalmic n.
optic n. (N.II, ON)
orbital optic n.
output n.
n. palsy
peripapillary retinal n.
peripheral oculomotor n.
petrosal n.
postganglionic short ciliary n.
prechiasmal optic n.
preganglionic oculomotor n.

prelaminar optic n.
regeneration of n.
n. regeneration
second cranial n.
secretomotor n.
sensory n.
seventh cranial n.
n. sheath
n. sheath meningioma
short ciliary n.
sixth cranial n.
supraorbital n.
supratrochlear n.
tentorial n.
third cranial n.
trigeminal n. (NV)
trochlear n. (N.IV)
tumor of optic n.
vascular circle of optic n.
vestibular n.
vidian n.
zygomatic n.
zygomaticofacial n.
zygomaticotemporal n.
nervea
tunica n.
nervi (*pl. of* nervus)
Nervocaine
N. with epinephrine
nervous asthenopia
nervus, pl. nervi
nervi ciliares breves
nervi ciliares longi
n. infraorbitalis
n. intermedius
n. lacrimalis
n. maxillaris
n. nasociliaris
n. oculomotorius
n. ophthalmicus
n. opticus
n. supraorbitalis
n. trigeminus
n. trochlearis
n. zygomaticus
Nesacaine
nests and strands of cells

net
neovascular n.
parafoveal capillary n.
Nettleship-Falls X-linked ocular albinism
Nettleship iris repositor
Nettleship-Wilder dilator
network
choriocapillaris vascular n.
peritarsal n.
trabecular n.
vascular n.
Neubauer forceps
Neuhann cystitome
Neumann razor blade fragment holder
Neumann-Shepard
N.-S. corneal marker
N.-S. oval optical center marker
neural
n. crest
n. crest cell
n. lesion
n. retina
n. rim
n. tube
neuralgia
nasociliary n.
postherpetic n.
Raeder paratrigeminal n.
supraorbital n.
trifacial n.
trigeminal n.
vidian n.
neurasthenic asthenopia
neurectomy
opticociliary n.
neurilemmosarcoma
neurilemoma
ameloblastic n.
eyelid n.
malignant n.
neuritic atrophy
neuritis, pl. neuritides
acute idiopathic demyelinating optic n.

N

NOTES

neuritis *(continued)*
anterior ischemic optic n.
asymptomatic optic n.
atherosclerotic ischemic n.
chronic demyelinating optic n.
idiopathic demyelinating
optic n.
idiopathic nongranulomatous
optic n.
idiopathic perioptic n.
inflammatory optic n.
intraocular optic n.
n. nodosa
optic demyelinating n.
orbital n.
parainfectious optic n.
paraneoplastic optic n.
perioptic n.
postocular n.
postvaccination optic n.
retrobulbar n.
retrobulbar optic n.
subclinical optic n.
neuro-Behçet disease
neuroblastic
neurochorioretinitis
neurochoroiditis
neurodealgia
neurodeatrophia
neurodegenerative syndrome
neurodermatica
cataracta n.
neuroectodermal
neuroepithelial layer of retina
neuroepithelioma
orbital n.
neuroepithelium
neurofibroma
eyelid n.
iris n.
limbal n.
orbital n.
plexiform n.
uveal n.
neurofibromatosis
neurofilament triplets antibody
neurogenic
n. acquired ptosis
n. iris atrophy
n. mesenchyme
n. tumor
neuroimaging
neuroleptic malignant syndrome

neurologic
n. deficit
n. disorder
n. dysfunction
n. examination
neuroloptic drug
neuroma
acoustic n.
facial n.
mucosal n.
orbital n.
plexiform n.
neuromuscular
n. blocking drug
n. disorder
n. disorder-causing drug
n. effect
n. eyelid retraction
n. ptosis
neuromyelitis
n. optica
neuromyotonia
ocular n.
neuron
abducens internuclear n.
cholinergic n.
Golgi I n.
Golgi II n.
retinal n.
sympathetic n.
third order n.
neuro-ophthalmic manifestation
neuro-ophthalmologic
n.-o. case history
n.-o. diagnosis
n.-o. examination
neuro-ophthalmological investigation
neuro-ophthalmology
neuropapillitis
neuroparalytic
n. keratitis
n. keratopathy
n. ophthalmia
neuropathic
n. disease
n. eyelid retraction
n. tonic pupil
neuropathy
anterior compressive optic n.
anterior ischemic optic n.
(AION)
arteriosclerotic ischemic
optic n.

arteritic anterior ischemic
optic n.
autosomal dominant hereditary
optic n.
autosomal recessive hereditary
optic n.
compressive optic n.
Cuban epidemic optic n.
demyelinating optic n.
distal optic n.
dysthyroid optic n.
giant axonal n.
glaucomatous optic n.
hereditary optic n.
hypertrophic interstitial n.
infiltrative optic n.
inflammatory optic n.
ischemic optic n. (ION)
Jamaican optic n.
Leber hereditary optic n.
(LHON)
luetic n.
myelo-optic n.
nonarteritic anterior ischemic
optic n. (NAION)
nutritional optic n.
onion bulb n.
optic n.
parainfectious optic n.
peripheral n.
posterior ischemic optic n.
(PION)
radiation-induced optic n.
radiation optic n. (RON)
retrobulbar compressive
optic n.
retrobulbar ischemic optic n.
shock optic n.
subacute myelo-optic n.
(SMON)
toxic optic n.
traumatic optic n.
tropical optic n.
uremic optic n.
neurophakomatosis
neuroradiologic
neuroretinal rim

neuroretinitis
   cat scratch disease n.
   diffuse unilateral subacute n.
   (DUSN)
neuroretinopathy
   acute macular n.
   hypertensive n.
   macular n.
neurosensory
   n. retina
   n. retinal detachment
neuro-specific enolase antibody
neurotomy
   opticociliary n.
neurotonic pupil
neurotransmitter
   retinal n.
neurotrophic
   n. keratitis
   n. keratopathy
neurovisual manifestation
neutral
   n. density filter
   n. density filter test
   n. point
   n. zone
neutrophils
nevi (*pl. of* nevus)
nevocyte
nevoid
nevoxanthoendothelioma
   juvenile n.
nevus, pl. **nevi**
   basal cell n.
   blue n.
   choroidal n.
   compound n.
   conjunctival pigmented n.
   cystic amelanotic n.
   dermal n.
   episcleral n.
   epithelial n.
   eyelid n.
   intradermal n.
   junctional n.
   melanocytic n.
   nonpigmented n.

N

NOTES

nevus *(continued)*
Ota n.
n. of Ota
n. sebaceus of Jadassohn
Spitz n.
strawberry n.
subepithelial n.
uveal n.
Nevyas
N. double sharp cystitome
N. lens forceps
N. retractor
new
N. England Eye Bank
N. Orleans Eye & Ear
fixation forceps
N. Orleans lens
N. Orleans lens loupe
n. vessel disk
N. York erysiphake
N. York Eye & Ear Hospital
fixation forceps
newborn conjunctivitis
Newcastle disease virus
Newsom side port nucleus cracker
Newton disk
newtonian aberration
NewVues lens
Nexacryl
N. cohesive product
N. tissue adhesive
NFL
nerve fiber layer
niacin maculopathy
Niamtu video imaging system
niBUT
not invasive break-up time
Nichamin
N. fixation ring
N. hydrodissection cannula
N. triple chopper
N. vertical chopper
nicking
arteriolar n.
arteriovenous n.
AV n.
n. of retinal vein
retinal venous n.
Nicol prism
nicotinic acid maculopathy
nictation
nictitans
membrana n.

nictitating
n. membrane
n. spasm
nictitation
Nida nicking operation
Nidek
N. AR-2000 Objective
Automatic refractor
N. Auto Refractometer NR-
1000F
N. 3Dx stereodisk camera
N. EC-1000 excimer laser
EchoScan by N.
N. EC-5000 refractive laser
system
N. Laser System laser
Nieden syndrome
night
n. blindness
n. myopia
n. sight
n. vision
night-vision goggles
nigra
cataracta n.
nigricans
acanthosis n.
pseudoacanthosis n.
nigroid body
nigrum
pigmentum n.
tapetum n.
N.II
optic nerve
N.III
oculomotor nerve
Nikolsky sign
Nikon
N. aspheric lens
N. Auto Refractometer NR-
1000F
N. FS-3 photo slit lamp
Biomicroscope
N. Retinomax K-Plus
autorefractor
N. Retinopan fundus camera
N. zoom photo slit lamp
ninety hue discrimination test
NIPH
no improvement with pinhole
niphablepsia
niphotyphlosis

nipper
House-Dieter n.
Nitra lamp
nitrate
cellulose n.
Grocott-Gomori methenamine
silver n. (GMS)
phenylmercuric n.
pilocarpine n.
silver n.
N.IV
trochlear nerve
nivalis
ophthalmia n.
n. ophthalmia
Nizetic operation
NLD
nasolacrimal duct
NLP
no light perception
193-nm
193-n. excimer laser
excimer laser, 193193-n.
no
n. faci
n. improvement
n. improvement with pinhole
(NIPH)
n. light perception (NLP)
Noble forceps
Nocardia
N. asteroides
N. brasiliensis
N. caviae
N. keratitis
nocardial endophthalmitis
nocardiosis
ocular n.
Nocito eye implant
N₂O cryosurgical unit
nocturnal amblyopia
nodal
n. plane
n. point
node
Rosenmüller n.

nodiformis
cataracta n.
nodosa
conjunctivitis n.
endophthalmitis ophthalmia n.
iritis n.
neuritis n.
ophthalmia n.
periarteritis n. (PAN, PN)
polyarteritis n.
nodular
n. conjunctivitis
n. corneal degeneration
n. episcleritis
n. fasciitis
n. iritis
n. melanoma
n. scleritis
nodule
Busacca n.
conjunctival n.
Dalen-Fuchs n.
epibulbar Fordyce n.
episcleral rheumatic n.
Fordyce n.
iris n.
Koeppe n.
lemon-drop n.
lentiform n.
Lisch n.
millet seed n.
pseudorheumatoid n.
rheumatic n.
Salzmann n.
n.'s in sparganosis
subepidermal calcified n.
nodulus
n. conjunctivalis
n. lymphaticus
n. syndrome
Nokrome
N. bifocal
N. bifocal lens
Nolahist
no-light-perception vision
nomogram
Casebeer-Lindstrom n.

N

NOTES

nomogram *(continued)*
    Harrison-Stein n.
    n. system
nonabsorbable suture
non-*Acanthamoeba* amebic keratitis
nonaccommodation
nonaccommodative
    n. esodeviation
    n. esophoria
    n. esotropia
nonarteritic
    n. anterior ischemic optic
        neuropathy (NAION)
nonaspirating ultrasonic phaco
    chopper tip
nonatopic allergic conjunctivitis
noncaseating conjunctival granuloma
noncentral ulcer
noncicatricial entropion
noncomitant
    n. heterotropia
    n. squint
    n. strabismus
nonconcomitant strabismus
nonconfluent plaque
noncongestive glaucoma
noncontact tonometer (NCT)
noncycloplegic distance static
    retinoscopy
nonepithelial tumor
nonfenestrated capillary
nonfixed tissue
nongranulomatous
    n. anterior uveitis
    n. choroiditis
    n. iridocyclitis
non-Hodgkin lymphoma
non-insulin-dependent diabetes
    mellitus
noninvasive
    n. corneal redox fluorometry
    n. tear film break-up time
nonischemic CRVO
nonleaking bleb
nonliquefaciens
    Moraxella n.
nonmechanical trephination
nonmydriatic retinal photography
non-neovascular age-related macular
    degeneration
nonocular muscle group
nonophthalmos
nonoptic reflex eye movement

nonorganic
    n. blepharospasm
    n. disorder diagnosis
    n. paresis
    n. visual loss
Nonoxynol
nonparalytic strabismus
nonpenetrant gene
nonpenetrating keratoplasty
nonperfusion
    capillary n.
    retinal capillary n.
nonphysiologic visual field loss
nonpigmented
    n. ciliary epithelium
    n. nevus
nonpreserved artificial tears
nonproliferative
    n. diabetic retinopathy (NPDR)
    n. retinopathy
nonrapid eye movement
nonrefractive accommodative
    esotropia
nonrhegmatogenous retinal
    detachment
nonseton
non-Sjögren keratoconjunctivitis
    sicca
nonsteroidal anti-inflammatory drug
nonulcerative
    n. blepharitis
    n. interstitial keratitis
Noonan syndrome
Nordin-Ruiz trapezoidal marker
normal
    n. distribution
    n. fundus
    n. retinal correspondence
        (NRC)
    n. tension (TN)
normal-finger tension
normal-pressure glaucoma
normal-tension glaucoma (NTG)
Norman-Wood syndrome
normocytic
    n. anemia
    n. hypochromic anemia
normokalemic periodic paralysis
Normol
Norrie disease
North Carolina macular dystrophy
Northern
    Tracor N.

no-stitch phacoemulsification surgery
notation
   Jaeger n.
   Snellen n.
   standard n.
notch
   cerebellar n.
   n. of iris
   lacrimal n.
   supraorbital n.
notch-and-roll maneuver
notching
   lid n.
note blindness
Nothnagel syndrome
not invasive break-up time (niBUT)
no-touch transepithelial
  photorefractive keratectomy
Nova
   N. Aid lens
   N. Curve broad C-loop
    posterior chamber lens
   N. Curve Omnicurve lens
   Dioptron N.
   N. Soft II lens
Novatec LightBlade
Novus
   N. Omni 2000 photocoagulator
   N. 2000 ophthalmoscope
novyi
   Borrelia n.
Noyes
   N. forceps
   N. iridectomy scissors
   N. iris scissors
NP-3S auto chart projector
NPA
   near point of accommodation
NPC
   near point of convergence
NPDR
   nonproliferative diabetic retinopathy
NRC
   normal retinal correspondence
NR-1000F
   Nidek Auto Refractometer N.
   Nikon Auto Refractometer N.

NS
   nuclear sclerosis
NSU
   necrotizing sclerocorneal ulceration
NTG
   normal-tension glaucoma
nubecula
Nuck
   canal of N.
nuclear
   n. antigen
   n. arc
   n. bronzing
   n. change
   n. cytoplasmic ratio
   n. developmental cataract
   n. expression
   n. external layer
   n. horizontal gaze paralysis
   n. inner layer
   n. internal layer
   n. ophthalmoplegia
   n. outer layer
   n. palsy
   n. ring
   n. sclerosis (NS)
   n. sclerosis of lens
   n. tissue
   n. zone
nuclear-fascicular trochlear nerve
  palsy
nucleus, pl. nuclei
   accessory n.
   brainstem motor n.
   n. cracker
   n. delivery loupe
   dense brunescent n.
   Edinger-Westphal n.
   n. expressor
   geniculate n.
   5195 n. hydrodissector/rotator
   n. hydrolysis needle
   inferior olivary n.
   inferior salivary n.
   lateral geniculate n. (LGN)
   n. of lens
   lenticular n.

N

NOTES

nucleus *(continued)*
  n. lentiform
  n. lentis
  medial vestibular n. (MVN)
  oculomotor n.
  Perlia n.
  n. of posterior commissure
  pretectal n.
  pyknotic nuclei
  n. removal loupe
  rostral interstitial n.
  salivary n.
  n. spatula
  superior salivary n.
  suprachiasmatic n. (SCN)
  trochlear nerve n.
  vestibular n.
nudge test
Nugent
  N. fixation forceps
  N. hook
  N. rectus forceps
  N. soft cataract aspirator
  N. superior rectus forceps
Nugent-Gradle scissors
Nugent-Green-Dimitry erysiphake
Nulicaine
null
  n. condition
  n. point
  n. zone
number
  Snellen n.
numerical
  n. aperture (NA)
  n. visual acuity
nummular
  n. atrophy
  n. keratitis
nummularis
  keratitis n.
Nurolon suture
nut
  retrocorneal n.
nutans
  spasmus n.
Nu-Tears
  N.-T. II Solution
  N.-T. Solution
NutraTear
nutritional
  n. amblyopia
  n. blindness

  n. deficiency cataract
  n. optic neuropathy
Nutrivision
Nuvita lens
NuVue
NV
  trigeminal nerve
Nv
  naked vision
NVA
  near visual acuity
NVD
  neovascularization of disk
NVE
  neovascularization of new vessels
  elsewhere
NVI
  neovascularization of the iris
N.VI
  abducent nerve
NVP
  near visual point
nyctalope
nyctalopia
  n. with congenital myopia
Nylen-Barany maneuver
nylon
  n. frame
  n. loop
  n. 66 suture
nystagmic
nystagmiform
nystagmogram
nystagmograph
nystagmography
nystagmoid-like oscillation
nystagmoid movement
nystagmus
  acquired jerk n.
  acquired pendular n.
  after-n.
  ageotropic n.
  amaurosis n.
  amaurotic n.
  arthrokinetic n.
  ataxic n.
  audiokinetic n.
  aural n.
  Baer n.
  Bekhterev n.
  blockage n.
  n. blockage syndrome
  Bruns n.

caloric n.
caloric-induced n.
central vestibular n.
centripetal n.
cervical n.
Cheyne n.
circular n.
compressive n.
congenital n.
conjugate n.
constant n.
convergence-evoked n.
convergence retraction n.
deviational n.
disjunctive n.
dissociated vertical n.
divergence n.
downbeat n.
drug-induced n.
elliptic n.
elliptical n.
end-gaze n.
end-point n.
end-position n.
epileptic n.
eyelid n.
fatigue n.
fixation n.
galvanic n.
gaze n.
gaze-evoked n.
gaze-paretic n.
geotropic n.
head n.
hemi-seesaw n.
horizontal n.
hysterical n.
incongruent n.
irregular n.
Jensen jerk n.
jerk n.
labyrinthine n.
latent n.
lateral n.

left-beating n.
lid n.
manifest latent n.
miner's n.
minimal amplitude n.
monocular n.
muscle paretic n.
myasthenic n.
myoclonus n.
oblique n.
occlusion n.
ocular n.
opticokinetic n.
optokinetic n. (OKN)
oscillating n.
paretic n.
pendular n.
periodic alternating n.
periodic alternating windmill n.
peripheral vestibular n.
perverted n.
physiologic n.
positional n.
pseudocaloric n.
railroad n.
rebound n.
retraction n.
right-beating n.
rotary n.
rotation n.
rotational n.
rotatory n.
see-saw n.
sensory deprivation n.
strabismal n.
n. test
torsional n.
undulatory n.
upbeat n.
vertical n.
vestibular n.
vibratory n.
voluntary n.
n. with demyelination

N

NOTES

OAD
overall diameter of contact lens
OAG
open-angle glaucoma
Oaks
O. double needle
O. double straight cannula
O. straight cannula
OAO
ophthalmic artery occlusion
Oasis feather microscalpel
obcecation
object
Berens test o.
o. blindness
o. displacement
o. distance
fixation o.
o. of regard
o. size
o. space
test o.
object/image
o. conjugacy
o. relationship
objective
achromatic o.
apochromatic o.
o. optometer
o. perimetry
o. prism-neutralized cover test
o. refractor
o. vertigo
object-space focus
obligate carrier
obligatory suppression
oblique
o. aberration
o. astigmatism
o. dysfunction
o. fiber
o. illumination
inferior o.
o. muscle
o. muscle hook
o. nystagmus
o. palsy
o. position
o. prism
o. prism device

o. ray of light
superior o.
obliterans
endarteritis o.
thromboangiitis o.
obliteration
ductal orifice o.
O'Brien
O. akinesia technique
O. anesthesia
O. cataract
O. fixation forceps
O. lid block
O. marker
O. spud
O. stitch scissors
O'Brien-Elschnig fixation forceps
obscura
camera o.
obscuration
transient visual o.
obscured fovea
obscure vision
Obstbaum
O. lens spatula
O. synechia spatula
obstruction
carotid o.
congenital nasolacrimal duct o.
meibomian gland o.
nasolacrimal duct o.
outflow o.
primary acquired nasolacrimal
duct o. (PANDO)
silent central retinal vein o.
obstructive
o. glaucoma
o. retinal vasculitis
obturans
iritis o.
obturator
Moria o.
occipital
o. apoplexy
o. cortex
o. lobe
o. lobe unilateral cerebral
hemisphere lesion
occipitofrontalis
venter frontalis musculi o.

O

occipitothalamica
  radiatio o.
occipitothalamic radiation
occluded pupil
occludens
  zonula o.
occluder
  black/white o.
  clip-on/tie-on o.
  eye o.
  Halberg trial clip o.
  long/short o.
  lorgnette o.
  Maddox rod o.
  pinhole o.
  Pram o.
  red lens o.
  Rumison side port fixation o.
  single/double o.
  thumb o.
occlusion
  branch retinal artery o.
    (BRAO)
  branch retinal vein o. (BRVO)
  o. of branch vein
  carotid artery o.
  central retinal artery o.
    (CRAO)
  central retinal vein o. (CRVO,
    nonischemic CRVO)
  choroidal vascular o.
  macular arteriole o.
  macular branch retinal vein o.
    (MBRVO)
  monocular o.
  o. nystagmus
  ophthalmic artery o. (OAO)
  peripheral branch retinal
    vein o. (PBRVO)
  punctal o.
  o. of pupil
  retinal arterial o.
  retinal artery o.
  retinal vascular o.
  retinal vein o.
  o. of retinal vein
  retinal venous o.
  o. therapy
  vascular o.
occlusive
  o. microangiopathy
  o. retinal arteritis
  o. vascular disease

occlusor
  Elastoplast eye o.
occult
  o. annular ciliary body
  o. choroidal neovascularization
  o. temporal arteritis of
    Simmons
occupational
  o. lens
  o. ophthalmology
Occusert-Pilo
ochre
  o. hemorrhage
  o. mass
  o. membrane
ochronosis
  exogenous o.
  ocular o.
Ochsner
  O. cartilage forceps
  O. hook
  O. tissue/cartilage forceps
  O. tissue forceps
OCI
  Ophthalmic Confidence Index
o'clock
  1-o. position
  2-o. position
  3-o. position
  4-o. position
  5-o. position
  6-o. position
  7-o. position
  8-o. position
  9-o. position
  10-o. position
  11-o. position
  12-o. position
O'Connor
  O. depressor
  O. flat hook
  O. iris forceps
  O. lid forceps
  O. marker
  O. muscle hook
  O. operation
  O. sharp hook
  O. sponge forceps
  O. tenotomy hook
O'Connor-Elschnig fixation forceps
O'Connor-Peter operation
OCP
  ocular cicatricial pemphigoid

OCT
optical coherence tomography
octofluoropropane gas
Octopus
O. 1-2-3
O. automated perimetry
O. 101 bowl perimeter
O. 500 EZ
O. 201 perimeter
O. 201 perimeter test
Ocu-Bath
Ocu-Caine
OcuCaps
Akorn O.
Ocu-Carpine
OcuChart
Ocu-Chlor
OcuClear Ophthalmic
OcuClenz
OcuCoat
O. PF Ophthalmic Solution
Ocu-Cort
Ocu-Dex
Ocudose
Timoptic O.
Ocu-Drop
Ocufen
O. Ophthalmic
ocufilcon
Ocufit SR
Ocuflox
O. ophthalmic
Ocugestrin
Ocu-Guard
OcuHist
Oculab Tono-Pen
Oculaid lens
ocular
o. adnexa
o. adnexal tumor
o. albinism
o. alignment
o. angle
o. ataxia
o. axis
o. ballottement
o. barrier

o. bartonellosis
o. blepharospasm
o. bobbing
o. capsule
o. cicatricial pemphigoid (OCP)
o. coherence tomography
o. coloboma
o. cone
o. crisis
o. cryptococcal infection
o. cul-de-sac
o. cup
o. dipping
o. dominance
o. dominance column
o. duction
o. dysmetria
o. echography
o. flora
o. flutter
O. Gamboscope lens
O. Gamboscope loupe
o. gymnastics
o. hemodynamic assessment
o. hemodynamic value
o. herpes
o. histoplasmosis
o. histoplasmosis syndrome (OHS)
o. humor
o. hypertelorism
o. hypertension (OHT)
o. hypertension glaucoma
o. hypertensive glaucoma
o. hypotelorism
o. hypotony
o. image
o. immunology
o. inflammation
o. injury
o. irritation
o. ischemic syndrome (OIS)
o. larva
o. larva migrans
o. lens
o. lymphomatosis

NOTES

ocular *(continued)*
  o. marker
  o. massage
  o. medium
  o. melanocytosis
  o. melanoma
  o. meningioma
  o. microtremor
  o. motility
  o. motility disorder
  o. motility effect
  o. motility test
  o. motoneuron
  o. motor apraxia
  o. motor syndrome
  o. motor system
  o. movement
  o. muscle
  o. muscle palsy
  o. muscle paralysis
  o. muscle transplant
  o. myasthenia
  o. myiasis
  o. myoclonus
  o. myopathy
  o. neuromyotonia
  o. nocardiosis
  o. nystagmus
  o. ochronosis
  o. onchocerciasis
  o. oscillation
  o. pathology
  o. pemphigus
  o. perfusion pressure (OPP)
  o. phthisis
  o. pressure reducer
  o. prosthesis
  o. refraction
  o. region
  o. rigidity
  o. rosacea
  o. saccade
  o. siderosis
  o. sign
  o. sparganosis
  o. spectrum
  o. surface
  o. surface disease (OSD)
  o. syphilis
  o. syphilitic disease
  o. tension (Tn)
  o. tilt reaction (OTR)
  o. torticollis

  o. toxicity
  o. toxocariasis
  o. toxoplasmosis
  o. trauma
  o. vaccinial conjunctivitis
  O. Vergance and Accommodation Sensor (OVAS)
  o. vertigo
  o. vesicle
ocularis
  angor o.
  foveola o.
  vitrina o.
ocularist
oculentum
Oculex drug delivery system
oculi (*pl. of* oculus)
OcuLight
  O. GL/GLx green laser photocoagulator
  O. GLx green laser photocoagulator
  O. SL diode laser
  O. SLx ophthalmic laser
Oculinum
oculist
oculistics
oculoauditory syndrome
oculoauricular dysplasia
oculoauriculovertebral dysplasia
oculobuccogenital syndrome
oculocalorie response
oculocardiac reflex
oculocephalic
  o. maneuver
  o. reflex
  o. synkinesis
  o. test
  o. vascular anomaly
oculocephalogyric reflex
oculocerebral
  o. lymphoma
  o. syndrome
oculocerebromucomycosis
oculocerebrorenal
  o. dystrophy
  o. syndrome
oculocerebrovasculometer
oculocutaneous
  o. albinism
  o. albinoidism
  o. hypopigmentation

o. laser
o. syndrome
oculodentodigital dysplasia
oculodermal
  o. disorder
  o. melanocytosis
  o. melanosis
oculodigital
  o. reflex
  o. sign of Franchesseti
oculofacial paralysis
oculoglandular
  o. conjunctivitis
  o. disease
  o. syndrome
  o. tularemia
oculography
  infrared o.
  photoelectric o.
  photosensor o.
oculogravic illusion
oculogyral illusion
oculogyration
oculogyria
oculogyric
  o. auricular reflex
  o. crisis
  o. mechanism
oculomandibulodyscephaly
oculomasticatory myorhythmia
oculometer
oculometroscope
oculomigraine
oculomotor
  o. apraxia
  o. cranial nerve palsy
  o. decussation
  o. disorder
  o. nerve (N.III)
  o. nerve fascicle
  o. nerve lesion
  o. nerve misdirection
  o. nerve synkinesis
  o. nucleus
  o. paresis with cyclic spasm
  o. root

o. root of ciliary ganglion
o. system
oculomotorius
  nervus o.
oculomucous membrane syndrome
oculomycosis
oculonasal
Ocu-Lone
oculopalatal
  o. myoclonus
  o. myoclonus syndrome
oculopathy
  hypertensive o.
  lupus o.
  pituitarigenic o.
oculopharyngeal
  o. dystrophy
  o. reflex
  o. syndrome
oculoplastic
Oculo-Plastik ePTFE ocular implant
oculoplasty corneal protector
oculoplethysmography
oculopneumoplethysmography (OPG)
oculopupillary reflex
oculoreaction
oculorenal syndrome
oculorespiratory reflex
oculorotatory muscle
oculosensory cell reflex
oculospinal
oculosympathetic
  o. dysfunction
  o. paresis
  o. pathway
oculotoxic
oculovertebral dysplasia
oculovestibular reflex
oculozygomatic
Ocu-Lube
oculus, pl. oculi
  adnexa oculi
  albuginea oculi
  aqua oculi
  bulbus oculi
  camera oculi
  congenital melanosis oculi

NOTES

oculus *(continued)*
deprimens oculi
o. dexter (right eye)
elephantiasis oculi
endothelium oculi
equator bulbi oculi
fascia lata musculares oculi
fascia musculares oculi
fiber orbicularis oculi
fundus oculi
hypertonia oculi
hypotonia oculi
melanosis oculi
meridiani bulbi oculi
motor oculi
musculi oculi
musculus obliquus inferior
  oculi
musculus obliquus superior
  oculi
musculus orbicularis oculi
musculus rectus inferior oculi
musculus rectus lateralis oculi
musculus rectus medialis oculi
pars caeca oculi
pars lacrimalis musculi
  orbicularis oculi
pars orbitalis musculi
  orbicularis oculi
pars palpebralis musculi
  orbicularis oculi
polus anterior bulbi oculi
polus posterior bulbi oculi
pseudotumor oculi
o. sinister (left eye)
sphincter oculi
tapetum oculi
tendo oculi
O. trial frame
trochlea musculi obliqui
  superioris oculi
tunica adnata oculi
tunica albuginea oculi
tunica conjunctiva bulbi oculi
tunica fibrosa oculi
tunica nervosa oculi
tunica vascularis oculi
tunica vasculosa oculi
tutamina oculi
oculi unitas (both eyes)
oculi uterque (each eye) (OU)
vaginae oculi
vena choroideae oculi

visio o.
vitrina oculi
white tunica fibrosa oculi
OcuMax solution
ocumeter
Ocu-Mycin
Ocu-Pentolate
Ocu-Phrin
Ocu-Pred
O.-P. A
O.-P. Forte
Ocupress
O. Ophthalmic
O. Ophthalmic Solution
Ocuscan
O. A-scan biometric ultrasound
Sonometric O.
O. 400 transducer
Ocusert
O. device
O. Pilo-20
O. Pilo-40
O. Pilo-20 Ophthalmic
O. Pilo-40 Ophthalmic
Ocusil
Ocusoft scrub
Ocu-Sol
Ocu-Spor B
Ocu-Spor G
Ocusporin
Ocusulf-10 Ophthalmic
Ocu-Tears
Ocutome
O. DIOP
O. II fragmentation system
O. probe
O. vitrectomy unit
ocutome
Berkeley Bioengineering o.
CooperVision o.
disposable o.
Ocutricin
Ocutricin HC
Ocu-Trol
Ocu-Tropic
Ocu-Tropine
Ocuvite
OCuZIN
Ocu-Zoline
OCVM system
OD
right eye

ODM
   ophthalmodynamometry
O'Donoghue
   O. angled DCR probe
   O. silicone intubation
Odyssey phacoemulsification system
Oestrus ovis
off-axis imaging
ofloxacin
   o. ophthalmic solution
O'Gawa
   O. cataract-aspirating cannula
   O. suture-fixation forceps
   O. two-way aspirating cannula
Ogston-Luc operation
Oguchi disease
Ogura
   O. cartilage forceps
   O. operation
   O. tissue/cartilage forceps
   O. tissue forceps
OHS
   ocular histoplasmosis syndrome
     macular OHS
OHT
   ocular hypertension
oil layer
oily secretion
ointment (ung)
   AK-Spore H.C. Ophthalmic O.
   anesthetic o.
   bland ophthalmic o.
   Cortisporin Ophthalmic O.
   Neosporin Ophthalmic O.
   Neotricin HC Ophthalmic O.
   ophthalmic o.
   Terak Ophthalmic O.
   Terramycin Ophthalmic O.
   Terramycin w/Polymyxin B
     Ophthalmic O.
   ticrynafen o.
OIS
   ocular ischemic syndrome
   OIS image digitizing system
Okamura technique
Oklahoma iris wire retractor

OKN
   optokinetic nystagmus
OKT3
   orthoclone
Okuma plate
old
   o. eye
   o. sight
oleosa
   blepharitis o.
Olivella-Garrigosa photocoagulator
olive-tip
   o.-t. cannula
   o.-t. capsule polisher
   o.-t. irrigator
olivopontocerebellar atrophy
   (OPCA)
Olk
   O. vitreoretinal pick
   O. vitreoretinal spatula
OLM
   ophthalmic laser microendoscope
olopatadine hydrochloride
   ophthalmic solution
Olson phaco chopper
Olympus fundus camera
OM
   O. 2000 operation microscope
   O. 4 ophthalmometer
O'Malley-Heintz
   O.-H. infusion cannula
   O.-H. vitreous cutter
O'Malley-Pearce-Luma lens
O'Malley self-adhering lens implant
OMM
   ophthalmomandibulomelic
   OMM syndrome
Omnifit intraocular lens
OmniMed argon-fluoride excimer
   laser
Omni-Park speculum
OMS
   O. Empac Irrigation/Aspiration
   unit
   O. Machemer/Parel VISC
ON
   optic nerve

NOTES

O

on-axis imaging
Onchocerca
  O. caecutiens
  O. volvulus
onchocercal sclerosing keratitis
onchocerciasis
  ocular o.
onchocercosis
one-and-a-half syndrome
one-piece
  o.-p. bifocal
  o.-p. multifocal lens
  o.-p. plate haptic silicone
    intraocular lens
one-plane lens
one-snip
  o.-s. punctum
  o.-s. punctum operation
One solution
one-stage reconstruction of eye
  socket and eyelids
on-eye predicted power
Ong capsulotomy scissors
ONH
  optic nerve head
onion
  o. bulb neuropathy
  o. skin-like membrane
ONSD
  optic nerve sheath decompression
ONSF
  optic nerve sheath fenestration
ONSM
  optic nerve sheath meningioma
ONTT
  Optic Neuritis Treatment Trial
OP
  oscillatory potential
opaca
  cornea o.
opacification
  o. cherry-red spot
  corneal o.
  cortical o.
  cyan o.
  posterior capsule o. (PCO)
opacified cuff
opacity, pl. opacities
  calcium-containing o.
  Caspar ring o.
  congenital lens o.
  corneal deep o.
  cortical o.

crystalline o.
deep corneal stromal o.
dense o.
disciform o.
dust-like o.
early lens o.
facetted avascular disciform o.
interface o.
lenticular o.
leukomatous corneal o.
media o.
mycotic snowball o.
nebular stromal o.
peripheral corneal o.
posterior subcapsular o.
posterior supine position
  capsular o.
pulverulent o.
punctate corneal o.
snowball o.
spotty corneal o.
striate o.
stromal o.
subepithelial corneal o.
vitreous o.
opalescent cornea
opaque medium
OPCA
  olivopontocerebellar atrophy
Opcon
  Muro O.
  O. Ophthalmic
Opcon-A
open
  o. lens
  o. loop
open-angle glaucoma (OAG)
open-funnel detachment
opening
  apraxia of eyelid o. (AEO)
  compulsive eye o.
  orbital o.
  o. of orbital cavity
  palpebral o.
  punctal o.
open-loop accommodation
open-sky
  o.-s. cataract wound
  o.-s. cryoextraction
  o.-s. cryoextraction operation
  o.-s. dissection
  o.-s. technique

o.-s. trephination
o.-s. vitrectomy
operating
  o. loupe
  o. microscope
  o. microscope-induced
  phototoxic maculopathy
operation
  ab externo filtering o.
  Adams o.
  Adler o.
  Agnew o.
  Agrikola o.
  Allen o.
  Allport o.
  Alsus o.
  Alsus-Knapp o.
  Alvis o.
  Ammon o.
  Amsler o.
  Anagnostakis o.
  Anel o.
  Angelucci o.
  annular corneal graft o.
  Argyll-Robertson o.
  Arion o.
  Arlt o.
  Arlt-Jaesche o.
  Arrowhead o.
  Arroyo o.
  Arruga o.
  Arruga-Berens o.
  Badal o.
  Bangerter pterygium o.
  Bardelli lid ptosis o.
  Barkan-Cordes linear
  cataract o.
  Barkan double cyclodialysis o.
  Barkan goniotomy o.
  Barraquer enzymatic
  zonulolysis o.
  Barraquer keratomileusis o.
  Barrie-Jones
  canaliculodacryorhinostomy o.
  Barrio o.
  Basterra o.
  Beard o.

Beard-Cutler o.
Beer o.
Benedict orbit o.
Beren pterygium transplant o.
Berens sclerectomy o.
Berens-Smith o.
Berke o.
Berke-Motais o.
Bethke o.
Bielschowsky o.
Birch-Hirschfeld entropion o.
Blair o.
Blasius lid flap o.
Blaskovics canthoplasty o.
Blaskovics dacryostomy o.
Blaskovics inversion of
  tarsus o.
Blaskovics lid o.
Blatt o.
Böhm o.
Bonaccolto-Flieringa scleral
  ring o.
Bonaccolto-Flieringa vitreous o.
Bonnet enucleation o.
Bonzel o.
Borthen iridotasis o.
Bossalino blepharoplasty o.
Bowman o.
Boyd o.
Brailey o.
Bridge o.
bridge pedicle flap o.
Briggs strabismus o.
Bromley foreign body o.
Bronson foreign body
  removal o.
Budinger blepharoplasty o.
Burch eye evisceration o.
Burow flap o.
Buzzi o.
Byron Smith ectropion o.
Cairns o.
Calhoun-Hagler lens
  extraction o.
Callahan o.
Campodonico o.
Carter o.

NOTES

O

operation *(continued)*
Casanellas lacrimal o.
Casey o.
Castroviejo o.
Castroviejo-Scheie
  cyclodiathermy o.
cataract extraction o.
cautery o.
Celsus-Hotz o.
Celsus spasmodic entropion o.
cerclage o.
Chandler-Verhoeff o.
Chandler vitreous o.
Cibis o.
cinching o.
Cleasby iridectomy o.
Collin-Beard o.
Comberg foreign body o.
Conrad orbital blowout
  fracture o.
Cooper o.
corneal graft o.
Crawford sling o.
crescent o.
Critchett o.
Crock encircling o.
cryoextraction o.
cryotherapy o.
Csapody orbital repair o.
Cupper-Faden o.
Cusick o.
Cusick-Sarrail ptosis o.
Custodis o.
Cutler o.
Cutler-Beard o.
cyclodiathermy o.
Czermak pterygium o.
dacryoadenectomy o.
dacryocystectomy o.
dacryocystorhinotomy o.
dacryocystostomy o.
dacryocystotomy o.
Dailey o.
Dalgleish o.
Daviel o.
decompression of orbit o.
de Grandmont o.
Deiter o.
De Klair o.
de Lapersonne o.
Del Toro o.
Derby o.
Desmarres o.

de Vincentiis o.
DeWecker o.
Dianoux o.
diathermy o.
Dickey o.
Dickey-Fox o.
Dickson-Wright o.
Dieffenbach o.
dilation of punctum o.
discission of lens o.
D'ombrain o.
drainage of lacrimal gland o.
drainage of lacrimal sac o.
Duke-Elder o.
Dunnington o.
Dupuy-Dutemps o.
Durr o.
Duverger-Velter o.
Elliot o.
Elschnig canthorrhaphy o.
Ely o.
encircling of globe o.
encircling of scleral buckle o.
enucleation of eyeball o.
equilibrating o.
Erbakan inferior fornix o.
Escapini cataract o.
Esser inlay o.
Eversbusch o.
evisceration o.
Ewing o.
excision of lacrimal gland o.
excision of lacrimal sac o.
exenteration of orbital
  contents o.
extracapsular cataract
  extraction o.
Faden o.
Fanta cataract o.
Fasanella o.
Fasanella-Servat ptosis o.
fascia lata sling for ptosis o.
Fergus o.
Filatov o.
Filatov-Marzinkowsky o.
filtering o.
Fink o.
Flajani o.
Förster o.
Fould entropion o.
Fox o.
Franceschetti coreoplasty o.
Franceschetti corepraxy o.

Franceschetti deviation o.
Franceschetti keratoplasty o.
Franceschetti pupil deviation o.
Fricke o.
Friede o.
Friedenwald o.
Friedenwald-Guyton o.
Frost-Lang o.
Fuchs canthorrhaphy o.
Fuchs iris bombe
  transfixation o.
Fukala o.
Gayet o.
Georgariou cyclodialysis o.
Gifford o.
Gifford delimiting
  keratotomy o.
Gillies scar correction o.
Girard keratoprosthesis o.
Goldmann-Larson foreign
  body o.
Gomez-Marquez lacrimal o.
Gonin o.
Gonin cautery o.
goniotomy o.
Gradle keratoplasty o.
Graefe o.
Greaves o.
Grimsdale o.
Grossmann o.
Gutzeit dacryostomy o.
Guyton ptosis o.
Halpin o.
Harman o.
Harms-Dannheim
  trabeculotomy o.
Hasner o.
Heine o.
Heisrath o.
Herbert o.
Hess eyelid o.
Hess ptosis o.
Hiff o.
Hill o.
Hippel o.
Hogan o.
Holth o.

Horay o.
Horvath o.
Hotz-Anagnostakis o.
Hotz entropion o.
Hughes o.
Hummelsheim o.
Hunt-Transley o.
Iliff o.
Iliff-Haus o.
Imre lateral canthoplasty o.
indentation o.
iridectomy o.
iridencleisis o.
iridodialysis o.
iridotasis o.
iridotomy o.
Irvine o.
Jaesche o.
Jaesche-Arlt o.
Jaime lacrimal o.
Jameson o.
Jensen o.
Johnson o.
Jones o.
Katzin o.
Kelman o.
keratectomy o.
keratocentesis o.
keratomileusis o.
keratoplasty o.
keratotomy o.
Key o.
King o.
Kirby o.
Knapp o.
Knapp-Imre o.
Knapp-Wheeler-Reese o.
Koffler o.
Kraupa o.
Kreiker o.
Krieberg o.
Krönlein o.
Krönlein-Berke o.
Kuhnt eyelid o.
Kuhnt-Helmbold o.
Kuhnt-Szymanowski o.
Kuhnt-Thorpe o.

O

NOTES

operation *(continued)*
Kwitko o.
LaCarrere o.
Lagleyze o.
Lagleyze-Trantas o.
Lagrange o.
laissez-faire lid o.
Lancaster o.
Lanchner o.
Landolt o.
Langenbeck o.
Leahey o.
Lester Jones o.
Lexer o.
Lincoff o.
Lindner o.
Lindsay o.
Löhlein o.
Londermann o.
Lopez-Enriquez o.
Löwenstein o.
Machek-Blaskovics o.
Machek-Brunswick o.
Machek-Gifford o.
Machek ptosis o.
Mack-Brunswick o.
Magitot keratoplasty o.
magnet o.
magnetic o.
Magnus o.
Majewsky o.
Malbec o.
Malbran o.
Marquez-Gomez o.
Mauksch o.
Mauksch-Maumenee-Goldberg o.
Maumenee-Goldberg o.
McGavic o.
McGuire o.
McLaughlin o.
McLean o.
McReynolds o.
Meek o.
Meller o.
Meyer-Schwickerath o.
Michaelson o.
Mikamo double-eyelid o.
Minsky o.
Moncrieff o.
Moran o.
Morax o.
Morel-Fatio-Lalardie o.
Mosher o.

Mosher-Toti o.
Moss o.
Motais o.
Mueller o.
Mules o.
Mustarde o.
myectomy o.
myotomy o.
Naffziger o.
Neher o.
Nehra-Mack o.
Nida nicking o.
Nizetic o.
O'Connor o.
O'Connor-Peter o.
Ogston-Luc o.
Ogura o.
one-snip punctum o.
open-sky cryoextraction o.
orbital implant o.
Pagenstecher o.
Panas o.
pars plana o.
pattern cut corneal graft o.
Paufique o.
peripheral iridectomy o.
Peters o.
Physick o.
Pico o.
plombage o.
pocket o.
Polyak o.
Poulard o.
Power o.
Preziosi o.
probing lacrimonasal duct o.
Putenney o.
Quaglino o.
Raverdino o.
Ray-Brunswick-Mack o.
Ray-McLean o.
reattachment of choroid o.
reattachment of retina o.
recession of ocular muscle o.
Redmond-Smith o.
Reese-Cleasby o.
Reese-Jones-Cooper o.
Reese ptosis o.
removal of foreign body o.
Richet o.
Rosenburg o.
Rosengren o.
Roveda o.

Rowbotham o.
Rowinski o.
Rubbrecht o.
Ruedemann o.
Rycroft o.
Saemisch o.
Safar o.
Sanders o.
Sato o.
Savin o.
Sayoc o.
Scheie o.
Schepens o.
Schimek o.
Schirmer o.
Schmalz o.
scleral buckling o.
scleral fistulectomy o.
scleral shortening o.
scleroplasty o.
sclerotomy o.
sector iridectomy o.
Selinger o.
seton o.
Shaffer o.
Shugrue o.
Sichi o.
Silva-Costa o.
Silver-Hildreth o.
slant o.
slant muscle o.
Smith eyelid o.
Smith-Indian o.
Smith-Kuhnt-Szymanowski o.
Snellen ptosis o.
Soria o.
Soriano o.
Sourdille keratoplasty o.
Sourdille ptosis o.
Spaeth cystic bleb o.
Spaeth ptosis o.
Speas o.
Spencer-Watson Z-plasty o.
splitting lacrimal papilla o.
Stallard eyelid o.
Stallard flap o.
Stallard-Liegard o.

step graft o.
Stock o.
Stocker o.
Straith eyelid o.
Strampelli-Valvo o.
Streatfield o.
Streatfield-Fox o.
Streatfield-Snellen o.
Suarez-Villafranca o.
Summerskill o.
suture of cornea o.
suture of eyeball o.
suture of iris o.
suture of muscle o.
suture of sclera o.
Szymanowski o.
Szymanowski-Kuhnt o.
Tansley o.
Tasia o.
tattoo of cornea o.
Teale-Knapp o.
tenotomy o.
Terson o.
Tessier o.
Thomas o.
three-snip punctum o.
Tillett o.
Toti o.
Toti-Mosher o.
Townley-Paton o.
trabeculectomy o.
Trainor o.
Trainor-Nida o.
transfixion of iris o.
transplantation of muscle o.
Trantas o.
trapdoor scleral buckle o.
Tripier o.
Troutman o.
Truc o.
Tudor-Thomas o.
tumbling technique o.
Ulloa o.
Uyemura o.
Van Milligen o.
Verhoeff o.
Verhoeff-Chandler o.

o

NOTES

operation *(continued)*
Verwey eyelid o.
Viers o.
Vogt o.
Von Ammon o.
von Blaskovics-Doyen o.
von Graefe o.
von Hippel o.
Waldhauer o.
Walter Reed o.
Watzke o.
Weeker o.
Weeks o.
Weisinger o.
Wendell Hughes o.
Werb o.
West o.
Weve o.
Wharton-Jones o.
Wheeler o.
Wheeler-Reese o.
Whitnall sling o.
Wicherkiewicz eyelid o.
Wiener o.
Wies o.
Wilmer o.
Wolfe ptosis o.
Worst o.
Worth ptosis o.
Wright o.
Young o.
Ziegler o.
Zylik o.
opercula
operculated
o. hole
o. tear
operculum, gen. **operculi,** pl. **opercula**
free o.
peripheral retinal o.
OPG
oculopneumoplethysmography
OPGR
OptiMed glaucoma pressure
regulator
Ophacet
ophryogene
ulerythema o.
Ophtec
O. Co. lens
O. occlusion implant
Ophthacet
Ophthaine

Ophthalas
O. argon/krypton laser
O. argon laser
O. krypton laser
Ophthalgan
O. Ophthalmic
ophthalmagra
ophthalmalgia
ophthalmatrophia
ophthalmectomy
ophthalmencephalon
Ophthalmetron
Safir O.
ophthalmia
actinic ray o.
Brazilian o.
catarrhal o.
caterpillar o.
caterpillar-hair o.
o. eczematosa
Egyptian o.
electric o.
o. electrica
flash o.
gonococcal o.
gonorrheal o.
granular o.
o. hepatica
jequirity o.
o. lenta
metastatic o.
migratory o.
mucous o.
neonatal o.
o. neonatorum
neuroparalytic o.
o. nivalis
nivalis o.
o. nodosa
periodic o.
phlyctenular o.
pseudotuberculous o.
purulent o.
reaper's o.
scrofulous o.
spring o.
strumous o.
sympathetic o.
transferred o.
ultraviolet ray o.
varicose o.
vegetable o.
ophthalmiatrics

ophthalmic
Absorbonac o.
Achromycin O.
Acular O.
Adsorbocarpine O.
Akarpine O.
AK-Chlor O.
AK-Cide O.
AK-Con o.
AK-Dex O.
AK-Homatropine O.
AK-Neo-Dex O.
AK-Poly-Bac O.
AK-Pred O.
AKPro O.
AK-Sulf O.
AKTob O.
AK-Tracin O.
Albalon-A O.
Albalon Liquifilm O.
Alomide O.
alpha2-adrenergic agonist
  agent, o.
Antazoline-V O.
o. artery
o. artery aneurysm
o. artery occlusion (OAO)
Betimol O.
Betoptic O.
Betoptic S O.
Bleph-10 O.
Blephamide O.
Carbastat O.
Carboptic O.
o. cautery
Cetamide O.
Cetapred o.
Chloroptic O.
Chloroptic-P O.
Ciloxan O.
Collyrium Fresh O.
Comfort O.
O. Confidence Index (OCI)
o. corticosteroid
o. cul-de-sac
o. cup
Cyclomydril O.

Degest 2 O.
o. disorder
o. drug
Econopred O.
o. electrocautery
o. endoscope
E-Pilo-x O.
Estivin II O.
o. examination
Eyesine O.
Floropryl O.
o. ganglion
Garamycin O.
Garamycin O.
Geneye O.
Genoptic S.O.P. O.
Gentacidin O.
Gentak O.
o. glucocorticoid
Herplex O.
o. hook
Humorsol O.
o. hyperthyroidism
Ilotycin O.
I-Naphline O.
Inflamase Forte O.
Inflamase Mild O.
Isopto Carbachol O.
Isopto Carpine O.
Isopto Cetamide O.
Isopto Cetapred o.
Isopto Homatropine O.
Isopto Hyoscine O.
o. laser microendoscope
  (OLM)
Metimyd O.
o. migraine
O. Moldite Powder
Murine Plus O.
Murocoll-2 O.
Nafazair O.
Naphcon O.
Naphcon-A O.
Naphcon Forte O.
NeoDecadron O.
Neo-Dexameth O.
o. nerve

NOTES

O

ophthalmic *(continued)*
OcuClear O.
Ocufen O.
Ocuflox o.
Ocupress O.
Ocusert Pilo-20 O.
Ocusert Pilo-40 O.
Ocusulf-10 O.
o. ointment
Opcon O.
Ophthalgan O.
Optigene O.
OptiPranolol O.
Osmoglyn O.
Paremyd O.
Phospholine Iodide O.
O. Photographers Society
    (OPS)
Pilagan O.
Pilocar O.
Pilopine HS O.
Piloptic O.
Pilostat O.
o. plexus
Polysporin O.
Polytrim O.
Pred Forte O.
Pred-G O.
Pred Mild O.
Profenal O.
Propine O.
PxEx O.
o. reaction
Sodium Sulamyd O.
o. solution
o. sponge
Sulf-10 O.
o. test
Tetrasine O.
Tetrasine Extra O.
Timoptic O.
Timoptic-XE O.
TobraDex O.
Tobrex O.
Vasocidin O.
VasoClear O.
Vasocon-A O.
Vasocon Regular O.
Vasosulf O.
o. vein
o. vesicle
Vira-A O.
Viroptic O.

Visine Extra O.
Visine L.R. O.
o. vitreous surgical technique
Voltaren O.
ophthalmica
vesicula o.
zona o.
ophthalmicus
caliculus o.
herpes o.
herpes zoster o.
nervus o.
varicella zoster o.
zoster o.
ophthalmitic
ophthalmitis
ophthalmoblennorrhea
ophthalmocarcinoma
ophthalmocele
ophthalmocopia
ophthalmodesmitis
ophthalmodiagnosis
ophthalmodiaphanoscope
ophthalmodiastimeter
ophthalmodonesis
ophthalmodynamometer
Bailliart o.
Reichert o.
suction o.
ophthalmodynamometry (ODM)
ophthalmodynia
ophthalmoeikonometer
ophthalmofunduscope
ophthalmogram
ophthalmograph
ophthalmography
ophthalmogyric
ophthalmoleukoscope
ophthalmolith
ophthalmologic
ophthalmologist
ophthalmology
American Academy of O.
Association of Technical
    Personnel in O. (ATPO)
Joint Commission on Allied
    Health Personnel in O.
    (JCAHPO)
Montana Academy of O.
    (MAO)
occupational o.
ophthalmomalacia
ophthalmomandibulomelic (OMM)

ophthalmomandibulomelic dysplasia
ophthalmomelanosis
ophthalmomeningea
    vena o.
ophthalmomeningeal vein
ophthalmometer
    Haag-Streit o.
    Javal o.
    Javal-Schiotz o.
    Micromatic o.
    mires of o.
    OM 4 o.
ophthalmometroscope
ophthalmometry
ophthalmomycosis
ophthalmomyiasis
    Cuterebra o.
ophthalmomyitis
ophthalmomyositis
ophthalmomyotomy
ophthalmoneuritis
ophthalmoneuromyelitis
ophthalmoparesis
    internuclear o.
ophthalmopathy
    dysthyroid o.
    endocrine o.
    external o.
    Graves o.
    internal o.
    thyroid o.
ophthalmophacometer
ophthalmophantom
ophthalmophlebotomy
ophthalmophthisis
ophthalmoplasty
ophthalmoplegia
    autosomal-dominant o.
    autosomal-recessive o.
    basal o.
    binocular internuclear o.
    (BINO)
    chronic progressive external o.
    (CPEO)
    exophthalmic o.
    o. externa
    external o.

    fascicular o.
    infectious o.
    infranuclear o.
    o. interna
    internal o.
    internuclear o. (INO)
    o. internuclearis
    migraine o.
    migrainous o.
    nuclear o.
    orbital o.
    painful o.
    Parinaud o.
    partial o.
    o. partialis
    posterior internuclear o.
    o. progressiva
    progressive external o. (PEO)
    pseudointernuclear o.
    Sauvineau o.
    sensory ataxic neuropathy with
      dysarthria and o. (SANDO)
    thyrotoxicosis o.
    total o.
    o. totalis
ophthalmoplegic
    o. exophthalmos
    o. migraine
    o. muscular dystrophy
ophthalmoptosis
ophthalmoreaction
    Calmette o.
ophthalmorrhagia
ophthalmorrhea
ophthalmorrhexis
ophthalmoscope
    Alcon indirect o.
    AO binocular indirect o.
    AO Reichert Instruments
      binocular indirect o.
    Bailliart o.
    binocular o.
    binocular indirect o.
    confocal laser scanning o.
    confocal scanning laser o.
    cordless monocular indirect o.
    demonstration o.

O

NOTES

ophthalmoscope *(continued)*
    direct o.
    Doran pattern stimulator o.
    Exeter o.
    Fison indirect binocular o.
    Friedenwald o.
    Ful-Vue o.
    ghost o.
    Gullstrand o.
    Halberg indirect o.
    halogen o.
    Helmholtz o.
    Highlight spectral indirect o.
    indirect o.
    Keeler o.
    Loring o.
    Mentor Exeter o.
    metric o.
    MK IV o.
    monocular indirect o.
    Neolyte laser indirect o.
    Nerve Fiber Analyzer laser o.
    Novus 2000 o.
    polarizing o.
    Polle pod attachment for o.
    Propper-Heine o.
    Propper indirect o.
    Reichert binocular indirect o.
    Reichert Ful-Vue binocular o.
    Rodenstock scanning laser o.
    scanning laser o. (SLO)
    Schepens binocular indirect o.
    Schepens-Pomerantzeff o.
    TopSS scanning laser o.
    Vantage o.
    Video Binocular indirect o.
    (VBIO)
    Visuscope o.
    Welch-Allyn o.
    Zeiss o.
ophthalmoscopic
    o. examination
ophthalmoscopy
    binocular indirect o.
    confocal scanning laser o.
    direct o.
    distant direct o.
    dynamic scanning laser o.
    indirect o.
    medical o.
    metric o.
    slit-lamp o.
    o. with reflected light

ophthalmospectroscope
ophthalmospectroscopy
ophthalmostasis
ophthalmostat
ophthalmostatometer
ophthalmosteresis
ophthalmosynchysis
ophthalmothermometer
ophthalmotomy
ophthalmotonometer
ophthalmotonometry
ophthalmotoxin
ophthalmotrope
ophthalmotropometer
ophthalmotropometry
ophthalmovascular
ophthalmoxerosis
ophthalmoxyster
Ophthalon
    O. suture
ophthalsonic pachometer
Ophtha P/S
Ophthascan
Ophthasonic Ultrasonic Biometer
Ophthas subjective optometer
Ophthel
Ophthetic
Ophthilon
Ophthimus
    O. High-Pass Resolution
      perimeter
    O. ring perimeter
Ophthochlor
Ophthocort
opiate analgesic
OPL
    outer plexiform layer
OPMI
    O. PRO magis microscope
    O. VISU 200 microscope
Opmilas 144 surgical laser
OPP
    ocular perfusion pressure
opponent
    o. color
    o. colors theory
Opraflex drape
OPS
    Ophthalmic Photographers Society
opsin
    cone o.
opsinosis
opsiometer

opsoclonia
opsoclonus
   paraneoplastic o.
Optacon
Optacryl
Opt-Ease
Optec 3000 contrast sensitivity test
Optef
Optelec
   O. Passport magnifier
   O. Spectrum Jr.
Op-Temp
   O.-T. disposable cautery
   O.-T. disposable electrocautery
optesthesia
Op-Thal-Zin
Opthascan Mini-A scan
Optho
   RO O.
Opti-Bon
optic
   o. agnosia
   o. angle
   o. aphasia
   o. artery
   o. ataxia
   o. axis
   bioconvex o.
   o. canal
   o. center
   o. chiasm
   o. chiasmal lesion
   o. chiasmal syndrome
   o. coloboma
   o. commissure
   o. cul-de-sac
   o. cup
   o. cup-to-disk ratio
   o. decussation
   o. demyelinating neuritis
   o. disk
   o. disk anomaly
   o. disk atrophy
   o. disk cupping
   o. disk dragging
   o. disk drusen
   o. disk drusen calcification

o. disk drusen retinopathy
o. disk dysplasia
o. disk edema
o. disk pallor
o. disk pit
o. disk swelling
o. disk topography
o. disk tubercle
o. evagination
o. foramen
o. ganglion
o. groove
o. hyperesthesia
o. implant
o. iridectomy
o. keratoplasty
o. lemniscus
o. muscle recession
o. nerve (N.II, ON)
o. nerve aplasia
o. nerve atrophy
o. nerve coloboma
o. nerve cupping
o. nerve disease
o. nerve disorder
o. nerve drusen
o. nerve dysfunction
o. nerve dysplasia
o. nerve fiber
o. nerve glioma
o. nerve head (ONH)
o. nerve hemangioblastoma
o. nerve hypoplasia
o. nerve injury
o. nerve lesion
o. nerve myelination
o. nerve pit
o. nerve sheath
o. nerve sheath decompression
   (ONSD)
o. nerve sheath fenestration
   (ONSF)
o. nerve sheath meningioma
   (ONSM)
o. nerve tumor
O. Neuritis Treatment Trial
   (ONTT)

NOTES

O

optic *(continued)*
   o. neuropathy
   o. papilla (p)
   o. papilla cavity
   o. perineuritis
   o. pit
   o. primordium
   o. radiation
   o. radiation lesion
   o. recess
   o. stalk
   o. strut
   o. sulcus
   o. thalamus
   o. tract
   o. tract compression
   o. tract damage
   o. tract lesion
   o. tract syndrome
   o. vesicle
optica
   hyperesthesia o.
   neuromyelitis o.
   radiatio o.
opticae
   commissurae o.
Opticaid
   Spring Clip O.
optical
   o. aberration
   o. alexia
   o. allachesthesia
   o. axis
   o. bench
   o. blur
   o. breakdown
   o. center
   o. centering instrument
   o. center of spectacle lens
   o. clarity
   o. coherence tomography
     (OCT)
   o. contact lens
   o. correction
   o. cross
   o. density method
   o. disk anomaly
   o. disk swelling
   o. fossa
   o. frame
   o. glass
   o. heterogeneity
   o. illusion

   o. image
   o. iridectomy
   o. keratoplasty
   o. nodal point
   o. pachymeter
   o. power
   O. Radiation lens
   o. raytracing
   o. rehabilitation
   o. system
   o. zone (OZ)
   o. zone centration
   o. zone of contact lens
   o. zone diameter
   o. zone marker
optically empty
Opticath
optic disk
optici
   circulus vasculosus nervi o.
   discus nervi o.
   evulsio nervi o.
   excavatio papillae nervi o.
   radix lateralis tractus o.
   radix medialis tractus o.
   vaginae externa nervi o.
   vaginae interna nervi o.
   vaginae nervi o.
optician
opticianry
opticist
Opti-Clean
Opti-Clean II
opticoacoustic nerve atrophy
opticocerebral syndrome
opticochiasmatic, optochiasmic
   o. arachnoiditis
opticociliary, optociliary
   o. neurectomy
   o. neurotomy
   o. shunt
   o. shunt vein
   o. shunt vessel
opticocinerea
opticocochleodentate degeneration
opticofacial winking reflex
opticokinetic nystagmus
opticomyelitis
opticonasion
opticopupillary
opticopyramidal syndrome
Opticrom
Opticrom 4%

optics
> Allergan Medical O. (AMO)
> American Medical O.
> confocal o.
> Fresnel o.
> gaussian o.
> geometric o.
> o. of intraocular lens
> physical o.
> physiologic o.
> reverse o.

opticum
> chiasma o.
> foramen o.

opticus
> axis o.
> canaliculus infraorbitalis o.
> canalis o.
> discus o.
> nervus o.
> porus o.
> recessus o.

Opticyl
Optiflex lens
Opti-Free
Optigene
> O. Ophthalmic

Optik
Optima
> O. contact lens
> O. diamond knife

OptiMed
> O. device
> O. glaucoma pressure regulator (OPGR)

Optimine
Optimmune
Optimum
> O. blade

OPTIMUM rigid gas permeable starter kit
Optimyd
OptiPranolol
> O. Ophthalmic

Optipress
Opti-Pure System

Optique 1 Eye Drops
Optised
Optisoap
Opti-Soft
Optisol
> O. GS
> O. medium

Optisol-GS
optist
Opti-Tears
Opti-Vu lens
Opti-Zyme enzymatic cleaner
optoblast
optochiasmatic
> o. arachnoiditis
> o. tuberculomas

optochiasmic (var. of opticochiasmatic)
optociliary (var. of opticociliary)
optogram
optokinesis
optokinetic
> o. drum
> o. nystagmus (OKN)
> o. reflex
> o. stimulator
> o. stimulus
> o. system
> o. tape

optomeninx
optometer
> automatic infrared o.
> infrared o.
> laser o.
> objective o.
> Ophthas subjective o.
> Vernier o.

optometrist
optometry
optomotor reflex
optomyometer
optophone
optostriate
optotype
> Snellen letter o.

Optrex

O

NOTES

Opt-Visor
  O.-V. lens
  O.-V. loupe
Optycryl 60 contact lens
Optyl frame
Opus III contact lens
OR
  overrefraction
ora
  o. globule
  o. serrata retinae
oral
  AllerMax O.
  Banophen O.
  Belix O.
  Benadryl O.
  Cartrol O.
  Cytoxan O.
  Dimetabs O.
  Kerlone O.
  Phendry O.
  Siladryl O.
  Toradol O.
orange
  o. dye laser
  o. punctate pigmentation
Oratrol
orbiculare
  Pityrosporum o.
orbiculare
  os o.
orbicularis
  alopecia o.
  o. ciliaris
  musculus o.
  o. myectomy
  o. oculi muscle
  o. oris muscle
  o. phenomenon
  o. pupillary reflex
  o. reaction
  o. sign
  o. strength
orbicular muscle of eye
orbiculoanterocapsular fiber
orbiculociliary fiber
orbiculoposterocapsular fiber
orbit
  aneurysm of o.
  o. blade
  blow-out fracture of o.
  contusion of o.
  CT scan of o.

dermoid of o.
emphysema of o.
fracture of o.
o. hamartoma
idiopathic sclerosing
  inflammation of the o.
intraorbital margin of o.
lateral margin of o.
lesion of o.
roof of o.
supraorbital margin of o.
orbitae
  aditus o.
  corpus adiposum o.
  exenteratio o.
  margo infraorbitalis o.
  margo lateralis o.
  margo medialis o.
  margo supraorbitalis o.
  paries interior o.
  paries lateralis o.
  paries medialis o.
  paries superior o.
orbital
  o. abscess
  o. adipose tissue
  o. akinesia
  o. amyloidosis
  o. anesthesia
  o. aneurysm
  o. angiography
  o. angioma
  o. angiosarcoma
  o. aperture
  o. apex
  o. apex syndrome
  o. arch
  o. arch of frontal bone
  o. arteriovenous malformation
  o. axis
  o. blow-out fracture
  o. bone
  o. border of sphenoid bone
  o. canal
  o. cavity
  o. cellulitis
  o. content
  o. crest
  o. CT scan
  o. cyst
  o. decompression
  o. depressor
  o. dermoid

o. dystopia
o. echography
o. emphysema
o. encephalocele
o. enlargement
o. enucleation compressor
o. exenteration
o. extension
o. fascia
o. fasciitis
o. fat
o. fat pad
o. fat suppression
o. fibroma
o. fibromatosis
o. fibrosarcoma
o. floor
o. floor fracture
o. floor implant
o. floor prosthesis
o. ganglion
o. glioma
o. granuloma
o. hamartoma
o. height
o. hemangioendothelioma
o. hemangioma
o. hemangiopericytoma
o. hematoma
o. hemorrhage
o. hernia
o. hypertelorism
o. hypotelorism
o. hypoxia
o. implant operation
o. infarction
o. inferior rim
o. lamina
o. lens
o. lesion
o. lipoma
o. lymphoma
o. margin
o. medulloepithelioma
o. melanoma
o. meningioma
o. mesenchyme

o. metastasis
o. muscle
o. myositis
o. neoplasm
o. neuritis
o. neuroepithelioma
o. neurofibroma
o. neuroma
o. opening
o. ophthalmoplegia
o. optic nerve
o. palsy
o. pathology
o. periosteum
o. periostitis
o. pit
o. plane
o. plane of frontal bone
o. plaque brachytherapy
o. plate of ethmoid bone
o. plate of frontal bone
o. polymyositis
o. portion of eyelid
o. pseudotumor
o. radiology
o. radiotherapy
o. region
o. resilience
o. rhabdomyosarcoma
o. rim fracture
o. roentgenogram
o. roof
o. section
o. septum
o. sulci of frontal bone
o. sulcus
o. superior fissure
o. surgery
o. tomography
o. trauma
o. tumor
o. varix
o. vasculitis
o. vein thrombosis
o. venography
o. vessel
o. wall fracture

O

NOTES

orbital *(continued)*
   o. width
   o. wing of sphenoid bone
   o. x-ray
orbitale
   planum o.
   septum o.
orbitales
   fasciae o.
orbitalia
   cribra o.
orbitalis
   margo o.
   musculus o.
orbitectomy
   radical o.
orbitocranial trauma
orbitography
   Graves o.
orbitomalar foramen
orbitonasal
orbitonometer
orbitonometry
orbitopalpebral
orbitopathy
   dysthyroid o.
   Graves o.
   thyroid o.
orbitorhinomucormycosis
orbitostat
orbitotemporal
orbitotomy
   Berke-Krönlein o.
   lateral o.
Orca surgical blade
ORC intraocular lens
ordered array
ordering
   Dyer nomogram system of
   lens o.
organ
   o. culture
   o. transplantation
   vestibular o.
   o. of vision
   visual o.
organic amblyopia
organism
   coliform o.
organized vitreous
organum
   o. visuale
   o. visus

orientation
   epithelial o.
   false o.
   limbal parallel o.
oriented
   radially o.
original Sweet eye magnet
oris
   pars marginalis musculi
   orbicularis o.
   sphincter o.
ornithine tolerance test
orodigitofacial dysplasia
orthoclone (OKT3)
Orthogon lens
orthokeratology
Ortho-Lite
orthometer
orthophoria
orthophoric
orthopia
orthoposition
orthoptic
orthoptist
orthoptoscope
Ortho-Rater
orthoscope
orthoscopic
   o. lens
   o. spectacles
orthoscopy
Or-Toptic M
OS
   left eye
os
   o. lacrimale
   o. orbiculare
   o. palatinum
   o. planum
   o. unguis
oscillating
   o. nystagmus
   o. vision
oscillation
   convergent-divergent
   pendular o.
   macrosaccadic o.
   nystagmoid-like o.
   ocular o.
   voluntary saccadic o.
oscillatory potential (OP)
oscillopsia
   monocular o.

OSD
    ocular surface disease
O'Shea lens
Osher
    O. foreign body forceps
    O. gonio/posterior pole lens
    O. hook
    O. pan-fundus lens
    O. surgical gonio/posterior pole
      lens
    O. surgical keratometer
Osher-Neumann corneal marker
Osmitrol
    O. Injection
osmium tetroxide solution
Osmoglyn Ophthalmic
osmolarity
    tear o.
osmotherapy
    hypertonic o.
osmotic
    o. cataract
    o. pressure
Osopto Tears
ossea
    bulla o.
    cataracta o.
osseous
    o. anomaly
    o. choristoma
    o. lesion
    o. system
osseus
    tarsus o.
ossis
    bulla ethmoidalis o.
ossium
    fragilitas o.
osteitis deformans
osteoma
    choroidal o.
    uveal o.
osteomyelitis
    maxillary o.
osteoporosis-pseudoglioma syndrome
osteosclerotic myeloma

osteotome
    lacrimal o.
osteotomy
ostium
    internal o.
Ota
    nevus of O.
    O. nevus
    O. nevus syndrome
oticus
    herpes zoster o.
otolithic-ocular reflex
OTR
    ocular tilt reaction
OU
    both eyes
    oculi uterque (each eye)
outer
    o. canthus
    o. limiting membrane
    o. nuclear layer
    o. plexiform layer (OPL)
    o. retina
    o. segment
outflow
    aqueous o.
    coefficient of facility of o.
    conventional o.
    o. disorder
    facility of o.
    lacrimal o.
    o. obstruction
    parasympathetic o.
    o. resistance
    trabecular o.
    unconventional o.
    uveoscleral o.
outgrowth
    extrascleral o.
    local o.
outpouching
output nerve
Ovadendron sulphureo-ochraceum
   endophthamitis
oval
    o. cornea
    o. cup erysiphake

O

NOTES

oval *(continued)*
    o. eye
    o. eye patch
ovale
    Pityrosporum o.
oval-shaped vernal ulcer
OVAS
    Ocular Vergance and
    Accommodation Sensor
overaction
    inferior oblique o.
overall diameter of contact lens
    (OAD)
overcorrection
overflow diabetes
overrefraction (OR)
overripe cataract
overt diabetes
overwear syndrome (OWS)
ovis
    Oestrus o.
ovoid mass
OWS
    overwear syndrome
oxidation of solution
oxide
    mercuric o.
oxidopamine

oximetry sensor
oxprenolol
Oxsoralen
oxyblepsia
oxycephaly
oxycodone
    acetaminophen with o.
oxygen
    o. flux
    o. permeability
oxymetazoline
oxymorphone hydrochloride
oxyopia
oxyopter
oxyphenbutazone
oxyphenonium
Oxysept
    Lens Plus O.
oxysporum
    Fusarium o.
oxytetracycline
    o. and hydrocortisone
oxytetracycline and polymyxin B
oxytoca
    Klebsiella o.
oyster shuckers' keratitis
OZ
    optical zone

p
optic papilla
pupil
   p value

p-
4p- syndrome
9p- syndrome
P55 Pachymetric Analyzer
Pachette
   DGH-500 P.
PachKnife
   Corneo-Gage P.
pachometer
   Alcon ultrasound p.
   corneal p.
   Humphrey ultrasonic p.
   ophthalsonic p.
   Packo pars plana cannula p.
   Sonogage ultrasound p.
   ultrasound p.
Pach-Pen
   P.-P. XL pachymeter
   P.-P. XL tonometer
pachyblepharon
pachyblepharosis
pachymeter
   Advent p.
   Compuscan-P p.
   corneal p.
   optical p.
   Pach-Pen XL p.
   Ultrasonic p.
   Villasensor ultrasonic p.
pachymetry
   cornea p.
   ultrasonic p.
Pack
   Barrier Phaco Extracapsular P.
Packer
   P. tunnel silicone sponge
   P. Wick extrusion handpiece
Packo
   P. pars plana cannula
   P. pars plana cannula
      pachometer
pad
   eye p.
   fat p.
   felt p.
   orbital fat p.

Pro-Ophtha eye p.
spectacle frame p.
Telfa p.
paddle
   Rosen nucleus p.
   p. temple
paddy keratitis
Paecilomyces lilacinus
Page medium
Pagenstecher operation
pagetoid melanoma
pain
   atypical facial p.
   boring p.
   facial p.
   jaw muscle p.
   lancing p.
   p. reaction
   trigeminal p.
painful ophthalmoplegia
Pak
   Akorn Intraoperative P.
   Hedges Corneal Wetting P.
palatine bone
palatini
   processus orbitalis ossis p.
palatinum
   os p.
palatoethmoidalis
   sutura p.
palatomaxillaris
   sutura p.
palatomaxillary suture
pale optic disk
palinopsia
palisades of Vogt
palisading orbital granuloma
palladium
   p. 103 ophthalmic plaque
      brachytherapy
   p. 103 ophthalmic plaque
      radiotherapy
pallidotomy
pallidus
   globus p. (GP)
Pallin lens spatula
Pallister-Hall syndrome
pallor
   discussion p.
   disk p.

P

pallor *(continued)*
  p. of disk
  horizontal band p.
  p. of optic disk
  optic disk p.
  sector p.
  temporal artery p.
  temporal optic disk p.
palpebra, pl. **palpebrae**
  inferior tarsus p.
  margo p.
  paraphimosis palpebrae
  palpebrae superioris muscle
  superior tarsus p.
  tertius p.
  tunica conjunctiva p.
palpebral
  p. adipose bag
  p. aperture
  p. cartilage
  p. commissure
  p. conjunctiva
  p. fascia
  p. fissure
  p. fissure widening
  p. fold
  p. furrow
  p. gland
  p. ligament
  p. lobe
  p. oculogyric reflex
  p. opening
  p. raphe
  p. slant
  p. vein
palpebrale
  coloboma p.
  sebum p.
palpebrales
  venae p.
palpebralis
  epicanthus p.
palpebrarum
  dermatolysis p.
  facies anterior p.
  facies posterior p.
  pediculosis p.
  phthiriasis p.
  raphe p.
  rima p.
  tendo p.
  xanthoma p.
palpebrate

palpebration
palpebritis
palpebromandibular reflex
palpebronasal fold
palpebronasalis
  plica p.
palsy, pl. **palsies**
  abducens nerve p.
  accommodative p.
  Bell p.
  brachial plexus p.
  cerebral p.
  complete p.
  congenital abducens nerve p.
  congenital oculomotor nerve p.
  conjugate gaze p.
  cranial nerve p.
  double elevator p.
  elevator p.
  external p.
  facial nerve p.
  Féréol-Graux p.
  fourth nerve p.
  gaze p.
  idiopathic facial p.
  inhibitional p.
  internal p.
  ischemic oculomotor p.
  lateral rectus p.
  medial rectus p.
  multiple ocular motor palsies
  p. of muscle
  p. of muscle
  nerve p.
  nuclear p.
  nuclear-fascicular trochlear
   nerve p.
  oblique p.
  ocular muscle p.
  oculomotor cranial nerve p.
  orbital p.
  progressive supranuclear p.
  pseudoabducens p.
  pseudobulbar p.
  saccade p.
  sector p.
  seventh nerve p.
  sixth cranial nerve p.
  stem p.
  subarachnoid oculomotor
   nerve p.
  superior division p.
  superior oblique p.

supranuclear ocular p.
third nerve p.
trochlear nerve p.
twelfth nerve p.
PAM
potential acuity meter
PAM procedure
pamoate
hydroxyzine p.
PAN
periarteritis nodosa
Panamax
Panas operation
panchamber UV lens
Pancoast
P. superior sulcus syndrome
P. tumor
pancreatic
p. diabetes
p. disease
pancuronium bromide
pancytokeratin antibody
PANDO
primary acquired nasolacrimal duct
obstruction
panel
Farnsworth D-15 p.
panencephalitis
subacute sclerosing p.
panfundoscope
Rodenstock p.
panfundus
Panmycin
panni (*pl. of* pannus)
Pannu
P. intraocular lens
P. type II lens
Pannu-Kratz-Barraquer speculum
pannus, pl. **panni**
allergic p.
p. carnosus
corneal p.
p. crassus
degenerative p.
p. degenerativus
p. eczematosus
eczematous p.

fibrovascular p.
glaucomatous p.
phlyctenular p.
p. siccus
p. tenuis
p. trachomatosus
trachomatous p.
panophthalmia
panophthalmitis
clostridial p.
Panoptic bifocal
panoramic loupe
PanoView Optics lens
panphotocoagulation
panretinal
p. ablation
p. argon laser photocoagulation
p. membrane
p. photocoagulation (PRP)
pansinusitis
panstromal
pantachromatic
pantankyloblepharon
pantoscope
Keeler p.
pantoscopic
p. angle
p. angling
p. effect
p. spectacles
p. tilt
Panum fusion area
panuveitis
granulomatous p.
herpes p.
PAOG
primary open-angle glaucoma
papaverine hydrochloride
paper
Schirmer filter p.
papilla, pl. **papillae**
p. of Bergmeister
Bergmeister p.
cobblestone p.
conjunctival p.
drusen of optic p.
giant p.

NOTES

P

papilla *(continued)*
    lacrimal p.
    limbal papillae
    optic p. (p)
    splitting of lacrimal p.
papillary
    p. area
    p. conjunctival hypertrophy
    p. conjunctivitis
    p. ruff
    p. stasis
papilledema
    asymmetric p.
    chronic p.
    unilateral p.
papilliform tumor
papillitis
    ischemic p.
    necrotizing p.
papilloma
    caruncular p.
    conjunctival p.
    eyelid p.
    intralacrimal p.
    mulberry-type p.
    pedunculated p.
    sessile p.
papillomacular
    p. nerve fiber bundle
papillomatosis
papillopathy
    diabetic p.
    ischemic p.
papillophlebitis
papilloretinitis
papillovitreal
papulosa
    iritis p.
papyracea
    lamina p.
PAR
    posterior apical radius
    PAR CTS corneal topography
      system
parablepsia
parabulbar anesthesia
paracentesis
    anterior chamber p.
    aqueous p.
paracentral
    p. cell
    p. defect
    p. nerve fiber bundle

    p. ring scotoma
    p. visual field
paracentric
paracetamol
parachroma
parachromatism
parachromatopsia
Paradigm ocular blood flow
    analyzer
paradoxic
    p. gustolacrimal reflex
    p. levator excitation
    p. levator inhibition
paradoxical
    p. darkness reaction
    p. diplopia
    p. movement of eyelids
    p. pupil
    p. pupillary phenomenon
    p. pupillary reflex
paraequilibrium
paraflocculus
    p. syndrome
parafovea
parafoveal
    p. capillary net
    p. cystic space
    p. fluorescein
    p. halo
    p. macula
    p. microvascular leakage
parafoveolar
paraganglioma
Paragraphs
    Gray Standardized Oral
      Reading P.
parainfectious
    p. optic neuritis
    p. optic neuropathy
parallactic
parallax
    binocular p.
    crossed p.
    direct p.
    heteronymous p.
    homonymous p.
    motion p.
    stereoscopic p.
    p. test
    vertical p.
parallel
    p. interface
    p. ray

parallelism of gaze
parallel-plate flow chamber
paralysis, pl. **paralyses**
    abducens facial p.
    abducens nerve p.
    p. of accommodation
    amaurotic pupillary p.
    bulbar p.
    congenital abducens facial p.
    congenital abduction p.
    congenital bulbar p.
    congenital oculofacial p.
    conjugate p.
    convergence p.
    divergence p.
    facial p.
    familial periodic p.
    p. of gaze
    hyperkalemic periodic p.
    hypokalemic periodic p.
    internuclear p.
    Klumpke p.
    Landry ascending p.
    normokalemic periodic p.
    nuclear horizontal gaze p.
    ocular muscle p.
    oculofacial p.
    periodic p.
    psychogenic p.
    pupillary p.
    sectoral iris p.
    Todd p.
    vagus nerve p.
    Weber p.
paralytic
    p. ectropion
    p. heterotropia
    p. miosis
    p. mydriasis
    p. pontine exotropia
    p. strabismus
paralyticum
    ectropion p.
paramacular
parameter
    stereometric p.
paramethasone acetate

paramyotonia congenita
paranasal
    p. sinus
    p. sinusitis
paraneoplastic
    p. cerebellar degeneration
    p. opsoclonus
    p. optic neuritis
    p. retinopathy
    p. syndrome
Paraperm O2 contact lens
paraphimosis
    p. palpebrae
parapsilosis
    Candida p.
parasellar
    p. lesion
    p. syndrome
parasitic
    p. blepharitis
    p. uveitis
parasitica
    blepharitis p.
parastriate area
parasympathetic
    p. fiber
    p. nerve system
    p. outflow
    p. pathway
parasympatholytic drug
parasympathomimetic drug
parathyroid
    p. adenoma
    p. disorder
paratrachoma
paraxial
    p. lighting
    p. mesoderm
    p. ray
    p. ray of light
PAR-C-Scan videokeratoscope
Paredrine
Parel-Crock vitreous cutter
Paremyd
    P. Ophthalmic
parenchymatosus
    xerosis p.

NOTES

P

parenchymatous
   p. corneal dystrophy
   p. keratitis
paresis
   accommodation p.
   complete but pupil-sparing
      oculomotor nerve p.
   cyclic oculomotor p.
   incomplete pupil-sparing
      oculomotor nerve p.
   nonorganic p.
   oculosympathetic p.
   vertical gaze p.
paretic nystagmus
parfocal
paries
   p. interior orbitae
   p. lateralis orbitae
   p. medialis orbitae
   p. superior orbitae
parietal
   p. eye
   p. lobe
   p. lobe bilateral cerebral
      hemisphere lesion
   p. lobe field defect
   p. lobe unilateral cerebral
      hemisphere lesion
parieto-occipital artery
parieto-occipitalis
   arcus p.-o.
parieto-occipital-temporal junction
Parinaud
   P. oculoglandular conjunctivitis
   P. oculoglandular syndrome
   P. ophthalmoplegia
Parinaud-plus syndrome
PARK
   photoastigmatic refractive
      keratectomy
Park
   P. speculum
   P. three-step test
Parker discission knife
Parker-Heath
   P.-H. anterior chamber syringe
   P.-H. cautery
   P.-H. electrocautery
   P.-H. piggyback probe
Park-Guyton-Callahan speculum
Park-Guyton-Maumenee speculum
Park-Guyton speculum
Park-Maumenee speculum

Parks-Bielschowsky three-step head-
   tilt test
p arm
paromomycin
parophthalmia
parophthalmoncus
paropsia, paropsis
Parrot sign
Parry disease
pars
   p. caeca oculi
   p. caeca retinae
   p. ciliaris retinae
   p. corneoscleralis
   p. iridica retinae
   p. lacrimalis musculi
      orbicularis oculi
   p. marginalis musculi
      orbicularis oris
   p. nervosa retinae
   p. optica hypothalami
   p. optica retinae
   p. orbitalis glandulae lacrimalis
   p. orbitalis gyri frontalis
      inferioris
   p. orbitalis musculi orbicularis
      oculi
   p. orbitalis ossis frontalis
   p. palpebralis glandulae
      lacrimalis
   p. palpebralis musculi
      orbicularis oculi
   p. pigmentosa retinae
   p. plana
   p. plana approach
   p. plana Baerveldt tube
      insertion with vitrectomy
   p. plana corporis ciliaris
   p. plana operation
   p. plana vitrectomy (PPV)
   p. planitis
   p. plicata
   p. plicata corporis ciliaris
   p. scleralis
   p. uvealis
partial
   p. albinism
   p. cataract
   p. conjunctival flap (PCF)
   p. keratoplasty
   p. ophthalmoplegia
   p. response

p. sclerectasia
p. throw surgeon's knot
partialis
   ophthalmoplegia p.
partially sighted
partial-thickness
   p.-t. corneal laceration
   p.-t. trephination
particulate
   p. matter
   p. retinopathy
parvocellular
   p. cell
   p. pathway
PAS
   peripheral anterior synechia
Pascheff conjunctivitis
passant
   boutons en p.
Passarelli one-pass capsulorrhexis
   forceps
passivated polymethyl methacrylate
passive
   p. duction
   p. forced duction test
   p. illusion
Passport disposable injection system
past ocular history (POH)
past-pointing
PAT
   prism adaptation test
Patanol
patch
   binocular eye p.
   Bitot p.
   Cogan p.
   cotton-wool p.
   Donaldson eye p.
   p. eye
   glue p.
   p. graft
   Histoacryl glue p.
   Hutchinson p.
   monocular p.
   oval eye p.
   salmon p.
   Snugfit eye p.

venous sheath p.
wicking glue p.
patching
   pressure p.
patchy
   p. anterior stromal infiltrate
   p. atrophy
   p. window defect
patency
   tear duct p.
patent iridectomy
PathFinder Corneal Analysis
   software
pathognomonic radial keratoneuritis
pathologic
   p. cupping
   p. myopia
pathology
   ocular p.
   orbital p.
pathometer attachment
pathway
   afferent visual p.
   anterior visual p.
   cAMP final common p.
   canalicular p.
   infranuclear p.
   magnocellular visual p.
   oculosympathetic p.
   parasympathetic p.
   parvocellular p.
   pregeniculate visual p.
   retinogeniculate p.
   retrochiasmal p.
   sensory visual p.
   supranuclear p.
   sympathetic p.
   visual p.
patient
   straight-eyed p.
Paton
   P. anterior chamber lens
    implant forceps
   P. capsule forceps
   P. corneal knife
   P. corneal transplant forceps
   P. corneal trephine

NOTES

P

Paton *(continued)*
P. double spatula
P. eye shield
P. line
P. needle holder
P. single spatula
P. single speculum
P. suturing forceps
P. transplant spatula
P. transplant speculum
P. tying/stitch removal forceps
pattern
A p.
abnormal staining p.
Antoni p.
p. arborization
arborization p.
arteriovenous p.
AV p.
blur p.
classic flower petal p.
comedo p.
contiguous p.
p. cut corneal graft operation
p. discrimination perimetry
p. dystrophy
p. dystrophy of pigment
epithelium of Byers and
Marmor
p. electroretinogram
flower petal p.
Harrington-Flocks multiple p.
map p.
morpheaform p.
Morse code p.
mosaic p.
petaloid p.
racquet-like p.
p. recognition
scatter p.
semi-circinate p.
shagreen p.
staining p.
stippled p.
umbrella-like p.
V p.
p. visual-evoked response
(PVER)
vortex p.
Zellballen p.
pattern-cut corneal graft
pattern-evoked electroretinogram
(PERG)

Paufique
P. graft knife
P. keratoplasty
P. keratoplasty knife
P. operation
P. suturing forceps
P. synechiotomy
P. trephine
Paul lacrimal sac retractor
Pautler infusion cannula
paving-stone degeneration
Pavlo-Colibri corneal forceps
Payne retractor
PBII blue loop lens
PBK
pseudophakic bullous keratopathy
PBRVO
peripheral branch retinal vein
occlusion
PBZ
PBZ-SR
PC
posterior chamber
PC EDO ophthalmic office
laser
P&C
prism and cover test
P-cell
PCF
partial conjunctival flap
PCIOL
posterior chamber intraocular lens
PCL
posterior collagenous layer
PCLI
posterior chamber lens implant
PCNSL
primary central nervous system
lymphoma
PCO
posterior capsule opacification
PD
pupillary distance
PDR
proliferative diabetic retinopathy
PDS
pigment dispersion syndrome
PE
pigment epithelium
PE-400 ERG/VEP system
Peacekeeper cannula
peaking
temporal p.

peak latencies of pattern electroretinogram
peanut implant
pear cataract
Pearce
  P. coaxial irrigating/aspirating cannula
  P. nucleus hydrodissector
  P. posterior chamber intraocular lens
  P. trabeculectomy
Pearce-Knolle irrigating lens loop
pearl
  p. cyst
  p. diver's keratopathy
  Elschnig p.
  iris p.
  p. white mounds
pear-shaped pupil
Pease-Allen Color test
peau de chagrin
pectinate
  p. ligament
  p. ligament of iris
  p. villi
pectineal ligament
Peczon
  P. I/A cannula
  P. I/A unit
  P. I/A vectis
PED
  pigment epithelial detachment
pedal
  Vit Commander foot p.
pediatric
  p. Karickhoff laser lens
  p. lid speculum
  p. myasthenia
  p. ocular sarcoidosis
  p. three-mirror laser lens
  p. vitrectomy lens set
pedicle
  p. cone
  p. flap
  tarsoconjunctival p.
pediculated flap
pediculosis palpebrarum

pediculous blepharitis
pedigree
  p. analysis
  p. chart
peduncular hallucination
pedunculated papilloma
peek sign
peeler-cutter
  membrane p.-c.
peeling
  membrane p.
pefloxacin
PEHO
  progressive encephalopathy with edema, hypsarrhythmia and optic atrophy
  PEHO syndrome
PEK
  punctate epithelial keratopathy
Pel crisis
pellet extrusion
Pelli-Robson
  P.-R. contrast sensitivity chart
  P.-R. letter chart
pellucid
  corneal p.
  p. marginal corneal degeneration
  p. marginal retinal degeneration
pellucidum
  septum cavum p.
pemphigoid
  benign mucosal p.
  Brunsting-Perry cicatricial p.
  bullous p.
  Cibis p.
  cicatricial p.
  mucosal p.
  ocular cicatricial p. (OCP)
pemphigus
  ocular p.
pen
  gentian violet marking p.
  marking p.
  Rhein reusable cautery p.
  skin marking p.
  surgical marking p.

NOTES

P

Penbriten
pencil
astigmatism of oblique p.'s
cataract p.
p. cautery
20-gauge straight bipolar p.
glaucoma p.
retinal detachment p.
vitreous p.
Wallach cryosurgical p.
pendular-jerk waveform
pendular nystagmus
penetrant gene
penetrating
p. corneal graft
p. corneal transplant
p. full-thickness corneal graft
p. injury
p. keratoplasty (PK, PKP)
p. keratoplasty astigmatism
p. keratoplasty button
p. keratoplasty and glaucoma
(PKPG)
penicillin
acid-resistant p.
synthetic p.
penicillinase
peninsula pupil
penlight
Heine p.
LICO disposable p.
Welch-Allyn halogen p.
Penn-Anderson scleral fixation
forceps
Penrose drain
pentachromic
pentafilcon A
pentagonal block excision
pentamidine isethionate
Penthrane
pentigetide
pentobarbital sodium
Pentolair
pentolinium
Pentothal
pentoxifylline
Pentyde
penumbra
PEO
progressive external
ophthalmoplegia
pepper-and-salt fundus

Pepper Visual Skills for Reading
Test
Peptococcus
Peptostreptococcus
Percepta progressive lens
perceptible acuity
perception
binocular depth p.
color p.
contrast threshold for
motion p. (CTMP)
depth p.
p. dissociation
dissociation of visual p.
facial p.
form p.
light p. (LP)
limbus of p.
monocular depth p.
no light p. (NLP)
shape p.
simultaneous foveal p. (SFP)
simultaneous macular p. (SMP)
visual p.
perennial rhinoconjunctivitis
perfilcon A
perfluorane
perfluorocarbon
p. gas
liquid p.
perfluorodecalin
Perfluoron
perfluoropropane gas (C3F8)
perforans
scleromalacia p.
perforating keratoplasty
perforation
corneal p.
globe p.
perfringens
Clostridium p.
perfusion
capillary p.
juxtapapillary p.
luxury p.
PERG
pattern-evoked electroretinogram
Periactin
periaqueductal
p. gray matter
p. syndrome

periarteritis
    p. nodosa (PAN, PN)
    regional p.
peribulbar
    p. injection
    p. needle
pericanalicular connective tissue
pericentral
    p. rod-cone dystrophy
    p. scotoma
perichiasmal
perichoroidal, perichorioidal
    p. space
perichoroideale
    spatium p.
periconchitis
pericorneal plexus
peridectomy
perifascicular myofiber necrosis
perifoveal arteriole
perifoveolar
perikeratic
perilenticular
perilimbal
    p. stroma
    p. suction
    p. suction cup
    p. ulceration
    p. vitiligo
perilimbic circulation
perimacular vasculature
perimeter
    Allergan Humphrey p.
    arc p.
    arc and bowl p.
    automated hemisphere p.
    Brombach p.
    Canon p.
    Cilco p.
    CooperVision imaging p.
    p. corneal reflex test
    Digilab p.
    Ferree-Rand p.
    Goldmann p.
    Goldmann manual projection p.
    Henson CFS 2000 p.
    Humphrey p.

    Interzeag bowl p.
    kinetic p.
    Marco p.
    Medmont M600 p.
    Octopus 201 p.
    Octopus 101 bowl p.
    Ophthimus High-Pass
      Resolution p.
    Ophthimus ring p.
    Peritest p.
    projection p.
    p. projection
    Schweigger hand p.
    static p.
    Topcon p.
    Tübinger p.
perimetric
perimetry
    achromatic automated p. (AAP)
    Aimark p.
    arc p.
    automated static threshold p.
    binocular p.
    chromatic p.
    color p.
    computed p.
    flicker p.
    frequency doubling p.
    Goldmann kinetic p.
    hemisphere projection p.
    high-pass resolution p.
    kinetic p.
    manual kinetic p.
    mesopic p.
    motion automated p.
    motion and displacement p.
    objective p.
    Octopus automated p.
    pattern discrimination p.
    profile p.
    quantitative p.
    quantitative threshold p.
    resolution acuity p.
    ring p.
    Scanning Laser
      Ophthalmoscope p.
    scotopic p.

NOTES

P

perimetry *(continued)*
  short wavelength automated p. (SWAP)
  static p.
  suprathreshold static p.
  tangent p.
  temporal modulation p.
  Tübinger p.
perineural cell
perineuritis
  optic p.
  syphilitic optic p.
perinuclear
  p. cataract
periocular
  p. depigmentation
  p. drug sensitivity
  p. injection
periodic
  p. alternating gaze deviation
  p. alternating nystagmus
  p. alternating windmill nystagmus
  p. esotropia
  p. exotropia
  p. ophthalmia
  p. paralysis
  p. strabismus
periophthalmia
periophthalmic
periophthalmitis
perioptic
  p. cerebrospinal fluid
  p. hygroma
  p. neuritis
  p. sheath meningioma
  p. subarachnoid space
perioptometry
periorbit
periorbita
periorbital
  p. cellulitis
  p. edema
  p. fat atrophy
  p. hemangioma
  p. leukoderma
  p. membrane
  p. volume augmentation
periorbitis
periosteum
  orbital p.
periostitis
  orbital p.

peripapillary
  p. central serous choroidopathy
  p. choroid
  p. choroidal arterial system
  p. choroidal atrophy
  p. coloboma
  p. nerve fiber layer
  p. retinal height
  p. retinal nerve
  p. retinal nerve fiber
  p. scar
  p. sclerosis
  p. scotoma
  p. staphyloma
  p. subretinal neovascularization
periphacitis
periphakitis
peripheral
  p. anterior synechia (PAS)
  p. branch retinal vein occlusion (PBRVO)
  p. cataract
  p. chorioretinal atrophic spot
  p. chorioretinal atrophy
  p. corneal opacity
  p. corneal ulcer
  p. curve on contact lens
  p. cystoid degeneration
  p. detection test
  p. endotheliitis
  p. fusion
  p. glare
  p. glioma
  p. granuloma
  p. intraretinal hemorrhage
  p. iridectomy (PI)
  p. iridectomy operation
  p. iris roll
  p. light scatter
  p. multifocal chorioretinitis (PMC)
  p. necrotizing retinitis
  p. neuropathy
  p. oculomotor nerve
  p. posterior curve (PPC)
  p. proliferation
  p. ray of light
  p. retina
  p. retinal ablation
  p. retinal operculum
  p. retinal vascular sheathing
  p. ring infiltrate
  p. rod function

p. scotoma
p. tapetochoroidal degeneration
p. ulcerative keratitis (PUK)
p. uveitis
p. vestibular nystagmus
p. vision
p. visual field
p. vitreoretinal traction
peripherin/RDS gene
periphery
nasal p.
posterior pole and p. (PP&P)
periphlebitis
p. retinae
retinal p.
periphoria
periretinal edema
periscleral space
periscleritis
perisclerotic
periscopic
p. concave lens
p. convex lens
p. meniscus
p. spectacles
peristaltic pump
peristriate visual cortex
peritarsal network
peritectomy
Peritest perimeter
peritomize
peritomy
perivascular
p. neutrophil infiltration
p. sheathing
p. stromal cell
perivasculitis
retinal p.
periventricular lesion
PERK
prospective evaluation of radial
keratotomy
Perkins
P. applanation tonometer
P. brailler

PERLA
pupils equal, reactive to light and
accommodation
Perlia nucleus
Permaflex lens
Permalens lens
permeability
oxygen p.
permeable
rigid gas-p.
pernicious
p. anemia
p. myopia
Per-Protocol-Observed Cases
Perritt double-fixation forceps
PERRLA
pupils equal, round, reactive to light
and accommodation
perseveration
visual p.
persistent
p. anterior hyperplastic primary
vitreous
p. epithelial defect
p. hyperplasia of primary
vitreous (PHPV)
p. hyperplastic primary vitreous
p. postdrainage hypotony
(PPH)
p. posterior hyperplastic
primary vitreous
p. primary hyperplastic vitreous
p. pupillary membrane remnant
Personnel
Joint Review Committee for
Ophthalmic Medical P.
(JRCOMP)
Perspex
P. CQ
P. CQ-Shearing-Simcoe-Sinskey
lens
P. CQ UV PMMA
P. frame
P. rod
pertussis
Bordetella p.

NOTES

P

perverted
 p. nystagmus
 p. ocular movement
P-ES
 Isopto P-ES
petaloid pattern
Peters
 P. anomaly
 P. operation
Petit canal
Petriellidum boydii
petrificans
 conjunctivitis p.
 keratitis p.
petrosal nerve
petrous
 p. apex
 p. bone
 p. ridge
Petrus single-mirror laser lens
Petzetakis-Takos syndrome
Petzval surface
PEXG
 pseudoexfoliative glaucoma
Peyman
 P. full-thickness eye-wall
 resection
 P. iridocyclochoroidectomy
 P. vitrectomy unit
 P. vitrector
 P. vitreophage unit
 P. wide-field lens
Peyman-Green
 P.-G. vitrectomy lens
 P.-G. vitreous forceps
Peyman-Tennant-Green lens
PF
 Acular P.
Pfeiffer-Komberg method
P.F. Lee pediatric goniolens
PGC
 pontine gaze center
PGTP
 primary glaucoma triple procedure
PH
 pinhole
phacitis
Phaco
 P. Cavitron irrigating/aspirating
 unit
 P. Emulsifier Cavitron unit
Phaco-4 diamond step knife

phacoallergica
 endophthalmitis p.
phacoanaphylactic
 p. endophthalmitis
 p. uveitis
phacoanaphylactica
 endophthalmitis p.
phacoanaphylaxis
phacoantigenic
 p. endophthalmitis
phacoaspiration
phacoblade
 Myocure p.
phacocele
phaco-chop
 p.-c. technique
phacocyst
phacocystectomy
phacocystitis
phacodonesis
phacoemulsification,
 phakoemulsification
 Alcon p.
 p. cautery
 endocapsular p.
 p. handpiece
 high-vacuum p.
 small-incision p.
phacoemulsifier
phacoemulsify
phacoerysis
phacoexcavation
phacoexcavator
PhacoFlex
 P. II SI30NB intraocular lens
 SingleStitch P.
phacofracture
phacofragmatome
phacofragmentation
phacogenetica
 endophthalmitis p.
phacogenic, phakogenic
 p. glaucoma
 p. uveitis
phacoglaucoma
phacogoniosynechialysis
phacohymenitis
phacoid
phacoiditis
phacoidoscope
Phacojack Phaco System
phacolysin

phacolysis
  calcific p.
phacolytic, phakolytic
  p. glaucoma
  p. uveitis
phacoma
phacomalacia
phacomatosis
phacometachoresis
phacometer
phacomorphic, phakomorphic
  p. glaucoma
phacopalingenesis
phacoplanesis
phacosclerosis
phacoscope
phacoscopy
phacoscotasmus
phaco sleeve
phacotoxic uveitis
phagocytosed cellular debris
Phakan
phakia
phakic
  p. cystoid macular edema
  p. eye
  p. glaucoma
  P. 6 lens
  p. pupillary block
phakitis
phakodonesis
phakoemulsification (*var. of*
  phacoemulsification)
phakofragmatome
  Girard p.
phakogenic (*var. of* phacogenic)
phakolytic (*var. of* phacolytic)
phakoma
phakomatous
  p. choristoma
  p. choristoma tumor
phakomorphic (*var. of*
  phacomorphic)
phalangosis
phantom vision
Pharmacia
  P. corneal trephine

P. Intermedics
P. intraocular lens
P. Visco J-loop lens
pharmacological
  p. blockade
  p. dilation
pharmacologic manipulation
phase difference haloscope
PHEMA
  P. core-and-skirt
  keratoprosthesis
  P. KPro implantation
phemfilcon A
phenacaine
  p. hydrochloride
phenacetin
Phenazine
phenazopyridine
phenbenicillin
phencyclidine hydrochloride
Phendry Oral
phenelzine sulfate
Phenergan
phengophobia
phenindamine
pheniramine maleate and
  naphazoline HCl
phenmetrazine hydrochloride
phenobarbital sodium
phenolphthalein
phenomenon, pl. phenomena
  Alder-Reilly p.
  aqueous-influx p.
  Ascher aqueous-influx p.
  Ascher glass-rod p.
  Aubert p.
  autokinetic visible light p.
  Bell p.
  Bezold-Brücke p.
  Bielschowsky p.
  blood-influx p.
  blue-field entoptic p.
  break p.
  breakup p.
  Brücke-Bartley p.
  click p.
  crowding p.

NOTES

P

phenomenon *(continued)*
doll's head p.
entoptic p.
escape p.
extinction p.
flicker p.
Galassi pupillary p.
glass-rod negative p.
glass-rod positive p.
Gunn jaw-winking p.
halo p.
hemifield slide p.
Hertwig-Magendie p.
interface phenomena
jack-in-the-box p.
jaw-winking p.
Le Grand-Geblewics p.
Marcus Gunn jaw-winking p.
misdirection p.
Mitzuo p.
Mizuo-Nakamura p.
negative visual p.
orbicularis p.
paradoxical pupillary p.
phi p.
Piltz-Westphal p.
positive visual p.
pseudo-Graefe p.
Pulfrich stereo p.
Purkinje p.
Riddoch p.
Schlieren p.
setting-sun p.
shot-silk p.
Tournay p.
Tulio p.
Tyndall p.
Uhthoff p.
Westphal p.
Westphal-Piltz p.
Phenoptic
phenothiazine keratopathy
phenoxybenzamine hydrochloride
phenylephrine
sulfacetamide p. h.
phenylephrine hydrochloride
phenylmercuric
p. acetate
p. nitrate
phenylpropanolamine hydrochloride
Phialophora

Philadelphia
Wills Eye Hospital/Children's
Hospital of P. (WEH/CHOP)
Phillips fixation forceps
phi phenomenon
phlebitis
retinal p.
phlebophthalmotomy
phlebosclerosis
phlegmatous conjunctivitis
phlegmonous
p. dacryocystis
p. dacryocystitis
phlorhizin diabetes
phlyctenar
phlyctenular
p. conjunctivitis
p. keratitis
p. keratoconjunctivitis
p. ophthalmia
p. pannus
phlyctenule
corneal p.
phlyctenulosis
allergic p.
conjunctival p.
corneal p.
tuberculous p.
PHM
posterior hyaloid membrane
PHNI
pinhole no improvement
phocomelia
Roberts-SC p.
phonometer
Tektronix digital p.
phoria
basal p.
decompensated p.
far p.
lateral p.
monofixational p.
nearpoint p.
vertical p.
phoriascope
phorometer
phorometry
phoro-optometer
phoroptor
p. retractor
Ultramatic Rx Master p.
p. vision tester
phoroscope

phorotone
phosphate
    Aralen P.
    Decadron P.
    dexamethasone sodium p.
    p. diabetes
    disodium hydrogen p.
    ganciclovir cyclic p.
    Hexadrol P.
    Hydrocortone P.
    naphazoline and antazoline p.
    potassium p.
    prednisolone sodium p.
    sodium p.
phosphate-buffered saline
phosphene
    accommodation p.
Phospholine
    Echothiophate P.
    P. Iodide
    P. Iodide Ophthalmic
photalgia
photerythrous
photesthesia
photic
    p. maculopathy
    p. retinal toxicity
photo
    fundus p. (FP)
photoablation
    excimer laser transepithelial p.
    transepithelial p.
photoablative
    p. laser goniotomy (PLG)
photoastigmatic refractive
  keratectomy (PARK)
photobrown lenses
photoceptor
photochemical
    p. process
    p. visual pigment
photochemistry
photochromic
    p. lens
    p. spectacles
photocoagulation
    argon laser p.

    focal laser p.
    grid laser p. (GLP)
    indirect ophthalmoscopic
      laser p.
    krypton p.
    laser panretinal p.
    macular p.
    panretinal p. (PRP)
    panretinal argon laser p.
    retinal laser p.
    retinal scatter p.
    scatter p.
    transscleral retinal p.
    xenon arc p.
photocoagulator
    Clinitex p.
    Coherent p.
    Ialo p.
    IOLAB I&A p.
    IOLAB irrigating/aspirating p.
    laser p.
    Mira p.
    Novus Omni 2000 p.
    OcuLight GL/GLx green
      laser p.
    OcuLight GLx green laser p.
    Olivella-Garrigosa p.
    Ultima p.
    Ultima 2000 p.
    VIRIDIS p.
    VIRIDIS-LITE p.
    xenon arc p.
    Zeiss p.
photocoreoplasty
photodisrupting laser
photodynamic therapy
photodynia
photodysphoria
photoelasticity
photoelectric oculography
photofrin
photogene
photogrammeter
    Raster p.
photograph
    fundus p.

NOTES

P

387

photograph *(continued)*
red free p.
stereoscopic fundus p.
photography
central endothelial p.
cross-polarization p.
fluorescence retinal p.
nonmydriatic retinal p.
Scheimpflug p.
photogray lens
photokeratitis
photo-kerato attachment
photokeratoscope
Allergan Humphrey p.
Allergan Medical Optics p.
computerized p.
CooperVision refractive
surgery p.
Corneascope nine-ring p.
Tomey TMS-1 p.
photokeratoscopy
digital subtraction p.
photolysis
Dodick p.
photometer
Bunsen grease spot p.
flame p.
flicker p.
Förster p.
Kowa laser flare p.
Kowa laser flare-cell p.
photometry
laser flare p.
laser flare-cell p.
photomydriasis
Clinitex p.
photopapillometry
photophobia
photophobic
photophthalmia
photopia
photopic
p. adaptation
p. eye
p. illumination
p. vision
photopigment
cone p.
PhotoPoint
P. laser
P. laser therapy
P. treatment

photopsia
transient p.
photopsin
photopsy
photoptarmosis
photoptometer
Förster p.
photoptometry
photoreception
photoreceptive
photoreceptor
p. cell
p. dysfunction
p. preservation
photoreceptor-bipolar synapse
photorefraction
eccentric p.
photorefractive
p. astigmatic keratectomy
p. keratectomy
p. keratoplasty (PRK)
p. surgery
photoretinitis
photoretinopathy
photoscopy
photosensitive lens
photosensitization
photosensor oculography
photostress
macular p.
p. recovery time (PRT)
p. test
photosun lens
phototherapeutic keratectomy (PTK)
phototherapy
Phototome System 2700
phototonus
phototoxic
p. lesion
p. maculopathy
phototoxicity
phototransduction cascade
photovaporation laser
photovaporization
photovaporizing laser
PHPV
persistent hyperplasia of primary
vitreous
phthalocyanide
phthiriasis palpebrarum
phthiriatica
blepharitis p.
phthisical eye

phthisis
    p. bulbi
    p. cornea
    essential p.
    ocular p.
phycomycosis
    cerebral p.
phylloquinone (K)
physical
    p. manipulation
    p. optics
Physick operation
physiologic
    p. anisocoria
    p. astigmatism
    p. blind spot
    p. cup
    p. excavation
    p. myopia
    p. nystagmus
    p. optics
    p. retina
    p. scotoma
physostigmine
    pilocarpine and p.
    p. and pilocarpine
    p. sulfate
PI
    peripheral iridectomy
pial
    p. arterial plexus
    p. sheath
    p. system
pick
    Burch p.
    Desmarres fixation p.
    fiberoptic p.
    fixation p.
    fixation/anchor p.
    light pipe p.
    Michel p.
    Olk vitreoretinal p.
    P. retinitis
    Rice p.
    scleral p.
    P. sign

    Sinskey p.
    P. vision
Pickford-Nicholson analmoscope
pickup
    Shoch foreign body p.
    p. spatula suture
Pico operation
pictograph
picture chart
piebald eyelash
pie-in-the-sky defect
pie-on-the-floor defect
Pierce
    P. coaxial irrigating/aspirating
      cannula
    P. I/A cannula
    P. I/A irrigating vectis
    P. I/A unit
    P. irrigating vectis
Pierre-Marie ataxia
Pierse
    P. corneal Colibri-type forceps
    P. eye speculum
    P. fixation forceps
Pierse-Hoskins forceps
Pierse-type Colibri forceps
piezoelectric transducer technique
piezometer
piggyback
    p. contact lens
    p. implant
    p. probe
pigment
    p. atrophy
    p. cell
    p. change
    clumped retinal p.
    p. clumping
    p. demarcation line
    p. deposition
    p. derangement
    p. dispersion
    p. dispersion syndrome (PDS)
    p. epithelial detachment (PED)
    p. epithelial detachment
      maculopathy
    p. epithelial dystrophy

NOTES

P

pigment *(continued)*
p. epithelial hypertrophy
p. epitheliitis
epitheliitis focal retinal p.
p. epitheliopathy
p. epithelium (PE)
p. floater
gold tattoo p.
p. granule
p. layer
p. layer ectropion
p. mottling
photochemical visual p.
placoid p.
platinum tattoo p.
p. precipitate
p. seam
silver tattoo p.
tattoo p.
trabecular membrane p.
visual p.
white p.
xanthophyll p.
pigmentary
p. deposits on lens
p. dilution
p. dispersion glaucoma
p. dispersion syndrome
p. dropout
p. halo
p. migration
p. perivenous chorioretinal
degeneration
p. rarefaction and clumping
p. retinopathy
pigmentation
clumped p.
congenital optic disk p.
hematogenous p.
Hudson-Stähli line of
corneal p.
orange punctate p.
p. rarefaction
pigmented
p. epithelium of iris
p. keratic precipitate
p. layer of ciliary body
p. layer of eyeball
p. layer of iris
p. layer of retina
p. lesion
p. line of cornea
p. macular pucker

p. paravenous chorioretinal
atrophy
p. paravenous retinochoroidal
atrophy
p. preretinal membrane
p. stroma
p. veil
pigmenti
incontinentia p.
pigmento
retinitis pigmentosa sine p.
RP sine p.
pigmentosa
autosomal dominant retinitis p.
pseudoretinitis p.
retinitis p. (RP)
sector retinitis p.
X-linked retinitis p. (XLRP)
pigmentosum
conjunctivitis xeroderma p.
xeroderma p.
pigmentum nigrum
pigtail
p. fixation
p. probe
Pilagan
P. Ophthalmic
PilaSite
Pillat dystrophy
pillow
Richard p.
Pilo-20
Ocusert P.
Pilo-40
Ocusert P.
Pilocar
P. Ophthalmic
pilocarpine
p. and epinephrine
epinephrine and p.
p. HCl
p. nitrate
physostigmine and p.
p. and physostigmine
p. test
timolol and p.
p. and timolol maleate
Pilocel
pilocyte
pilocytic astrocytoma
Pilofrin
Pilokair
pilomatrixoma tumor

Pilomiotin
Pilopine
    P. gel 4%
    P. HS
    P. HS gel
    P. HS Ophthalmic
Piloptic
    P. Ophthalmic
Pilostat
    P. P.
pilot application
Piltz sign
Piltz-Westphal phenomenon
pimaricin
pimelopterygium
pin
    p. cushion distortion
    Pischel p.
    Walker micro p.
pince-nez
pineal
    p. blastoma
    p. eye
    p. gland
pinealoblastoma
pinealoma
ping-pong gaze
pinguecula, pinguicula
pingueculae
pinhole (PH)
    p. accommodation
    p. disk
    p. and dominance test
    p. goggles
    p. no improvement (PHNI)
    no improvement with p.
    (NIPH)
    p. occluder
    p. pupil
    p. vision
pink
    p. eye
    p. eye conjunctivitis
    p. eye disk
    sharp and p. (S&P)
Pinky ball

pinocytotic vesicle
pinpoint pupil
PION
    posterior ischemic optic neuropathy
pipe light
piperacillin
piperazine
piperocaine hydrochloride
piqûre diabetes
Pischel
    P. electrode
    P. micropins
    P. pin
    P. scleral rule
pisciform cataract
pit
    congenital optic nerve p.
    Gaule p.
    Herbert peripheral p.
    Herbit p.
    iris p.
    lens p.
    optic p.
    optic disk p.
    optic nerve p.
    orbital p.
    temporal p.
pituitarigenic
    p. oculopathy
pituitary
    p. ablation
    p. adenoma
    apoplexy of p.
    p. apoplexy
    p. body
    p. gland
    p. tumor
Pityrosporum
    P. orbiculare
    P. ovale
pivot point
pixel
PK
    penetrating keratoplasty
PKP
    penetrating keratoplasty

NOTES

P

PKPG
  penetrating keratoplasty and
    glaucoma
placebo eye drops
placement
  implant p.
placido
  P. disk
  P. disk image
  p. ring
placido-based axial curvature
  mapping
Placido-disk videokeratoscopy system
Placidyl
placode
  lens p.
  p. lens
placoid
  p. pigment
  p. pigmentation of epithelium
  p. pigment epitheliopathy
pladaroma, pladarosis
Plain
  Isopto P.
plain
  p. catgut suture
  p. collagen suture
  p. gut suture
plaited frill
plana
  cornea p.
  pars p.
  trans pars p.
Planar blade
Planarm Haag Streit attachment
plane
  Broca visual p.
  Daubenton p.
  equivalent refracting p.
  eye/ear p.
  Frankfort horizontal p.
  horizontal p.
  p. of incidence
  lens p.
  Listing p.
  nodal p.
  orbital p.
  p. parallel plate
  principal p.
  p. of regard
  spectacle p.
  unity conjugacy p.'s

  vertical p.
  visual p.
plane-surface refraction
Plange spud
planitis
  cyclitis in pars p.
  pars p.
planned extracapsular cataract
  extraction
Planner
  VISX Refractive P.
plano
  p. lens
  P. T lens
planoconcave lens
planoconvex
  p. nonridge lens
  p.-shaped disk
planum
  p. orbitale
  os p.
  xanthoma p.
plaque
  avascular p.
  cholesterol p.
  demyelinating p.
  endothelial p.
  episcleral eye p.
  eye p.
  eyelid p.
  gold eye p.
  gray p.
  Hollenhorst p.
  hyaline p.
  hyperkeratotic p.
  p. keratopathy
  nonconfluent p.
  preretinal p.
  radioactive eye p.
  p. radiotherapy
  red scaly p.
  scaly p.
  subcapsular p.
  subepithelial p.
Plaquenil
plasma
  p. cell
  p. cell tumor
plasmacytoid infiltrate
Plasmodium
plasmoid
  p. agglutination

p. aqueous
p. aqueous humor
plaster shell
plastic
    p. bifocal
    p. cyclitis
    p. disposable irrigating vectis
    p. eye shield
    p. frame
    p. iritis
    p. lens
    p. prism
    p. repair of eyelid
    p. sphere implant
plate
    American Optical Hardy-Rand-
      Rittler color p.
    base p.
    depth p.
    embryonic p.
    Gelfilm p.
    Hardy-Rand-Ritter
      pseudoisochromatic p.
    Hardy-Rand-Ritter screening p.
    Ishihara pseudoisochromatic p.
    isochromatic p.
    Jaeger lid p.
    lid p.
    Okuma p.
    plane parallel p.
    pseudoisochromatic color p.
    reticular p.
    scar p.
    Silastic p.
    Stahl caliper p.
    Storz lid p.
    tarsal p.
    Teflon p.
    Thayer-Martin p.
plateau
    p. iris
    p. iris configuration
    p. iris syndrome
Plateau-Talbot law
plate-haptic silicone lens
Platform
    Ladarvision P.

Platina
    P. clip
    P. clip lens
    P. intraocular lens implant
platinum
    p. probe spatula
    p. tattoo pigment
platysmal reflex
pleomorphic adenoma
pleoptic exercise
pleoptics
    Bangerter method of p.
    Cüppers method of p.
pleoptophor
plesiopia
plethysmographic goggles
plethysmography
plexiform
    p. external layer
    p. inner layer
    p. internal layer
    p. neurofibroma
    p. neuroma
    p. outer layer
Plexiglas
    P. frame
    P. implant
plexus
    angular aqueous sinus p.
    annular p.
    capillary p.
    ciliary ganglionic p.
    epithelial nerve p.
    Hovius p.
    intraepithelial p.
    intrascleral p.
    ophthalmic p.
    pericorneal p.
    pial arterial p.
    scleral p.
    stroma p.
    subepithelial p.
    sympathetic carotid p.
    vascular p.
Pley extracapsular forceps
PLG
    photoablative laser goniotomy

NOTES

P

Pliagel
plica, gen. and pl. **plicae**
    plicae ciliares
    plicae iridis
    p. lacrimalis
    p. lunata
    p. palpebronasalis
    p. semilunaris
    p. semilunaris conjunctivae
plicata
    pars p.
plication
    retractor p.
Plitz reflex
plombage operation
plug
    Berkeley Bioengineering brass scleral p.
    brass scleral p.
    collagen p.
    Dohlman p.
    EaglePlug tapered-shaft punctum p.
    EagleVision Freeman punctum p.
    epithelial p.
    Freeman punctum p.
    Herrick lacrimal p.
    Micro punctum p.
    punctal p.
    punctum p.
    Super punctum p.
    Tapered-Shaft punctum p.
    TearSaver punctum p.
    Teflon p.
    Umbrella punctum p.
plugging
    follicular p.
plumes
    corneal ablation p.
plus
    Amvisc P.
    cyclophoria p.
    p. cyclophoria
    cyclotropia p.
    p. disease
    Duramist P.
    Econopred P.
    ICaps P.
    Lens P.
    Murine P.
    Refresh P.

    p. spectacle lens
    Tears P.
    Unisol P.
    Wet-N-Soak P.
plus-minus syndrome
PM
    psammomatous meningioma
PMC
    peripheral multifocal chorioretinitis
PMMA
    polymethyl methacrylate
    Blue core PMMA
    Perspex CQ UV PMMA
PN
    periarteritis nodosa
PNET
    primitive neuroectodermal tumor
pneumatic
    p. retinopathy
    p. retinopexy
    p. tonometer
    p. trabeculoplasty
pneumatonograph
    Alcon applanation p.
pneumatonometer
    Micro One p.
    Modular One p.
pneumococcal
    p. bacillus
    p. conjunctivitis
    p. endophthalmitis
    p. ulcer
pneumococcus ulcer
pneumoencephalography
pneumoniae
    Klebsiella p.
    Streptococcus p.
pneumonitis
    interstitial p.
    lymphocytic interstitial p.
pneumotomography
pneumotonometer
pneumotonometry
POAG
    primary open-angle glaucoma
pocket
    corneal p.
    detachment p.
    p. operation
    stromal p.
POH
    past ocular history

POHS
  presumed ocular histoplasmosis
  syndrome
    pseudo POHS
poikiloderma
  p. atrophicans and cataract
  p. congenitale
point
  anterior focal p.
  axial p.
  blur p.
  break p.
  central yellow p.
  congruent p.
  conjugate p.
  convergence p.
  p.'s of convergence
  correspondence p.
  corresponding retinal p.
  diathermy p.
  disparate retinal p.
  p. of dispersion
  p. of divergence
  eye p.
  far p.
  p. of fixation
  fixation p.
  fixed p.
  focal image p.
  identical p.
  image p.
  incident p.
  lacrimal p.
  lustrous central yellow p.
  near visual p. (NVP)
  neutral p.
  nodal p.
  null p.
  optical nodal p.
  pivot p.
  posterior focal p.
  principal p.
  p. of regard
  restoration p.
  retinal p.'s
  secondary focal p.
  p. source

  sphere end p.
  stereo-identical p.
  supraorbital p.
  p. system test type
  virtual p.
  visual p.
  yellow p.
points
Poiseuille law
poisoning degenerative cataract
Polack keratoscope
Poladex
Polaramine
polar cataract
polarimeter
  confocal scanning laser p.
  scanning laser p.
polarimetry
  scanning laser p.
polariscope
polariscopic
polariscopy
polarization
  angle of p.
polarized light
polarizing
  p. lens
  p. ophthalmoscope
Polaroid
  P. filter
  P. vectograph slide
Polaron sputter coater
pole
  anterior p.
  inferior p.
  posterior p.
  superior p.
polioencephalitis
  superior p.
poliosis
polisher
  Buedding squeegee cortex
    extractor and p.
  capsule p.
  Drews capsule p.
  felt disk p.
  Gills-Welsh capsule p.

NOTES

P

polisher *(continued)*
    Holladay posterior capsule p.
    Knolle capsule p.
    Kraff capsule p.
    Kratz p.
    Look capsule p.
    olive tip capsule p.
    Terry silicone capsule p.
polisher/scratcher
    Jensen p./s.
    Kratz p./s.
    Kratz-Jensen p./s.
polishing
    diamond-bur p.
    posterior capsular p.
Polle pod attachment for ophthalmoscope
Pollock
    P. forceps
    P. punch
Polocaine
polus
    p. anterior bulbi oculi
    p. anterior lentis
    p. posterior bulbi oculi
    p. posterior lentis
Polyak operation
polyarteritis nodosa
polycarbonate lens
polychondritis
    atrophic p.
    relapsing p.
polychromatic
    p. light
    p. luster
Polycon
    P. I contact lens
    P. II contact lens
polycoria
    p. spuria
    p. vera
Polycycline
polycythemicus
    fundus p.
Polydek suture
polydystrophy
    pseudo-Hurler p.
polyester suture
polyethylene
    p. glycol
    p. implant
    p. T-tube
    p. tube

polyglactin suture
polyglycolate suture
polyglycolic acid suture
polygonal pigmented cell
polyhedral cells
polyhexamethylene biguanide
Polymacon lens
polymegalism
polymegathism
polymerase chain reaction
polymer ring
polymethyl
    p. methacrylate (PMMA)
    p. methacrylate contact lens
    p. methacrylate frame
polymorphic
    p. macular degeneration of Brayley
    p. superficial keratitis
polymorphonuclear
    p. reaction
    p. response
polymorphous dystrophy
polymyositis
    orbital p.
polymyxin
    p. B
    bacitracin, neomycin, and p. B
    p. B sulfate
    p. B and Terramycin
    p. E
    oxytetracycline and p. B
    trimethoprim and p. B
polyopia, polyopsia
    binocular p.
    cerebral p.
    p. monophthalmica
polyphaga
    Acanthamoeba p.
Poly-Pred
    P.-P. Ophthalmic Suspension
polypropylene
    p. suture
polypseudophakia
Polyquad
Polysporin
    P. Ophthalmic
polystichia
polytome x-ray
Polytrim
    P. Ophthalmic
pons lesion

pontine
p. gaze center (PGC)
p. lesion
Pontocaine Eye
pontomesencephalic dysfunction
pool
tear p.
pooling of dye
poparacaine ophthalmic drops
porcupine lymphoma
PORN
progressive outer retinal necrosis
porofocon
porous
p. hydroxyapatite sphere
p. orbital implant
port
Berkeley Bioengineering
infusion terminal p.
butterfly needle infusion p.
Gills-Welsh guillotine p.
3-p. pars plana vitrectomy
sclerotomy p.
self-sealing side p.
side p.
p. vitrectomy
porus opticus
position
p. accommodation
p. ametropia
Bertel p.
cardinal p.
convergence p.
p. cyclophoria
dissociated p.
p. error
p. eyepiece
face-down p.
fusion-free p.
heterophoric p.
midline p.
oblique p.
1-o'clock p.
2-o'clock p.
3-o'clock p.
4-o'clock p.
5-o'clock p.

6-o'clock p.
7-o'clock p.
8-o'clock p.
9-o'clock p.
10-o'clock p.
11-o'clock p.
12-o'clock p.
primary p.
Rhese p.
p. scotoma
secondary p.
sulcus fixated p.
tertiary p.
vertical divergence p.
positional
p. abnormalities of retina
p. nystagmus
positive
p. accommodation
p. afterimage
p. convergence
cyclophoria p.
cyclotropia p.
p. eyepiece
p. meniscus
p. meniscus lens
p. scotoma
p. vertical divergence
p. visual phenomenon
Posner
P. diagnostic gonioprism
P. diagnostic lens
P. slit lamp
P. surgical gonioprism
post
p. chamber
p. chiasmal
p. occlusion measurement
p. saccadic drift
postbasic stare
postcanalicular system
postcataract bleb
postequatorial retina
posterior
p. amorphous corneal
dysgenesis

NOTES

P

posterior *(continued)*
p. amorphous corneal dystrophy
p. angle
p. apical radius (PAR)
camera bulbi p.
camera oculi p.
p. capsular polishing
p. capsular zonular barrier
p. capsular zonular disruption
p. capsule opacification (PCO)
p. capsulotomy
p. central curve
p. cerebral artery
p. chamber (PC)
p. chamber intraocular lens (PCIOL)
p. chamber lens implant (PCLI)
p. chiasmatic commissure
p. choroiditis
p. ciliary artery
p. ciliary vein
p. collagenous layer (PCL)
p. conical cornea
p. conjunctival artery
p. conjunctival vein
p. corneal depression
p. discission
p. dislocation
p. embryotoxon
p. epithelium of cornea
p. explant
p. fixation suture
p. focal point
p. hyaloid membrane (PHM)
p. hydrophthalmia
p. incision
p. inferior cerebellar artery syndrome
p. intermediate curve
p. internuclear ophthalmoplegia
p. ischemic optic neuropathy (PION)
p. keratoconus
p. lamellar disk
lamina elastica p.
p. lamina raphe
p. lenticonus
p. limiting lamina
p. limiting ring
membrana capsularis lentis p.
p. optical zone (POZ)

p. peribulbar block
p. peripheral curve
p. pigment epitheliopathy
p. pituitary ectopia
p. polar cataract
p. pole
p. pole of eye
p. pole of eyeball
p. pole of lens
p. pole and periphery (PP&P)
p. polymorphic dystrophy
p. polymorphous corneal dystrophy
p. scleritis
p. sclerochoroiditis
p. sclerotomy
p. segment
p. staphyloma
p. subcapsular cataract (PSC)
p. subcapsular opacity
p. sub-Tenon injection
p. supine position capsular opacity
p. symblepharon
p. synechia
p. thermal sclerostomy
p. tube shunt implant
p. uveal melanoma
p. uveitis
p. visual pathway imaging
p. vitreal detachment (PVD)
p. vitrectomy
p. vitreous
posteriores
limbus palpebrales p.
postganglionic
p. fiber
p. fiber regeneration
p. Horner syndrome
p. short ciliary nerve
postgeniculate congenital homonymous hemianopia
Post-Harrington erysiphake
postherpetic
p. headache
p. neuralgia
posticum
staphyloma p.
postinfectious epithelial keratopathy
postinflammatory
p. atrophy
p. cataract
postkeratoplasty

postlensectomy
postmarital amblyopia
postocular neuritis
postoperative
  p. adjustment
  p. amblyopia
  p. blindness
  p. endophthalmitis
  p. iritis
  p. mydriasis
postorbital
postpapilledema atrophy
postplaced suture
postsurgical hyphema
postsynaptic congenital myasthenic
  disorder
posttraumatic
  p. headache
  p. iridocyclitis
postural exophthalmos
postvaccination optic neuritis
postvitrectomy
  p. cataract
  p. fibrin
potassium
  p. acetate
  p. hydroxide (KOH)
  p. iodide
  p. phosphate
potential
  p. acuity meter (PAM)
  compound muscle action p.
  (CMAP)
  early receptor p.
  evoked p.
  flash visual evoked p.
  oscillatory p. (OP)
  receptor p.
  S p.
  p. visual acuity
  visual-evoked p. (VEP)
  visual-evoked cortical p.
  (VECP)
POTF
  preocular tear film
Potter-Bucky diaphragm
Potter syndrome

pouch
  Rathke p.
Poulard
  P. entropion
  P. operation
Pourcelot ratio
Powder
  Ophthalmic Moldite P.
Powell wand
power
  add p.
  back vertex p. (BVP)
  bending p.
  p. calculation
  contact lens vertex p.
  dioptric p.
  equivalent p.
  intraocular lens p. (IOLP)
  keratometric p. (K)
  lacrimal p.
  lens p.
  magnifying p.
  mean corneal p.
  p. of mirror
  on-eye predicted p.
  P. operation
  optical p.
  Prentice position p.
  radiant p.
  refractive p.
  resolving p.
  topographic simulated
    keratometric p. (TOPO)
  p. vergence
  vertex of p.
  zero optical p.
POZ
  posterior optical zone
PP
  punctum proximum of convergence
p.p.
  punctum proximum
PPC
  peripheral posterior curve
PPDR
  preproliferative diabetic retinopathy

NOTES

P

PPH
persistent postdrainage hypotony
PP&P
posterior pole and periphery
PPV
pars plana vitrectomy
PR
presbyopia
p.r.
punctum remotum
practolol
Praeger iris hook
prairie conjunctivitis
Pram occluder
Prausnitz-Kustner reaction
pre-bleached dark-adapted threshold
precancerous lesion
prechiasmal
p. compression
p. disorder
p. optic nerve
p. optic nerve compression
syndrome
prechopper
Akahoshi phaco p.
Akahoshi universal p.
precipitate
keratic p. (KP)
keratitic p.
mutton-fat keratic p.
pigment p.
pigmented keratic p.
punctate keratic p.
precision
p. astigmatism reduction
p. astigmatism reduction
procedure
P. Cosmet intraocular lens
implant
P. Cosmet lens
P. refractor
p. suture tome
PreClean soak system
precorneal tear film
Pred
P. Forte
P. Forte Ophthalmic
Liquid P.
P. Mild
P. Mild Ophthalmic
Ocu-P. A
Predair A
Predair Forte

Predamide
Predate
Predcor-TBA Injection
Pred-G
P.-G. Ophthalmic
Pred-G S.O.P
predictive value
predisposing condition
Prednefrin Forte
prednisolone
p. acetate
atropine and p.
p. and atropine
chloramphenicol and p.
p. and gentamicin
Isopto P.
neomycin, polymyxin B,
and p.
p. sodium phosphate
sulfacetamide and p.
prednisone
Predsulfair
Predulose
preferential looking
preferential-looking technique
preferred retinal locus (PRL)
Preflex for Sensitive Eyes
Prefrin
P. Ophthalmic Solution
P. Z Liquifilm
Prefrin-A
preganglionic
p. Horner syndrome
p. lesion
p. oculomotor nerve
p. parasympathetic axon
pregeniculate visual pathway
prelaminar optic nerve
preliminary iridectomy
premacular
p. gliosis
p. subhyaloid hemorrhage
premature presbyopia
prematurity
cataract of p.
cicatricial retinopathy of p.
p. myopia
retinopathy of p. (ROP)
p. retinopathy
threshold stage III of
retinopathy of p. (TS III
ROP)
premelanosome

Premiere
P. irrigation-aspiration unit
P. SmallPort phaco system
P. vitreous cutter
Prentice
P. position power
P. rule
preocular tear film (POTF)
preorbita
prepapillary
p. arterial loop
p. hemorrhage
p. vascular loop
preparatory iridectomy
preplaced suture
preponderance
directional p.
prepresbyopia
preproliferative diabetic retinopathy (PPDR)
preretinal
p. gliosis
p. hemorrhage
p. macular fibrosis
p. membrane
p. neovascularization
p. plaque
presbyope
presbyopia (PR)
p. glasses
premature p.
presbyopic
presbytia
presbytism
presenile
p. cataract
p. melanosis
preseptal
p. cellulitis
p. orbicularis muscle
p. space
Presert
preservation
photoreceptor p.
visual p.
preservatives in solution

pressing
eye p.
molded p.
press-on
p.-o. Fresnel lens
p.-o. prism
pressure
p. amaurosis
applanation p.
p. bandage
digital p.
episcleral venous p. (EVP)
exophthalmos due to p.
eye restored to
normotensive p.
intracranial p. (ICP)
intraluminar p.
intraocular p. (IOP)
mercury p.
Michaelson counter p.
ocular perfusion p. (OPP)
osmotic p.
p. patch dressing
p. patching
p. phosphene tonometer
p. shield
white without p.
presumed
p. ocular histoplasmosis
p. ocular histoplasmosis
syndrome (POHS)
presynaptic congenital myasthenic disorder
pretectal
p. area
p. nucleus
p. region
p. syndrome
Prevost sign
Preziosi operation
prezonular space
Price corneal transplant system
Priestley-Smith retinoscope
Prima KTP/532 laser
primary
p. acetylcholine receptor
deficiency

NOTES

P

primary *(continued)*
p. acquired melanosis
p. acquired nasolacrimal duct obstruction (PANDO)
p. action
p. angle-closure glaucoma
p. anophthalmia
p. cataract
p. central nervous system lymphoma (PCNSL)
p. color
p. cone dysfunction
p. demyelinating disease
p. deviation
p. dye test
p. dysgenesis mesodermalis
p. eye
p. familial amyloidosis
p. focal length
p. gaze alignment
p. glaucoma triple procedure (PGTP)
p. graft failure
p. infantile glaucoma
p. infantile glaucoma blepharospasm
p. lens
p. lens implant
p. line of sight
p. mechanism
p. myopia
p. ocular disease
p. ocular lymphoma
p. open-angle glaucoma (PAOG, POAG)
p. optic atrophy
p. perivasculitis of retina
p. persistent hyperplastic vitreous
p. pigmentary degeneration
p. position
p. position of gaze
p. retinal fold
p. visual cortex
Primbs suturing forceps
primitive neuroectodermal tumor (PNET)
primordium, pl. **primordia**
optic p.
Prince
P. cautery
P. electrocautery
P. muscle clamp
P. muscle forceps
P. rule
principal
p. fiber
p. focus
p. line
p. line of direction
p. optic axis
p. plane
p. point
p. visual direction
principle
Fresnel p.
Imbert-Fick p.
Mackay-Marg p.
Scheimpflug p.
Scheiner p.
printers' point system
Prio video display terminal vision tester
prism
p. adaptation test (PAT)
Allen-Thorpe gonioscopic p.
AO rotary p.
apex of p.
p. ballast
ballast p.
p. ballast contact lens
p. bar
bar p.
base-down p. (BD)
Becker gonioscopic p.
Berens p.
p. cover measurement
p. and cover test (P&C)
p. cover test
p. degree
diopter p.
p. diopter
dispersion p.
p. dissociation test
Drews inclined p.
Fresnel press-on p.
Goldmann contact lens p.
Goldmann three-mirror p.
gonioscopic p.
hand-held rotary p.
Jacob-Swann gonioscopic p.
Keeler p.
Maddox p.
Nicol p.
oblique p.
plastic p.

press-on p.
reflecting p.
refracting angle of p.
right-angle p.
Risley rotary p.
rotary p.
scanning p.
p. segment
p. shift test
p. spectacles
square p.
temporary p.
three-mirror p.
p. vergence test
Wolff-Eisner p.
prismatic
   p. contact lens
   p. dioptric value
   p. effect
   p. effect by lens
   p. fundus
   p. gonioscopic lens
   p. gonioscopy lens
   p. goniotomy lens
   p. spectacle lens
   p. spectacles
prism-neutralized cover test
prismoptometer
prismosphere
prisoptometer
Pritikin punch
PRK
   photorefractive keratoplasty
PRL
   preferred retinal locus
probe
   Alcon vitrectomy p.
   Anel p.
   angled p.
   Bodian lacrimal pigtail p.
   Bodian mini lacrimal p.
   Bowman lacrimal p.
   Castroviejo lacrimal sac p.
   p. cataract
   Clinitex Charles
     endophotocoagulator p.
   cryopexy p.

cryotherapy p.
curved retinal p.
Dodick photolysis p.
Ellis foreign body spud
   needle p.
French lacrimal p.
Frigitronics freeze-thaw
   cryopexy p.
Harms trabeculotomy p.
Hertzog pliable p.
Ilg p.
Iliff lacrimal p.
Josephberg p.
Keeler-Amoils curved
   cataract p.
Keeler-Amoils glaucoma p.
Keeler-Amoils long-shank
   retinal p.
Keeler-Amoils microcurved
   cataract p.
Keeler-Amoils ophthalmic
   curved cataract p.
Keeler-Amoils ophthalmic long-
   shank p.
Keeler-Amoils ophthalmic
   Machemer retinal p.
Keeler-Amoils ophthalmic
   microcurved cataract p.
Keeler-Amoils ophthalmic
   retinal p.
Keeler-Amoils ophthalmic
   straight cataract p.
Keeler-Amoils ophthalmic
   vitreous p.
Keeler-Amoils straight
   cataract p.
Keeler-Amoils vitreous p.
Knapp iris p.
lacrimal intubation p.
Linde cryogenic p.
Manhattan Eye & Ear p.
Mannis p.
Microvit p.
nasolacrimal duct p.
p. needle
needle p.
Ocutome p.

NOTES

P

probe *(continued)*
O'Donoghue angled DCR p.
Parker-Heath piggyback p.
piggyback p.
pigtail p.
Quickert-Dryden p.
Quickert lacrimal intubation p.
Ritleng p.
Rolf lacrimal p.
Rollet lacrimal p.
Simpson lacrimal p.
spatula p.
p. spatula
straight retinal p.
p. syringe
Theobald p.
trabeculotomy p.
Vygantas-Wilder retinal
drainage p.
Werb right-angle p.
Williams p.
Worst pigtail p.
Ziegler p.
probing
p. lacrimonasal duct
p. lacrimonasal duct operation
procaine hydrochloride
procedure
acuity card p.
advancement p.
Anderson-Kestenbaum p.
artificial divergence p.
Baerveldt filtering p.
Bick p.
Cairns p.
Cibis liquid silicone p.
ciliary p.
Custodis nondraining p.
cyclodestructive p.
Donders p.
Faden p.
Fasanella-Servat p.
filtering p.
Girard p.
hamular p.
Harada-Ito p.
hex p.
Hill p.
Hummelsheim p.
Ito p.
Jannetta p.
Jensen transposition p.
Jones tube p.

keratorefractive p.
Kestenbaum p.
Knapp p.
Krönlein p.
Kuhnt-Szymanowski p.
lathing p.
lower lid sling p.
modified corncrib (inverted
T) p.
modified Wies p.
PAM p.
precision astigmatism
reduction p.
primary glaucoma triple p.
(PGTP)
Quickert p.
Ruiz p.
Sato p.
Savin p.
Sayoc p.
scleral buckling p.
situ keratomileusis p.
sling p.
strip p.
surgical decompression p.
tarsal strip p.
Thal p.
Toti p.
triple p.
tuck p.
tumbling p.
uncinate p.
up-and-down staircases p.
Wheeler p.
Wies p.
PRO CEM-4 microscope
procerus
musculus p.
process
ciliary p.
disciform p.
fine iris p.
iris p.
lacrimal p.
photochemical p.
replamineform p.
Sand p.
spin-cast p.
visual p.
zygomatico-orbital p.
processus
p. ciliares

p. frontosphenoidalis ossis
  zygomatici
p. orbitalis ossis palatini
p. zygomaticus maxillae
procyonis
  Baylisascaris p.
prodromal
  p. glaucoma
  p. myopia
product
  Katena p.
  Nexacryl cohesive p.
  Xomed Surgical P.'s
production
  reflex tear p.
Profenal
  P. Ophthalmic
profile
  p. analyzer
  p. perimetry
ProFinesse II ultrasonic handpiece
**ProFree/GP weekly enzymatic
  cleaner**
profunda
  keratitis p.
  keratitis punctata p.
  keratitis pustuliformis p.
prognosis
  visual p.
program
  Casebeer keratorefractive
    planning p.
  diagnostic p.
  Rabinowitz-Klyce/Maeda
    keratoconus screening p.
progressiva
  ophthalmoplegia p.
progressive
  p. addition lens
  p. cataract
  p. choroidal atrophy
  p. cone degeneration
  p. cone dystrophy
  p. cone-rod dystrophy
  p. encephalopathy with edema,
    hypsarrhythmia and optic
    atrophy (PEHO)

p. external ophthalmoplegia
  (PEO)
p. fluorescein leakage
p. foveal dystrophy
p. hearing loss
p. hemifacial atrophy
p. herpetic corneal
  endotheliopathy
p. macular dystrophy
p. multifocal lens
p. myopia
p. myopic degeneration
p. optic atrophy
p. outer retinal necrosis
  (PORN)
p. outer retinal necrosis
  syndrome
p. supranuclear palsy
p. systemic sclerosis
p. tapetochoroidal dystrophy
p. vaccinia
progressive-add bifocal
project
  Cataract PPO p.
  P. Research Ophthalmic
    specular microscope
projecting staphyloma
projection
  erroneous p.
  false p.
  light p.
  perimeter p.
  p. perimeter
  retinocortical p.
  retinogeniculostriate p.
  visual p.
Project-O-Chart
  AO Reichert Instruments P.-O.-
  C.
  Ultramatic P.-O.-C.
projector
  acuity visual p.
  fiberoptic light p.
  Lancaster red-green p.
  Marco chart p.
  NP-3S auto chart p.
  Topcon chart p.

NOTES

P

405

projector *(continued)*
  Ultramatic Project-O-Chart p.
    (UPOC)
Pro-Koester wide-field SCM
  microscope
prolactin-secreting adenoma
prolapse
  iris p.
  p. of iris
  vitreous p.
Prolene suture
proliferans
  fibrous p.
proliferating retinitis
proliferation
  anterior hyaloidal
    fibrovascular p.
  conjunctival lymphoid p.
  epimacular p.
  epiretinal membrane p. (EMP)
  fibrovascular p.
  glial p.
  hyaloidal fibrovascular p.
  massive periretinal p. (MPP)
  peripheral p.
proliferative
  p. choroiditis
  p. diabetic retinopathy (PDR)
  p. lupus retinopathy
  p. retinitis
  p. sickle-cell retinopathy
  p. vitreoretinopathy (PVR)
prolonged-wear
  p.-w. contact lens
promethazine
prominence
  Ammon scleral p.
prominent
  p. buckle
  p. indentation
  p. Schwalbe ring
Pro-Ophtha
  P.-O. drape
  P.-O. dressing
  P.-O. eye pad
  P.-O. sponge
  P.-O. stick
propamidine isethionate
proparacaine
  p. HCl
  p. hydrochloride
prophylactic antibiotic

prophylaxis
  Credé p.
  retinal p.
Propine
  P. Ophthalmic
propionate
  clobetasol p.
  sodium p.
Propionibacterium
  P. acnes
  P. propionicus
propionicus
  Propionibacterium p.
Propper-Heine ophthalmoscope
Propper indirect ophthalmoscope
propria
  substantia p.
proprioception
proprioceptive
  p. head-turning reflex
  p. oculocephalic reflex
  p. stimulus
proptometer
proptosis
  axial p.
  ipsilateral p.
  Moran p.
  unilateral p.
proptotic
propylene glycol
Prorex
PROSHIELD collagen corneal
  shield
prosopagnosia
  apperceptive p.
  associative p.
  developmental p.
prosopantritis
prospective
  p. evaluation of radial
    keratotomy (PERK)
  p. study
prostaglandin analog
prosthesis, pl. prostheses
  ocular p.
  orbital floor p.
  shell p.
  socket p.
prosthetic
  p. lens
  P. Orthotic Associates
prosthetophacos
prosthokeratoplasty

Prostigmin test
protan color blindness
protanomal
protanomalopia
protanomalous
    protanope p.
protanomaly
protanope
    p. protanomalous
protanopia
protanopic
protanopsia
protective
    p. lens
    p. spectacles
protector
    Arroyo p.
    Arruga p.
    eye p.
    oculoplasty corneal p.
protein
    p. deposit
    silver p.
proteinaceous
    p. aqueous exudation
    p. coating
    p. cyst
proteinolipidic film
proteolytic enzyme
Proteus syndrome
protometer
proton
    p. beam
ProTon portable tonometer
protozoan uveitis
protriptyline hydrochloride
protruding eyes
protrusion
    conical p.
    corneal p.
Provisc
provocative
    p. test
    p. testing
Prowazek-Greeff body
Prowazek-Halberstaedter body
Prowazek inclusion body

proximal
    p. convergence
    p. myotonic myopathy
proximum
    punctum p. (p.p.)
PRP
    panretinal photocoagulation
PRRE
    pupils round, regular, and equal
PRT
    photostress recovery time
psammoma body
psammomatous meningioma (PM)
PSC
    posterior subcapsular cataract
Pseudallescheria boydii
pseudoabducens palsy
pseudoacanthosis nigricans
pseudoaccommodation
pseudo-Argyll-Robertson pupil
pseudobaggy eyelid
pseudoblepsia, pseudoblepsis
pseudobulbar palsy
pseudocaloric nystagmus
pseudocancerous lesion
pseudochiasmal
pseudocoloboma
pseudo-CSF signal
pseudodendritic keratitis
pseudodiphtheriticum
    Corynebacterium p.
pseudodoubling
pseudodrusen
pseudoephedrine
    carbinoxamine and p.
pseudoepitheliomatous hyperplasia
pseudoesotropia
pseudoexfoliation (PXF)
    p. of lens capsule
    p. syndrome
pseudoexfoliative
    p. capsular glaucoma
    p. glaucoma (PEXG)
pseudoexophoria
pseudoexophthalmos
pseudoexotropia
pseudo-Foster Kennedy syndrome

NOTES

P

pseudoglaucoma
pseudoglaucomatous macrocupping
pseudoglioma
pseudo-Graefe
　　p.-G. phenomenon
　　p.-G. sign
pseudohemianopsia
pseudohistoplasmosis
pseudohole
pseudo-Hurler polydystrophy
pseudohypopyon
pseudoinflammatory
　　p. macular dystrophy
　　p. macular dystrophy of
　　　Sorsby
pseudointernuclear ophthalmoplegia
pseudoiritis
pseudoisochromatic
　　p. color plate
　　p. color test
pseudomembrane
　　conjunctival p.
pseudomembranous
　　p. conjunctivitis
　　p. rhinitis
Pseudomonas
　　P. aeruginosa
　　P. cepacia
　　P. pyocyanea
　　P. stutzeri
pseudomycosis
pseudomyopia
pseudonystagmus
pseudo-operculum
pseudopannus
pseudopapilledema
pseudopapillitis
pseudopemphigoid
pseudophacos, pseudophakos
pseudophake implant
pseudophakia
　　p. adiposa
　　p. fibrosa
pseudophakic
　　p. bullous keratopathy (PBK)
　　p. detachment
　　p. eye
pseudophakodonesis
pseudophakos (*var. of* pseudophacos)
pseudopolycoria
pseudopresumed ocular
　　histoplasmosis syndrome (pseudo
　　POHS)

pseudoprolactinoma
pseudoproptosis
pseudopseudohypoparathyroidism
pseudopsia
pseudopterygia
pseudopterygium
pseudoptosis
pseudoretinitis pigmentosa
pseudoretinoblastoma
pseudorheumatoid nodule
pseudosarcomatous endothelial
　　hyperplasia
pseudosclerosis
　　spastic p.
pseudoscopic vision
pseudostereo image
pseudostrabismus
pseudotabes
　　pupillotonic p.
pseudotemporal arteritis
pseudotrachoma
pseudotuberculous ophthalmia
pseudotumor
　　p. cerebri (PTC)
　　idiopathic inflammatory p.
　　lymphoid p.
　　p. oculi
　　orbital p.
pseudovernal conjunctivitis
pseudoxanthoma
　　elastic p.
　　p. elasticum (PXE)
psittaci
　　Chlamydia p.
psoriatic corneal abscess
psorophthalmia
psychic blindness
psychogenic
　　p. microsopia
　　p. paralysis
psychophysics
　　visual p.
PTC
　　pseudotumor cerebri
pterion
pterygial tissue
pterygium, pl. pterygia
　　active p.
　　Arlt p.
　　belly of p.
　　congenital p.
　　conjunctival p.
　　epitarsus p.

p. scissors
p. unguis
pterygium-induced astigmatism
pterygoid levator synkinesis
pterygomaxillary fissure
pterygopalatine ganglion
ptilosis
PTK
  phototherapeutic keratectomy
ptosis, pl. **ptoses**
  acquired myopathic p.
  p. adiposa
  age-related p.
  aponeurotic p.
  Berke p.
  Blaskovics-Berke p.
  botulism-induced p.
  cerebral p.
  congenital dystrophic p.
  congenital myopathic p.
  cortical p.
  p. crutch spectacles
  developmental p.
  drug-induced p.
  p. of eyelid
  eyelid p.
  false p.
  p. forceps
  Hiff p.
  Horner p.
  involutional senile p.
  p. knife
  p. lipomatosis
  mechanical acquired p.
  midbrain p.
  morning p.
  myogenic acquired p.
  myopathic p.
  neurogenic acquired p.
  neuromuscular p.
  p. scissors
  senescent p.
  snake bite-induced p.
  p. sympathetica
  traumatic p.
  upside-down p.
  waking p.

ptotic
pucker
  macular p.
  pigmented macular p.
puckering
  macular p.
puddler's cataract
puff of loose vitreous
PUK
  peripheral ulcerative keratitis
Pulfrich stereo phenomenon
pulpit spectacles
Pulsair tonometer
pulsatile exophthalmos
pulsating exophthalmos
pulsation
  spontaneous retinal venous p.
  spontaneous venous p. (SVP)
  venous p.
pulse
  choroidal p.
  p. mode
  radiofrequency p.
  retinal venous p.
  saccadic p.
  square-wave p.
pulseless disease
pulverulenta
  cataracta centralis p.
  cataracta zonularis p.
pulverulent opacity
pump
  AMO HPF 500 p.
  peristaltic p.
  tear p.
  TurboStaltic p.
pump-leak system
punch
  Barron donor corneal p.
  Berens corneoscleral p.
  p. block
  bone p.
  bone-biting p.
  Castroviejo corneoscleral p.
  corneal p.
  corneoscleral p.
  Descemet membrane p.

NOTES

P

punch *(continued)*
 Gass corneoscleral p.
 Gass scleral p.
 Gass sclerotomy p.
 Hardy p.
 Holth scleral p.
 Kelly-Descemet membrane p.
 Klein p.
 Luntz-Dodick p.
 Pollock p.
 Pritikin p.
 Reiss punctal p.
 Rothman Gilbard cornea p.
 Rubin-Holth p.
 scleral p.
 sclerectomy p.
 sclerotomy p.
 Storz corneoscleral p.
 Tanne corneal p.
 Tanne guillotine-style p.
 p. trephine
 Troutman p.
 Walser corneoscleral p.
 Walton p.
punched-out
 p.-o. chorioretinal scar
 p.-o. lesion
puncta (*pl. of* punctum)
punctal
 p. cautery
 p. dilator
 p. ectropion
 p. lens
 p. occlusion
 p. opening
 p. plug
 p. stenosis
punctata
 p. albescens retinopathy
 chondrodystrophia calcificans
  congenita p.
 hyalitis p.
 keratitis p.
punctate
 p. cataract
 p. corneal epithelial defect
 p. corneal opacity
 p. epithelial erosion
 p. epithelial keratitis
 p. epithelial keratopathy (PEK)
 p. epithelial keratoplasty
 p. epithelial microcyst
 p. hemorrhage

 p. hyalitis
 p. hyalosis
 p. inner choroiditis
 p. keratic precipitate
 p. oculocutaneous albinism
 p. oculocutaneous albinoidism
 p. outer retinal toxoplasmosis
 p. retinitis
 p. staining
puncti (*gen. of* punctum)
punctiform
punctograph
punctoplasty
punctum, gen. **puncti**, pl. **puncta**
 p. aplasia
 p. caecum
 p. cecum
 dilation of p.
 p. dilator
 eversion of p.
 everted p.
 inferior p.
 lacrimal p.
 p. lacrimale
 lower p.
 p. luteum
 one-snip p.
 p. plug
 p. proximum (p.p.)
 p. proximum of
  accommodation
 p. proximum of convergence
  (PP)
 p. remotum (p.r.)
 p. stenosis
 superior p.
 three-snip p.
 upper p.
punctumeter
puncture
 anterior p.
 p. diabetes
 diathermy p.
 lumbar p.
 p. needle
 self-sealing scleral p.
 p. wound
 Ziegler p.
puncture-tip needle
Puntenney forceps
pupil (p)
 Adie tonic p.
 amaurotic p.

Argyll-Robertson p.
artificial p.
Behr p.
p. block
p. block glaucoma
"blown p."
bounding p.
Bumke p.
catatonic p.
cat's eye p.
cholinergic p.
cogwheel p.
constricted p.
contraction of p.
cornpicker's p.
p. cycle induction test
diabetic Argyll-Robertson p.
dilated p.
p. dilation
p. dilator
dilator muscle of p.
p. disorder
elliptic p.
entrance p.
p.'s equal, reactive to light
  and accommodation (PERLA)
p.'s equal, round, reactive to
  light and accommodation
  (PERRLA)
exit p.
fixed dilated p.
Gunn p.
hammock p.
Holmes-Adie p.
Horner p.
Hutchinson p.
iris and p. (I/P)
irregular p.
isolated fixed dilated p.
keyhole p.
light response of p.
local tonic p.
Marcus Gunn p. (MG)
p. miosis
miotic p.
myotonic p.
neuropathic tonic p.

neurotonic p.
occluded p.
occlusion of p.
paradoxical p.
pear-shaped p.
peninsula p.
pinhole p.
pinpoint p.
pseudo-Argyll-Robertson p.
reverse Marcus Gunn p.
rigid p.
Robertson p.
p.'s round, regular, and equal
  (PRRE)
Saenger p.
scalloped p.
seclusion of p.
p. size
skew p.
sphincter muscle of p.
p. spreader/retractor forceps
spring p.
square p.
stiff p.
p. stretching
tadpole p.
teardrop p.
tonic p.
updrawn p.
Wernicke p.
white p.
pupilla, pl. **pupillae**
caligo p.
pupillae muscle of iris
musculus dilator p.
musculus sphincter p.
sphincter pupillae
synizesis pupillae
synkinesis p.
pupillaris
membrana p.
pupillary
p. aperture
p. areflexia
p. athetosis
p. axis
p. block

NOTES

P

pupillary *(continued)*
  p. block glaucoma
  p. capture
  p. center
  p. disorder
  p. distance (PD)
  p. effect
  p. entrapment
  p. escape
  p. floater
  p. iris cyst
  p. lens
  p. light reflex
  p. line
  p. margin of iris
  p. membrane
  p. membrane remnant
  p. miosis
  p. near response
  p. paradoxic reflex
  p. paralysis
  p. sparing
  p. sphincter akinesis
  p. sphincter contraction
  p. sphincter muscle
  p. zone
pupilloconstrictor fiber
pupillograph
pupillography
pupillometer
  Colvard p.
  reflex p.
pupillometry
  infrared p.
pupillomotor
  p. fiber
pupilloplegia
pupilloscope
pupilloscopy
pupillostatometer
pupillotonia
pupillotonic pseudotabes
pupil-to-root iridectomy
Puralube
  P. Tears
  P. Tears Solution
pure
  p. alexia
  p. color
  p. cyclitis
Purisol
Purkinje
  P. effect

  P. image
  P. image tracker
  P. phenomenon
  P. shadow
  P. shift
Purkinje-Sanson mirror image
Purlytin
purple
  visual p.
purpurea
  Digitalis p.
purpuriferous
purpuriparous
purpurogenous membrane
pursuit
  cogwheel p.
  p. mechanism
  p. movement
  saccadic p.
  p. testing
  p. tracking
Purtscher
  P. angiopathic retinopathy
  P. disease
purulent
  p. conjunctivitis
  p. cyclitis
  p. iritis
  p. keratitis
  p. ophthalmia
  p. retinitis
  p. rhinitis
pusher
  Aker lens p.
  De LaVega lens p.
  Martin Surefit lens p.
  Visitec lens p.
push plus refraction technique
push/pull
  Ilg p./p.
  Kuglein p./p.
push-up method
pustular blepharitis
Putenney operation
Putterman
  P. levator resection clamp
  P. ptosis clamp
**Putterman-Chaflin ocular
  asymmetry device**
**Putterman-Mueller blepharoptosis
  clamp**

P.V.
    P. Carpine
    P. Carpine Liquifilm
PVD
    posterior vitreal detachment
PVER
    pattern visual-evoked response
PVR
    proliferative vitreoretinopathy
PXE
    pseudoxanthoma elasticum
PxEx Ophthalmic
PXF
    pseudoexfoliation
pyknotic
    p. keratitis
    p. nuclei
pyocyanea
    Pseudomonas p.

pyocyaneal ulcer
pyocyaneus
    Bacillus p.
pyogenes
    Streptococcus p.
pyogenic
    p. granuloma
    p. metastasis
Pyopen
pyophthalmia
pyophthalmitis
pyramidal
    p. cataract
    p. system
Pyrex
    P. eye sphere
    P. T-tube
    P. tube

NOTES

P

q arm
Q-banding
Q-switched
    Q.-s. Er:YAG laser
    Q.-s. neodymium:YAG laser
    Q.-s. ruby laser
13q- syndrome
Quad cutting tip
QuadPediatric fundus lens
quadrantanopsia, quadrantanopia
    homonymous q.
    superior q.
quadrant hemianopsia
quadrantic
    q. defect
    q. hemianopsia
    q. sclerectomy with internal
      drainage
    q. scotoma
Quaglino operation
quality
    tear q.
quantitative
    q. echography
    q. haze assessment
    q. perimetry
    q. static threshold
    q. threshold perimetry
quantity
    tear q.
Quantum enhancement knife
quaternary
    q. ammonium chloride
    q. ammonium compound
Questek laser tube

questionnaire
    National Eye Institute Visual
    Function Q.
    VF-14 q.
    Visual Activities Q.
Quevedo
    Q. fixation forceps
    Q. suturing forceps
Quickert
    Q. lacrimal intubation probe
    Q. procedure
    Q. suture
    Q. three-suture technique
Quickert-Dryden
    Q.-D. probe
    Q.-D. tube
quick left/right component
QuickRinse automated instrument
  rinse system
Quickswitch irrigation/aspiration
  ophthalmic system
quiescent stromal scarring
quiet
    q. chamber
    eye was q.
    q. iritis
Quiet-Vac
quinacrine hydrochloride
quinaquine
quinine
    q. amblyopia
    q. sulfate
Quire mechanical finger forceps
QYS

Rabinowitz-Klyce/Maeda keratoconus
  screening program
Rabinowitz-McDonnell test
Rabl lamella
raccoon eyes
racemose
  r. aneurysm
  r. angioma
  r. hemangioma
  r. hemangiomatosis
racemosum
  staphyloma corneae r.
rack
  Luneau retinoscopy r.
racquet body
racquet-like pattern
radial
  r. astigmatism
  r. cells of Mueller
  r. dilator muscle
  r. fiber
  r. infiltration
  r. iridotomy
  r. iridotomy scissors
  r. keratotomy (RK)
  r. keratotomy knife
  r. keratotomy marker
  r. sponge
  r. transillumination defect
  r. vessel array
radially oriented
radiance
radiant
  r. absorptance
  r. emittance
  r. energy
  r. flux
  r. intensity
  r. and luminous flux
  r. power
  r. reflectance
radiata
  corona r.
radiatio
  r. occipitothalamica
  r. optica
radiation
  artificial UV r.
  beta r.
  r. burn

  r. cataract
  r. effect
  electromagnetic r.
  geniculocalcarine r.
  Goldmann Coherent r.
  heavy ion r.
  infrared r.
  r. injury
  ionizing r.
  r. keratitis
  natural UV r.
  occipitothalamic r.
  optic r.
  r. optic neuropathy (RON)
  r. retinopathy
  solar r.
  r. therapy
  ultraviolet r.
  visual r.'s
radiation-induced
  r.-i. carcinoma
  r.-i. optic neuropathy
radical
  r. astigmatism
  r. orbitectomy
radicans
  Rhus r.
radices (pl. of radix)
radii (pl. of radius)
Radin-Rosenthal eye implant
radioactive
  r. eye plaque
  r. plaque brachytherapy
radiofrequency pulse
radiogenic vasculopathy
radioisotope scan
radiology
  orbital r.
radioscope
  Lombart r.
radiotherapy
  orbital r.
  palladium 103 ophthalmic
    plaque r.
  plaque r.
radius, pl. radii
  apical r.
  back optic zone r. (BOZR)
  r. of curvature
  front optic zone r. (FOZR)

R

radius *(continued)*
  r. gauge
  r. of lens
  r. of lentis
  posterior apical r. (PAR)
radix, pl. **radices**
  r. lateralis tractus optici
  r. medialis tractus optici
  r. oculomotoria ganglii ciliaris
  r. sympathica ganglii ciliaris
radon
  r. ring brachytherapy
  r. seed implantation
Raeder paratrigeminal neuralgia
ragged-red fiber
rag-wheel method
railroad nystagmus
rainbow
  r. symptom
  r. syndrome
  r. vision
raindrop-shaped keratometric reflection
Rainen clip-bending spatula
Rainin lens spatula
Raji cell assay
raking
  endoscopic r.
Raman
  R. effect
  R. spectrum
ramollitio retinae
Ramsden eyepiece
ramus
  tentorii r.
Randolph
  R. cyclodialysis cannula
  R. irrigator
random-dot
  r.-d. kinematogram
  r.-d. kinematography
random-dot stereogram
Randot
  R. chart
  R. circle
  R. Dot E stereo test
  R. Stereo Smile test
range
  r. of accommodation
  r. of convergence
  vertical fusion r.
RAPD
  relative afferent pupillary defect

raphe
  canthal r.
  horizontal r.
  lateral palpebral r.
  palpebral r.
  r. palpebralis lateralis
  r. palpebrarum
  r. plica semilunaris
  posterior lamina r.
  temporal r.
rapid eye movement (REM)
Rappazzo intraocular manipulator
rare earth intraocular magnet
rarefaction
  pigmentation r.
rasp
  Lundsgaard r.
  Lundsgaard-Burch corneal r.
Raster photogrammeter
rastersteriography
rastersteriography-based elevation map
Rathke
  R. cleft cyst
  R. pouch
  R. pouch tumor
ratio
  accommodation-convergence r.
  accommodative convergence/accommodation r. (AC/A)
  AL/CR r., axial length/corneal radius ratio
    axial length/corneal radius ratio
  aperture r.
  arteriovenous r.
  artery-to-vein r. (A/V)
  axial length/corneal radius r. (AL/CR ratio, axial length/corneal radius ratio)
  CA/C r.
    convergence accommodation ratio
  convergence accommodation r. (CA/C ratio)
  cup-disk r.
  cup-to-disk r. (C/D)
  L/D r.
    light/dark amplitude ratio
  light/dark amplitude r. (L/D ratio)
  light-peak to dark-trough r.

nuclear cytoplasmic r.
optic cup-to-disk r.
Pourcelot r.
rim-to-disk r.
Raven Progressive Matrices test
Raverdino operation
ray
convergent r.
converging r.
divergent r.
emergent r.
r. incident
r. of light
medullary r.
monochromatic r.
parallel r.
paraxial r.
r. tracing
Ray-Brunswick-Mack operation
Rayleigh
R. color matching test
R. limit
R. scattering
R. test
Ray-McLean operation
Raymond-Cestan syndrome
Raymond syndrome
Rayner-Choyce implant
Rayner lens
raytracing
optical r.
razor
Bard-Parker r.
r. blade
r. bladebreaker
r. blade knife
r. needle
razor-blade trephine
razor-tip needle
RBRVS
Resource-Based Relative Value
Scale
RC-2 fundus camera
RCL
recurrent corneal lesion
RD
retinal detachment

reaction
adverse r.
anaphylactic r.
anterior chamber r.
Arthus r.
basophilic r.
conjunctival r.
consensual r.
direct pupillary light r.
eosinophilic r.
hemiopic pupillary r.
hypersensitivity r.
immune r.
immunologic r.
indirect pupillary r.
Jarisch-Herxheimer r.
lid closure r.
light r.
Loewi r.
Mazzotti r.
mononuclear r.
near r.
ocular tilt r. (OTR)
ophthalmic r.
orbicularis r.
pain r.
paradoxical darkness r.
polymerase chain r.
polymorphonuclear r.
Prausnitz-Kustner r.
toxic r.
vestibular pupillary r.
Weil-Felix r.
Wernicke r.
reader
bar r.
reading
r. card
r. chart
r. glasses
K r.'s
keratometric reading
keratometric readings
keratometric r.'s (K readings)
r. rectangle
reagent strip

NOTES

real
    r. focus
    r. image
reaper's
    r. keratitis
    r. ophthalmia
reattachment
    r. of choroid
    r. of choroid operation
    hydraulic retinal r.
    r. of retina
    r. of retina operation
rebound nystagmus
receptacle
    dome r.
receptive field
receptor
    r. amblyopia
    r. potential
recess
    Arlt-Jaesche r.
    canthal r.
    optic r.
recessed-angle glaucoma
recession
    angle r.
    bimedial r.
    conjunctival r.
    r. forceps
    lateral rectus r.
    left inferior oblique r.
    r. of muscle
    r. of ocular muscle operation
    optic muscle r.
    tendon r.
    traumatic angle r.
recession-angle glaucoma
recession-resection (R&R)
recessive dystrophic epidermolysis bullosa
recess-resect (R&R)
recessus
    r. opticus
rechutes
    iritis blenorrhagique à r.
recipient bed
reciprocal innervation
reciprocity law
Recklinghausen
    R. disease
    R. syndrome
reclination

recognition
    pattern r.
reconstruction
    r. of eyelid
    socket r.
    V-Y advancement myotarsocutaneous flap for upper eyelid r.
recovery
    fluid-attenuated inversion r.
rectangle
    reading r.
rectangular blade
rectifier
    delayed r.
    inward r.
rectus
    inferior r. (IR)
    lateral r. (LR)
    r. lateralis muscle
    medial r. (MR)
    r. medialis muscle
    superior r. (SR)
recurrent
    r. central retinitis
    r. choroiditis
    r. corneal erosion
    r. corneal erosion syndrome
    r. corneal lesion (RCL)
    r. epithelial erosion
    r. erosion of cornea
    r. exophthalmos
    r. hypopyon
    r. pupillary sparing
recurrentis
    Borrelia r.
red
    r. blindness
    r. cone degeneration
    r. desaturation
    r. eye
    r. filter
    r. flash stimulus
    r. free photograph
    r. glare test
    r. glass test
    r. lens occluder
    r. reflex
    R. Reflex Lens Systems lens
    r. rubber catheter
    r. scaly plaque
    r. vision
redeepening

red-eyed shunt syndrome
red-filter
    r.-f. test
    r.-f. therapy
red-free filter
red-green
    r.-g. axis
    r.-g. blindness
    r.-g. glasses
Reditron refractometer
Redmond-Smith operation
reduced
    r. eye
    r. eye model
    r. Snellen card
    r. vergence
reducer
    McCannel ocular pressure r.
    ocular pressure r.
reducing body myopathy
reductase
    aldose r.
reduction
    chemo r.
    precision astigmatism r.
reduplicated cataract
reduplication
    r. cataract
    r. of Descemet membrane
Reed-Sternberg cell
Reeh scissors
reel aspiration cannula
re-epithelialization
Reese
    R. muscle forceps
    R. ptosis knife
    R. ptosis operation
    R. syndrome
Reese-Cleasby operation
Reese-Ellsworth
    R.-E. classification
    R.-E. group Va disease
    R.-E. group Vb disease
    R.-E. group V retinoblastoma
    R.-E. stage IIIA retinoblastoma
Reese-Jones-Cooper operation
refined refraction

refixation
reflectance
    radiant r.
reflected
    r. color
    r. light
reflecting
    r. prism
    r. retinoscope
    r. surface
reflection
    angle of r.
    corneal r.
    D-shaped keratometric r.
    raindrop-shaped keratometric r.
    shiny cellophane r.
    specular r.
reflective scattering
reflectivity
    internal r.
reflectometer
reflectometry
reflex
    r. accommodation
    accommodation r.
    acquired gustolacrimal r.
    r. amaurosis
    r. amblyopia
    Aschner r.
    attention r.
    auditory oculogyric r.
    Bekhterev r.
    Bell r.
    black r.
    r. blepharospasm
    blind spot r.
    blink r.
    cat's eye r.
    cellophane macular r.
    cerebral cortex r.
    cerebropupillary r.
    cervico-ocular r. (COR)
    Charleaux oil droplet r.
    choked r.
    ciliary r.
    ciliospinal r.
    circumpapillary light r.

NOTES

R

421

reflex *(continued)*

coaxially sighted corneal r.
cochleopupillary r.
congenital paradoxic
gustolacrimal r.
conjunctival r.
consensual light r.
convergency r.
copper-wire r.
corneal light r.
corneomandibular r.
corneomental r.
corneopterygoid r.
corticopupillary r.
crescentic circumpapillary
light r.
crossed r.
cutaneous pupillary r.
dazzle r.
direct r.
direct-light r.
doll's eye r.
emergency light r.
eye r.
eyeball compression r.
eyeball-heart r.
eye-closure r.
eyelid-closure r.
r. eye movement
eye-popping r.
fixation r.
foveal r.
foveolar r.
fundal r.
fundus r.
fusion r.
Gault r.
Gifford r.
Gifford-Galassi r.
Gunn pupillary r.
gustatolacrimal r.
Haab r.
head-turning r.
Hirschberg r.
iridoplegia r.
iris contraction r.
juvenile r.
lacrimal r.
lacrimation r.
lid closure r.
light optometer r.
Lockwood light r.
McCarthy r.

myopic r.
nasolacrimal r.
near light r.
oculocardiac r.
oculocephalic r.
oculocephalogyric r.
oculodigital r.
oculogyric auricular r.
oculopharyngeal r.
oculopupillary r.
oculorespiratory r.
oculosensory cell r.
oculovestibular r.
opticofacial winking r.
optokinetic r.
optomotor r.
orbicularis pupillary r.
otolithic-ocular r.
palpebral oculogyric r.
palpebromandibular r.
paradoxical pupillary r.
paradoxic gustolacrimal r.
platysmal r.
Plitz r.
proprioceptive head-turning r.
proprioceptive oculocephalic r.
pupillary light r.
pupillary paradoxic r.
r. pupillometer
red r.
reversed pupillary r.
Ruggeri r.
senile r.
shot-silk r.
silver-wire r.
skin pupillary r.
spasm of the near r.
stretch r.
supraorbital r.
synkinetic near r.
tapetal light r.
r. tear production
r. tear secretion
threat r.
trigeminal r.
trigeminus r.
r. trigeminus
utricular r.
vestibulo-ocular r.
visual orbicularis r.
water-silk r.
Weiss r.
Westphal-Piltz r.

R

Westphal pupillary r.
white pupillary r.
wink r.
yellow light r.
reflux
r. of tears
r. vergence
reformation
r. of chamber
fornix r.
inferior fornix r.
refracted light
refractile
r. body
r. crystal
r. deposit
refracting
r. angle of prism
r. medium
refraction
angle of r.
r. angle
cycloplegic r. (CR)
cylindric r.
direct-light r.
double r.
dynamic r.
fogging system of r.
homatropine r.
index of r. (n)
law of r.
manifest r. (MR)
ocular r.
plane-surface r.
refined r.
r. spectacles
spherical r.
static r.
unrefined r.
refractionist
refractionometer
Hartinger Coincidence r.
vertex r.
Zeiss vertex r.
refractive
r. accommodative esotropia
r. amblyopia

r. ametropia
r. anisometropia
r. astigmatism
r. contact lens
r. error
r. hyperopia
r. keratoplasty
r. keratotomy
r. medium
r. myopia
r. power
r. state
r. surgery
refractivity
refractometer
Abbe r.
Canon auto r.
Hoya HDR objective r.
Hoya MRM objective r.
meridional r.
Reditron r.
Rodenstock eye r.
Speedy-1 Auto r.
8000 Supra Series auto r.
Topcon eye r.
Topcon RM-A2300 auto r.
refractometry
laser r.
urine r.
refractor
Agrikola r.
Allergan Humphrey r.
Amoils r.
AR 1000 r.
automated r.
automatic r.
Barraquer-Krumeich Swinger r.
Berens r.
Brawley r.
Bronson-Turtz r.
Campbell r.
Canon r.
Castallo r.
Castroviejo r.
Coburn r.
CooperVision Diagnostic
Imaging r.

NOTES

refractor *(continued)*
    Desmarres r.
    Elschnig r.
    Ferris-Smith r.
    Ferris-Smith-Sewall r.
    Fink r.
    Goldstein r.
    Gradle r.
    Graether r.
    Green r.
    Groenholm r.
    Hartstein r.
    Hillis r.
    Humphrey automatic r.
    Kirby r.
    Knapp r.
    Kronfeld r.
    Kuglein r.
    Leland r.
    Marco r.
    McGannon r.
    Meller r.
    Mueller r.
    Nidek AR-2000 Objective Automatic r.
    objective r.
    Precision r.
    Reichert r.
    Remote Vision electronic r.
    Rizzuti r.
    Rollet r.
    Schepens r.
    SR-IV Programmed Subjective r.
    Stevenson r.
    subjective r.
    Topcon r.
    Wilmer r.
Refresh
    R. Ophthalmic Solution
    R. Plus
    R. Plus lubricant eye drops
    R. Plus Ophthalmic Solution
    R. PM
    R. Tears eye drops
refringence
refringent
Refsum disease
Regan-Lancaster dial
Regan low-contrast acuity chart
regard
    area of conscious r.
    object of r.

    plane of r.
    point of r.
regeneration
    aberrant r.
    r. aberration
    r. of innervation
    nerve r.
    r. of nerve
    postganglionic fiber r.
region
    ciliary r.
    ethmoidal r.
    infraorbital r.
    ocular r.
    orbital r.
    pretectal r.
    retrochiasmatic r.
    scutum r.
    third framework r. (FR3)
regional
    r. block
    r. periarteritis
Registry
    Australian Corneal Graft R.
regression
    myopic r.
    univariate polytomous logistic r.
regular astigmatism
regulator
    OptiMed glaucoma pressure r. (OPGR)
rehabilitation
    optical r.
Reichert
    R. binocular indirect ophthalmoscope
    R. camera
    R. Ful-Vue binocular ophthalmoscope
    R. Ful-Vue spot retinoscope
    R. Lenschek advanced logic lensometer
    R. membrane
    R. noncontact tonometer
    R. ophthalmodynamometer
    R. radius gauge
    R. refractor
    R. slit lamp
Reichling corneal scissors
reimplantation
Reinecke-Carroll lacrimal tube

reinforcement
scleral r.
Reinverting Operating Lens System (ROLS)
Reis-Bücklers
R.-B. disease
R.-B. ring-shaped dystrophy
R.-B. superficial corneal dystrophy
Reisinger lens-extracting forceps
Reisman sign
Reiss punctal punch
Reiter
R. conjunctivitis
R. disease
R. syndrome
rejection
allograft corneal r.
r. line
Rekoss disk
relapsing polychondritis
relationship
agonist-antagonist r.
object/image r.
relative
r. accommodation
r. afferent pupillary defect (RAPD)
r. amblyopia
r. convergence
r. divergence
first-degree r.
r. hemianopsia
r. hyperopia
near-point r.
r. scotoma
second-degree r.
r. size
r. spectacle magnification
r. strabismus
relaxing incision
relay
retino-tecto-pulvino-cortical r.
releasable suture
release
r. hallucination

r. of traction for hypotony and vitreoretinopathy
Relief
R. Ophthalmic Solution
relucency
REM
rapid eye movement
remnant
persistent pupillary membrane r.
pupillary membrane r.
remodeling
corneal stromal r.
Remote Vision electronic refractor
remotum
punctum r. (p.r.)
removal
r. of foreign body
r. of foreign body operation
lens r.
remover
Alger brush rust ring r.
Bailey foreign body r.
DMV II contact lens r.
frog cortex r.
Soft Mate protein r.
Remy separator
renal
r. diabetes
r. retinitis
r. retinopathy
r. ultrasound
Renewed
Tears R.
renin-angiotensin system
ReNu
R. Effervescent enzymatic cleaner
R. Multi-Purpose
R. Thermal enzymatic cleaner
repair
Arlt epicanthus r.
Arlt eyelid r.
Blair epicanthus r.
blepharochalasis r.
blepharoptosis r.
Jones r.

R

NOTES

425

repair *(continued)*
  Kuhnt-Junius r.
  lacrimal gland r.
  levator aponeurosis r.
  medial canthal r.
  trichiasis r.
  Wheeler halving r.
reparative giant cell granuloma
repens
  Dirofilaria r.
replaceable blade
replacer
  Green iris r.
  Smith-Fisher iris r.
replamineform process
reposited
repositioning
repositor
  iris r.
  Knapp iris r.
  Nettleship iris r.
Rescula
resection
  levator r.
  Mohs microsurgical r.
  muscle r.
  r. of muscle
  Peyman full-thickness eye-
    wall r.
  scleral r.
  wedge r.
reserve
  base-in r.
  base-out r.
  divergence r.
  fusional r.
residual
  r. accommodation
  r. astigmatism
  r. cortex
  r. vision
resilience
  orbital r.
resistance
  impact r.
  insulin r.
  outflow r.
resistive index
resistor
  Guardian scalpel with
    myoguard depth r.
Resochin

resolution
  r. acuity
  r. acuity perimetry
  logarithmic Minimum Angle
    of R. (logMAR)
Resolve/GP
resolving power
resorption
  spontaneous r.
**Resource-Based Relative Value
  Scale (RBRVS)**
response
  accommodation r.
  accommodative r.
  acquired immune r.
  allergic r.
  cone r.
  consensual light r.
  consensual pupillary r.
  curve r.
  direct-light r.
  direct pupillary r.
  eosinophilic r.
  flare r.
  immune r.
  mononuclear r.
  near r.
  oculocalorie r.
  partial r.
  pattern visual-evoked r.
    (PVER)
  polymorphonuclear r.
  pupillary near r.
  rod b-wave r.
  synkinetic near r.
  trabecular meshwork-inducible
    glucocorticoid r. (TIGR)
  vestibulo-ocular r. (VOR)
  visual-evoked r. (VER)
  visual-vestibulo-ocular r.
restoration
  Berens-Smith cul-de-sac r.
  r. point
restricting strand
restrictive syndrome
result
  false-negative r.
  false-positive r.
reticle
  hand-held magnifying r.
reticular
  r. cystoid degeneration
  r. dystrophy

r. haze
r. keratitis
r. plate
reticulum
r. cell
r. cell lymphoma
r. cell sarcoma
endoplasmic r.
extraconal fat r.
fat r.
rough endoplasmic r.
retina
angiomatosis of r.
arteriosclerosis of r.
avascular peripheral r.
central r.
central fovea of r.
cerebral layer of r.
cerebral stratum of r.
cholesterol emboli of r.
coloboma of r.
concussion of the r.
r. cyanosis
deep r.
demarcation line of r.
detached r.
detachment of r.
disciform degeneration of r.
disinserted r.
disinsertion of r.
dragged r.
dysplastic r.
falciform fold of r.
fat embolism of r.
flecked r.
ganglionic layer of r.
ganglionic stratum of r.
ganglion layer of r.
giant cyst of r.
glioma of r.
inferior zone of r.
inflammatory changes of r.
inner r.
ischemic r.
juxtapapillary r.
lattice degeneration of r.
leopard r.

lipemic r.
lower r.
medial arteriole of r.
medial venulae of r.
murine r.
nasal arteriole of r.
nasal venule of r.
neovascularization of r.
nerve layer of r.
neural r.
neuroepithelial layer of r.
neurosensory r.
outer r.
peripheral r.
physiologic r.
pigmented layer of r.
positional abnormalities of r.
postequatorial r.
primary perivasculitis of r.
reattachment of r.
rivalry of r.
sensory r.
separation of r.
shot-silk r.
R. Society classificationo
stiff r.
superior zone of r.
tear of r.
temporal arteriole of r.
temporal venule of r.
temporal zone of r.
tented-up r.
thrombosis in r.
tigroid r.
upper r.
vascularization elsewhere in the r. (VNE)
vessel abnormalities of r.
watered-silk r.
yellow spot of r.
retinae
albedo r.
angiomatosis r.
arteriola medialis r.
atrophia choroideae et r.
coloboma r.
commotio r.

NOTES

retinae *(continued)*
cyanosis r.
dialysis r.
ischemia r.
limbal luteus r.
macula r.
macula flava r.
macula lutea r.
ora serrata r.
pars caeca r.
pars ciliaris r.
pars iridica r.
pars nervosa r.
pars optica r.
pars pigmentosa r.
periphlebitis r.
ramollitio r.
rubeosis r.
stratum cerebrale r.
striae r.
sublatio r.
torpor r.
vasa sanguinea r.
vasculitis r.
vena centralis r.
venula medialis r.
retinal
r. abiotrophy
r. abnormality
r. adaptation
r. angiography
r. angiomatosis
r. anlage tumor
r. aplasia
r. apoplexy
r. arterial filling
r. arterial occlusion
r. arteriole
r. arteriovenous malformation
r. artery
r. artery aneurysm
r. artery occlusion
r. asthenopia
r. astrocytoma
r. atresia
r. axon
r. blood
r. blur spot
r. break
r. burn
r. camera
r. capillaritis
r. capillary bed

r. capillary nonperfusion
r. circinate
r. circulation
r. cone
r. cone dystrophy
r. correspondence
r. cryopexy
r. cryotherapy
r. crystal
r. cyst
r. degeneration slow (RDS) gene
r. dehiscence
r. demarcation band
r. detachment (RD)
r. detachment hook
r. detachment pencil
r. detachment syringe
r. dialysis
r. disease
r. disorder
r. disparity
r. dragging
r. dysplasia
r. edema
r. element
r. ellipsometer
r. embolism
r. epithelial pigment hyperplasia
r. error
r. excavation
r. exudate
r. fixed fold
r. flap
r. foveola
r. ganglion
r. ganglion cell layer
r. Gelfilm implant
r. gliocyte
r. glioma
r. gliosarcoma
r. gliosis
r. hemorrhage
r. hole
r. horseshoe tear
r. hypoxia
r. ice ball
r. image
r. image size
r. imbrication
r. ischemia
r. isomerase

R

r. laser photocoagulation
r. lattice degeneration
r. lesion
r. macroaneurysm
r. microcirculation
r. microembolism
r. micropsia
r. migraine
r. montage
r. necrosis
r. necrosis syndrome
r. nerve fiber layer (RNFL)
r. nerve fiber myelination
r. neuron
r. neurotransmitter
r. periphlebitis
r. perivasculitis
r. phlebitis
r. pigmentary dystrophy
r. pigment epithelial atrophy
r. pigment epithelial defect
r. pigment epithelial
  hypertrophy
r. pigment epitheliitis
r. pigment epitheliopathy
r. pigment epithelium (RPE)
r. pigment epithelium dropout
r. pigment epithelium mottling
r. pigment epithelium serous
  detachment
r. points
r. probe sleeve
r. prophylaxis
r. quadrant neovascularization
r. rivalry
r. rod
r. scatter photocoagulation
r. spike
r. staphyloma
r. stress line
r. striation
r. surgery
r. tack
r. telangiectasia
r. telangiectasis
r. thrombosis
r. toxicity

r. translocation
r. tuft
r. vascular occlusion
r. vasculature
r. vasculitis
r. vein
r. vein occlusion
r. vein sheathing
r. venous beading
r. venous nicking
r. venous occlusion
r. venous pulse
r. venule
r. vessel
r. visual cell
r. whitening
r. wrinkling
r. zone

retinalis
  lipemia r.
retinal-slip velocity
retinascope
retinectomy
retinene isomerase
retinitis
  acquired toxoplasmosis r.
  actinic r.
  AIDS-related r.
  albuminuric r.
  apoplectic r.
  azotemic r.
  central angioplastic r.
  central angiospastic r.
  r. centralis serosa
  central serous r.
  r. circinata
  circinate r.
  Coats r.
  cytomegalovirus r.
  diabetic r.
  r. disciformans
  r. exudativa
  exudative r.
  foveomacular r.
  gravid r.
  r. gravidarum
  gravidic r.

NOTES

429

retinitis *(continued)*
r. haemorrhagica
herpes simplex r.
hypertensive r.
Jacobson r.
Jensen r.
leukemic r.
metastatic r.
necrotizing r.
r. nephritica
peripheral necrotizing r.
Pick r.
r. pigmentosa (RP)
r. pigmentosa GTPase regulator
gene (RPGR)
r. pigmentosa inversa
r. pigmentosa sine pigmento
r. proliferans
proliferating r.
proliferative r.
r. punctata albescens
punctate r.
purulent r.
recurrent central r.
renal r.
rubella r.
r. sclopetaria
secondary r.
septic r.
serous r.
simple r.
solar r.
splenic r.
r. stellata
striate r.
suppurative r.
syphilitic r.
r. syphilitica
uremic r.
Wagener r.
X-linked r.
retinoblastoma
bilateral sporadic r.
r. cell
familial r.
intraocular r.
r. locus
macular r.
Reese-Ellsworth group V r.
Reese-Ellsworth stage IIIA r.
trilateral r.
unilateral sporadic r.
retinocerebellar angiomatosis

retinochiasmatic
retinochoroid
retinochoroidal
r. atrophy
r. coloboma
r. infarction
r. layer
retinochoroidectomy
retinochoroiditis
birdshot r.
infectious r.
r. juxtapapillaris
toxoplasmic r.
retinochoroidopathy
birdshot r.
central serous r.
retinocortical
r. projection
retinocytoma
retinodialysis
Rétinofocomètre
retinogeniculate pathway
retinogeniculostriate projection
retinograph
retinography
retinoid
retinoillumination
retinoma
retinomalacia
Retinomax
R. cordless hand-held
autorefractor
R. K-Plus
autorefractor/keratometer
R. refractometry instrument
retinometer
Heine Lambda 100 r.
retinomigraine
Retinopan 45 camera
retinopapillitis of premature infants
retinopathy
acute zonal occult outer r.
(AZOOR)
angiopathic r.
arteriosclerotic r.
background diabetic r. (BDR)
birdshot r.
blood-and-thunder r.
bull's eye r.
cancer-associated r. (CAR,
CAR syndrome)
canthaxanthine crystalline r.
carbon monoxide r.

carotid occlusive disease r.
cellophane r.
central angioplastic r.
central angiospastic r.
central disk-shaped r.
central serous r. (CSR)
chloroquine r.
chloroquine/hydroxychloro-
quine r.
circinate r.
CMV r.
compression r.
crystalline r.
diabetic r. (DR)
drug abuse r.
dysoric r.
dysproteinemic r.
eclamptic r.
eclipse r.
electric r.
external exudative r.
exudative r.
foveomacular r.
gold dust r.
gravidic r.
r. hemorrhage
hemorrhagic r.
herpetic necrotizing r.
hypertensive r. (HR)
hypotensive r.
inflammatory r.
ischemic r.
Keith-Wagener r.
Leber idiopathic stellate r.
leukemic r.
lipemic r.
macular r.
melanoma-associated r.
necrotizing r.
nonproliferative r.
nonproliferative diabetic r.
(NPDR)
optic disk drusen r.
paraneoplastic r.
particulate r.
pigmentary r.
pneumatic r.

r. of prematurity (ROP)
prematurity r.
preproliferative diabetic r.
(PPDR)
proliferative diabetic r. (PDR)
proliferative lupus r.
proliferative sickle-cell r.
punctata albescens r.
Purtscher angiopathic r.
radiation r.
renal r.
rubella r.
salt-and-pepper r.
serous r.
sickle cell r.
solar r.
stellate r.
surface wrinkling r.
syphilitic r.
tamoxifen r.
tapetoretinal r.
toxemic r. of pregnancy
toxic r.
traumatic r.
Valsalva r.
Van Heuven r.
vascular r.
venous stasis r. (VSR)
venous stenosis r.
vitrectomy for proliferative r.
Wisconsin Epidemiologic Study
of Diabetic R. (WESDR)
X-linked juvenile r.

retinopexy
cyanoacrylate r.
pneumatic r.
transscleral r.

retinopiesis
retinoschisis
acquired r.
age-related r.
bullous r.
congenital r.
degenerative r.
familial foveal r.
juvenile r.
senescent r.

R

NOTES

retinoschisis *(continued)*
senile r.
X-linked juvenile r.
retinoscope
Copeland streak r.
Ful-Vue spot r.
Ful-Vue streak r.
Keeler r.
luminous r.
Priestley-Smith r.
reflecting r.
Reichert Ful-Vue spot r.
spot r.
streak r.
retinoscopy
Copeland r.
cylinder r.
dark r.
fogging r.
monocular-estimate-method
dynamic r.
noncycloplegic distance
static r.
static r.
streak r.
retinosis
retino-tecto-pulvino-cortical relay
retinotomy
retinotopic
r. stimulus
retinotoxic
retraction
congenital myopathic eyelid r.
endocrine lid r.
eyelid r.
flap r.
lid r.
mechanical lid r.
mesencephalic lid r.
myopathic eyelid r.
neuromuscular eyelid r.
neuropathic eyelid r.
r. nystagmus
spontaneous eyelid r.
r. syndrome
thyroid lid r.
vitreous r.
retractor
Agrikola lacrimal sac r.
Alexander-Ballen r.
Amenabar iris r.
Amoils r.
angled iris r.

Arruga elevator r.
Arruga orbital r.
Ballen-Alexander orbital r.
Barraquer-Krumeich-Swinger r.
Bechert-Kratz cannulated
nucleus r.
Berens lid r.
Blair r.
Brawley r.
Bronson-Turtz r.
Campbell r.
Castallo r.
Castroviejo lid r.
Coleman r.
conjunctiva r.
Converse double-ended alar r.
Conway lid r.
Coston-Trent iris r.
deep blunt rake r.
Desmarres lid r.
Drews-Rosenbaum iris r.
Duane r.
Eliasoph lid r.
Elschnig r.
eyelid r.
Fasanella r.
Ferris-Smith r.
Ferris-Smith-Sewall r.
Fink lacrimal r.
Fisher lid r.
flexible translimbal iris r.
Forker r.
Fullerview iris r.
Givner lid r.
Goldstein lacrimal sac r.
Good r.
Gradle r.
Graether collar-button micro-
iris r.
Grieshaber flexible iris r.
Groenholm r.
Gross r.
Harrington r.
Harrison r.
Hartstein irrigating iris r.
Helveston Great Big Barbie r.
Hill r.
Hillis r.
Jaeger r.
Jaffe-Givner lid r.
Jaffe lid r.
Kaufman type II r.
Keeler-Fison tissue r.

Keeler-Rodger iris r.
Keizer-Lancaster lid r.
Kelman iris r.
Kirby lid r.
Knapp lacrimal sac r.
Kronfeld r.
Kuglein r.
lacrimal sac r.
lower lid r.
MacVicar double-end
 strabismus r.
McCool capsule r.
McGannon r.
Meller lacrimal sac r.
Mueller lacrimal sac r.
Nevyas r.
Oklahoma iris wire r.
Paul lacrimal sac r.
Payne r.
phoroptor r.
r. plication
Rizzuti iris r.
Rollet r.
Rosenbaum-Drews r.
Sanchez-Bulnes lacrimal sac r.
Sato lid r.
Schepens orbital r.
Schultz iris r.
self-adhering lid r.
self-retaining r.
Senn r.
Sewall r.
Stevens muscle hook r.
Stevenson lacrimal sac r.
Teflon iris r.
Thomas r.
Tiko pliable iris r.
Ultramatic Rx Master
 phoroptor r.
Vaiser-Cibis muscle r.
Vasco-Posada orbital r.
Visitec iris r.
Welsh iris r.
Wilder scleral r.
Wilmer r.
retrieval device

retriever
 Utrata r.
retroauricular complex graft
retrobulbar
 r. abscess
 r. akinesia
 r. alcohol injection
 r. anesthesia
 r. artery
 r. compressive lesion
 r. compressive optic
  neuropathy
 r. hemorrhage
 r. hemorrhage glaucoma
 r. ischemic optic neuropathy
 r. lid block
 r. needle
 r. neuritis
 r. optic neuritis
 r. space
retrochiasmal
 r. pathway
 r. visual field defect
 r. visual field loss
retrochiasmatic region
retrocorneal
 r. membrane
 r. nut
retrodisplacement
retroflexion of iris
retrogeniculate lesion
retrograde transsynaptic
 degeneration
retrohyaloid premacular hemorrhage
retroilluminate
retroillumination
retroiridian
retrolaminar
retrolental fibroplasia (RLF)
retrolenticular
retromembranous
retroocular space
retroorbital
 r. headache
retroplacement
retropupillary
retroscopic lens

NOTES

433

retrospective study
retrotarsal fold
Reuss
    R. color chart
    R. color table
Reverdin suture needle
reverse
    r. amblyopia
    r. bobbing
    r. dipping
    r. Marcus Gunn pupil
    r. optics
    r. pupillary block
reverse-cutting needle
reversed
    r. astigmatism
    r. ophthalmic artery flow
    (ROAF)
    r. pupillary reflex
reverse-shape implant
reversible
    r. amblyopia
    r. lid speculum
Rēv-Eyes
Revolution lens
Rey-Osterreith Complex Figure
RGP
    rigid gas-permeable contact lens
rhabdoid tumor
rhabdomyosarcoma
    orbital r.
rhegmatogenous retinal detachment
    (RRD)
Rhein
    R. Advantage diamond knife
    R. capsulorrhexis cystotome
    forceps
    R. clear corneal diamond knife
    R. 3-D trapezoid diamond
    blade
    R. fine foldable lens-insertion
    forceps
    R. reusable cautery pen
Rhese position
rheumatic nodule
rheumatoid
    r. related ulceration
    r. sclerouveitis
rheumatoid-associated nuclear
  antigen
rhinitis
    acute catarrhal r.
    allergic r.

atrophic r.
r. caseosa
chronic catarrhal r.
croupous r.
dyscrinic r.
fibrinous r.
gangrenous r.
hypertrophic r.
membranous r.
pseudomembranous r.
purulent r.
scrofulous r.
r. sicca
syphilitic r.
tuberculous r.
rhinocanthectomy
rhinoconjunctivitis
    perennial r.
    seasonal r.
rhinodacryolith
rhino-orbital mucormycosis
rhinophyma
rhinoplasty
rhinoscleroma
rhinosporidiosis
Rhinosporidium seeberi
rhinotomy
rhodogenesis
rhodophylactic
rhodophylaxis
rhodopsin
Rhus
    R. radicans
    R. toxicodendron
rhytids
    eyelid r.
ribbon gauze dressing
ribbon-like keratitis
Riccò law
Rice pick
Richard pillow
Richet operation
rickettsial blepharitis
Riddoch
    R. phenomenon
    R. syndrome
ridge
    laser r.
    r. lens
    mesenchymal r.
    petrous r.
    supraorbital r.
    synaptic r.

riding bow temple
Ridley
    R. anterior chamber lens
      implant
    R. lens
    R. Mark II lens implant
Riedel
    R. needle
    R. thyroiditis
Rieger
    R. anomaly
    R. syndrome
Rifkind sign
rifle
    air r.
right
    r. deorsumvergence
    r. deviation
    r. esotropia
    r. exotropia
    r. eye (OD)
    r. gaze
    r. gaze verticals
    r. hyperphoria
    r. hypertropia
    r. sursumvergence
right-angle
    r.-a. deflected venule
    r.-a. prism
right-beating nystagmus
right-handed cornea scissors
right/left corneoscleral scissors
rigid
    r. contact lens
    r. gas-permeable
    r. gas-permeable contact lens
    (RGP)
    r. pupil
rigidity
    mydriatic r.
    ocular r.
    scleral r.
Riley-Smith syndrome
rim
    inferior orbital r.
    neural r.
    neuroretinal r.

    orbital inferior r.
    saucering of r.
rima
    r. cornealis
    r. palpebrarum
rimexolone ophthalmic suspension
rimless frame
rim-to-disk ratio
ring
    abscess r.
    r. abscess
    annular r.
    anterior limiting r.
    Bloomberg SuperNumb
      anesthetic r.
    Bonaccolto-Flieringa scleral r.
    Bonaccolto scleral r.
    Bores twist fixation r.
    Burr corneal r.
    Caspar r.
    cataract mask r.
    r. cataract mask eye shield
    centering r.
    choroidal r.
    ciliary r.
    Coats white r.
    collagenolytic trabecular r.
    collagenous trabecular r.
    common tendinous r.
    conjunctival r.
    corneal transplant centering r.
    R. D chromosome syndrome
    Döllinger tendinous r.
    Donders r.
    Fine-Thornton scleral
      fixation r.
    fixation r.
    fixation/anchor r.
    Fleischer keratoconus r.
    Fleischer-Strumpell r.
    Flieringa fixation r.
    Flieringa-Kayser copper r.
    Flieringa-Kayser fixation r.
    Flieringa-LeGrand fixation r.
    Flieringa scleral r.
    r. forceps
    Girard scleral-expander r.

R

NOTES

435

ring *(continued)*
glaucomatous r.
glial r.
immune Wessely r.
r. infiltrate
Intacs r.
intracorneal r.
intrastromal corneal r.
r. of iris
iris r.
iron Fleischer r.
Kayser-Fleischer corneal r.
r. keratitis
KeraVision r.
Klein-Tolentino r.
Landers irrigating vitrectomy r.
Landers vitrectomy r.
Landolt broken r.
Landolt C r.
LED-illuminated r.
r. lens expressor
lenticular r.
light reflex r.
Lowe r.
Martinez corneal transplant
  centering r.
Maxwell r.
McKinney fixation r.
McNeill-Goldmann r.
Nichamin fixation r.
nuclear r.
r. perimetry
placido r.
polymer r.
posterior limiting r.
prominent Schwalbe r.
rust r.
Saturn r.
Schwalbe anterior border r.
scleral expander r.
r. scotoma
scotoma r.
Soemmering r.
r. of Soemmering
suction r.
symblepharon r.
Tano r.
tantalum "O" r.
Thornton-Fine r.
Thornton fixating r.
Tolentino r.
r. ulcer

r. ulcer of cornea
Villasenor-Navarro fixation r.
Vossius lenticular r.
Weiss r.
Wessely r.
white r.
Zinn r.
Ringer lactate solution
ring-form congenital cataract
ring-like corneal dystrophy
ring-shaped
  r.-s. cataract
  r.-s. dystrophy
  r.-s. stromal infiltrate
ring-tip forceps
Riolan muscle
Ripault sign
rip-cord suture
ripe cataract
Risley rotary prism
Ritch
  R. contact lens
  R. nylon suture laser lens
  R. trabeculoplasty laser lens
**Ritch-Krupin-Denver eye valve-
  insertion forceps**
Ritleng probe
Ritter fiber
rivalry
  binocular r.
  r. of retina
  retinal r.
river blindness
rivus lacrimalis
Rizzuti
  R. fixation forceps
  R. graft carrier spoon
  R. iris retractor
  R. lens expressor
  R. rectus forceps
  R. refractor
  R. scleral fixation forceps
Rizzuti-Bonaccolto instrument
Rizzuti-Fleischer instrument
**Rizzuti-Furniss cornea-holding
  forceps**
Rizzuti-Kayser-Fleischer instrument
Rizzuti-Lowe instrument
Rizzuti-Maxwell instrument
**Rizzuti-McGuire corneal section
  scissors**
Rizzuti-Soemmering instrument

Rizzuti-Spizziri
R.-S. cannula knife
R.-S. knife
RK
radial keratotomy
RK marker
RLF
retrolental fibroplasia
RLX
R. coating
R. lens
RNFL
retinal nerve fiber layer
ROAF
reversed ophthalmic artery flow
Roaf syndrome
ROAM
roaming optical access multiscope
roaming optical access multiscope (ROAM)
Robertson
R. pupil
R. sign
Roberts-SC phocomelia
Robin chalazion clamp
Robinow syndrome
Rochat test
Rochon-Duvigneaud
bouquet of R.-D.
R.-D. bouquet of cones
rod
r. achromatopsia
bipolar r.
r. b-wave amplitude
r. b-wave response
r. cell
r. and cone dystrophy
r.'s and cones
r. electroretinogram
r. fiber
r. function
graceful swirling r.
r. granule
Maddox r.
Mira silicone r.
r. monochromasy
r. monochromat

r. monochromatism
r. myopathy
Perspex r.
retinal r.
scleral sponge r.
silicone r.
Viers r.
vision r.
r. vision
rod-cone
r.-c. amplitude
r.-c. degeneration
r.-c. dysfunction
r.-c. dystrophy
Rodenstock
R. eye refractometer
R. panfundoscope
R. panfundus lens
R. scanning laser ophthalmoscope
R. slit lamp
R. system
rodent ulcer
Rodin orbital implant
roentgenogram
orbital r.
Rolf
R. dilator
R. forceps
R. lacrimal probe
R. lance
roll
FLUFTEX gauze r.
iris r.
peripheral iris r.
scleral r.
rolled-up epithelium with wavy border
roller forceps
Rollet
R. irrigating/aspirating unit
R. lacrimal probe
R. refractor
R. retractor
R. rougine
R. syndrome

NOTES

437

rolling
    counter r.
    r. of eyes
ROLS
    Reinverting Operating Lens System
Romaña sign
Romberg
    R. sign
    R. syndrome
Rommel
    R. cautery
    R. electrocautery
Rommel-Hildreth
    R.-H. cautery
    R.-H. electrocautery
RON
    radiation optic neuropathy
Rondec
    R. Drops
    R. Filmtab
    R. Syrup
Rondec-TR
rongeur
    Belz lacrimal sac r.
    biting r.
    bone r.
    Citelli r.
    Kerrison mastoid r.
    lacrimal sac r.
    Lempert r.
    single-action r.
Ronne nasal step
roof
    r. fracture
    r. of orbit
    orbital r.
RO Optho
root
    iris r.
    motor r.
    oculomotor r.
    sensory r.
ROP
    retinopathy of prematurity
Roper alpha-chymotrypsin cannula
Roper-Hall
    R.-H. localizer
    R.-H. locator
ropy mucus
Rosa-Berens orbital implant
rosacea
    acne r.

    blepharitis r.
    blepharoconjunctivitis r.
    keratitis r.
    r. keratitis
    ocular r.
Roscoe-Bunsen law
roseata
    iritis r.
rose bengal red solution
Rosen
    R. nucleus paddle
    R. phaco splitter
Rosenbach sign
Rosenbaum
    R. card
    R. pocket vision screener
Rosenbaum-Drews retractor
Rosenblatt scissors
Rosenburg operation
Rosengren operation
Rosenmüller
    R. body
    R. gland
    R. node
    R. valve
    valve of R.
Rosets
rosette
    Flexner-Wintersteiner r.
    Homer-Wright r.
    Wintersteiner r.
Rosner tonometer
rostral
    r. interstitial medial
        longitudinal fasciculus
    r. interstitial nucleus
rotary
    r. cutting tip
    r. nystagmus
    r. prism
rotating brush
rotating-type cutter
rotation
    center of r.
    r. center
    eye r.
    r. nystagmus
    suture r.
    wheel r.
rotational
    r. nystagmus
    r. test

rotator
Bechert nucleus r.
Jaffe-Bechert nucleus r.
rotatory nystagmus
Roth
R. spot
R. spot syndrome
Roth-Bielschowsky
R.-B. deviation
R.-B. syndrome
Rothman Gilbard cornea punch
Rothmund syndrome
Rothmund-Thomson syndrome
rotoextractor
Douvas r.
rotundum foramen
Rouget muscle
rough endoplasmic reticulum
rougine
Rollet r.
round
r. hemorrhage
r. top bifocal
route
canalicular r.
external r.
transconjunctival r.
Roveda
R. lid everter
R. operation
roving eye movement
Rowbotham operation
Rowen spatula
Rowinski operation
Rowland keratome
Rowsey fixation cannula
RP
retinitis pigmentosa
RP hypertrophy
RP sine pigmento
RPE
retinal pigment epithelium
hemorrhagic RPE
RPGR
retinitis pigmentosa GTPase
regulator gene

R&R
recession-resection
recess-resect
RRD
rhegmatogenous retinal detachment
Rubbrecht operation
rubella
r. cataract
r. retinitis
r. retinopathy
rubeola
r. conjunctivitis
r. keratitis
rubeosis
iridis r.
r. iridis
r. iridis diabetica
r. retinae
rubeotic glaucoma
Rubin-Holth punch
Rubinstein
R. cryoextractor
R. cryophake
R. cryoprobe
ruby
r. diamond knife
r. laser
Rucker body
rudimentary eye
rudiment lens
Ruedemann
R. eye implant
R. lacrimal dilator
R. operation
R. tonometer
Ruedemann-Todd tendon tucker
ruff
papillary r.
ruffed canal
Ruggeri reflex
Ruiz
R. fundus contact lens
R. fundus laser lens
R. microkeratome
R. plano fundus lens implant
R. procedure
R. trapezoidal keratotomy

R

NOTES

Ruiz-Nordan trapezoidal marker
rule
    accommodation r.
    astigmatism with the r.
    Behren r.
    Kestenbaum r.
    Knapp r.
    Kollner r.
    Krimsky-Prince
      accommodation r.
    Luedde transparent r.
    Pischel scleral r.
    Prentice r.
    Prince r.
ruler
    biometric r.
    Bio-Pen biometric r.
    Helveston scleral marking r.
    Hyde astigmatism r.
    Hyde-Osher keratometric r.
    Scott No. 2 curved r.
    Weck astigmatism r.
Rumex titanium instrument
Rumison side port fixation occluder
running nylon penetrating
   keratoplasty suture
rupture
    choroidal r.
    indirect choroidal r.

    scleral r.
    traumatic choroidal r.
ruptured globe
Rushton ocular measurement
Russell
    R. body
    R. syndrome
Russian
    R. forceps
    R. four-pronged fixation hook
rust
    r. ring
    r. ring of cornea
    r. spot
Rutherford syndrome
Ruysch
    R. membrane
    R. tunic
ruyschiana
    membrana r.
ruyschian membrane
RV275
    Tracoustic R.
Rycroft
    R. cannula
    R. needle
    R. operation
    R. tying forceps

S
spherical lens
S cone excitation
S potential
S-100 protein antibody
S5-1804-HUMER lens-folding forceps
Sabin-Feldman dye test
Sabouraud medium
Sabreloc needle
saburral
s. amaurosis
s. amaurosis fugax
sac
conjunctival s.
diverticulum of lacrimal s.
drainage of lacrimal s.
Förster lacrimal s.
lacrimal s.
nasolacrimal s.
tear s.
saccade
hypometric s.
ocular s.
s. palsy
scanning s.
slow-to-no s.
saccadic
s. abnormality
s. contrapulsion
s. dysmetria
s. eccentric target
s. eye movement
s. intrusion
s. movements of eye
s. pulse
s. pursuit
s. velocity
saccadomania
saccular aneurysm
sacculus lacrimalis
saccus
s. conjunctivae
s. conjunctivalis
s. lacrimalis
Sachs tissue forceps
saddle
s. bridge
Turkish s.

Saemisch
S. operation
S. section
S. ulcer
Saenger
S. pupil
S. sign
Safar operation
safety
s. glasses
s. lens
s. spectacles
Safil synthetic absorbable surgical suture
Safir Ophthalmetron
sagittal
s. axis
s. axis of eye
s. axis of Fick
s. depth
s. height
SAI
surface asymmetry index
Sainton sign
Sakler erysiphake
saline
Blairex sterile s.
Hydrocare preserved s.
hypertonic s.
Lens Plus s.
Murine sterile s.
phosphate-buffered s.
s.-saturated wool dressing
Soft Mate s.
s. solution
sorbic acid Sorbi-Care s.
salivary
s. gland
s. nucleus
salmon
s. patch
s. patch hue
salmon-patch hemorrhage
salt-and-pepper
s.-a.-p. appearance
s.-a.-p. fundus
s.-a.-p. retinopathy
Salus
S. arch
S. sign

S

Salzmann
S. nodular corneal degeneration
S. nodular corneal dystrophy
S. nodule
Salz nuclear splitter
Samoan conjunctivitis
Sampaoelesi line
sampling error
Sanchez-Bulnes lacrimal sac
retractor
Sanchez-Salorio syndrome
Sanders
S. disease
S. disorder
S. operation
Sanders-Castroviejo suturing forceps
Sanders-Retzlaff-Kraff formula
(SRK)
SANDO
sensory ataxic neuropathy with
dysarthria and ophthalmoplegia
Sand process
Sandt forceps
sanguineous cataract
Sanson image
Sanyal conjunctivitis
Sappey fiber
sapphire knife
saprophytic bacteria
saprophyticus
Staphylococcus s.
saquinavir sulfate
sarcoid
Boeck s.
s. uveitis
sarcoidosis
s. infiltration
pediatric ocular s.
sarcoidosis-associated uveitis
sarcoma, pl. sarcomata
Ewing s.
granulocytic s.
hemorrhagic s.
Kaposi s.
melanotic s.
multifocal hemorrhagic s.
reticulum cell s.
sarcomatosum
ectropion s.
glioma s.
s. senilis
s. spasticum
s. uveae

satellite
s. cell
s. lesion
SatinCrescent implant knife
SatinShortCut implant knife
SatinSlit implant knife
Sato
S. cataract needle
S. corneal knife
S. keratoconus
S. lid retractor
S. operation
S. procedure
Satoyoshis syndrome
Sattler
S. layer
S. veil
saturated color
saturation
color s.
SaturEyes contact lens
Saturn
S. II contact lenses
S. ring
saturninus
halo s.
saucering of rims
saucerization
saucer-shaped cataract
Sauer
S. corneal debrider
S. infant speculum
S. suture forceps
Sauflon
S. lens
S. PW lens
Sauvineau ophthalmoplegia
Saverburger irrigation/aspiration tip
Savin
S. operation
S. procedure
saw
Stryker s.
Sayoc
S. operation
S. procedure
SBV
single binocular vision
SC
stem cell
s̄c
without correction

scaffolding
    capillary s.
scale

    Activities of Daily Vision S.
    Esterman s.
    Fitzpatrick sun-sensitivity s.
    Klyce/Wilson s.
    Resource-Based Relative
      Value S. (RBRVS)
    Snell-Sterling visual
      efficiency s.
scalloped
    s. border
    s. contours
    s. pupil
scalloping
scalpel
    s. guard
    Guyton-Lundsgaard s.
    Microcap s.
    Myocure blade s.
ScalpelTec
    S. phaco keratome slit blade
    S. wound-enlargement blade
scalp flap
scaly plaque
scan
    A-s.
    axial CT s.
    choroidal s.
    computed tomography s.
    Contact A-s.
    contact B-s.
    coronal CT s.
    cross-vector A-s.
    duplex s.
    gallium s.
    isotope s.
    limited gallium s.
    magnetic resonance imaging s.
    MRI s.
    Opthascan Mini-A s.
    orbital CT s.
    radioisotope s.
    technetium s.
    Ultra-Image A-s.

scanner
    Dine digital s.
    Heidelberg laser tomographic s.
    laser tomography s. (LST)
scanning
    s. excimer laser
    gallium s.
    s. laser glaucoma test
    s. laser ophthalmoscope (SLO)
    S. Laser Ophthalmoscope
      perimetry
    s. laser polarimeter
    s. laser polarimetry
    s. prism
    s. saccade
    s. slit confocal microscope
scar
    corneal s.
    disciform macular s.
    facetted corneal s.
    gray-white corneal s.
    herpes simplex s.
    linear s.
    peripapillary s.
    s. plate
    punched-out chorioretinal s.
    vascularized s.
scarification
scarifier
    Desmarres s.
    s. knife
    Kuhnt corneal s.
Scarpa staphyloma
scarring
    bulbar conjunctival s.
    conjunctival s.
    corneal s.
    episcleral s.
    ghost s.
    gossamer s.
    linear s.
    quiescent stromal s.
    stromal ghost s.
    subretinal s.
scatter
    beam s.
    forward light s.

NOTES

S

scatter *(continued)*
 light s.
 s. pattern
 peripheral light s.
 s. photocoagulation
 sclerotic s.
scattergram
scattering
 light s.
 Rayleigh s.
 reflective s.
scatterplot
SCH
 suprachoroidal hemorrhage
Schaaf foreign body forceps
Schachar lens
Schacher ganglion
Schachne-Desmarres lid everter
Schaedel cross-action towel clamp
Schaefer
 S. fixation forceps
 S. sponge holder
Schaffer sign
Scharf lens
Schaumann inclusion body
Scheie
 S. akinesia
 S. anterior chamber cannula
 S. blade
 S. cataract-aspirating cannula
 S. cataract-aspirating needle
 S. classification
 S. electrocautery
 S. goniopuncture knife
 S. goniotomy knife
 S. operation
 S. ophthalmic cautery
 S. syndrome
 S. technique
 S. thermal sclerostomy
 S. trephine
Scheie-Graefe fixation forceps
Scheie-Westcott corneal section
 scissors
Scheimpflug
 S. photography
 S. principle
 S. slit image
 S. videophotography system
Scheiner
 S. experiment
 S. principle
Scheiner theories

schematic eye
schenckii
 Sporothrix s.
Schepens
 S. binocular indirect
 ophthalmoscope
 S. electrode
 S. forceps
 S. Gelfilm
 S. hollow hemisphere implant
 S. operation
 S. orbital retractor
 S. refractor
 S. retinal detachment unit
 S. scleral depressor
 S. spoon
 S. technique
 S. thimble depressor
Schepens-Pomerantzeff
 ophthalmoscope
scheroma
Schillinger suture support
Schimek operation
Schiötz
 S. tonofilm
 S. tonometer
Schirmer
 S. filter paper
 S. operation
 S. syndrome
 S. tear quality test
 S. tear test strip
 S. 1 test
 S. test I
 S. test II
schisis
 s. cavity
schisis-related detachment
schistosa
 Enhydrina s.
Schlegel lens
schleiferi
 Staphylococcus s.
Schlemm
 canal of S.
 S. canal
Schlichting dystrophy
Schlieren phenomenon
Schmalz operation
Schmid-Fraccaro syndrome
Schmidt keratitis
Schmincke tumor

Schnabel
S. cavern
S. optic atrophy
Schnaitmann bifocal
Schnidt clamp
Schnyder crystalline corneal
dystrophy
Schöbl scleritis
Schocket
S. anterior chamber tube shunt
S. scleral depressor
S. tube implant
Schöler treatment
Schön theory
school myopia
Schott lid speculum
Schultz
S. fiber basket
S. iris retractor
Schumann giant type eye magnet
Schwalbe
S. anterior border ring
S. line (SL)
S. space
Schwann
S. cell
cords of S.
schwannoma
malignant s.
melanotic s.
Schwartz-Jampel syndrome
Schwartz syndrome
Schweigger
S. capsule forceps
S. extracapsular forceps
S. hand perimeter
scieropia
scimitar scotoma
scintillans
synchesis s.
scintillating
s. granule
s. scotoma
s. vision loss
scintillation
scintillography
lacrimal s.

scirrhencanthis
scirrhophthalmia
scissors
Aebli corneal section s.
alligator s.
anterior chamber synechia s.
Atkinson corneal s.
bandage s.
Barraquer-DeWecker s.
Barraquer iris s.
Barraquer vitreous strand s.
Becker corneal section
spatulated s.
Berens corneal transplant s.
Berens iridocapsulotomy s.
Berkeley Bioengineering
mechanized s.
Birks Mark II Instruments
micro trabeculectomy s.
Bonn iris s.
canalicular s.
capsulotomy s.
Castroviejo anterior synechia s.
Castroviejo corneal section s.
Castroviejo corneal
transplant s.
Castroviejo iridocapsulotomy s.
Castroviejo keratoplasty s.
Castroviejo synechia s.
Castroviejo-Vannas
capsulotomy s.
Cohan-Vannas iris s.
Cohan-Westcott s.
conjunctival s.
corneal section spatulated s.
corneal spatulated s.
corneoscleral right/left hand s.
curved iris s.
curved tenotomy s.
DeWecker iris s.
DeWecker-Pritikin s.
dissecting s.
enucleation s.
eye suture s.
Fine suture s.
Frost s.
Giardet corneal transplant s.

S

NOTES

scissors *(continued)*
Gill s.
Gill-Hess s.
Gills-Welsh s.
Gills-Welsh-Vannas angled
  micro s.
Girard corneoscleral s.
Glasscock s.
Grieshaber vertical cutting s.
Grieshaber vitreous s.
Guist enucleation s.
Haenig irrigating s.
Halsted strabismus s.
Harrison s.
Hoskins-Castroviejo corneal s.
Hoskins-Westcott tenotomy s.
House-Bellucci alligator s.
Huey s.
Hunt chalazion s.
iridectomy s.
iridocapsulotomy s.
iridotomy s.
iris s.
Irvine probe-pointed s.
Karakashian-Barraquer s.
Katzin s.
Keeler intravitreal s.
keratectomy s.
keratoplasty s.
Kirby s.
Knapp iris s.
Kramp s.
Kreiger-Spitznas vibrating s.
Lagrange sclerectomy s.
Lambert-Heiman s.
Lawton corneal s.
left-handed cornea s.
Lister s.
Littauer dissecting s.
Littler dissecting s.
Manson-Aebli corneal
  section s.
Mattis corneal s.
Maunoir iris s.
Max Fine s.
Mayo s.
McClure iris s.
McGuire corneal s.
McLean capsulotomy s.
McPherson-Castroviejo corneal
  section s.
McPherson corneal section s.
McPherson-Vannas microiris s.

McPherson-Westcott
  conjunctival s.
McPherson-Westcott stitch s.
McReynolds pterygium s.
mechanized s.
micro s.
micro Westcott s.
mini-keratoplasty stitch s.
Moore-Troutman corneal s.
s. movement
MPC automated intravitreal s.
Nadler superior radial s.
Noyes iridectomy s.
Noyes iris s.
Nugent-Gradle s.
O'Brien stitch s.
Ong capsulotomy s.
pterygium s.
ptosis s.
radial iridotomy s.
Reeh s.
Reichling corneal s.
right-handed cornea s.
right/left corneoscleral s.
Rizzuti-McGuire corneal
  section s.
Rosenblatt s.
Scheie-Westcott corneal
  section s.
Shield iridotomy s.
Smart s.
Spencer eye suture s.
Spring iris s.
Stevens eye s.
Stevens tenotomy s.
Storz-Westcott conjunctival s.
strabismus s.
straight tenotomy s.
superior radial tenotomy s.
Sutherland s.
Sutherland-Grieshaber s.
Thomas s.
Thorpe s.
Thorpe-Castroviejo s.
Thorpe-Westcott s.
Troutman-Castroviejo corneal
  section s.
Troutman conjunctival s.
Troutman-Katzin corneal
  transplant s.
Troutman microsurgical s.
Troutman suture s.
Vannas capsulotomy s.

Vannas iridocapsulotomy s.
Verhoeff s.
vibrating s.
vitreous strand s.
Walker s.
Walker-Apple s.
Walker-Atkinson s.
Werb s.
Westcott conjunctiva s.
Westcott stitch s.
Westcott tenotomy s.
Westcott utility s.
Wilmer conjunctival s.
Wincor enucleation s.
scissors-shadow
SCL
  soft contact lens
sclera, pl. **scleras, sclerae**
  bared s.
  baring of s.
  blue s.
  buckling s.
  ectasia of s.
  foramen of s.
  lamina cribrosa sclerae
  lamina fusca sclerae
  limbus of s.
  massive granuloma of s.
  melanosis sclerae
  sinus venosus s.
  sulcus s.
  white s.
scleral
  s. band
  s. blade
  s. buckle
  s. buckling
  s. buckling operation
  s. buckling procedure
  s. canal
  s. cautery
  s. channel
  s. contact lens
  s. crescent
  s. cyst
  s. degeneration
  s. depression

s. depressor
s. ectasia
s. exoplant
s. expander
s. expander ring
s. explant
s. explant surgery
s. fistula
s. fistulectomy operation
s. flap
s. flap suture
s. framework
s. furrow
s. grip
s. hook
s. icterus
s. implant
s. indentation
s. lamina cribrosa
s. lip
s. marker
s. miniflap
s. patch graft
s. pick
s. plexus
s. punch
s. reinforcement
s. resection
s. resection knife
s. rigidity
s. roll
s. rupture
s. search coil
s. search coil technique
s. shell
s. shell glaucoma
s. shortening clip
s. shortening operation
s. show
s. sponge rod
s. spur (SS)
s. staphyloma
s. substance
s. sulcus
s. supporter
s. tissue
s. trabecula

S

NOTES

scleral *(continued)*
  s. tunnel
  s. tunnel abscess
  s. tunnel incision
  s. twist
  s. twist-grip forceps
  s. venous sinus
  s. window
scleralis
  pars s.
scleralization
scleral-limbal-corneal incision
scleras (*pl. of* sclera)
scleratitis
sclerectasia
  partial s.
  total s.
sclerectasis
sclerectoiridectomy
sclerectoiridodialysis
sclerectome
sclerectomy
  holmium YAG laser s.
  Holth s.
  Iliff-House s.
  s. punch
  thermal s.
scleriasis
scleriritomy
scleritis
  annular s.
  anterior s.
  brawny s.
  deep s.
  diffuse anterior s.
  gelatinous s.
  herpes simplex s.
  idiopathic s.
  malignant s.
  s. necroticans
  necrotizing nodular s.
  posterior s.
  Schöbl s.
  syphilitic s.
sclerocataracta
sclerochoroiditis
  anterior s.
  posterior s.
scleroconjunctival
scleroconjunctivitis
sclerocornea

sclerocorneal
  s. junction
  s. sulcus
scleroiritis
sclerokeratectomy
sclerokeratitis
sclerokeratoiritis
sclerokeratoplasty
sclerokeratosis
sclerolimbus
scleromalacia perforans
scleronyxis
sclero-optic
sclerophthalmia
scleroplasty operation
sclerosing
  s. keratitis
  s. orbital granuloma
  s. panencephalitis chorioretinitis
sclerosis, *pl.* **scleroses**
  arteriolar s.
  central areolar choroidal s.
  central choroidal s.
  choroidal primary s.
  diffuse choroidal s.
  multiple s.
  nuclear s. (NS)
  peripapillary s.
  progressive systemic s.
  systemic s.
  tuberous s.
sclerostomy
  enzymatic s.
  holmium laser s.
  s. needle
  posterior thermal s.
  Scheie thermal s.
  thermal s.
  trabecuphine laser s.
sclerotic
  s. cataract
  s. coat
  s. scatter
  s. stroma
sclerotica
  tunica s.
scleroticectomy
scleroticochoroidal canal
scleroticochoroiditis
scleroticonyxis
scleroticopuncture
scleroticotomy
sclerotitis

sclerotome
  Alvis-Lancaster s.
  Atkinson s.
  Castroviejo s.
  Curdy s.
  Guyton-Lundsgaard s.
  Lundsgaard s.
  Lundsgaard-Burch s.
  Walker-Lee s.
sclerotomy
  anterior s.
  deep s.
  DeWecker anterior s.
  foreign body s.
  Lindner s.
  s. operation
  s. port
  posterior s.
  s. punch
  s. removal of foreign body
  s. with drainage
  s. with exploration
sclerouveitis
  rheumatoid s.
sclopetaria
  chorioretinitis s.
  retinitis s.
SCN
  suprachiasmatic nucleus
Scobee oblique muscle hook
scoop
  Arlt s.
  Daviel s.
  enucleation s.
  Kirby intraocular lens s.
  Knapp s.
  Lewis s.
  Mules s.
  Wilder s.
scope
  Bjerrum s.
  tangent s.
  Welch-Allyn Pocket s.
scopolamine hyoscine
scoria
scoterythrous vision
scotodinia

scotograph
scotoma, pl. **scotomata**
  absolute s.
  altitudinal s.
  annular s.
  arc s.
  arcuate Bjerrum s.
  aural s.
  bitemporal hemianopic s.
  Bjerrum s.
  cecocentral s.
  central s.
  centrocecal s.
  color s.
  comet s.
  congruous homonymous
    hemianopic s.
  cuneate-shaped s.
  double arcuate s.
  eclipse s.
  equatorial ring s.
  flittering s.
  focal s.
  frame s.
  glaucomatous nerve-fiber
    bundle s.
  hemianopic s.
  homonymous hemianopic s.
  insular s.
  ipsilateral centrocecal s.
  s. junction
  junction s.
  junctional s.
  Mariotte s.
  motile s.
  s. for motion
  negative s.
  paracentral ring s.
  pericentral s.
  peripapillary s.
  peripheral s.
  physiologic s.
  position s.
  positive s.
  quadrantic s.
  relative s.
  s. ring

NOTES

scotoma *(continued)*
ring s.
scimitar s.
scintillating s.
Seidel s.
sickle s.
superior arcuate s.
suppression s.
thin-rim s.
s. of Traquair
unilateral altitudinal s.
zonular s.
scotomagraph
scotomameter
scotomata (*pl. of* scotoma)
scotomatous
scotometer
Bjerrum s.
scotometry
scotomization
scotopia
scotopic
s. adaptation
s. eye
s. perimetry
s. sensitivity
s. sensitivity loss
s. stimulus
s. vision
scotopsin
scotoscope
scotoscopy
Scott
S. lens-insertion forceps
S. No. 2 curved ruler
scraper
epithelial s.
Knolle capsule s.
Kratz capsule s.
Tano membrane s.
scraping
conjunctival s.
corneal epithelial s.
epithelial s.
scratched contact lens
scratcher
Jensen capsule s.
Knolle capsule s.
Kratz capsule s.
Kratz-Jensen s.
scratch-resistant spectacle lens
screen
Bernell tangent s.

Bjerrum s.
Grey-Hess s.
Hess diplopia s.
Hess-Lee s.
tangent s.
screener
Rosenbaum pocket vision s.
scrofulous
s. conjunctivitis
s. keratitis
s. ophthalmia
s. rhinitis
scrub
lid s.
Ocusoft s.
s. typhus
scrubber
Simcoe anterior chamber
capsule s.
scurf
lid s.
scutum region
sea
s. fan sign
s. frond
seam
pigment s.
Searcy
S. anchor/fixation
S. chalazion trephine
S. oval cup erysiphake
seasonal rhinoconjunctivitis
sebaceous
s. adenoma
s. cell
s. cell carcinoma
s. cyst
s. gland of conjunctiva
s. glands of conjunctiva gland
sebaceum
adenoma s.
seborrhea
seborrheic
s. blepharitis
s. keratosis
sebum palpebrale
seclusion
s. of pupil
secobarbital sodium
second
s. cranial nerve
s. sight

secondary
  s. action
  s. amyloidosis
  s. anophthalmia
  s. axis
  s. cataract
  s. curve on contact lens
  s. deviation
  s. dye test
  s. exotropia
  s. eye
  s. focal length
  s. focal point
  s. keratitis
  s. lens
  s. lens implant
  s. malignant neoplasm
  s. mechanism
  s. membrane
  s. neovascular glaucoma
  s. neovascularization
  s. optic atrophy
  s. position
  s. retinitis
  s. strabismus
  s. vitreous
second-degree relative
second-grade fusion
secretion
  basal tear s.
  meibomian s.
  oily s.
  reflex tear s.
  tear s.
secretomotor nerve
secretory epithelial cell
section
  nerve cross s.
  orbital s.
  Saemisch s.
  trigeminal nerve root s.
sector
  s. cut
  s. defect
  s. iridectomy
  s. iridectomy operation
  s. pallor

  s. palsy
  s. retinitis pigmentosa
sectoral iris paralysis
sectoranopia
  congruous homonymous
    horizontal s.
  congruous homonymous
    quadruple s.
sector-shaped defect
sedimentary cataract
SEE
  Surgical Eye Expeditions
seeberi
  Rhinosporidium s.
seeding
  vitreous s.
Seeligmüller sign
see-saw
  s.-s. anisocoria
  s.-s. nystagmus
segment
  anterior s.
  anterior ocular s.
  bifocal s.
  compensated s.
  dissimilar s.
  extramedullary s.
  Fenhoff external and
    anterior s.
  inner s.
  intramedullary s.
  intratemporal s.
  outer s.
  posterior s.
  prism s.
segmental
  s. explant
  s. hypoplasia
  s. implant
  s. iris atrophy
  s. lens
segmentation
  neodymium:yttrium-lithium-
    fluoride laser s.
Seibel nucleus chopper
Seidel
  S. scotoma

S

NOTES

Seidel *(continued)*
   S. sign
   S. test
Seiff frontalis suspension set
seizure
   visual s.
Seldane
selective
   s. facial myectomy
   s. laser trabeculoplasty (SLT)
self-adhering lid retractor
self-centering micromanipulator
self-retaining
   s.-r. infusion cannula
   s.-r. irrigating cannula
   s.-r. retractor
self-sealing
   s.-s. scleral puncture
   s.-s. side port
self-stabilizing vitrectomy lens
Selinger operation
sella, pl. **sellae**
   empty s.
   J-shaped s.
   tilt of s.
   s. turcica
sellar calcification
SEM
   slow eye movement
semi-circinate pattern
semicircular canal
semifinished
   s. blank
   s. contact lens
   s. glass
   s. lens
semilunar
   s. fold
   s. folds of conjunctiva
semilunaris
   plica s.
   raphe plica s.
semiscleral contact lens
semishell implant
senescent
   s. cortical degenerative cataract
   s. disciform macular
    degeneration
   s. ectropion
   s. elastosis
   s. enophthalmus
   s. entropion
   s. halo

   s. keratosis
   s. macular exudative choroiditis
   s. macular hole
   s. miosis
   s. nuclear degenerative cataract
   s. ptosis
   s. retinoschisis
senile
   s. atrophy
   s. cataract
   s. chorioretinitis
   s. choroidal change
   s. disciform macular
    degeneration
   s. ectropion
   s. elastosis
   s. entropion
   s. exudative macular
    degeneration
   s. furrow degeneration
   s. guttate choroidopathy
   s. halo
   s. keratosis
   s. lenticular myopia
   s. macular degeneration (SMD)
   s. macular exudative choroiditis
   s. miosis
   s. nuclear sclerotic cataract
   s. reflex
   s. retinoschisis
   s. sclerotic cataract
   s. vitritis
senilis
   arcus s.
   cataract s.
   choroiditis guttata s.
   circus s.
   ectropion s.
   linea corneae s.
   sarcomatosum s.
Senior-Loken syndrome
Senn retractor
senopia
sensation
   corneal s.
   decreased corneal s.
   s. disturbance
   foreign-body s.
   s. impairment
   light s.
   threshold of visual s.
   s. time

sense
    color s.
    form s.
    light s.
    stereognostic s.
Sensitive
    S. Eyes
    S. Eyes daily cleaner
    S. Eyes drops
    S. Eyes saline/cleaning solution
sensitivity
    contrast s.
    cornea s.
    corneal s.
    increment threshold spectral s.
    light s.
    periocular drug s.
    scotopic s.
    spatial-contrast s.
    spectral s.
    s. threshold
sensor
    Ocular Vergance and
      Accommodation S. (OVAS)
    oximetry s.
    Shell s.
Sensorcaine with epinephrine
sensorimotor disorder
sensory
    s. amblyopia
    s. ataxic neuropathy with
      dysarthria and
      ophthalmoplegia (SANDO)
    s. correspondence
    s. deprivation nystagmus
    s. detachment
    s. elevation
    s. esotropia
    s. exotropia
    s. fiber
    s. fusion
    s. nerve
    s. retina
    s. root
    s. root of ciliary ganglion
    s. system
    s. visual pathway

separable acuity
separate image test
separation
    s. of retina
    vitreofoveal s.
    vitreomacular s.
    vitreous s.
separator
    Allen stereo s.
    Kirby cylindrical zonal s.
    Kirby flat zonal s.
    Remy s.
septic
    s. retinitis
    s. thrombosis
septica
    iridocyclitis s.
Septicon
septo-optic
    s.-o. dysplasia
    s.-o. dysplasia syndrome
septum
    s. cavum pellucidum
    intermuscular s.
    orbital s.
    s. orbitale
    s. sequela
    tarsus orbital s.
sequela, pl. sequelae
    septum s.
sequence
    linear sebaceous nevus s.
sequestered space
Serdarevic
    S. Circle of Light
    S. speculum
    S. suture adjuster
Sereine
series
    s. five forceps
    Kurova Shursite lens s.
    Zeiss slit-lamp s.
serosa
    choroiditis s.
    s. choroiditis
    retinitis centralis s.

S

NOTES

serous
s. chorioretinopathy
s. cyclitis
s. cyst
s. detachment maculopathy
s. iritis
s. macular detachment
s. membrane
s. pigment epithelial
    detachment
s. pigment epithelium
s. retinitis
s. retinopathy
Serpasil
serpent ulcer of cornea
serpiginous
s. choroiditis
s. choroidopathy
s. corneal ulcer
s. keratitis
serrated conjunctival forceps
Serratia
S. liquefaciens
S. marcescens ·
serrefine
s. clamp
Dieffenbach s.
Lemoine s.
serum lysozyme
Service
Lighthouse Low Vision S.
sessile papilloma
set
Bloomberg trabeculotome s.
British Standards Institution
    optotype s.
Catalano intubation s.
Crawford lacrimal s.
diagnostic fitting s.
DORC subretinal instrument s.
Jackson lacrimal intubation s.
Jaffe laser blepharoplasty and
    facial resurfacing s.
Jaffe lid retractor s.
McIntyre infusion s.
Mentanium vitreoretinal
    instrument s.
pediatric vitrectomy lens s.
Seiff frontalis suspension s.
Simcoe lens positioning s.
Tolentino vitrectomy lens s.
Volk Superfield multi-adapter
    transformer lens s.

seton
Ahmed drainage s.
S. drainage device
s. operation
setting
field diaphragm s.
luminance s.
lux s.
setting-sun
s.-s. phenomenon
s.-s. sign
Set-Up
AMO S.-U.
seventh
s. cranial nerve
s. nerve palsy
Severin
S. implant
S. lens
Sewall
S. forceps
S. retractor
sex-linked recessive optic atrophy
SF6 gas
SFP
simultaneous foveal perception
SH
suprachoroidal hemorrhage
shadow
s. graph
Purkinje s.
s. test
shadowing
acoustical s.
hollowing and s.
Shafer sign
Shaffer operation
Shaffer-Weiss classification
shaft vision
shagreen
anterior capsule s.
anterior mosaic crocodile s.
crocodile s.
s. pattern
shallow
s. chamber
s. detachment
shallowing
anterior chamber s.
s. of chamber
sham-movement vertigo
shaped cataract
shape perception

shaper
    automated corneal s.
    Chiron automated corneal s.
sharp
    s. hook
    s. and pink (S&P)
Sharplan argon laser
Sharpoint
    S. microsurgical knife
    S. ophthalmic microsurgical
      suture
    S. slit knife
    S. spoon blade
    S. Ultra-Guide ophthalmic
      needle
    V-lance S.
    S. V-lance blade
Sharvelle side port splitter
shear force
Shearing
    S. intraocular lens
    S. planar posterior chamber
      intraocular lens
    S. posterior chamber
      intraocular lens implant
    S. suction kit
shearing
    s. injury
Shea syndrome
sheath
    arachnoid s.
    bulbar s.
    dural s.
    eyeball s.
    fetal fibrovascular s.
    fibrovascular s.
    muscle s.
    nerve s.
    optic nerve s.
    pial s.
    s. syndrome
sheathing
    arteriolar s.
    halo s.
    peripheral retinal vascular s.
    perivascular s.
    retinal vein s.

    s. of retinal vessel
    vascular s.
    venous s.
    vessel s.
    s. of vessel
sheathotomy
Sheehy-Urban sliding lens adapter
sheen dystrophy
sheet
    Barrier s.
    Eye-Pak II s.
    foil s.
    glassy s.
    ground glass s.
    Silastic s.
    Supramid s.
    Teflon s.
sheeting
    micromesh s.
Sheets
    S. irrigating vectis
    S. lens
    S. lens glide
    S. lens-inserting forceps
    S. lens spatula
    S. microiris hook
Sheets-McPherson tying forceps
shelf-type implant
shell
    s. implant
    plaster s.
    s. prosthesis
    scleral s.
    S. sensor
Shepard
    S. incision depth gauge
    S. incision irrigating cannula
    S. intraocular lens forceps
    S. intraocular utility forceps
    S. lens-inserting forceps
    S. microiris hook
    S. optical center marker
    S. radial keratotomy irrigating
      cannula
    S. reversed iris hook
    S. tying forceps
Shepard-Reinstein forceps

S

NOTES

455

Sheridan-Gardiner isolated letter-matching test
Sherman card
Sherrington
  S. law
  S. law of reciprocal innervation
shield
  aluminum eye s.
  Barraquer eye s.
  Buller eye s.
  Cartella eye s.
  cataract mask s.
  collagen s.
  corneal light s.
  Cox II ocular laser s.
  Durette external laser s.
  Expo Bubble eye s.
  eye s.
  face s.
  S.'s forceps
  Fox aluminum s.
  Fox eye s.
  Grafco eye s.
  Green eye s.
  Guibor s.
  Hessburg corneal s.
  Hessburg eye s.
  S. iridotomy scissors
  Jardon eye s.
  Mueller eye s.
  Paton eye s.
  plastic eye s.
  pressure s.
  PROSHIELD collagen corneal s.
  ring cataract mask eye s.
  Soft Shield collagen corneal s.
  trigeminal s.
  s. ulcer
  Universal eye s.
  Visitec corneal s.
  Weck eye s.
shield-shaped
shift
  criterion s.
  eye-head s.
  hyperopic s.
  Purkinje s.
Shigella
  S. flexneri
  S. sonnei
shiny cellophane reflection

shipyard
  s. conjunctivitis
  s. disease
  s. eye
  s. keratoconjunctivitis
Shirmer basal secretion test
Shoch
  S. foreign body pickup
  S. suture
shock optic neuropathy
shoelace stitch
Shoemaker intraocular lens forceps
short
  s. ciliary artery
  s. ciliary nerve
  s. C-loop lens
  s. posterior ciliary artery
  s. root of ciliary ganglion
  s. sight
  s. wavelength automated perimetry (SWAP)
  s. wavelength autoperimetry
ShortCut A-OK small-incision knife
short-scale contrast
shortsightedness
shot-silk
  s.-s. phenomenon
  s.-s. reflex
  s.-s. retina
show
  scleral s.
Shprintzen syndrome
shredded iris
Shugrue operation
shunt
  aqueous tube s.
  Baerveldt s.
  dural s.
  opticociliary s.
  Schocket anterior chamber tube s.
  s. vessel
  White glaucoma pump s.
shunting
  left-to-right s.
sialylated chain
sicca
  blepharitis s.
  keratitis s.
  keratoconjunctivitis s. (KCS)
  non-Sjögren keratoconjunctivitis s.
  rhinitis s.

s. syndrome
transplantation of submandibular
 gland for
 keratoconjunctivitis s.
siccus
pannus s.
Sichel
  S. blade
  S. disease
  S. knife
Sichi
  S. operation
  S. orbital implant
sickle
  s. cell anemia
  s. cell retinopathy
  s. scotoma
side-biting spatula
side-cutting spatulated needle
side port
side-port cannula
siderophone
sideroscope
siderosis
  s. bulbi
  s. cataract
  s. conjunctivae
  s. lentis
  ocular s.
siderotic cataract
sidewall infusion cannula
Sidler-Huguenin endothelioma
Sieger streak
Siegrist
  S. spot
  S. streak
Siegrist-Hutchinson syndrome
**Siemens Quantum 2000 Color
 Doppler**
sight
  day s.
  far s.
  line of s.
  long s.
  near s.
  night s.
  old s.

primary line of s.
second s.
short s.
sighted
partially s.
sign
Abadie s.
Argyll-Robertson pupil s.
Arroyo s.
Ballet s.
Bárány s.
Bard s.
Barré s.
Battle s.
Bekhterev s.
Berger s.
Bianchi s.
Bielschowsky s.
Bjerrum s.
black dot s.
black sunburst s.
Bonnet s.
Boston s.
Braley s.
Brickner s.
Cantelli s.
cerebellar eye s.
Charcot s.
Charleaux oil droplet s.
Chvostek s.
Cogan s.
Cogan lid-twitch s.
Collier s.
Cowen s.
Dalrymple s.
digito-ocular s.
doll's eye s.
s. of edema of lower eyelid
Elliot s.
Enroth s.
Gianelli s.
Gifford s.
Goppert s.
Gower s.
Graefe s.
Griffith s.
Grocco s.

S

NOTES

sign *(continued)*
Gunn s.
Hoaglund s.
Hutchinson s.
Jellinek s.
Jendrassik s.
Joffroy s.
Knies s.
Kocher s.
Larcher s.
Loewi s.
Lotze local s.
Macewen s.
Magendie s.
Magendie-Hertwig s.
Mann s.
Marcus Gunn pupillary s.
Maxwell-Lyons s.
May s.
Means s.
Metenier s.
Möbius s.
Möbius-von Graefe-Stellway s.
Munson s.
Nikolsky s.
ocular s.
orbicularis s.
Parrot s.
peek s.
Pick s.
Piltz s.
Prevost s.
pseudo-Graefe s.
Reisman s.
Rifkind s.
Ripault s.
Robertson s.
Romaña s.
Romberg s.
Rosenbach s.
Saenger s.
Sainton s.
Salus s.
Schaffer s.
sea fan s.
Seeligmüller s.
Seidel s.
setting-sun s.
Shafer s.
Skeer s.
Stellwag s.
Stimson s.
Suguira s.

Suker s.
Summerskill s.
swinging flashlight s.
Tellais s.
Theimich lip s.
Topolanski s.
Tournay s.
Trousseau s.
Uhthoff s.
von Graefe s.
Watzke-Allen s.
Weber s.
Weber-Rinne s.
Wernicke s.
Widowitz s.
Wilder s.
Woods s.
signal
pseudo-CSF s.
Signet Optical lens
signet-ring
s.-r. carcinoma
s.-r. lymphoma
Sila Clean
Siladryl Oral
silafilcon A
silafocon A
Silastic
S. intubation
S. plate
S. scleral buckler implant
S. sheet
S. T-tube
silent
s. central retinal vein
obstruction
s. sinus syndrome
silica gel
silicone
s. acrylate
s. acrylate contact lens
s. band
s. button
s. conformer
s. elastomer lens
s. eye sphere
s. hemisphere
s. introducer
s. intubation
s. lubricant
s. mesh implant
s. oil injection

s. oil tamponade
s. rod
s. rod and sleeve forceps
s. sponge explant
s. sponge forceps
s. strip
s. tire
s. tube
s. tubing
siliculose, siliquose
s. cataract
Silikon 1000 retinal tamponade
silk traction suture
Silsoft contact lens
Silva-Costa operation
silver
s. compound
s. nitrate
s. nitrate solution
s. protein
s. tattoo pigment
Silver-Hildreth operation
silver-wire
s.-w. arteriole
s.-w. reflex
s.-w. vessel
Simcoe
S. anterior chamber capsule scrubber
S. aspirating needle
S. corneal marker
S. double cannula
S. double-end lens loupe
S. I&A system
S. II PC aspirating needle
S. II PC double cannula
S. II PC lens
S. II PC nucleus delivery loupe
S. interchangeable tip
S. irrigation-aspiration system
S. lens implant forceps
S. lens-inserting forceps
S. lens positioning set
S. notched spatula
S. nucleus delivery loupe
S. nucleus erysiphake

S. nucleus forceps
S. nucleus lens loupe
S. posterior chamber lens forceps
S. reverse aperture cannula
S. reverse irrigating-aspirating cannula
S. suture needle
S. upeop
S. wire speculum
Simmons
occult temporal arteritis of S.
simple
s. acute conjunctivitis
s. anisocoria
s. color
s. diplopia
s. episcleritis
s. glaucoma
s. heterochromia
s. hyperopic astigmatism
s. myopia
s. myopic astigmatism
s. optic atrophy
s. plus lens
s. retinitis
simplex glaucoma
Simpson
S. lacrimal probe
S. test
simulans
Staphylococcus s.
Simulantest
simulator
video display terminal s. (VDTS)
simultanagnosia
simultaneous
s. contrast
s. foveal perception (SFP)
s. macular perception (SMP)
s. prism cover test (SPC)
Sinarest 12 Hour nasal solution
Singapore epidemic conjunctivitis
single
s. binocular vision (SBV)

S

NOTES

459

single *(continued)*
  s. cover test
  s. lid eversion
single-action rongeur
single-armed suture
single-cut
  s.-c. contact lens
single/double occluder
single-mirror goniolens
single-running suture
single-stitch aponeurotic tuck
  technique
SingleStitch PhacoFlex
sinister
  oculus s. (left eye)
  tension oculus s. (tension of
    left eye) (TOS)
  visio oculus s. (vision of left
    eye) (VOS)
sinistrality
sinistrocular
sinistrocularity
sinistrogyration
sinistrotorsion
Sinskey
  S. intraocular lens
  S. lens hook
  S. lens-manipulating hook
  S. microiris hook
  S. microlens hook
  S. micro-tying forceps
  S. pick
Sinskey-Wilson foreign body forceps
sinus
  anterior chamber s.
  Arlt s.
  Arlt-Jaesche s.
  s. catarrh
  cavernous s.
  s. circularis iridis
  ethmoid s.
  ethmoidal s.
  frontal s.
  s. headache
  s. of Maier
  Maier s.
  s. mucocele
  paranasal s.
  scleral venous s.
  sphenoid s.
  s. venosus sclera
  venous s.

sinusitis
  frontal s.
  maxillary s.
  paranasal s.
sinusoidal
  s. grating
Sipple-Gorlin syndrome
Sipple syndrome
SITA
  Swedish interactive thresholding
  algorithm
SITE
  SITE irrigating/aspirating needle
  SITE macrobore plus needle
  SITE Phaco I/A needle
  SITE Phaco II handpiece
  SITE TXR diaphragmatic
    microsurgical system
  SITE TXR 2200 microsurgical
    unit
  SITE TXR peristaltic
    microsurgical system
  SITE TXR phacoemulsification
    system
site
in situ
  i. s. DNA nick end labeling
    (TUNEL)
  i. s. DNA nick end labeling
    staining
situ keratomileusis procedure
sixth
  s. cranial nerve
  s. cranial nerve palsy
size
  burn spot s.
  dark-adapted pupil s. (DAPS)
  eye s.
  lens s.
  object s.
  pupil s.
  relative s.
  retinal image s.
  spot s.
  Thornton guide for optical
    zone s.
Sjögren
  S. disease
  S. reticular dystrophy
  S. syndrome
Sjögren-Larsson syndrome
Skeele curette
Skeer sign

skein
- Holmgren s.
- test s.
- s. test

skeletal abnormality
Skeleton fine forceps
skew
- s. deviation
- s. motion
- s. pupil

skiameter
skiametry
skiascope
skiascopy bar
skiascotometry
skin
- s. autograft
- s. change
- s. diabetes
- s. flap
- s. graft
- s. hook
- s. marking pen
- s. pupillary reflex

ski needle
skirt
- vitreous s.

Sklar-Schiötz tonometer
skull
- exophthalmos due to tower s.
- s. temple

sky-blue spot
SL
- Schwalbe line

slab-off
- s.-o. grinding
- s.-o. lens

slant
- antimongoloid s.
- S. haptic
- S. haptic single-piece intraocular lens
- mongoloid s.
- s. muscle operation
- s. operation
- palpebral s.

SLE
- slit-lamp examination

sleep test
sleeve
- anterior segment s.
- Charles anterior segment s.
- Charles infusion s.
- Charles vitrector with s.
- clear keratin s.
- implant s.
- s. implant
- phaco s.
- retinal probe s.
- s. spreading forceps
- Stevens-Charles s.
- SupraSLEEVES nylon s.
- Watzke s.

slide
- AO Vectographic Project-O-Chart s.
- epithelial s.
- Polaroid vectograph s.

sliding flap
slimcut blade
SlimFit
- S. ovoid intraocular lens
- S. small-incision ovoid lens

sling
- Arion s.
- fascia lata frontalis s.
- frontalis muscle s.
- s. for implant
- s. procedure
- suture s.
- tarsoligamentous s.

slit
- s. blade knife
- s. illumination

slit-beam test
slit-lamp
- s.-l. biomicroscopy
- s.-l. cup
- s.-l. examination (SLE)
- s.-l. fluorophotometer
- s.-l. microscope
- s.-l. ophthalmoscopy

Slit Lamp 900 BQ

NOTES

461

SLK
    superior limbic keratoconjunctivitis
SLO
    scanning laser ophthalmoscope
Sloan
    S. letters
    S. M system
    S. reading card
sloping isopters
slough
    conjunctival s.
sloughing base
slow
    s. conjugate roving eye
    movement
    s. eye movement (SEM)
slow-channel syndrome
slow-to-no saccade
10 SL/O Zeiss keratometer
SLT
    selective laser trabeculoplasty
sludging of circulation
sluggish movements of eyes and
    eyelids
Sly syndrome
small
    s. aperture Steri-Drape
    s. incision trabeculectomy
small-incision
    s.-i. cataract surgery
    s.-i. phacoemulsification
SmallPort phaco system
Smart
    S. forceps
    S. scissors
Smart-Leiske cross-action
    intraocular lens forceps
SMD
    senile macular degeneration
smear
    conjunctival s.
smegmatis
    Mycobacterium s.
Smirmaul
    S. nucleus extractor
    S. technique
Smith
    S. expressor
    S. expressor hook
    S. eyelid operation
    S. intraocular capsular
    amputator
    S. knife

S. lid hook
S. modification
S. modification of Van Lint
    lid block
S. orbital floor implant
S. speculum
S. trabeculectomy
Smith-Fisher
    S.-F. iris replacer
    S.-F. knife
    S.-F. spatula
Smith-Green cataract knife
Smith-Indian
    S.-I. operation
    S.-I. technique
Smith-Kuhnt-Szymanowski operation
Smith-Leiske cross-action intraocular
    lens forceps
Smith-Lemli-Optiz syndrome
Smith-Magenis syndrome
Smith-Riley syndrome
SMON
    subacute myelo-optic neuropathy
smooth cannula
smooth-pursuit movement
SMP
    simultaneous macular perception
SMZ-10A zoom stereo microscope
snail tracks
snake bite-induced ptosis
snare
    Banner enucleation s.
    Castroviejo enucleation s.
    enucleation wire s.
    s. enucleator
    Förster enucleation s.
    Foster enucleation s.
    wire enucleation s.
Snell law
Snellen
    S. chart
    S. conventional reform implant
    S. entropion forceps
    S. fraction
    S. lens loupe
    S. letter optotype
    S. letters
    S. line
    S. notation
    S. number
    S. ptosis operation
    S. reading card
    S. reform eye

S. soft contact lens
S. test
S. test type
S. vectis
S. visual acuity
Snell-Sterling visual efficiency scale
Sno Strips
snow
  s. blindness
  s. conjunctivitis
  s. glasses
snowball opacity
snowflake cataract
snowstorm cataract
Snugfit eye patch
Snyder corneal spring forceps
Soac-Lens
soaking solution
Society
  Ophthalmic Photographers S.
  (OPS)
socket
  anophthalmic s.
  contracted s.
  s. contracture
  s. discharge
  s. prosthesis
  s. reconstruction
sodium
  s. acetate
  s. bicarbonate
  s. borate
  carboxymethylcellulose s.
  cefamandole s.
  s. chloride
  s. chloride in solution
  s. cromoglycate
  cromolyn s.
  cromolyn s. 46
  dantrolene s.
  diclofenac s.
  flomoxef s.
  fluorescein s.
  s. fluorescein (NaFl)
  flurbiprofen s.
  fomivirsen s.
  foscarnet s.

ganciclovir s.
s. hexametaphosphate
hyaluronate s.
s. hyaluronate and chondroitin
  sulfate
s. hyaluronate 1% solution
s. hydroxide
s. lauryl sulfate
naproxen s.
S. Oulamyd ophthalmic
pentobarbital s.
phenobarbital s.
s. phosphate
s. propionate
secobarbital s.
sterile acetazolamide s.
S. Sulamyd
S. Sulamyd Ophthalmic
sulfacetamide s.
suramin s.
thiopental s.
valproate s.
warfarin s.
Soemmering
  S. crystalline swelling
  S. foramen
  ring of S.
  S. ring
  S. ring cataract
  S. spot
SOF
  superior orbital fissure
Soflens
  S. 66
  S. contact lens
  S. enzymatic contact lens
  cleaner
  SofLens 66 lens
SoFlex series lenses
Sof/Pro-Clean
Sofsilk nonabsorbable silk suture
soft
  s. cataract
  s. contact lens (SCL)
  s. contact lens solution
  s. drusen
  s. exudate

S

NOTES

soft *(continued)*
   s. intraocular lens
   S. Mate
   S. Mate Comfort Drops for
     Sensitive Eyes
   S. Mate Consept
   S. Mate daily cleaning
     solution
   S. Mate disinfection and
     storage solution
   S. Mate Enzyme Alternative
   S. Mate Enzyme Plus cleaner
   S. Mate Hands Off daily
     cleaner
   S. Mate protein remover
   S. Mate saline
   S. Mate Saline for Sensitive
     Eyes
   S. Shield collagen corneal
     shield
   s. silicone sponge
   s. tissue swelling
Softcon
soft-finger tension
SoftSITE high add aspheric
  multifocal contact lens
soft-tipped
   s.-t. cannula
   s.-t. extrusion handpiece
Soft-Touch A-Probe
software
   PathFinder Corneal Analysis s.
   Visulas 532 Combi s.
   VISULAS InterChange s.
solani
   Fusarium s.
Sola Optical USA Spectralite high
  index lens
solar
   s. blindness
   s. burn
   s. damage
   s. keratoma
   s. keratosis
   s. maculopathy
   s. radiation
   s. retinitis
   s. retinopathy
solid
   s. color
   s. silicone with Supramid
     mesh implant
   s. vision

solium
   Taenia s.
Soll suture and incision marker
Solurex L.A.
solution
   Adsorbotear Ophthalmic S.
   AK-Dilate Ophthalmic S.
   AK-Nefrin Ophthalmic S.
   Akwa Tears S.
   Alomide ophthalmic s.
   AMO Vitrax viscoelastic s.
   Amvisc s.
   Amvisc Plus s.
   apraclonidine ophthalmic s.
   AquaSite Ophthalmic S.
   balanced saline s.
   balanced salt s. (BSS)
   Barnes-Hind contact lens
     cleaning and soaking s.
   Barnes-Hind wetting s.
   BioLon 1% s.
   Bion Tears S.
   boric acid s.
   Boston Advance
     conditioning s.
   Boston conditioning s.
   brimonidine tartrate
     ophthalmic s. 0.2%
   BSS sterile irrigating s.
   Comfort Tears S.
   ContaClair multi-purpose
     contact lens s.
   CooperVision balanced salt s.
   Cosopt ophthalmic s.
   Crolom Ophthalmic S.
   cromolyn sodium ophthalmic s.
   Dakrina Ophthalmic S.
   dexamethasone s.
   Dey-Drop Ophthalmic S.
   disinfecting s.
   Domeboro s.
   dorzolamide hydrochloride
     ophthalmic s.
   dorzolamide hydrochloride-
     timolol maleate ophthalmic s.
   Dry Eyes S.
   Dry Eye Therapy S.
   Dwelle Ophthalmic S.
   emedastine difurmarate
     ophthalmic s.
   eye irrigating s.
   Eye-Lube-A S.
   Eye-Sed s.

Eyesine s.
Eye Stream s.
Eye Wash s.
Feldman buffer s.
fluorescein dye and stain s.
Freeman s.
graft preservation s.
Healon s.
hydrolysis of s.
hypertonic s.
HypoTears S.
HypoTears PF S.
hypotonic s.
Indocin ophthalmic s.
Iocare balanced salt s.
I-Phrine Ophthalmic S.
irrigating s.
Isopto Plain S.
Isopto Tears S.
isotonic s.
Just Tears S.
ketorolac tromethamine
  ophthalmic s., 0.5%
K Sol preservation s.
Lacril Ophthalmic S.
latanoprost s. 0.005%
latanoprost ophthalmic s.
Liquifilm Forte S.
Liquifilm Tears S.
lodoxamide tromethamine
  ophthalmic s.
loteprednol etabonate
  ophthalmic s. 0.5%
LubriTears S.
Miochol s.
Murine S.
Murocel Ophthalmic S.
Mydfrin Ophthalmic S.
Nature's Tears S.
Neosporin Ophthalmic S.
Neo-Synephrine Ophthalmic S.
Nu-Tears S.
Nu-Tears II S.
OcuCoat PF Ophthalmic S.
OcuMax s.
Ocupress Ophthalmic S.
ofloxacin ophthalmic s.

olopatadine hydrochloride
  ophthalmic s.
One s.
ophthalmic s.
osmium tetroxide s.
oxidation of s.
Prefrin Ophthalmic S.
preservatives in s.
Puralube Tears S.
Refresh Ophthalmic S.
Refresh Plus Ophthalmic S.
Relief Ophthalmic S.
Ringer lactate s.
rose bengal red s.
saline s.
Sensitive Eyes
  saline/cleaning s.
silver nitrate s.
Sinarest 12 Hour nasal s.
soaking s.
sodium chloride in s.
sodium hyaluronate 1% s.
soft contact lens s.
Soft Mate daily cleaning s.
Soft Mate disinfection and
  storage s.
solvent s.
Soquette contact lens
  soaking s.
sterility of s.
Tear Drop S.
TearGard Ophthalmic S.
Teargen Ophthalmic S.
Tearisol S.
Tears Naturale S.
Tears Naturale Free S.
Tears Naturale II S.
Tears Plus S.
Tears Renewed S.
timolol maleate ophthalmic gel-
  forming s.
Trump s.
Ultra Tears S.
Unicare blue and green all-in-
  one cleaning s.
Visalens contact lens cleaning
  and soaking s.

S

NOTES

465

solution *(continued)*
   Viscoat s.
   viscoelastic s.
   Viva-Drops S.
   wetting s.
   zinc sulfate s.
solvent solution
somatic cell
Sondermann canal
sonnei
   Shigella s.
Sonogage
   S. System Corneo-Gage 20
   MHz center frequency
   transducer
   S. ultrasound pachometer
sonolucent
   acoustical s.
   s. cleft
   s. lesion
Sonomed
   S. A/B-Scan system
   S. A-Scan system
   S. B-1500 system
Sonometric Ocuscan
sonoreflective
Soothe eye
S.O.P.
   Bleph-10 S.O.P.
   Blephamide S.O.P.
   Chloroptic S.O.P.
   FML S.O.P.
   Genoptic S.O.P.
   Lacri-Lube S.O.P.
Soper
   S. cone contact lens
   S. cone lens
Soquette contact lens soaking solution
sorbic acid Sorbi-Care saline
Sorbi-Care
Soriano operation
Soria operation
Sorsby
   S. maculopathy
   S. pseudoinflammatory macular degeneration
   pseudoinflammatory macular dystrophy of S.
   S. pseudoinflammatory macular dystrophy
   S. syndrome
soul blindness

sound
   lacrimal s.
source
   point s.
Sourdille
   S. forceps
   S. keratoplasty
   S. keratoplasty operation
   S. ptosis operation
Southern
   S. blot hybridization assay
   S. blot technique
Sovereign bifocal lens
S&P
   sharp and pink
space
   Berger s.
   circumlental s.
   episcleral s.
   Fontana s.
   s. of Fontana
   intercellular s.
   interfascial s.
   interlamellar s.
   s. of iridocorneal angle
   Kuhnt s.
   s. myopia
   object s.
   parafoveal cystic s.
   perichoroidal s.
   perioptic subarachnoid s.
   periscleral s.
   preseptal s.
   prezonular s.
   retrobulbar s.
   retroocular s.
   Schwalbe s.
   sequestered s.
   subarachnoid s.
   subpigment epithelial s.
   subretinal s.
   suprachoroidal s.
   Tenon s.
   zonular s.
space-occupying lesion
spacer
   eyelid s.
Spaeth
   S. block
   S. cystic bleb operation
   S. ptosis operation
Spaleck forceps
Spanish silk suture

Spanlang-Tappeiner syndrome
sparganosis
> nodules in s.
> ocular s.

sparing
> foveal s.
> macular s.
> pupillary s.
> recurrent pupillary s.

Sparta microforceps
spasm
> accommodation s.
> s. of accommodation
> accommodative s.
> ciliary s.
> convergence s.
> cyclic ocular motor s.
> facial s.
> hemifacial s.
> near-reflex s.
> s. of the near reflex
> near reflex s.
> nictitating s.
> oculomotor paresis with
>   cyclic s.
> winking s.

spasmodic
> s. mydriasis
> s. strabismus

spasmus nutans
spastic
> s. ectropion
> s. entropion
> s. lagophthalmia
> s. miosis
> s. mydriasis
> s. paretic facial contracture
> s. pseudosclerosis

spasticity of conjugate gaze
spasticum
> ectropion s.
> entropion s.
> sarcomatosum s.

spatia
> s. anguli iridis
> s. anguli iridocornealis
> s. zonularia

spatial
> s. acuity
> s. discrimination
> s. interaction
> s. localization
> s. perception disorder
> s. summation

spatial-contrast sensitivity
spatiotopic stimulus
spatium
> s. episclerale
> s. interfasciale
> s. intervaginale
> s. perichoroideale

spatula
> angled iris s.
> angulated iris s.
> Bangerter iris s.
> Barraquer irrigator s.
> Berens s.
> Birks Mark II micro
>   push/pull s.
> capsule fragment s.
> Castroviejo cyclodialysis s.
> Castroviejo double-ended s.
> Castroviejo synechia s.
> Cleasby s.
> corneal fascia lata s.
> corneal graft s.
> Culler iris s.
> cyclodialysis s.
> double s.
> Drews-Sato suture-pickup s.
> Elschnig cyclodialysis s.
> Fisher-Smith s.
> French hook s.
> French lacrimal s.
> French pattern s.
> Fukusaku s.
> Gills-Welsh s.
> Green double s.
> Green lens s.
> Green replacer s.
> Guimaraes ophthalmic s.
> Hersh LASIK retreatment s.
> Hertzog lens s.
> Hirschman s.

S

NOTES

spatula *(continued)*
  hook s.
  s. hook
  iridodialysis s.
  iris s.
  Jaffe intraocular s.
  Jaffe lens s.
  Katena iris s.
  Kimura platinum s.
  Kirby angulated iris s.
  Kirby iris s.
  Knapp iris s.
  Knolle lens cortex s.
  Knolle lens nucleus s.
  Laird s.
  Lindner s.
  Maddox LASIK s.
  Manhattan Eye & Ear s.
  Maumenee vitreous sweep s.
  McIntyre s.
  McPherson s.
  McReynolds s.
  microvitreoretinal s.
  needle s.
  nucleus s.
  Obstbaum lens s.
  Obstbaum synechia s.
  Olk vitreoretinal s.
  Pallin lens s.
  Paton double s.
  Paton single s.
  Paton transplant s.
  platinum probe s.
  s. probe
  probe s.
  Rainen clip-bending s.
  Rainin lens s.
  Rowen s.
  Sheets lens s.
  side-biting s.
  Simcoe notched s.
  Smith-Fisher s.
  s. spoon
  spoon s.
  suture pickup s.
  synechia s.
  Tan s.
  Thornton malleable s.
  Tooke s.
  vitreous sweep s.
  Wheeler iris s.
spatulated needle
spatule temple

SPC
  simultaneous prism cover test
spear
  s. developmental cataract
  Merocel surgical s.
  Weck-cel surgical s.
Speas operation
special
  s. sense vertigo
  s. spectacle lens
speckled corneal dystrophy
spectacle-induced aniseikonia
spectacles
  aphakic s.
  Bartel s.
  bifocal s.
  s. blur
  bridge of s.
  cataract s.
  clerical s.
  compound s.
  s. correction
  s. crown
  decentered s.
  divers' s.
  divided s.
  folding s.
  s. frame
  s. frame pad
  Franklin s.
  half-glass s.
  Hallauer s.
  hemianopic s.
  industrial s.
  s. lens
  s. magnifier
  Masselon s.
  mica s.
  orthoscopic s.
  pantoscopic s.
  periscopic s.
  photochromic s.
  s. plane
  prism s.
  prismatic s.
  protective s.
  ptosis crutch s.
  pulpit s.
  refraction s.
  safety s.
  stenopaic s.
  stenopeic s.
  telescopic s.

temples of s.
tinted s.
wire frame s.
spectacular image
spectra (*pl. of* spectrum)
spectral
  s. sensitivity
Spectralite Transitions lens
spectrocolorimeter
spectroscopy
  magnetic resonance s. (MRS)
spectrum, pl. **spectra, spectrums**
  chromatic s.
  color s.
  electromagnetic s.
  facio-auriculovertebral s.
  fortification s.
  ocular s.
  Raman s.
  visible s.
specula (*pl. of* speculum)
specular
  s. attachment
  s. glare
  s. image
  s. microscope
  s. microscopy
  s. reflection
specularity
Specular reflex slit lamp
speculum, pl. **specula**
  Alfonso pediatric eyelid s.
  Azar lid s.
  Barraquer-Colibri s.
  Barraquer wire s.
  basket-style scleral supporter s.
  Becker-Park s.
  Bercovici wire lid s.
  Berens s.
  Bronson-Park s.
  Burch-Lester s.
  Castallo s.
  Castroviejo s.
  Clark s.
  Cook s.
  Culler s.
  Douvas-Barraquer s.

eye s.
eyelid s.
Fanta s.
fine-wire s.
Floyd-Barraquer wire s.
Fox s.
Gaffee s.
Guist s.
Guist-Bloch s.
Guyton-Maumenee s.
Guyton-Park eye s.
Guyton-Park lid s.
Hirschman s.
Iliff-Park s.
Jaffe lid s.
Kaiser s.
Katena s.
Keeler-Pierse s.
Keeler-Pierse eye s.
Keizer-Lancaster s.
Keizer-Lancaster eye s.
Knapp-Culler s.
Knapp eye s.
Knolle lens s.
Kratz s.
Kratz-Barraquer wire eye s.
Lancaster eye s.
Lancaster lid s.
Lancaster-O'Connor s.
Lang s.
Lange s.
Lester-Burch s.
lid s.
LidFix s.
Lieberman K-Wire s.
Lindstrom-Chu aspirating s.
Manche LASIK s.
Maumenee-Park eye s.
McKee s.
McKinney eye s.
McPherson s.
Mellinger s.
Metcher s.
Moria one-piece s.
Mueller s.
Murdock eye s.
Murdock-Wiener eye s.

NOTES

speculum *(continued)*
 Murdoon eye s.
 nasal s.
 Omni-Park s.
 Pannu-Kratz-Barraquer s.
 Park s.
 Park-Guyton s.
 Park-Guyton-Callahan s.
 Park-Guyton-Maumenee s.
 Park-Maumenee s.
 Paton single s.
 Paton transplant s.
 pediatric lid s.
 Pierse eye s.
 reversible lid s.
 Sauer infant s.
 Schott lid s.
 Serdarevic s.
 Simcoe wire s.
 Smith s.
 stop s.
 Sutherland-Grieshaber s.
 Weeks s.
 Weiss s.
 Wiener s.
 Williams pediatric eye s.
 wire lid s.
 Ziegler s.
 Zirm LASIK aspiration s.
Speedy-1 Auto refractometer
Spencer
 S. chalazion forceps
 S. eye suture scissors
 S. silicone subimplant
Spencer-Watson
 S.-W. Z-plasty
 S.-W. Z-plasty operation
Spero forceps
spersapolymyxin
sph.
 sphere
 spherical
 spherical lens
sphenocavernous syndrome
sphenoccipital fissure
sphenofrontal suture
sphenoid
 s. bone
 s. door jamb
 greater wing of s.
 lesser wing of s.
 s. sinus
 s. wing meningioma

sphenoidal fissure
sphenoidalis
 ala minor ossis s.
 foramen s.
sphenomaxillary fissure
spheno-orbital suture
sphenopalatine ganglion
sphenorbital
sphere (sph.)
 Carter s.
 diopter s. (DS)
 Doherty s.
 s. end point
 s. implant
 s. introducer
 method of the s.
 Morgagni s.
 Mules vitreous s.
 porous hydroxyapatite s.
 Pyrex eye s.
 silicone eye s.
spherical (sph.)
 s. aberration
 s. cornea
 s. equivalent
 s. equivalent lens
 s. implant
 s. lens (S, sph.)
 s. lens aberration
 s. refraction
 s. refractive error
Spherical Twirl
spherocylinder
spherocylindrical lens
spherocylindric lens
spheroid degeneration
spherometer
spherophakia
spherophakia-brachymorphia
 syndrome
spheroprism
sphincter
 s. erosion
 s. fiber
 s. iridis
 iris s.
 s. muscle
 s. muscle of pupil
 s. oculi
 s. oris
 s. pupillae
 s. tear

spider
    s. angioma
    s. telangiectasia
    s. vasculature
Spielmeyer-Sjögren disease
Spielmeyer-Stock disease
Spielmeyer-Vogt disease
spike
    blue s.
    intraocular pressure s.
    retinal s.
spillover cell
spinal
    s. canal tumor
    s. miosis
    s. mydriasis
spina trochlearis
spin-cast
    s.-c. lens
    s.-c. process
spindle
    s. A melanoma
    Axenfeld-Krukenberg s.
    s. B melanoma
    cataract s.
    s. cataract
    s. cell
    s. cell melanoma
    Krukenberg corneal s.
    Krukenberg pigment s.
spindle-cell tumor
spindle-shaped
    s.-s. area
    s.-s. cell
spinocerebellar
    s. ataxia
    s. degeneration
spiral
    s. field
    Tillaux s.
    s. of Tillaux
spiralis
    Trichinella s.
spirochetiform cataract
Spitz nevus
Spizziri cannula knife

SPK
    superficial punctate keratitis
splaytooth forceps
splenic retinitis
splenium of corpus callosum
splinter disk hemorrhage
split-calvarial bone graft
split fixation
splitter
    Brierley nucleus s.
    Goldberg side port s.
    Koch-Salz nucleus s.
    Kraff nucleus s.
    Rosen phaco s.
    Salz nuclear s.
    Sharvelle side port s.
    Wan side port s.
split-thickness autograft
splitting
    foveal s.
    s. of lacrimal papilla
    s. lacrimal papilla operation
    macular s.
    Minsky intramarginal s.
    stromal s.
spoke-like sutural cataract
sponge
    cellulose surgical s.
    Custodis s.
    s. explant
    Fuller silicone s.
    grooved silicone s.
    implant s.
    s. implant
    Krukenberg s.
    lens s.
    Lincoff lens s.
    lint-free s.
    Masciuli silicone s.
    Merocel s.
    Microsponge Teardrop s.
    ophthalmic s.
    Packer tunnel silicone s.
    Pro-Ophtha s.
    radial s.
    soft silicone s.
    Vaiser s.

S

NOTES

471

sponge *(continued)*
  Visi-Spear eye s.
  vitrectomy s.
  Weck s.
  Weck-cel s.
spongy
  s. appearance
  s. iritis
spontaneous
  s. congenital iris cyst
  s. ectopia lentis
  s. extrusion of lens
  s. extrusion of vitreous
  s. eyelid retraction
  s. hyphema
  s. intracranial hypotension
  s. resorption
  s. retinal venous pulsation
  s. venous pulsation (SVP)
spoon
  Bunge evisceration s.
  Castroviejo lens s.
  cataract s.
  Culler lens s.
  Cutler lens s.
  Daviel lens s.
  Elschnig s.
  enucleation s.
  evisceration s.
  Fisher s.
  graft carrier s.
  Hess s.
  Kalt s.
  Kirby intracapsular lens s.
  Knapp lens s.
  lens s.
  needle s.
  s. needle
  Rizzuti graft carrier s.
  Schepens s.
  s. spatula
  spatula s.
  Wells enucleation s.
sporadic aniridia
Sporothrix schenckii
spot
  acoustic s.
  ash leaf s.
  baring of blind s.
  birdshot s.
  Bitot s.
  blank s.
  blind s.

blue s.
blur s.
Brushfield s.
cherry-red s.
chorioretinal atrophic s.
cluster of pigmented s.'s
corneal s.
cotton-wool s. (CWS)
cribriform s.
depigmented s.
dry s.
Elschnig s.
eye s.
flame s.
Förster-Fuchs s.
Förster-Fuchs black s.
Fuchs black s.
Gaule s.
histo s.
Horner-Trantas s.
iridescent s.
Lisch s.
Mariotte blind s.
Maxwell s.
mongolian s.
opacification cherry-red s.
peripheral chorioretinal
  atrophic s.
physiologic blind s.
retinal blur s.
s. retinoscope
Roth s.
rust s.
Siegrist s.
s. size
sky-blue s.
Soemmering s.
Tay cherry-red s.
white s.
Wies s.
Wölfflin-Krückmann s.
yellow s.
spotty corneal opacity
Spratt mastoid curette
spread
  s. function
  illusory visual s.
  visual s.
spreader
  Athens suture s.
  conjunctiva s.
  Costenbader incision s.
  Gill incision s.

incision s.
Kwitko conjunctival s.
Suarez s.
Wilder band s.
spring
s. catarrh
S. Clip Opticaid
s. conjunctivitis
S. iris scissors
s. ophthalmia
s. pupil
spring-hinge temple
springing mydriasis
springtime conjunctivitis
spud
Alvis foreign body s.
Bahn s.
Corbett s.
curved needle eye s.
Davis s.
Dix foreign body s.
Ellis foreign body s.
eye s.
Fisher s.
flat eye s.
foreign body s.
Francis s.
Goldstein golf-club s.
golf-club eye s.
s. gouge
gouge s.
Hosford s.
LaForce knife s.
Levine s.
needle s.
s. needle
O'Brien s.
Plange s.
Storz folding-handle eye s.
s. tool
Walter s.
Walton s.
spur
Fuchs s.
Grunert s.
Michel s.
scleral s. (SS)

spuria
polycoria s.
spurious cataract
Sputnik Russian razor blade
squamosa
blepharitis s.
squamous
s. cell
s. cell carcinoma
s. cell carcinoma of eyelid
s. metaplasia
s. seborrheic blepharitis
square
s. prism
s. pupil
square-wave
s.-w. jerks
s.-w. pulse
squashed-tomato appearance
Squid instrument/apparatus
squint
accommodative s.
angle s.
angle of s.
s. angle
comitant s.
convergent s.
deviation s.
s. deviation
divergent s.
downward s.
Duane classification of s.
external s.
s. hook
internal s.
latent s.
noncomitant s.
upward s.
squinting eye
squirrel plague conjunctivitis
SR
superior rectus
Ocufit SR
SRI
surface regularity index
**SR-IV Programmed Subjective
refractor**

NOTES

S

SRK
    Sanders-Retzlaff-Kraff formula
    SRK formula
    Sanders-Retzlaff-Kraff
SRM
    subretinal membrane
SRNV
    subretinal neovascularization
SRNVM
    subretinal neovascular membrane
⁹⁰Sr-plaque irradiation
SS
    scleral spur
Staar
    S. AA 4207 lens
    S. implantable contact lens
    S. intraocular lens
    S. toric lens
    S. 4203VF lens
    S. 4207VF lens
stability
    tear-film s.
stabilizer
    mast cell s.
    Stamler corneal transplant s.
Stableflex anterior chamber lens
stable vision
stage
Stahl
    S. caliper block
    S. caliper plate
    S. calipers
    S. lens gauge
    S. nucleus expressor
Stähli pigment line
staining
    arc s.
    arcuate s.
    blotchy positive s.
    bright s.
    coarse punctate s.
    conjunctival s.
    corneal s.
    corneal blood s.
    fluorescein s.
    focal s.
    immunofluorescent s.
    immunoperoxidase s.
    s. pattern
    punctate s.
    in situ DNA nick end
        labeling s.
    stippling and s.

three o'clock s.
    TUNEL s.
stalk
    optic s.
Stallard
    S. eyelid operation
    S. flap operation
Stallard-Liegard
    S.-L. operation
    S.-L. suture
Stamler
    S. corneal transplant stabilizer
    S. side-port fixation hook
stand
    Mayo s.
standard
    s. deviation
    s. near card
    s. notation
    s. thickness
stand-off
    edge s.-o.
Stangel modified Barraquer
    microsurgical needle holder
staphylococcal
    s. allergic keratoconjunctivitis
    s. blepharitis
    s. blepharoconjunctivitis
    s. conjunctivitis
Staphylococcus
    S. aureus
    S. epidermidis
    S. haemolyticus
    S. hominis
    S. hyicus
    S. intermedius
    S. lugdunensis
    S. saprophyticus
    S. schleiferi
    S. simulans
    S. warneri
staphyloma
    annular s.
    anterior s.
    anterior corneal s.
    ciliary s.
    congenital anterior s. (CAS)
    s. corneae racemosum
    corneal s.
    equatorial s.
    intercalary s.
    peripapillary s.
    posterior s.

s. posticum
projecting s.
retinal s.
Scarpa s.
scleral s.
uveal s.
staphylomatous
staphylotomy
star
epicapsular lens s.
s. fold
lens s.
s. lens
Lindstrom S.
macular s.
Winslow s.
stare
hyperthyroid s.
postbasic s.
thyroid s.
Stargardt
S. and Best disease
S. disease
S. dystrophy
S. maculopathy
S. syndrome
Star-Optic eye wash
Starr fixation forceps
star-shaped field
STAR S2 SmoothScan excimer laser system
startle myoclonus
stasis, pl. **stases**
axoplasmic s.
papillary s.
venous s.
Stat
S. aspirator
S. machine
S. Scrub handwasher machine
state
deturgescent s.
dissociative s.
refractive s.
static
s. accommodation insufficiency
s. countertorsion

s. perimeter
s. perimetry
s. refraction
s. retinoscopy
stationary
s. cataract
s. night blindness
statometer
Statpac test
Statrol
Stay-Brite
Stay-Wet
Stay-Wet 3
steady-state accommodation
steal syndrome
Stealth
S. DBO diamond blade
S. DBO free-hand diamond knife
Steclin
Steele-Richardson-Olszewski
S.-R.-O. disease
S.-R.-O. syndrome
steep
s. contact lens
steepening
corneal s.
inferior s.
videokeratographic corneal s.
steepest meridian
Stefan law
Steiger curve
Steinert-Deacon incision gauge
Steinert double-ended claw chopper
Steinhauser electromucotome
stella
s. lentis hyaloidea
s. lentis iridica
stellata
retinitis s.
stellate
s. cataract
s. retinopathy
Stellwag
S. brawny edema
S. sign
S. symptom

S

NOTES

stem
  brain s.
  s. cell (SC)
  s. palsy
stenochoria
stenocoriasis
stenon duct
stenopaic
  s. disk
  s. spectacles
stenopeic
  s. disk
  s. iridectomy
  s. spectacles
stenophotic
stenosis
  aqueductal s.
  s. canaliculus
  carotid artery s.
  involutional s.
  lacrimal punctal s.
  punctal s.
  punctum s.
Stenstrom ocular measurement
stent
  lacrimal s.
  Supramid occluding s.
step
  corneal graft s.
  s. graft operation
  nasal s.
  Ronne nasal s.
Stephenson needle holder
Stephens soft IOL-inserting forceps
Step-Knife diamond blade knife
stepwise fashion
Sterane
stereo
  s. reindeer test
  s. x-ray
stereoacuity
stereocampimeter
  Lloyd s.
stereognostic sense
stereogram
  random-dot s.
stereo-identical point
stereometric parameter
stereo-ophthalmoscope
stereo-optic disk diapositive
stereo-orthopter
stereophantoscope
stereophorometer

stereophoroscope
stereophotography
stereopsis
  Gross s.
  macular s.
  s. test
stereoscope
stereoscopic
  s. acuity
  s. diplopia
  s. fundus photograph
  s. imaging
  s. parallax
  s. vision
stereoscopy
stereotest
  Lang s.
stereoviewer
  Donaldson s.
Steri-Drape
  S.-D. drape
  3M small aperture S.-D.
  small aperture S.-D.
sterile
  s. acetazolamide sodium
  s. adhesive bubble chamber
  s. adhesive bubble dressing
  s. corneal ulcer
  s. endophthalmitis
  s. hypopyon
  s. melt
sterility of solution
Steriseal disposable cannula
Stern-Castroviejo
  S.-C. locking forceps
  S.-C. suturing forceps
Sterofrin
  Isopto S.
steroid
  s. diabetes
  s. glaucoma
  s. therapy
steroid-induced
  s.-i. cataract
  s.-i. glaucoma
steroidogenic diabetes
Stevens
  S. eye scissors
  S. iris forceps
  S. muscle hook retractor
  S. needle holder
  S. tenotomy hook
  S. tenotomy scissors

Stevens-Charles sleeve
Stevens-Johnson syndrome
Stevenson
  S. lacrimal sac retractor
  S. refractor
stick
  fluorescein s.
  needle s.
  Pro-Ophtha s.
Stickler syndrome
sties (*pl. of* sty)
Stifel figure
stiff
  s. pupil
  s. retina
  s. retinal fold
stigmatic
  s. image
  s. lens
stigmatometer
stigmatometric test card
stigmatoscope
stigmatoscopy
Stiles-Crawford effect
stiletto
  Berkeley Bioengineering s.
  Blair s.
  s. knife
stillicidium lacrimarum
Stilling
  canal of S.
  S. color table
  S. color test
Stilling-Turk-Duane syndrome
Stimson sign
stimulator
  CAM s.
  optokinetic s.
stimulatory antibody
stimulus, pl. **stimuli**
  auditory s.
  blue flash s.
  body-referenced s.
  bright-white flash s.
  s. deprivation
  eye-referenced s.
  flash s.

flicker fusion s.
light s.
optokinetic s.
proprioceptive s.
red flash s.
retinotopic s.
scotopic s.
spatiotopic s.
Vernier s.
stippled
  s. hyperfluorescence
  s. pattern
stippling and staining
stitch
  bow-tie s.
  cuticular s.
  shoelace s.
  triple-throw square knot s.
  s. with twists
  zipper s.
stitch-removal forceps
stitch-removing knife
St. Martin-Franceschetti cataract
  hook
Stocker
  S. line
  S. needle
  S. operation
Stocker-Holt dystrophy
Stocker-Holt-Schneider dystrophy
Stock operation
Stock-Spielmeyer-Vogt syndrome
Stokes lens
Stolte capsulorrhexis forceps
stone
  S. implant
  tear s.
Stone-Jordan implant
stony-hard eye
stop
  Bowman needle s.
  Castroviejo corneal scissors
    with inside s.
  s. speculum
Storz
  S. band
  S. calipers

S

NOTES

Storz *(continued)*
S. capsule forceps
S. CAPSULORBLUE
   intraocular lens
S. cataract knife
S. cilia forceps
S. corneal bur
S. corneal forceps
S. corneal trephine
S. corneoscleral punch
S. DiaPhine trephine
S. folding-handle eye spud
S. handle
S. handpiece
S. keratome
S. keratometer
S. lid plate
S. microscope
S. MicroSeal
S. Microvit magnet
S. Microvit vitrector
S. Millennium microsurgical
   system
S. Premiere Microvit
S. radial incision marker
S. tonometer
Storz-Atlas hand eye magnet
Storz-Bell erysiphake
Storz-Bonn suturing forceps
Storz-Duredge steel cataract knife
Storz-Utrata forceps
**Storz-Walker retinal detachment
unit**
Storz-Westcott conjunctival scissors
Stoxil
strabismal, strabismic
s. amblyopia
s. deviation
s. nystagmus
strabismometer
strabismus
A-s.
absolute s.
accommodative s.
alternate day s.
alternating s.
A-pattern s.
Bielschowsky s.
bilateral s.
binocular s.
Braid s.
cicatricial s.
comitant s.

concomitant s.
constant s.
convergent s.
cyclic s.
s. deorsum vergens
s. divergence
divergent s.
dynamic s.
external s.
s. fixus
s. forceps
Graves s.
s. hook
incomitant vertical s.
intermittent s.
internal s.
kinetic s.
latent s.
manifest s.
mechanical s.
mixed s.
monocular s.
monolateral s.
muscular s.
noncomitant s.
nonconcomitant s.
nonparalytic s.
paralytic s.
periodic s.
relative s.
s. scissors
secondary s.
spasmodic s.
suppressed s.
s. surgery
s. sursum vergens
unilateral s.
uniocular s.
variable s.
vertical s.
X-s.
strabometer
strabometry
strabotome
strabotomy
straight
s. mosquito clamp
s. retinal probe
s. temple
s. tenotomy scissors
s. tying forceps
straight-eyed patient
straight-line bifocal

straight-tip bipolar forceps
strain
    eye s.
Straith eyelid operation
Strampelli
    S. lens
    S. lens implant
Strampelli-Valvo operation
strand
    fibrin s.
    glassine s.
    iris s.
    lysis of restricting s.
    mucin s.
    mucous-like s.
    mucus s.
    restricting s.
    stromal s.
    vitreous s.
strap
    Velcro head s.
stratified squamous epithelium
stratum cerebrale retinae
Straus curved retrobulbar needle
strawberry
    s. hemangioma
    s. nevus
straylight meter
streak
    angioid retinal s.
    Knapp s.
    lightning s.
    Moore lightning s.
    s. retinoscope
    s. retinoscopy
    Sieger s.
    Siegrist s.
    Verhoeff s.
Streatfield-Fox operation
Streatfield operation
Streatfield-Snellen operation
strength
    orbicularis s.
strephosymbolia
streptococcal
    s. bacillus
    s. blepharitis

Streptococcus
    S. faecalis
    S. pneumoniae
    S. pyogenes
    S. viridans
Streptomyces
    S. caespitosum
    S. caespitosus
    S. tsukubaensis
stretching
    pupil s.
stretch reflex
stria, gen. and pl. **striae**
    striae ciliaris
    concentric s.
    corneal s.
    Haab s.
    Knapp s.
    striae retinae
    vertical s.
    Vogt s.
striascope
striatal nigral degeneration
striate
    s. keratitis
    s. keratopathy
    s. melanokeratosis
    s. opacity
    s. retinitis
    s. visual cortex
striated glasses
striation
    retinal s.
stringy mucus
strip
    Color Bar Schirmer s.
    EyeClose Adhesive s.
    Ful-Glo-s.'s
    gliotic s.
    marginal tear s.
    s. procedure
    reagent s.
    Schirmer tear test s.
    silicone s.
    Sno S.'s
    tear s.

S

NOTES

stripe
   central reflex s.
stripper
   Crawford fascial s.
   fascia lata s.
   zonular s.
   zonule s.
stripping
   cortical s.
   s. membrane
stroboscopic disk
stroke-like episode
stroma
   avascular corneal s.
   corneal s.
   iris s.
   s. of iris
   limbal s.
   perilimbal s.
   pigmented s.
   s. plexus
   sclerotic s.
   vitreous s.
   s. vitreum
stromal
   s. annular infiltrate
   s. bed
   s. blood vessel
   s. corneal dystrophy
   s. derma
   s. disease
   s. ectasia
   s. edema
   s. ghost scarring
   s. haze
   s. hydration
   s. ingrowth
   s. keratitis
   s. keratouveitis
   s. line
   s. matrix
   s. melt
   s. necrosis
   s. neovascularization
   s. opacity
   s. pocket
   s. ring infiltrate
   s. splitting
   s. strand
   s. thickness
   s. thinning
   s. ulcer
   s. vascularization

Stromberg curve
Strow corneal forceps
Struble lid everter
structure
   angle s.
   Kolmer crystalloid s.
strumous ophthalmia
strut
   optic s.
Stryker
   S. frame
   S. saw
STTOdx ophthalmic surgery system
Student unpaired *t*-test
study
   Beaver Dam Eye S.
   Blue Mountain Eye S.
   case-control s.
   cohort s.
   Collaborative Initial Glaucoma
     Treatment S. (CIGTS)
   double-blind s.
   Early Treatment Diabetic
     Retinopathy S. (ETDRS)
   family s.
   Herpetic Eye Disease S.
   Lens Opacities Case-Control S.
   Macular Photocoagulation S.
     (MPS)
   prospective s.
   retrospective s.
   vectographic s.
Sturge-Weber
   S.-W. disease
   S.-W. syndrome
Sturge-Weber-Dimitri syndrome
Sturm
   conoid of S.
   S. conoid
   interval of S.
   S. interval
stutzeri
   Pseudomonas s.
sty, stye, pl. sties, styes
   meibomian s.
   zeisian s.
Style S2 clear-loop lens
styrene contact lens
Suarez spreader
Suarez-Villafranca operation
sub-2 incision

subacute
- s. myelo-optic neuropathy (SMON)
- s. necrotizing encephalomyelopathy
- s. sclerosing panencephalitis

subarachnoid
- s. bleed
- s. fluid
- s. hemorrhage
- s. oculomotor nerve lesion
- s. oculomotor nerve palsy
- s. space

subcapsular
- s. cataract
- s. epithelium
- s. plaque

subchoroidal
subciliary incision
subclinical
- s. diabetes
- s. optic neuritis

Subco needle
subconjunctival
- s. cyst
- s. edema
- s. emphysema
- s. foreign body
- s. hemorrhage
- s. injection
- s. needle

subconjunctivitis
subcortical alexia
subcutaneous
- s. amyloid
- s. fat atrophy

subdural hematoma
subepidermal calcified nodule
subepithelial
- s. corneal haze
- s. corneal opacity
- s. fibrosis
- s. keratitis
- s. nevus
- s. plaque
- s. plexus
- s. punctate corneal infiltrate

subepithelialis
- keratitis punctata s.

subfoveal
- s. choroidal neovascularization
- s. neovascular membrane

subhyaloid
- s. blood
- s. hemorrhage

subimplant
- Spencer silicone s.

subinternal limiting membrane hemorrhage
subjective
- S. Autorefractor-7
- s. prism-neutralized cover test
- s. refraction test
- s. refractor
- s. testing
- s. vertigo
- s. vision

subjectoscope
subjunctival hemorrhage
sublatio retinae
subluxated lens
subluxation of lens
subluxed lens
submacular surgery
submembrane fluid
subnormal
- s. accommodation
- s. vision

suboptimal vision
suborbital
subperiosteal
- s. abscess
- s. implant

subpigment epithelial space
subretinal
- s. fluid
- s. fluid cuff
- s. fluid drainage
- s. hemorrhage
- s. membrane (SRM)
- s. neovascularization (SRNV)
- s. neovascular membrane (SRNVM)

NOTES

481

subretinal *(continued)*
    s. scarring
    s. space
subscleral
subsclerotic
substance
    corneal s.
    s. exophthalmos
    exophthalmos-producing s.
    (EPS)
    s. of lens
    s. P
    scleral s.
    toxic s.
substantia
    s. corticalis lentis
    s. propria
    s. propria corneae
sub-Tenon
    s.-T. anesthesia cannula
    s.-T. corticosteroid injection
subterminale
    Clostridium s.
subtilis
    Bacillus s.
subtotal thyroidectomy
subtraction topography
subvolution
Sucaryl
successive contrast
succnate
succulent vessel
succus cineraria Maritima
suction
    s. ophthalmodynamometer
    perilimbal s.
    s. ring
    s. trephine
    Vactro perilimbal s.
sudden visual loss
sudoriferous cyst
sugar cataract
sugar-induced cataract
sugar-loaf cornea
Suguira sign
suis
    Brucella s.
Suker sign
Sulamyd
    Sodium S.
sulcus
    chiasmal s.
    ciliary s.

corneoscleral s.
s. fixated position
s. fixation
s. infraorbitalis maxillae
infrapalpebral s.
s. infrapalpebralis
intramarginal s.
iridociliary s.
lacrimal s.
optic s.
orbital s.
s. orbitales lobi frontalis
s. sclera
scleral s.
sclerocorneal s.
superior s.
s. support
supraorbital s.
Sulf-10
    S. Ophthalmic
Sulfacel 15
sulfacetamide
    s. phenylephrine
    s. and prednisolone
    s. sodium
    s. sodium and fluorometholone
sulfa drug
Sulfair 10
Sulfair Forte
Sulfamide
Sulfasuxidine
sulfate
    alkyl ether s.
    atropine s.
    chondroitin s.
    dermatan s.
    dimethyl s.
    eserine s.
    ferrous s.
    gentamicin s.
    heparan s.
    hydroxychloroquine s.
    indinavir s.
    keratan s.
    neomycin s.
    phenelzine s.
    physostigmine s.
    polymyxin B s.
    quinine s.
    saquinavir s.
    sodium hyaluronate and
      chondroitin s.
    sodium lauryl s.

tranylcypromine s.
zinc s.
sulfur
s. gas
s. hexafluoride
sulfurhexafluoride gas
Sulphrin
Sulpred
Sulten-10
summation
spatial s.
Summerskill
S. operation
S. sign
Summit
S. Apex laser
S. excimer laser
S. OmniMed excimer laser
S. SVS Apex laser
S. UV 200 Excimed laser
sunburst
black s.
s. dial
s. dial chart
s. effect
sunburst-type lesion
sunflower cataract
sunglasses
Sung reverse nucleus chopper
sunrise syndrome
sunset syndrome
Super
S. Field NC slit lamp lens
S. Pinky ball
S. punctum plug
Superblade
Bishop-Harman S.
S. No. 75 blade
supercilia (*pl. of* supercilium)
superciliaris
arcus s.
superciliary
s. arch
s. muscle

supercilii
musculus corrugator s.
musculus depressor s.
supercilium, pl. supercilia
superduction
superficial
s. congestion
s. corneal line
s. keratectomy
s. lamellar keratoplasty
s. linear keratitis
s. line of cornea
s. punctate keratitis (SPK)
s. punctate keratopathy
s. reticular degeneration of Koby
superficialis
keratitis ramificata s.
xerosis s.
superinfection
bacterial s.
corneal s.
superior
s. arcuate bundle
s. arcuate scotoma
arcus palpebralis s.
arteriola macularis s.
arteriola nasalis retinae s.
arteriola temporalis retinae s.
s. canaliculus
s. cervical ganglion
s. colliculus
s. commissura of Meynert
s. conjunctival fornix
s. cornea
s. corneal shield ulcer
s. division palsy
s. eyelid crease
fissura orbitalis s.
s. gaze
glandula lacrimalis s.
s. homonymous quadrantic defect
s. lacrimal gland
s. limbic keratoconjunctivitis (SLK)
s. macular arteriole

S

NOTES

superior *(continued)*
musculus tarsalis s.
s. myokymia
s. nasal artery
s. nasal vein
s. oblique
s. oblique extraocular muscle
s. oblique microtremor
s. oblique muscle and
trochlear luxation
s. oblique myokymia
s. oblique palsy
s. oblique tack surgery
s. oblique tendon
s. oblique tendon sheath
syndrome
s. oblique transposition
s. ophthalmic vein
s. orbital fissure (SOF)
s. orbital fissure syndrome
s. palpebral furrow
s. palpebral vein
s. pole
s. polioencephalitis
s. punctum
s. quadrantanopsia
s. radial tenotomy scissors
s. rectus (SR)
s. rectus extraocular muscle
s. rectus forceps
s. salivary nucleus
s. sector iridectomy
s. sulcus
s. tarsal muscle
s. tarsus
s. tarsus palpebrae
s. temporal artery
s. temporal vein
temporal venulae retina s.
s. tendon of Lockwood
s. vascular arcade
vena ophthalmica s.
venula macularis s.
venula nasalis retinae s.
venula temporalis retinae s.
s. zone of retina
superiores
venae palpebrales s.
superioris
levator palpebrae s.
musculus levator palpebrae s.
superoccipital

superonasal
s. macula
s. paracentral visual field
supertemporal
supertraction
conus s.
s. conus
supplement
ICaps TR dietary s.
MaxiVision dietary s.
support
capsular s.
iris s.
Schillinger suture s.
sulcus s.
supporter
scleral s.
suppressant
aqueous s.
cycloplegios s.
suppressed
s. amblyopia
s. strabismus
suppression
s. amblyopia
central s.
facultative s.
macular s.
obligatory s.
orbital fat s.
s. scotoma
suppressor T cell
suppurativa
hyalitis s.
suppurative
s. choroiditis
s. hyalitis
s. keratitis
s. retinitis
s. ulcer
SupraCAPS quarter-globe cap
suprachiasmatic nucleus (SCN)
suprachoroid
s. lamina
s. layer
suprachoroidal
s. hemorrhage (SCH, SH)
s. space
suprachoroidea
lamina s.
supraciliaris
epicanthus s.
supraciliary canal

supraduction
Supramid
  S. bridle collagen suture
  S. lens implant
  S. lens implant suture
  S. occluding stent
  S. sheet
Supramid-Allen implant
supranuclear
  s. cataract
  s. control
  s. deficiency
  s. deviation
  s. disorder
  s. input
  s. lesion
  s. ocular palsy
  s. paresis of vertical gaze
  s. pathway
supraocular
supraoptic
  s. canal
  s. commissure
supraorbital
  s. akinesia
  s. arch
  s. arch of frontal bone
  s. artery
  s. canal
  s. foramen
  s. incisure
  s. margin of frontal bone
  s. margin of orbit
  s. nerve
  s. neuralgia
  s. notch
  s. point
  s. reflex
  s. ridge
  s. sulcus
  s. vein
supraorbitale
  foramen s.
supraorbitalis
  incisura s.
  nervus s.
suprascleral

suprasellar
  s. aneurysm
  s. lesion
  s. meningioma
  s. tumor
8000 Supra Series auto refractometer
SupraSLEEVES nylon sleeve
supratemporally
supratentorial arteriovenous malformation
suprathreshold static perimetry
supratrochlear nerve
supravergence
supraversion
suprofen
suramin sodium
Surefit AC 85J lens
Surevue contact lens
surface
  s. analgesia
  s. asymmetry index (SAI)
  s. breakdown
  concave reflecting s.
  convex reflecting s.
  curved reflecting s.
  s. dyslexia
  ellipsoidal back s.
  s. implant
  s. irregularity
  s. lamellar keratoplasty
  s. lubrication
  ocular s.
  Petzval s.
  s. photorefractive keratectomy
  reflecting s.
  s. regularity index (SRI)
  s. tension
  toric s.
  s. wrinkling retinopathy
Surgamid
surgeon
  vitreoretinal s.
surgery
  American Society of Ophthalmic Plastic and Reconstruction S.

NOTES

485

surgery *(continued)*
antiglaucoma s.
artificial divergency s.
asymmetric s.
cataract s.
ciliodestructive s.
closed-eye s.
corneal s.
cranio-orbital s.
decompression s.
decompressive s.
eyelid s.
eye muscle s.
eye plaque s.
filtration s.
fistulizing s.
foldable intraocular lens s.
glaucoma filtering s.
glaucoma filtration s.
intraoperative adjustable
   suture s.
lacrimal s.
laser s.
laser-filtering s.
macular hole s.
no-stitch phacoemulsification s.
orbital s.
photorefractive s.
refractive s.
retinal s.
scleral explant s.
small-incision cataract s.
strabismus s.
submacular s.
superior oblique tack s.
sutureless cataract s.
symmetric s.
vitreous s.
Surg-E-Trol
S.-E.-T. I/A System
S.-E.-T. System
   irrigating/aspirating unit
surgical
s. calipers
s. decompression procedure
S. Eye Expeditions (SEE)
s. gut suture
s. keratometry
s. marking pen
s. patch grafting
surgically induced refractive change
Surgicraft suture needle

Surgidev
S. intraocular lens
S. PC BUV 20-24 intraocular
   lens
S. suture
Surgikos disposable drape
SurgiMed suture
SurgiScope
Marco S.
Surgisol
Surgistar
S. corneal trephine
S. ophthalmic blade
Surodex
surplus field
sursumduction
alternating s.
sursumvergence
left s.
right s.
sursumversion
Survey
Baltimore Eye S.
Susac syndrome
suspect
glaucoma s.
suspension
AK-Spore H.C. Ophthalmic S.
Alrex ophthalmic s.
brinzolamide ophthalmic s.
Cortisporin Ophthalmic S.
fluorometholone 0.1%
   ophthalmic s. (FML)
FML-S Ophthalmic S.
frontalis fascia lata s.
hydrocortisone s.
Lotemax ophthalmic s.
Poly-Pred Ophthalmic S.
rimexolone ophthalmic s.
Terra-Cortril Ophthalmic S.
transconjunctival frontalis s.
Vexol Ophthalmic S.
suspensory
s. ligament
s. ligament of eye
Sussman
S. four-mirror gonioscope
S. lens
sustainer
Akahoshi nucleus s.
sustentacular
s. fiber
s. tissue

Sutcliffe laser shield and retracting instrument
Sutherland
  S. lens
  S. rotatable microsurgery instrument
  S. scissors
Sutherland-Grieshaber
  S.-G. scissors
  S.-G. speculum
sutura
  s. ethmoidolacrimalis
  s. ethmoidomaxillaris
  s. frontolacrimalis
  s. infraorbitalis
  s. lacrimoconchalis
  s. lacrimomaxillaris
  s. palatoethmoidalis
  s. palatomaxillaris
sutural developmental cataract
suture
  absorbable s.
  adjustable s.
  s. adjustment
  Alcon s.
  anchor s.
  anchoring s.
  antitorque s.
  Arroyo encircling s.
  Arruga encircling s.
  Atraloc s.
  16-bite nylon s.
  black braided nylon s.
  black braided silk s.
  black silk sling s.
  Bondek s.
  braided silk s.
  braided Vicryl s.
  bridge s.
  bridle s.
  buried s.
  canaliculus rod and s.
  cardinal s.
  catgut s.
  cheesewiring of s.'s
  chromic catgut s.
  chromic collagen s.

chromic gut s.
clove-hitch s.
coated Vicryl s.
compression s.
s. of cornea operation
Custodis s.
Dacron s.
Davis-Geck s.
Deknatel silk s.
Dermalon s.
Dexon s.
double-armed s.
double-running penetrating keratoplasty s.
Ethicon-Atraloc s.
Ethicon micropoint s.
Ethicon Sabreloc s.
s. of eyeball operation
Faden s.
fetal Y s.
figure-of-eight s.
fixation s.
Foster s.
frontolacrimal s.
frontosphenoid s.
Frost s.
Gaillard-Arlt s.
groove s.
guy s.
Guyton-Friedenwald s.
horizontal mattress s.
infraorbital s.
interrupted nylon s.
intracameral s.
intraluminal s.
iris s.
s. of iris operation
juxtalimbal s.
lacrimoconchal s.
lacrimoethmoidal s.
lacrimomaxillary s.
lacrimoturbinal s.
s. lancet
lancet s.
s. of lens
Look s.
Mannis s.

S

NOTES

suture *(continued)*
   mattress s.
   McCannel s.
   McLean s.
   Mersilene s.
   Micro-Glide corneal s.
   micropoint s.
   mild chromic s.
   monofilament nylon s.
   s. of muscle operation
   nonabsorbable s.
   Nurolon s.
   nylon 66 s.
   Ophthalon s.
   palatomaxillary s.
   s. pickup spatula
   pickup spatula s.
   plain catgut s.
   plain collagen s.
   plain gut s.
   Polydek s.
   polyester s.
   polyglactin s.
   polyglycolate s.
   polyglycolic acid s.
   polypropylene s.
   posterior fixation s.
   postplaced s.
   preplaced s.
   Prolene s.
   Quickert s.
   releasable s.
   rip-cord s.
   s. rotation
   s. rotation technique
   running nylon penetrating
     keratoplasty s.
   Safil synthetic absorbable
     surgical s.
   scleral flap s.
   s. of sclera operation
   Sharpoint ophthalmic
     microsurgical s.
   Shoch s.
   silk traction s.
   single-armed s.
   single-running s.
   s. sling
   Sofsilk nonabsorbable silk s.
   Spanish silk s.
   sphenofrontal s.
   spheno-orbital s.
   Stallard-Liegard s.

   Supramid bridle collagen s.
   Supramid lens implant s.
   surgical gut s.
   Surgidev s.
   SurgiMed s.
   Swiss silk s.
   Tevdek s.
   traction s.
   transscleral s.
   twisted virgin silk s.
   Verhoeff s.
   Vicryl s.
   virgin silk s.
   white braided silk s.
   Worst s.
   Y s.
   zygomatic s.
sutureless cataract surgery
"suture-out" astigmatism
suture-pickup hook
suturing
   s. of eyelid
   s. forceps
   s. needle
   temporary keratoprosthesis s.
suturolysis
Svedberg unit
SVP
   spontaneous venous pulsation
swab
   calcium alginate s.
   wooden s.
Swan
   S. discission knife
   S. incision
   S. lancet
   S. needle
   S. syndrome
Swan-Jacob gonioprism
SWAP
   short wavelength automated
     perimetry
**Swedish interactive thresholding
   algorithm (SITA)**
sweep
   Barraquer s.
   eye s.
   iris s.
   s. view
sweeper
   Tiko zonule s.
Sweet
   S. locator

S. method
S. original magnet
swelling
    chronic optic disk s.
    corneal s.
    s. of disk
    optical disk s.
    optic disk s.
    Soemmering crystalline s.
    soft tissue s.
Swets goniotomy knife cannula
swift-cut phaco incision knife
swimmer's goggles
swimming pool conjunctivitis
Swim'n Clear
swinging
    s. flashlight sign
    s. flashlight test
    s. lid flap
    s. light test
Swiss
    S. bladebreaker
    S. silk suture
Swiss-cheese visual field
sycosiform
sycosis tarsi
syllabic blindness
Sylva
    S. anterior chamber irrigator
    S. irrigating/aspirating unit
Sylvian aqueduct syndrome
symblepharon
    anterior s.
    s. lysis
    posterior s.
    s. ring
    total s.
symblepharopterygium
symbol
    test s.
symmetric surgery
sympathetic
    s. carotid plexus
    s. heterochromia
    s. hyperactivity
    s. iridoplegia
    s. iritis

    s. nervous system
    s. neuron
    s. ophthalmia
    s. pathway
    s. uveitis
sympathetica
    ptosis s.
sympathizing eye
sympatholytic drug
symptom
    afferent visual s.
    Anton s.
    Berger s.
    Epstein s.
    Haenel s.
    halo s.
    Liebreich s.
    Magendie s.
    rainbow s.
    Stellwag s.
    Uhthoff s.
    Wernicke s.
symptomatic blepharospasm
synaphymenitis
synapse
    photoreceptor-bipolar s.
synaptic
    s. body
    s. connection
    s. ridge
synaptophysin antibody
synathroisis
syncanthus
synchesis
    s. corporis vitrei
    s. scintillans
syndectomy
syndermatotic cataract
syndesmitis
syndrome
    13q- s.
    4p- s.
    9p- s.
    A s.
    Aarskog s.
    Aase s.
    accommodative effort s.

S

NOTES

syndrome *(continued)*
acquired Horner s.
acquired immunodeficiency s.
(AIDS)
acute retinal necrosis s. (ARN)
adherence s.
adhesive s.
Adie s.
Ahlström s.
AICA s.
Aicardi s.
Alezzandrini s.
Alport s.
Alström s.
Alström-Hallgren s.
Alström-Olsen s.
alternating Horner s.
amniotic band s.
Andersen s.
Andosky s.
Angelman s.
Angelucci s.
anterior chamber cleavage s.
anterior cleavage s.
anterior optic chiasmal s.
anti-elevation s. (AES)
Antley-Bixler s.
Anton s.
Anton-Babinski s.
Apert s.
ARN s.
arteriovenous strabismus s.
Ascher s.
ataxia-telangiectasia s.
AV strabismus s.
Axenfeld s.
Axenfeld-Fieger s.
Axenfeld-Reiger s.
Backhaus s.
Balint s.
Baller-Gerold s.
Bamatter s.
Bannayan s.
Bardet-Biedl s.
bare lymphocyte s.
Barlow s.
Baron-Bietti s.
Bartholin s.
basal cell nevus s.
Bassen-Kornzweig s.
Batten s.
Batten-Mayou s.
battered-baby s.

battered-child s.
Béal s.
Behçet s.
Behr s.
Benedikt s.
Bernard s.
Bernard-Horner s.
Bielschowsky-Jansky s.
Bielschowsky-Lutz-Cogan s.
Biemond s.
Bietti s.
big blind spot s.
bilateral uveal effusion s.
blepharophimosis ptosis s.
blepharospasm-oromandibular
dystonia s.
blind spot s.
Bloch-Stauffer s.
Bloch-Sulzberger s.
blue rubber bleb nevus s.
Bonnet-DeChaume-Blanc s.
Bonnier s.
brachial arch s.
brittle cornea s.
Brown s.
Brown-McLean s.
Brown tendon sheath s.
Brown vertical retraction s.
Brueghel s.
Brushfield-Wyatt s.
capsular exfoliation s.
capsule contraction s.
CAR s.
Carpenter s.
cataract with Down s.
cat's eye s.
cavernous sinus s.
central scotoma s.
Centurion s.
cerebrohepatorenal s.
cervico-oculo-acoustic s.
Cestan s.
Cestan-Chenais s.
Chandler s.
CHARGE s.
Charles-Bonnet s.
Charlin s.
Chédiak-Higashi s.
cherry-red spot myoclonus s.
chiasma s.
chiasmal s.
chiasmatic s.
Churg-Strauss s.

Claude s.
Claude Bernard s.
Claude-Bernard-Horner s.
cleavage s.
cleft s.
Coats s.
Cockayne s.
co-contraction s.
Coffin-Lowry s.
Cogan s.
Cogan-Reese s.
Cohen s.
Collins s.
competition swimmer's
  eyelid s.
computer vision s. (CVS)
congenital adherence s.
congenital fibrous s.
congenital Horner s.
congenital juxtafoveolar s.
congenital rubella s.
congenital tilted disk s.
Conn s.
conotruncal anomalies face s.
Conradi s.
contact lens overwearing s.
Cornelia de Lange s.
cranial stenosis s.
craniofacial s.
CREST s.
cri du chat s.
Crouzon s.
Cushing s.
cutaneomucouveal s.
DAF s.
D chromosome ring s.
Degos s.
DeGrouchy s.
Dejean s.
de Lange s.
de Morsier s.
DeMosier s.
DIDMOAD s.
diencephalic s.
DiGeorge s.
dispersion s.
distal optic nerve s.

dorsal midbrain s.
Down s.
Doyne s.
Drews s.
dry eye s.
D trisomy s.
Duane retraction s.
dural shunt s.
dyscephalic s.
E s.
Eaton-Lambert s.
Edwards s.
Ehlers-Danlos s.
Ellingson s.
Elschnig s.
embryonic fixation s.
empty sella s.
exfoliation s.
extrapyramidal s.
Fabry s.
Falls-Kertesz s.
Fanconi s.
fetal hydantoin s.
fetal trimethadione s.
fetal warfarin s.
fibrosis s.
Fiessinger-Leroy-Reiter s.
Fisher s.
Fitz-Hugh-Curtis s.
flaccid canaliculus s.
flecked retina s.
flocculus s.
floppy eyelid s.
Foix s.
Forsius-Eriksson s.
Forssman carotid s.
Foster Kennedy s.
foveomacular cone
  dysfunction s.
Foville s.
Foville-Wilson s.
Franceschetti s.
Franceschetti-Klein s.
François s.
Fraser s.
Freeman-Sheldon s.

S

NOTES

syndrome *(continued)*
Frenkel anterior ocular
traumatic s.
Frey s.
Friedenwald s.
Friedreich s.
Fuchs s.
Fuchs-Kraupa s.
GAPO s.
Gardner s.
Gerstmann s.
Goldberg s.
Goldenhar s.
Goldenhar-Gorlin s.
Goldmann-Favre s.
Goltz s.
Goltz-Gorlin s.
Gradenigo s.
Graefe s.
Greig s.
Grönblad-Strandberg s.
Gruber s.
Gunn s.
Hagberg-Santavuori s.
half-moon s.
Hallermann-Streiff s.
Hallermann-Streiff-Francois s.
Hallervorden-Spatz s.
Hallgren s.
Haltia-Santavuori type of
Batten s.
Harada s.
Hay-Wells s.
Heerfordt s.
Heidenhain s.
hereditary benign intraepithelial
dyskeratosis s.
hereditary optic atrophy s.
heredodegenerative
neurologic s.
Hermansky-Pudlak s.
Hertwig-Magendie s.
HHH s.
Hippel-Lindau s.
histoplasmosis s.
Holmes-Adie tonic pupil s.
Holt-Oram s.
Homén s.
Horner s.
Horner-Bernard s.
Horton s.
Hunter s.
Hunter-Hurler s.

Hurler s.
Hurler-Scheie s.
Hutchinson s.
hyperophthalmopathic s.
hyperviscosity s.
hypoxic eyeball s.
ICE s.
idiopathic orbital
inflammatory s. (IOIS)
infantile strabismus s.
internal capsule s.
iridocorneal endothelial s.
(ICE)
iridocorneal epithelial s.
iridocyclitis masquerade s.
iridoendothelial s.
iris-nevus s.
iris retraction s. of Campbell
Irvine-Gass s.
ischemic chiasmal s.
ischemic ocular s.
Jacod s.
Jahnke s.
Jansky-Bielschowsky s.
jaw-winking s.
Jeune s.
Johnson s.
Joubert s.
Kasabach-Merritt s.
Kearns-Sayre s. (KSS)
Kennedy s.
Kiloh-Nevin s.
Kimmelstiel-Wilson s.
Koeppe s.
Koerber-Salus-Elschnig s.
Krause s.
Kufs s.
Kurz s.
lacrimo-auriculo-dento-digital s.
Lambert-Eaton myasthenic s.
Langer-Giedion
trichorhinophalangeal s.
Larsen s.
lateral medullary s.
Laurence-Biedl s.
Laurence-Moon s.
Laurence-Moon-Bardet-Biedl s.
Laurence-Moon-Biedl s.
Lawford s.
Leber s.
Leber plus s.
lens-induced UGH s.
Lenz s.

LEOPARD s.
Letterer-Siwe s.
lid imbrication s.
Löfgren s.
Lowe oculocerebrorenal s.
Lowe-Terrey-MacLachlan s.
Lyle s.
Lytico-Bodig s.
macular ocular
  histoplasmosis s.
Magendie-Hertwig s.
Marcus Gunn jaw-winking s.
Marinesco-Sjögren s.
Marshall s.
masquerade s.
McCune-Albright s.
Meige s.
Melkersson s.
Melkersson-Rosenthal s.
microtropic s.
Mietens s.
milk-alkali s.
Millard-Gubler s.
Miller s.
Miller-Fisher s.
Milles s.
Möbius s.
Monakow s.
monofixation s.
morning glory s.
Morquio s.
Morquio-Brailsford s.
multiple evanescent white-
  dot s.
multiple lentigines s.
myasthenia s.
myasthenia-like s.
Naegeli s.
Nager s.
neurodegenerative s.
neuroleptic malignant s.
Nieden s.
nodulus s.
Noonan s.
Norman-Wood s.
Nothnagel s.
nystagmus blockage s.

ocular histoplasmosis s. (OHS)
ocular ischemic s. (OIS)
ocular motor s.
oculoauditory s.
oculobuccogenital s.
oculocerebral s.
oculocerebrorenal s.
oculocutaneous s.
oculoglandular s.
oculomucous membrane s.
oculopalatal myoclonus s.
oculopharyngeal s.
oculorenal s.
OMM s.
one-and-a-half s.
optic chiasmal s.
opticocerebral s.
opticopyramidal s.
optic tract s.
orbital apex s.
osteoporosis-pseudoglioma s.
Ota nevus s.
overwear s. (OWS)
Pallister-Hall s.
Pancoast superior sulcus s.
paraflocculus s.
paraneoplastic s.
parasellar s.
Parinaud oculoglandular s.
Parinaud-plus s.
PEHO s.
periaqueductal s.
Petzetakis-Takos s.
pigmentary dispersion s.
pigment dispersion s. (PDS)
plateau iris s.
plus-minus s.
posterior inferior cerebellar
  artery s.
postganglionic Horner s.
Potter s.
prechiasmal optic nerve
  compression s.
preganglionic Horner s.
presumed ocular
  histoplasmosis s. (POHS)
pretectal s.

S

NOTES

493

syndrome *(continued)*
progressive outer retinal
  necrosis s.
Proteus s.
pseudoexfoliation s.
pseudo-Foster Kennedy s.
pseudopresumed ocular
  histoplasmosis s. (pseudo
  POHS)
rainbow s.
Raymond s.
Raymond-Cestan s.
Recklinghausen s.
recurrent corneal erosion s.
red-eyed shunt s.
Reese s.
Reiter s.
restrictive s.
retinal necrosis s.
retraction s.
Riddoch s.
Rieger s.
Riley-Smith s.
Ring D chromosome s.
Roaf s.
Robinow s.
Rollet s.
Romberg s.
Roth-Bielschowsky s.
Rothmund s.
Rothmund-Thomson s.
Roth spot s.
Russell s.
Rutherford s.
Sanchez-Salorio s.
Satoyoshis s.
Scheie s.
Schirmer s.
Schmid-Fraccaro s.
Schwartz s.
Schwartz-Jampel s.
Senior-Loken s.
septo-optic dysplasia s.
Shea s.
sheath s.
Shprintzen s.
sicca s.
Siegrist-Hutchinson s.
silent sinus s.
Sipple s.
Sipple-Gorlin s.
Sjögren s.
Sjögren-Larsson s.

slow-channel s.
Sly s.
Smith-Lemli-Optiz s.
Smith-Magenis s.
Smith-Riley s.
Sorsby s.
Spanlang-Tappeiner s.
sphenocavernous s.
spherophakia-brachymorphia s.
Stargardt s.
steal s.
Steele-Richardson-Olszewski s.
Stevens-Johnson s.
Stickler s.
Stilling-Turk-Duane s.
Stock-Spielmeyer-Vogt s.
Sturge-Weber s.
Sturge-Weber-Dimitri s.
sunrise s.
sunset s.
superior oblique tendon
  sheath s.
superior orbital fissure s.
Susac s.
Swan s.
Sylvian aqueduct s.
tectal midbrain s.
tegmental s.
temporal crescent s.
tendon sheath s.
Terry s.
Terson s.
tight lens s. (TLS)
tilted disk s.
Tolosa-Hunt s.
tonic pupil s.
top-of-the-basilar s.
Touraine s.
toxic Strep s.
Treacher Collins s.
UGH s.
UGH+ s.
Uhthoff s.
Ullrich s.
uncal s.
Usher s.
uveal effusion s.
uveitis-vitiligo-alopecia-
  poliosis s.
uveocutaneous s.
uveoencephalitic s.
uveomeningeal s.
uveomeningitis s.

Uyemura s.
V s.
velocardiofacial s.
vertical retraction s.
visceral larva migrans s.
visual deprivation s.
visual paraneoplastic s.
vitreomacular traction s.
vitreoretinal choroidopathy s.
vitreoretinal traction s.
vitreous wick s.
V-K-H s.
  Vogt-Koyanagi-Harada
  syndrome
Vogt s.
Vogt-Koyanagi s.
Vogt-Koyanagi-Harada s. (V-K-
  H syndrome)
Vogt-Spielmeyer s.
von Graefe s.
von Hippel-Lindau s.
von Recklinghausen s.
Waardenburg s.
Waardenburg-Klein s.
Wagner s.
Wagner-Stickler s.
Walker-Warburg s.
Wallenberg lateral medullary s.
Warburg s.
Weber s.
Weber-Gubler s.
Weill-Marchesani s.
Werner s.
Wernicke s.
Weyers-Thier s.
white dot s.
Wildervanck s.
Wilson s.
windshield wiper s.
wipe-out s.
Wolf s.
Wolfram s.
Wyburn-Mason s.
Zellweger s.
synechia, pl. **synechiae**
annular s.
anterior s.

Castroviejo anterior s.
circular s.
congenital anterior s.
iridocorneal s.
iris s.
peripheral anterior s. (PAS)
posterior s.
s. spatula
total anterior s.
total posterior s.
synechial closure
synechialysis
synechiotomy
  Paufique s.
synechotome
synechotomy
synephris
syneresis of vitreous
syneretic vitreous
synergistic divergence
synizesis
  s. pupillae
synkinesia
  congenital oculopalpebral s.
  lid-triggered s.
synkinesis
  external pterygoid levator s.
  facial s.
  oculocephalic s.
  oculomotor nerve s.
  pterygoid levator s.
  s. pupilla
  trigemino-oculomotor s.
synkinetic
  s. movement
  s. near reflex
  s. near response
synophrys
synophthalmia, synophthalmos,
  synophthalmus
synoptophore
synoptoscope
syntenic gene
synthetic
  S. Optics random dot butterfly
  test
  s. penicillin

S

NOTES

syphilis
  acquired s.
  congenital s.
  ocular s.
syphilitic
  s. cataract
  s. chorioretinitis
  s. choroiditis
  s. dacryocystis
  s. dacryocystitis
  s. episcleritis
  s. iritis
  s. keratitis
  s. ocular disease
  s. optic perineuritis
  s. retinitis
  s. retinopathy
  s. rhinitis
  s. scleritis
syphilitica
  retinitis s.
syringe
  Anel s.
  Fink-Weinstein two-way s.
  Fragmatome flute s.
  Fuchs retinal detachment s.
  Fuchs two-way s.
  Goldstein anterior chamber s.
  Goldstein lacrimal s.
  lacrimal s.
  Luer-Lok s.
  Parker-Heath anterior
    chamber s.
  probe s.
  retinal detachment s.
  tuberculin s.
  two-way s.
  Yale Luer-Lok s.
syringoma
  eyelid s.
  s. tumor
syrup
  Carbodec S.
  Cardec-S S.
  Rondec S.
system
  Accurus vitreoretinal surgical s.
  Aesculap Meditec MEL60 s.
  afocal optical s.
  Alcon Closure S. (ACS)
  Alcon EyeMap EH-290 corneal
    topography s.

AMO Prestige advanced
  cataract extraction s.
AMO Prestige Phaco S.
Anterior Eye Segment
  Analysis S.
autonomic nervous s.
Autoswitch S.
Badal stimulus s.
Bio-Optics Bambi Cell
  Analysis S.
Bio-Optics Bambi image
  analysis s.
Bio-Optics telescope s.
bioptic amorphic lens s.
BKS Refractive S.
Blairex S.
British N s.
Buzard Diamond
  Barraqueratome
  Microkeratome S.
Candela videoimaging s.
Catarex cataract removal s.
Cavitron irrigation/aspiration s.
Cavitron-Kelman
  irrigation/aspiration s.
central nervous s. (CNS)
Chromos imager s.
closed-loop s.
CMS AccuProbe 450 s.
Coburn irrigation/aspiration s.
Combiline S.
complement s.
Computed Anatomy Corneal
  Modeling S.
Corneal Modeling S.
corneal topography s. (CTS)
CorneaSparing LTK s.
C-Scan corneal topography s.
delivery s.
Digital B S.
Dioptimum S.
dioptric s.
DORC fast freeze
  cryosurgical s.
DuoVisc viscoelastic s.
EAS-1000 anterior eye segment
  analysis s.
ErgoTec vitreoretinal
  instrument s.
extrapyramidal s.
eyeFix speculum s.
EyeMap EH-290 corneal
  tomography s.

EyeSys S. 2000
EyeSys corneal analysis s.
EyeSys 2000 corneal
topographic mapping s.
EyeSys corneal topography s.
EyeSys surface topography s.
EZE-FIT IOL s.
FlapMaker microkeratome s.
full-field s.
gaussian optical s.
Grieshaber power injector s.
Grolman photographic s.
Hessburg subpalpebral
lavage s.
Hexon illumination s.
Humphrey ATLAS Eclipse
corneal topography s.
Humphrey Instruments vision
analyzer overrefraction s.
Humphrey Mastervue corneal
topography s.
hyaloid s.
ImageNet image digitizing s.
immune s.
INNOVA S. 920
Inverter vitrectomy s.
IRIS OcuLight SLx indirect
ophthalmoscope delivery s.
irrigation-aspiration s.
IVEX s.
Jaeger s.
Jaeger grading s.
Katena quick switch I/A s.
Kellan capsular sparing s.
Keratome excimer laser s.
Koeller illumination s.
Konan SP8000 image
analysis s.
Kowa fluorescein s.
lacrimal s.
LADARVision excimer laser s.
Langerman diamond knife s.
Lens Opacification
Classification S. (LOCS)
Lens Plus Oxysept S.
Mackool s.

Malis bipolar
coagulating/cutting s.
Massachusetts XII
vitrectomy s. (MVS)
Mastel compass-guided arcuate
keratotomy s.
Materials Testing S.
McGuire I/A s.
McIntyre coaxial irrigating-
aspirating s.
McIntyre I/A s.
McIntyre irrigation/aspiration s.
Medi-Duct ocular fluid
management s.
micropigmentation s.
Microprobe integrated laser and
endoscope s.
Microvit probe s.
midget s.
Millennium CX
microsurgical s.
Millennium LX
microsurgical s.
MiraSept S.
Monarch IOL delivery s.
Mot-R-Pak vitrectomy s.
Mport lens insertion s.
M-TEC 2000 Surgical S.
nasolacrimal drainage s.
Nelson grading s.
Niamtu video imaging s.
Nidek EC-5000 refractive
laser s.
nomogram s.
ocular motor s.
Oculex drug delivery s.
oculomotor s.
Ocutome II fragmentation s.
OCVM s.
Odyssey phacoemulsification s.
OIS image digitizing s.
optical s.
Opti-Pure S.
optokinetic s.
osseous s.
parasympathetic nerve s.

S

NOTES

497

system *(continued)*
PAR CTS corneal
topography s.
Passport disposable injection s.
PE-400 ERG/VEP s.
peripapillary choroidal
arterial s.
Phacojack Phaco S.
Phototome S. 2700
pial s.
Placido-disk videokeratoscopy s.
postcanalicular s.
PreClean soak s.
Premiere SmallPort phaco s.
Price corneal transplant s.
printers' point s.
pump-leak s.
pyramidal s.
QuickRinse automated
instrument rinse s.
Quickswitch irrigation/aspiration
ophthalmic s.
Reinverting Operating Lens S.
(ROLS)
renin-angiotensin s.
Rodenstock s.
Scheimpflug
videophotography s.
sensory s.
Simcoe irrigation-aspiration s.
SITE TXR diaphragmatic
microsurgical s.
SITE TXR peristaltic
microsurgical s.
SITE TXR
phacoemulsification s.
Sloan M s.
SmallPort phaco s.
Sonomed A/B-Scan s.
Sonomed A-Scan s.
Sonomed B-1500 s.
STAR S2 SmoothScan excimer
laser s.
Storz Millennium
microsurgical s.
STTOdx ophthalmic surgery s.
Surg-E-Trol I/A S.
sympathetic nervous s.

T s.
tear drainage s.
tear duct s.
TMS corneal topography s.
Tomey topographic modeling s.
Tomey topography s.
Topcon CM-1000 corneal
mapping s.
Topcon IMAGEnet digital
imaging s.
Topographic Modeling S.-1
(TMS-1)
Topographic Scanning S.
(TopSS)
TopSS topographic scanning s.
Ultrascan Digital B s.
Unfolder implantation s.
Unipulse CO_2 surgical laser s.
UniPulse 1040 Surgical CO_2
laser s.
United Sonics J shock phaco
fragmentor s.
Veatch ophthalmic ReSeeVit s.
Venturi-Flo valve s.
vertebrobasilar s.
vestibular s.
Vision
Analyzer/Overrefraction S.
visual sensory s.
Visulab S.
VISX Star excimer laser s.
VISX STAR S2 excimer
laser s.
VISX Twenty/Twenty s.
Vit Commander S.
vortex s.
Wheeler cyclodialysis s.
Wilmer Cataract Photo-
grading S.
Wisconsin age-related
maculopathy grading s.
YC 1400 Ophthalmic YAG
laser s.
Zaldivar limbal relaxing
incision s.
Zeiss DAS-1 hydrophobic s.
Zeiss fiberoptic illumination s.
zoom s.

systemic
- s. amyloidosis
- s. bacterial endophthalmitis
- s. corticosteroid therapy
- s. drug
- s. glucocorticoid

- s. myopathy
- s. myositis
- s. sclerosis

Szymanowski-Kuhnt operation
Szymanowski operation

NOTES

S

T
  T. lens
  T. system
TA
  temporal arteritis
tab
  vitrectomy prism lens t.
tabes dorsalis
tabetic optic atrophy
table
  Reuss color t.
  Stilling color t.
tablet
  Carbiset T.
  Carbiset-TR T.
  Carbodec T.
  Carbodec TR T.
Tac-40
tachistesthesia
tachistoscope
tack
  retinal t.
taco test
tacrolimus
tactile tension
tadpole pupil
Taenia solium
tag
  vitreoretinal t.
Taillefer valve
Takahashi iris retractor forceps
Takata laser
Takayasu
  idiopathic arteritis of T.
talantropia
Talbot
  T. law
  T. unit
tamoxifen retinopathy
tamponade
  gas t.
  intraocular silicone oil t.
  silicone oil t.
  Silikon 1000 retinal t.
tandem scanning confocal microscope
tangent
  t. perimetry
  t. scope

  t. screen
  t. screen testing
Tangier disease
Tanne
  T. corneal cutting block
  T. corneal punch
  T. guillotine-style punch
Tano
  T. device
  T. double mirror peripheral vitrectomy lens
  T. eraser
  T. membrane scraper
  T. ring
Tansley operation
Tan spatula
tantalum
  t. clip
  t. mesh
  t. mesh implant
  t. "O" ring
TAP
  tension by applanation
tap
  anterior chamber t.
  choroidal t.
  vitreous t.
tap-biopsy
tape
  Blenderm t.
  brow t.
  optokinetic t.
  Transpore eye t.
taper-cut needle
Tapered-Shaft punctum plug
taper-point needle
tapetal light reflex
tapetochoroidal
  t. degeneration
  t. dystrophy
tapetoretinal
  t. degeneration
  t. retinopathy
tapetoretinopathy
tapetum
  t. choroideae
  t. lucidum
  t. nigrum
  t. oculi

T

501

taping
eyelid t.
tapioca iris melanoma
tapir
bouche de t.
target
accommodative t.
fixation t.
saccadic eccentric t.
tarsadenitis
tarsal
t. artery
t. asthenopia
t. canal
t. cartilage
t. conjunctiva
t. cyst
t. ectropion
t. gland
t. laceration
t. membrane
t. muscle
t. plate
t. portion of eyelid
t. strip procedure
tarsales
glandulae t.
tarsalis
epicanthus t.
tarsectomy
Blaskovics t.
Kuhnt t.
tarsi
sycosis t.
tinea t.
tarsitis
tuberculous t.
tarsocheiloplasty
tarsoconjunctival
t. composite graft
t. flap
t. gland
t. pedicle
tarsoligamentous sling
tarsomalacia
tarso-orbital
tarsophyma
tarsoplasia
tarsoplasty
tarsorrhaphy
tarsotomy
transverse t.

tarsus
inferior t.
t. orbital septum
t. osseus
superior t.
Tasia operation
tattoo
t. of cornea operation
t. pigment
tattooing
medical t.
t. needle
Tauranol
Tavist
Tavist-1
tax double needle
Tay
T. cherry-red spot
T. choroiditis
T. disease
Tay-Sachs disease
TBUT
tear break-up test
T-cell lymphoma
TCF
total conjunctival flap
Teale-Knapp operation
tear
Akwa T.'s
Artificial T.'s
artificial t.'s
Bion T.'s
bloody t.'s
t. break-up test (TBUT)
breakup time of t.
Comfort T.'s
conjunctival t.
crocodile t.
t. drainage
t. drainage system
T. Drop Solution
t. duct
t. duct patency
t. duct system
t. film
t. film break-up time
t. film debris
t. film disorder
t. film instability
t. film test
fishmouth t.
flap t.
t. flow

t. function test
t. gas
giant retinal t. (GRT)
horseshoe t.
iatrogenic retinal t.
I-Liqui T.'s
iris sphincter t.
Isopto T.'s
Just T.'s
t. lake
t. layer
Liquifilm T.'s
t. of meniscus
Milroy Artificial T.'s
mucin of t.
t. mucus ferning
Muro T.'s
Natural T.'s
T.'s Naturale
T.'s Naturale Free Solution
T.'s Naturale II
T.'s Naturale II Solution
nonpreserved artificial t.
operculated t.
t. osmolarity
Osopto T.'s
T.'s Plus
T.'s Plus Solution
t. pool
t. protein deposit
t. pump
Puralube T.'s
t. quality
t. quantity
reflux of t.
T.'s Renewed
T.'s Renewed Solution
t. of retina
retinal horseshoe t.
t. sac
t. secretion
t. secretion classification
sphincter t.
t. stone
t. strip
traction-related t.
t. turnover

Ultra T.'s
Visine T.'s
vitreous cells as indicator of
  retinal t.
t. volume
teardrop pupil
Tear-Efrin
Tearfair
tear-film
  t.-f. disturbance
  t.-f. stability
TearGard Ophthalmic Solution
Teargen
  T. Ophthalmic Solution
tear-induced retinal detachment
tearing
Tearisol
  T. Solution
TearSaver punctum plug
Tearscope
  Keeler T.
  T. Plus tear film kit
technetium scan
technique
  Armaly-Drance t.
  Atkinson t.
  bare scleral t.
  blind-spot projection t.
  Boyden chamber t.
  Brockhurst t.
  Brown-Beard t.
  capsule forceps t.
  chip-and-flip
    phacoemulsification t.
  closed-dissection t.
  crack-and-flip
    phacoemulsification t.
  Crawford t.
  divide-and-conquer t.
  erysiphake t.
  feeder-frond t.
  flicher-fusion frequency t.
  Fraunfelder "no touch" t.
  frontalis sling t.
  Goldmann kinetic t.
  Goldmann static t.
  high-tension suturing t.

T

NOTES

technique *(continued)*
    Hughes modification of
      Burch t.
    immunohistochemical t.
    iris-fixation t.
    Knoll refraction t.
    laser-scrape t.
    letterbox t.
    masquerade t.
    Maurice corneal depot t.
    McCannel suture t.
    McLean t.
    McReynolds t.
    Miyake t.
    mustache t.
    O'Brien akinesia t.
    Okamura t.
    open-sky t.
    ophthalmic vitreous surgical t.
    phaco-chop t.
    piezoelectric transducer t.
    preferential-looking t.
    push plus refraction t.
    Quickert three-suture t.
    Scheie t.
    Schepens t.
    scleral search coil t.
    single-stitch aponeurotic tuck t.
    Smirmaul t.
    Smith-Indian t.
    Southern blot t.
    suture rotation t.
    transillumination t.
    transocular t.
    transpupillary t.
    transscleral suture fixation t.
    tumbling t.
    Van Lint modified t.
    Van Milligen eyelid repair t.
    von Graefe t.
technology
    Catarex t.
    imaging t.
TechnoMed
    T. C-Scan
    T. C-Scan videokeratoscope
tectal midbrain syndrome
tectonic
    t. corneal graft
    t. epikeratoplasty
    t. keratoplasty
Teflon
    T. block

    T. implant
    T. injection catheter
    T. iris retractor
    T. plate
    T. plug
    T. sheet
tegmental syndrome
teichopsia
Tektronix digital phonometer
tela
    t. cellulosa
    t. conjunctiva
Telachlor
telangiectasia
    calcinosis cutis, Raynaud
      phenomenon, esophageal
      motility disorder,
      sclerodactyly, and t. (CREST)
    essential t.
    idiopathic acquired retinal t.
    retinal t.
    spider t.
telangiectasis
    idiopathic juxtafoveal retinal t.
    retinal t.
telangiectatic glioma
Teldrin
telebinocular
telecanthus
telecentric fundus camera
teleopsia
telephoto effect
telescope
    afocal t.
    Galilean t.
    Hopkins rod lens t.
    monocular t.
telescopic
    t. lens
    t. spectacles
Telfa
    T. pad
    T. plastic film dressing
Tellais sign
Teller
    T. acuity card
    T. visual acuity
TE MOO mode beam laser
template
temple
    cable t.
    curl t.
    hockey-end t.

t. length
library t.
loafer t.
paddle t.
riding bow t.
skull t.
spatule t.
t.'s of spectacles
spring-hinge t.
straight t.

temporal
t. arcade
t. arteriole of retina
t. arteritis (TA)
t. artery
t. artery biopsy
t. artery pallor
t. bone
t. bulbar conjunctiva
t. crescent
t. crescent syndrome
t. hemianopsia
t. island of visual field
t. lobe
t. lobe field defect
t. lobe unilateral cerebral
hemisphere lesion
t. loop
t. macula
medial t. (MT)
medial superior t. (MST)
t. modulation perimetry
t. optic disk pallor
t. peaking
t. pit
t. raphe
t. self-sealing clear corneal
incision
t. venulae retina superior
t. venule of retina
t. wedge
t. zone of retina

temporalis
commissura palpebrarum t.
t. muscle

temporary
t. balloon buckle

t. diabetes
t. intracanalicular collagen
implant
t. keratoprosthesis suturing
t. prism

temporo-occipital artery
temporoparietal lobe
tenacious
t. distance fusion
t. proximal fusion

tendinous insertion
tendo
t. oculi
t. palpebrarum

tendon
t. advancement
Brown t.
canthal t.
lateral canthal t.
Lockwood t.
medial canthal t.
t. recession
t. sheath syndrome
superior oblique t.
tenotomy of ocular t.
t. tucker
Zinn t.

tendotome
tendotomy
tenectomy
Tennant
T. Anchorflex AC lens
T. anchor lens-insertion hook
T. implant
T. lens-inserting forceps
T. lens-manipulating hook
T. titanium suturing forceps
T. tying forceps

Tennant-Colibri corneal forceps
Tennant-Troutman superior rectus
forceps
Tenner
T. lacrimal cannula
T. titanium suturing forceps

Tenon
T. capsule
T. fascia bulbi

NOTES

T

505

Tenon *(continued)*
   T. fascia lata
   T. flap
   T. membrane
   T. patch graft
   T. space
tenonectomy
tenonitis
   brawny t.
tenonometer
tenontotomy
Tenormin
tenosynovitis
tenotome
tenotomist
tenotomize
tenotomy
   Arroyo t.
   Arruga t.
   curb t.
   free t.
   graduated t.
   t. hook
   intrasheath t.
   t. of ocular tendon
   t. operation
   Z marginal t.
tensile strength of vessel
Tensilon
   T. implant
   T. test
tension
   applanation t. (AT)
   t. by applanation (TAP)
   t. of eye
   finger t.
   hard-finger t.
   intraocular t.
   normal t. (TN)
   normal-finger t.
   ocular t. (Tn)
   t. oculus dextra (tension of right eye) (TOD)
   t. oculus sinister (tension of left eye) (TOS)
   soft-finger t.
   surface t.
   tactile t.
   t. test
   zonular t.
tensor insertion
tented-up retina
tentorial nerve

tentorii ramus
tenuis
   pannus t.
Tenzel
   T. elevator
   T. forceps
   T. rotational cheek flap
Terak Ophthalmic Ointment
teratogenic association
terfanadine
Terg-A-Zyme
terminal bulb
terminaux
   boutons t.
termini
   carboxy t.
terminus
   incision t.
Terra-Cortril
   T.-C. Ophthalmic Suspension
Terramycin
   T. Ophthalmic Ointment
   polymyxin B and T.
   T. w/Polymyxin B Ophthalmic Ointment
terreus
   Aspergillus t.
Terrien
   T. marginal degeneration
   T. ulcer
Terry
   T. astigmatome
   T. keratometer
   T. silicone capsule polisher
   T. syndrome
Terson
   T. capsule forceps
   T. extracapsular forceps
   T. operation
   T. syndrome
tertiary
   t. position
   t. vitreous
tertius palpebra
tessellated fundus
Tessier
   T. classification
   T. clefting
   T. operation
test
   afterimage t.
   alternate cover t. (ACT)
   alternate cover-uncover t.

alternating light t.
Amsler grid t.
anaglyph t.
Arabic eye t.
a-wave t.
Bagolini striated glasses t.
Bailey-Lovie Near T.
Bárány caloric t.
Barraquer-Krumeich t.
4Δ base-out t.
basic secretion t.
Behçet skin puncture t.
Benton Facial Recognition T.
Berens pinhole and
  dominance t.
Berens three-character t.
Bielschowsky-Parks head-tilt
  three-step t.
Bielschowsky three-step, head-
  tilt t.
Binocular Visual Acuity T.
biochrome t.
biometry t.
biopter t.
blindness t.
breakup time t.
Brightness Acuity T. (BAT)
Bruchner t.
butterfly t.
caloric irrigation t.
t. card
cardinal field t.
Catford visual acuity t.
chi-squared test
cocaine t.
color bar Schirmer tear t.
color comparison t.
color vision t.
complement fixation t.
confrontation visual field t.
contour stereo t.
contrast sensitivity t.
corneal impression t. (CIT)
corneal staining t.
cotton thread tear t.
cover t.
cover-uncover t.

cross cover t.
Cuignet t.
D-15 t.
dark-room t.
DEM t.
denervation supersensitivity t.
Developmental Eye
  Movement t.
D-15 Hue Desaturated Panel t.
dissimilar image t.
dissimilar target t.
DIVA t.
Dix-Hallpike t.
double Maddox rod t.
duction t.
duochrome t.
Dupuy-Dutemps
  dacryocystorhinostomy dye t.
dye disappearance t. (DDT)
E t.
edrophonium chloride t.
Ehrmann t.
Farnsworth-Munsell 100-hue
  color vision t.
Farnsworth Panel D-15 t.
Fastpac 24-2 t.
F2 Color Vision t.
Fisher t.
fistula t.
flashlight t.
flicker perimetry t.
fluorescein angiogram t.
fluorescein clearance t. (FCT)
fluorescein dilution t.
fluorescein dye
  disappearance t.
fluorescein instillation t.
fluorescein strip t.
fluorescent antibody t.
fly t.
FM-100 t.
forced-duction t.
forced generation t.
forward traction t.
four-dot t.
Frequency Doubling
  Perimeter t.

T

NOTES

test *(continued)*
Fridenberg stigmatometric t.
Friedman t.
Functional Acuity Contrast T.
(FACT)
glare t.
glaucoma hemifield t.
Haidinger brush t.
hair bulb incubation t.
hand-motion visual acuity t.
hand-movement visual acuity t.
haploscopic t.
Hardy-Rand-Ritter t.
Harrington-Flocks t.
head-tilt t.
Hemifield glaucoma t.
Hering t.
Hering-Bielschowsky after-
image t.
Hess screen t.
higher visual function t.
Hirschberg t.
Holladay contrast acuity t.
Holmgren color t.
Holmgren wool skein t.
Hooper Visual Organization T.
(HVOT)
100 hue t.
28 Hue de Roth t.
Humphrey glaucoma
hemifield t.
ice t.
interference visual acuity t.
intravenous thyrotropin-releasing
hormone t.
Jaeger visual t.
Jenning t.
Jones dye t.
Jones I t.
Jones II t.
Keystone view stereopsis t.
Kirby-Bauer disk sensitivity t.
Kirsch t.
Kodak Surecell Chlamydia t.
Kolmogorov-Smirnov t.
Krimsky prism t.
Kruskal-Wallis t.
Kveim t.
lacrimal irrigation t.
Lancaster red/green t.
Lancaster-Regan t.
Lancaster screen t.
Landolt broken-ring t.

Lang stereo t.
lantern t.
t. letter
letter t.
Lighthouse Distance Visual
Acuity T.
light projection t.
light-stress t.
line t.
linear visual acuity t.
lupus erythematosus cell t.
Maddox rod t.
Maddox wing t.
magnetic field-search coil t.
major amblyoscope t.
Mann-Whitney U t.
Marcus Gunn t.
Marlow t.
Mauthner t.
McNemar t.
Mecholyl t.
Mentor B-VAT II BVS
contour circles distance
stereoacuity t.
Mentor B-VAT II BVS
random dot E distance
stereoacuity t.
microhemagglutination t.
MicroTrac Direct Specimen T.
Mira Pola t.
mirror rocking t.
Modified Clinical Technique t.
monocular confrontation visual
field t.
Mr. Color t.
mydriatic provocative t.
Nagel t.
near vision t.
neostigmine t.
neutral density filter t.
ninety hue discrimination t.
nudge t.
nystagmus t.
t. object
objective prism-neutralized
cover t.
Octopus 201 perimeter t.
ocular motility t.
oculocephalic t.
ophthalmic t.
Optec 3000 contrast
sensitivity t.
ornithine tolerance t.

parallax t.
Parks-Bielschowsky three-step head-tilt t.
Park three-step t.
passive forced duction t.
Pease-Allen Color t.
Pepper Visual Skills for Reading T.
perimeter corneal reflex t.
peripheral detection t.
photostress t.
pilocarpine t.
pinhole and dominance t.
primary dye t.
prism adaptation t. (PAT)
prism and cover t. (P&C)
prism dissociation t.
prism-neutralized cover t.
prism shift t.
prism vergence t.
Prostigmin t.
provocative t.
pseudoisochromatic color t.
pupil cycle induction t.
Rabinowitz-McDonnell t.
Randot Dot E stereo t.
Randot Stereo Smile t.
Raven Progressive Matrices t.
Rayleigh t.
Rayleigh color matching t.
red-filter t.
red glare t.
red glass t.
Rochat t.
rotational t.
Sabin-Feldman dye t.
scanning laser glaucoma t.
Schirmer 1 t.
Schirmer t. I
Schirmer tear quality t.
secondary dye t.
Seidel t.
separate image t.
shadow t.
Sheridan-Gardiner isolated letter-matching t.
Shirmer basal secretion t.

Simpson t.
simultaneous prism cover t. (SPC)
single cover t.
skein t.
t. skein
sleep t.
slit-beam t.
Snellen t.
Statpac t.
stereopsis t.
stereo reindeer t.
Stilling color t.
subjective prism-neutralized cover t.
subjective refraction t.
swinging flashlight t.
swinging light t.
t. symbol
Synthetic Optics random dot butterfly t.
t t.
taco t.
tear break-up t. (TBUT)
tear film t.
tear function t.
Tensilon t.
tension t.
three-character t.
three-step t.
thyroid function t. (TFT)
thyrotropin-releasing hormone t.
Titmus stereo t.
Titmus stereoacuity t.
Titmus vision t.
TNO stereo t.
traction t.
transillumination t.
TRH t.
triiodothyronine suppression t.
Tukey HSD t.
tumbling E t.
tyrosinase t.
vertical prism t.
Vistech 6500 contrast t.
Visuscope motor t.
Visuscope sensory t.

NOTES

T

test (*continued*)
    water-drinking t.
    water provocative t.
    Watzke-Allen t.
    W4D t.
    Welland t.
    Werner t.
    Westcott t.
    Wilbrand prism t.
    Wilcoxon matched pairs t.
    Wilcoxon signed rank t.
    Wirt stereo t.
    Wirt stereopsis t.
    Wirt vision t.
    Wolff-Eisner t.
    Worth four-dot t.
    Worth four-dot near
      flashlight t.
    χ^2 t.
χ^2 test
tester
    Mentor B-VAT II video
      acuity t.
    Miller-Nadler glare t.
    phoroptor vision t.
    Prio video display terminal
      vision t.
    Topcon vision t.
    Vistech Multivision Contrast T.
      8000
testing
    Brückner reflex t.
    confrontation visual field t.
    cranial nerve t.
    dark-room t.
    extraocular muscle t.
    forced-duction t.
    four base-out prism t.
    hypothesis t.
    kinetic visual field t.
    lacrimal t.
    levator function t.
    near acuity t.
    near vision t.
    provocative t.
    pursuit t.
    subjective t.
    tangent screen t.
    visual acuity t.
    visual field t.
    Zone Quick tear volume t.
tetani
    Clostridium t.

tetany
    t. cataract
    zonular t.
tetartanope
tetartanopia
tetartanopic
tetartanopsia
tetracaine hydrochloride
Tetracon
tetracycline
tetrad
    Konoto t.
tetraethylammonium chloride
tetrafilcon A
tetrahydrozoline
    t. hydrochloride
tetranopsia
Tetrasine
    T. Extra Ophthalmic
    T. Ophthalmic
tetrastichiasis
Tevdek suture
text blindness
TFT
    thyroid function test
TG-140 needle
thalamolenticular
thalamus
    optic t.
Thal procedure
thaw-freeze
Thayer-Martin plate
THC:YAG laser
Theimich lip sign
Thelazia
    T. callipaeda
thelaziasis
Theobald probe
theobromae
    Lasiodiplodia t.
Theodore keratoconjunctivitis
theory
    Alhazen t.
    Barkan t.
    color t.
    Ladd-Franklin t.
    migration t.
    molecular dissociation t.
    opponent colors t.
    Scheiner t.'s
    Schön t.
    trichromatic color t.
    Unna abtropfung t.

von Frisch t.
Wollaston t.
Young-Helmholtz t. of color
  vision
therapeutic
  t. contact lens
  t. iridectomy
therapy
  cidofovir t.
  cobalt t.
  corticosteroid t.
  cytokine t.
  external beam radiation t.
  ganciclovir t.
  hyperbaric oxygen t. (HBO)
  immunoadsorption t.
  laser t.
  maximum tolerated medical t.
  miotic t.
  mydriatic-cycloplegic t.
  occlusion t.
  photodynamic t.
  PhotoPoint laser t.
  radiation t.
  red-filter t.
  steroid t.
  systemic corticosteroid t.
TheraTears
thermal
  t. adhesion
  t. burn
  t. cataract
  t. keratoplasty (TKP)
  t. sclerectomy
  t. sclerostomy
thermocautery
thermokeratoplasty
  laser t.
thermosclerectomy
thermosclerostomy
thermosclerotomy
thermotherapy
  adjuvant microwave t.
  microwave plaque t.
  transpupillary t. (TT, TTT)
thick lens

thickness
  central corneal t. (CCT)
  contact lens t.
  t. of contact lens
  standard t.
  stromal t.
Thill Aniseikonia Worksheet
thimerosal
thin lens
thinning
  choroidal t.
  corneal t.
  stromal t.
thin-rim scotoma
thiopental sodium
thioridazine
  t. hydrochloride
  t. retinal toxicity
third
  t. cranial nerve
  t. framework region (FR3)
  t. nerve palsy
  t. order neuron
third-grade fusion
Thomas
  T. brush
  T. calipers
  T. cryoextractor
  T. cryoprobe
  T. cryoptor
  T. cryoretractor
  T. fixation forceps
  T. irrigating-aspirating cannula
  T. Kapsule instrument
  T. operation
  T. retractor
  T. scissors
  T. subretinal instrument set II
Thornton
  T. arcuate blade
  T. 360 degree arcuate marker
  T. fixating ring
  T. fixation forceps
  T. guide for optical zone size
  T. K3-7991 360 degree
    arcuate marker
  T. malleable spatula

T

NOTES

Thornton *(continued)*
    T. needle
    T. optical center marker
    T. tri-square blade
Thornton-Fine ring
Thorpe
    T. calipers
    T. conjunctival forceps
    T. corneal forceps
    T. foreign body forceps
    T. four-mirror goniolaser
    T. four-mirror goniolaser lens
    T. four-mirror goniolens
    T. four-mirror vitreous fundus
       laser lens
    T. scissors
    T. slit lamp
    T. surgical gonioscope
Thorpe-Castroviejo
    T.-C. calipers
    T.-C. corneal forceps
    T.-C. fixation forceps
    T.-C. goniolens
    T.-C. scissors
    T.-C. vitreous foreign body
       forceps
Thorpe-Westcott scissors
Thrasher lens implant forceps
thread
    mucous t.
threat reflex
three-character test
three-mirror
    t.-m. contact lens
    t.-m. prism
three o'clock staining
three-piece
    t.-p. acrylic intraocular lens
    t.-p. silicone intraocular lens
three-point touch
three-snip
    t.-s. punctum
    t.-s. punctum operation
three-step test
three-toothed forceps
three-wall decompression
threshold
    achromatic t.
    brightness difference t.
    color-contrast t.
    displacement t.
    t. effect

    final t.
    light differential t.
    t. limit value (TLV)
    minimum light t.
    pre-bleached dark-adapted t.
    quantitative static t.
    sensitivity t.
    t. stage III of retinopathy of
       prematurity (TS III ROP)
    tolerance t.
    visual t.
    t. of visual sensation
thromboangiitis obliterans
thrombosed artery
thrombosis
    carotid artery t.
    cavernous sinus t.
    orbital vein t.
    t. in retina
    retinal t.
    septic t.
thromboxane receptor antagonist
thrombus
    fibrin t.
through-the-lid contact ultrasound
thrush
    lid t.
thumb occluder
Thurmond nucleus-irrigating
    cannula
Thygeson
    T. chronic follicular
       conjunctivitis
    T. disease
    T. superficial punctate keratitis
    T. superficial punctate
       keratopathy
thymic hypoplasia
thymidine analog
thymoxamine hydrochloride
Thymoxid
thyroid
    t. exophthalmos
    t. eye disease
    t. function test (TFT)
    t. gland disorder
    t. lid retraction
    t. ophthalmopathy
    t. orbitopathy
    t. stare
thyroidectomy
    subtotal t.

thyroiditis
Hashimoto t.
Riedel t.
thyroid-releasing hormone (TRH)
thyrotoxic exophthalmos
thyrotoxicosis
t. ophthalmoplegia
thyrotropic exophthalmos
thyrotropin-releasing hormone (TRH)
t.-r. h. test
thyroxine, thyroxin
TIA
transient ischemic attack
tiapride
Tiapridex
tic
t. douloureux
local t.
motor t.
ticrynafen ointment
tie-over Sellotape dressing
tight
t. contact lens
t. lens syndrome (TLS)
TIGR
trabecular meshwork-inducible glucocorticoid response
tigré
fundus t.
TIGR **gene**
tigroid
t. background
t. fundus
t. retina
Tiko
T. pliable iris retractor
T. zonule sweeper
Tilderquist needle holder
Tillaux
extraocular muscles of T.
spiral of T.
T. spiral
Tillett operation
Tillyer bifocal lens
tilt
pantoscopic t.

t. of sella
visual t.
tilted
t. disk
t. disk syndrome
t. vision
tilting
t. lens
t. lens atresia
time
breakup t. (BUT)
death-to-preservation t.
edge-light pupil cycle t.
fading t.
implicit t.
lacrimal transit t.
noninvasive tear film break-up t.
not invasive break-up t. (niBUT)
photostress recovery t. (PRT)
sensation t.
tear film break-up t.
timolol
t. maleate
t. maleate ophthalmic gel-forming solution
t. and pilocarpine
Timoptic
T. Ocudose
T. Ophthalmic
Timoptic-XE
T.-X. Ophthalmic
Timpilo
tinea tarsi
tinnitus
gaze-evoked t.
tinted
t. contact lens
t. spectacles
tinting of spectacle lens
tip
Binkhorst t.
diathermy t.
endolaser probe t.
Girard irrigating t.
guillotine cutting t.

NOTES

513

tip *(continued)*
Keeler lancet t.
Keeler micro round t.
Keeler micro spear t.
Keeler puncture t.
Keeler razor t.
Keeler triple facet t.
Kelman t.
MicroTip phaco t.
nonaspirating ultrasonic phaco
chopper t.
Quad cutting t.
rotary cutting t.
Saverburger
irrigation/aspiration t.
Simcoe interchangeable t.
TurboSonic t.
Welsh flat olive-t.

tire
276 t.
implant t.
t. implant
silicone t.
Watzke t.

tisiris
tissue
t. adhesive
adipose t.
conjunctiva-associated
lymphoid t.
connective t.
cutaneous t.
donor t.
ectopic t.
epibulbar t.
episcleral t.
t. forceps
frozen t.
hypergranulation t.
hyperreflective t.
limbal t.
mesoblastic t.
mucosal associated lymphoid t.
nonfixed t.
nuclear t.
orbital adipose t.
pericanalicular connective t.
t. plasminogen activator (tPA)
pterygial t.
scleral t.
sustentacular t.
uveal t.

Titan

titanium
t. miniplate
t. needle
t. suturing forceps
Titmus
T. stereoacuity test
T. stereo fly
T. stereo test
T. vision test
TKP
thermal keratoplasty
TLS
tight lens syndrome
TLV
threshold limit value
TM
trabecular meshwork
TMS-1
Topographic Modeling System-1
TMS corneal topography system
TN
normal tension
Tn
ocular tension
TNO stereo test
tobacco/alcohol amblyopia
tobacco amblyopia
TobraDex Ophthalmic
tobramycin
tobramycin and dexamethasone
Tobrex
T. Ophthalmic
Toctron EA-290
TOD
tension oculus dextra (tension of
right eye)
Todd
T. cautery
T. electrocautery
T. gouge
T. paralysis
Tolentino
T. prism lens
T. ring
T. vitrectomy lens
T. vitrectomy lens set
T. vitreous cutter
tolerance threshold
Tolman micrometer
Tolosa-Hunt syndrome
Tomas
T. iris hook
T. suture hook

tomato-ketchup fundus
tome
Laschal precision suture t.
precision suture t.
Tomey
T. autorefractor
T. autotopographer
T. refractive workstation
T. retinal function analyzer
T. TMS-1 photokeratoscope
T. topographic modeling
system
T. topography system
T. Trooper AutoLensmeter
tomograph
Heidelberg retina t. (HRT)
tomography
axial t.
complex motion t.
computed t. (CT)
confocal scanning laser t.
Heidelberg retinal t.
ocular coherence t.
optical coherence t. (OCT)
orbital t.
tonic
t. accommodation
t. convergence
t. downward deviation
t. lid
t. pupil
t. pupil syndrome
t. upward deviation
t. vergence
tonicity
tonofilm
crescent t.
Schiötz t.
tonogram
tonograph
tonography
Tonomat applanation tonometer
tonometer
air-puff contact t.
air-puff noncontact t.
Alcon t.
Allen-Schiötz t.

AO Reichert Instruments
applanation t.
Aus Jena-Schiötz t.
Barraquer applanation t.
Barraquer operating room t.
Berens t.
Bigliano t.
biprism applanation t.
Carl Zeiss t.
Challenger digital
applanation t.
Coburn t.
Digilab t.
Draeger t.
Durham t.
electronic t.
Goldmann applanation t.
Harrington t.
impression t.
indentation t.
Intermedics intraocular t.
Keeler Pulsair t.
Krakau t.
Lombart t.
Mackay-Marg electronic t.
Maklakoff t.
McLean t.
Mueller electronic t.
noncontact t. (NCT)
Pach-Pen XL t.
Perkins applanation t.
pneumatic t.
pressure phosphene t.
ProTon portable t.
Pulsair t.
Reichert noncontact t.
Rosner t.
Ruedemann t.
Schiötz t.
Sklar-Schiötz t.
Storz t.
Tonomat applanation t.
Tono-Pen t.
Tono-Pen XL t.
tonometry
applanation t.
automatic t.

NOTES

T

tonometry *(continued)*
  digital t.
  indentation t.
Tono-Pen
  Oculab T.-P.
  T.-P. tonometer
  T.-P. XL tonometer
tonsil
  cerebellar t.
Tooke
  T. corneal knife
  T. cornea-splitting knife
  T. spatula
Tooke-Johnson corneal knife
tool
  spud t.
Topcon
  T. aspheric lens
  T. chart projector
  T. CM-1000 corneal mapping
  system
  T. eye refractometer
  T. 50IA camera
  T. IMAGEnet digital imaging
  system
  T. keratometer
  T. KR-7500 auto-kerato-
  refractometer
  T. LM P5 digital lensometer
  T. noncontact morphometric
  analysis
  T. perimeter
  T. refractor
  T. RM-A2300 auto
  refractometer
  T. SL-7E photo slip lamp
  T. SL-E Series slit lamp
  T. SL-1E slit lamp
  T. SP-1000 non-contact
  specular microscope
  T. TRC-50VT retinal camera
  T. TRC-50X retinal camera
  T. TRV-50VT fundus camera
  T. vision tester
Topia lentis
topical
  t. anesthesia
  t. anesthetic
  t. cycloplegic
  t. drug
  t. glucocorticoid
  NeoDecadron T.

TOPO
  topographic simulated keratometric
  power
top-of-the-basilar syndrome
topogometer
topographer
  Keratron corneal t.
topographic
  t. agnosia
  t. anatomy
  t. astigmatism
  t. disorientation
  t. echography
  t. electroretinography
  T. Modeling System-1 (TMS-
  1)
  t. scanning/indocyanine green
  angiography combination
  instrument
  T. Scanning System (TopSS)
  T. Scanning System/indocyanine
  green (TopSS/ICG)
  t. simulated keratometric power
  (TOPO)
topographical electroretinogram
topography
  computer-assisted corneal t.
  computerized corneal t.
  confocal laser scanning t.
  corneal t.
  elevation t.
  EyeSys Technologies corneal t.
  optic disk t.
  subtraction t.
Topolanski sign
TopSS
  Topographic Scanning System
  TopSS scanning laser
  ophthalmoscope
  TopSS topographic scanning
  system
TopSS/ICG
  Topographic Scanning
  System/indocyanine green
Toradol
  T. Injection
  T. Oral
Toric
  T. intraocular lens
toric
  t. ablation
  t. contact lens

t. spectacle lens
t. surface
toricity
Toric-Optima series lens
torn iris
toroidal
t. contact lens
torpor
t. retinae
torsional
t. deviation
t. diplopia
t. movement
t. nystagmus
torticollis
ocular t.
tortuosity
familial arteriolar t.
t. of retinal vessel
vascularized t.
venous t.
Torulopsis glabrata
TOS
tension oculus sinister (tension of left eye)
total
t. anterior synechia
t. astigmatism
t. blindness
t. cataract
t. conjunctival flap (TCF)
t. hydrophthalmia
t. hyperopia (Ht)
t. hyphema
t. keratoplasty
t. ophthalmoplegia
t. posterior synechia
t. sclerectasia
t. symblepharon
totale
ankyloblepharon t.
totalis
ophthalmoplegia t.
Toti
T. operation
T. procedure
Toti-Mosher operation

toto
eye removed in t.
touch
corneal endothelial t.
iridocorneal t.
three-point t.
vitreous t.
Touchlite zoom lens
Touraine syndrome
Tournay
T. phenomenon
T. sign
Touton giant cell
Toweletts
DisCide Disinfecting T.
Townley-Paton operation
toxemic retinopathy of pregnancy
toxic
t. amaurosis
t. amblyopia
t. cataract
t. diabetes
t. follicular conjunctivitis
t. maculopathy
t. optic neuropathy
t. reaction
t. retinopathy
t. Strep syndrome
t. substance
toxicity
light t.
ocular t.
photic retinal t.
retinal t.
thioridazine retinal t.
toxic-nutritional disease
toxicodendron
Rhus t.
toxicogenic conjunctivitis
toxin
botulinum A t.
toxin-induced myopathy
Toxocara
toxocariasis
t. endophthalmitis
ocular t.

NOTES

517

Toxoplasma
T. chorioretinitis
T. gondii
toxoplasmic
t. choroiditis
t. retinochoroiditis
t. uveitis
toxoplasmosis
t. chorioretinitis
congenital t.
fulminant ocular t.
ocular t.
punctate outer retinal t.
Toynbee corpuscle
tPA
tissue plasminogen activator
intravitreal tPA
T-PRK
tracker-assisted photorefractive
keratectomy
T-PRK laser
trabecula, gen. and pl. **trabeculae**
anterior chamber t.
scleral t.
trabecular
t. fiber
t. membrane
t. membrane pigment
t. meshwork (TM)
t. meshwork-inducible
glucocorticoid response
(TIGR)
t. network
t. outflow
trabeculectomy
ab externo t.
Cairns t.
t. operation
Pearce t.
small incision t.
Smith t.
trabeculitis
t. glaucoma
trabeculodysgenesis
trabeculopexy
argon laser t. (ALT)
trabeculoplasty
argon laser t. (ALTP)
diode laser t. (DLT)
laser t.
pneumatic t.
selective laser t. (SLT)
trabeculopuncture

trabeculotome
Allen-Burian t.
Harms t.
McPherson t.
trabeculotomy
t. probe
trabeculotomy-trabeculectomy
combined t.-t.
trabeculum
corneoscleral t.
trabecuphine laser sclerostomy
trachoma, pl. **trachomata**
Arlt t.
Arlt-Jaesche t.
t. body
brawny t.
cicatrizing t.
follicular t.
gland t.
t. gland
granular t.
inactive t.
t. inclusion conjunctivitis
trachomatis
Chlamydia t.
trachomatosus
pannus t.
trachomatous
t. conjunctivitis
t. dacryocystis
t. dacryocystitis
t. keratitis
t. pannus
tracing
ray t.
track
bear t.'s
corneal paracentesis t.
snail t.'s
tracker
Purkinje image t.
tracker-assisted
t.-a. photorefractive keratectomy
(T-PRK)
t.-a. PRK laser (T-PRK laser)
tracking
pursuit t.
Tracor Northern
Tracoustic RV275
tract
geniculocalcarine t.
leiomyoma of uveal t.

optic t.
uveal t.
traction
anterior loop t.
t. band
diabetic t.
foveal t.
macular t.
t. macular detachment
Moss t.
peripheral vitreoretinal t.
t. suture
t. test
vessel t.
vitreomacular t.
vitreopapillary t.
vitreoretinal t.
vitreous t.
tractional
t. retinal degeneration
t. retinal detachment (TRD)
traction-related tear
trained retinal locus
training
vision t.
Trainor-Nida operation
Trainor operation
Tramacort
transantral decompression
transcaruncular-transconjunctival approach
transcleral
transconjunctival
t. cryopexy
t. frontalis suspension
t. lower eyelid blepharoplasty
t. route
transducer
Ocuscan 400 t.
Sonogage System Corneo-Gage 20 MHz center frequency t.
vector array t.
transducin
transepithelial photoablation
transfer function
transferred ophthalmia

transfixion
t. of iris
t. of iris operation
transformed migraine
transient
t. ametropia
t. blindness
t. congestion
t. early exophthalmos
t. ischemia
t. ischemic attack (TIA)
t. layer of Chievitz
t. myopia
t. obscuration of vision
t. photopsia
t. unilateral dilation
t. unilateral mydriasis
t. vertebrobasilar ischemia
t. visual loss
t. visual obscuration
transillumination
t. technique
t. test
transilluminator
Finnoff t.
halogen Finhoff t.
transitional zone
transition zone
translimbal
translocation
macular t.
t. needle
retinal t.
translucent
transmission
t. electron microscope
light t.
transmitted light
transneuronal degeneration
transocular
t. technique
transorbital leukotomy
transparency
corneal t.
transparent ulcer of the cornea
trans pars plana

NOTES

transplant
    corneal t.
    lamellar corneal t.
    McReynolds pterygium t.
    ocular muscle t.
    penetrating corneal t.
transplantation
    amniotic membrane t.
    t. antigen
    autologous chondrocyte t.
    t. of cornea
    corneal t.
    epithelial t.
    limbal autograft t. (LAT)
    limbal stem-cell t.
    t. of muscle operation
    organ t.
    t. of submandibular gland for keratoconjunctivitis sicca
Transpore eye tape
transposition
    medial rectus t.
    muscle t.
    superior oblique t.
transpunctal endocanalicular approach
transpupillary
    t. cyclophotocoagulation
    t. laser
    t. technique
    t. thermotherapy (TT, TTT)
transscleral
    t. cryopexy
    t. cryotherapy
    t. laser cyclophotocoagulation
    t. neodymium:yttrium-aluminum-garnet cyclophotocoagulation for glaucoma
    t. retinal photocoagulation
    t. retinopexy
    t. suture
    t. suture fixation
    t. suture fixation technique
transsclerally sutured posterior chamber lens (TS-SPCL)
transsphenoidal encephalocele
transsynaptic degeneration
transverse
    t. axis of Fick
    t. suture of Krause
    t. tarsotomy
transvitreal

Trantas
    T. dot
    T. operation
tranylcypromine sulfate
TranZgraft
trapdoor scleral buckle operation
trapezoidal keratotomy
trapezoid single-plane clear corneal incision
trap incision
Traquair
    T. island
    junctional scotoma of T.
    scotoma of T.
trauma
    blunt t.
    corneal t.
    ocular t.
    orbital t.
    orbitocranial t.
traumatic
    t. amblyopia
    t. angle recession
    t. aniridia
    t. atrophy
    t. choroidal rupture
    t. choroiditis
    t. corneal abrasion
    t. corneal cyst
    t. degenerative cataract
    t. glaucoma
    t. gliosis
    t. hyphema
    t. mydriasis
    t. myopathy
    t. optic neuropathy
    t. ptosis
    t. pupillary miosis
    t. retinopathy
    t. scleral cyst
tray
    I-tech cannula t.
Trbinger detachment
TRC-50IX ICG-capable fundus camera
TRC-SS2 stereoscopic fundus camera
TRD
    tractional retinal detachment
Treacher Collins syndrome
treatment
    external beam radiation t.
    Imre t.

PhotoPoint t.
Schöler t.
tree
vascular t.
trematode infection
trematodiasis
tremor
head t.
tremulous
t. cataract
t. iris
trepanation
t. of cornea
corneal t.
trephination
elliptical t.
excimer laser t.
host t.
nonmechanical t.
open-sky t.
partial-thickness t.
trephine
Arroyo t.
Arruga lacrimal t.
automated t.
automatic t.
Bard-Parker t.
Barraquer t.
Barron epikeratophakia t.
Barron-Hessburg corneal t.
Barron radial vacuum t.
t. blade
Bonaccolto t.
bone t.
bone-biting t.
Boston t.
Brown-Pusey corneal t.
Cardona corneal prosthesis t.
Castroviejo corneal transplant t.
Castroviejo improved t.
chalazion t.
corneal prosthesis t.
Davis t.
DiaPhine t.
Dimitry chalazion t.
disposable t.
Elliot corneal t.

Elschnig t.
Gradle corneal t.
Green t.
Grieshaber calibrated t.
Grieshaber corneal t.
Guyton corneal transplant t.
hand-held t.
Hanna t.
Hessburg-Barron suction t.
Hessburg-Barron vacuum t.
Iliff lacrimal t.
Katena t.
Katzin t.
King corneal t.
lacrimal t.
Lichtenberg corneal t.
lid t.
Londermann corneal t.
Lopez-Enriquez scleral t.
Martinez disposable corneal t.
Moria t.
Mueller electric corneal t.
Paton corneal t.
Paufique t.
Pharmacia corneal t.
punch t.
razor-blade t.
Scheie t.
Searcy chalazion t.
Storz corneal t.
Storz DiaPhine t.
suction t.
Surgistar corneal t.
Troutman t.
Troutman tenotomy t.
Walker t.
Weck t.
treponemal antibody
TRH
thyroid-releasing hormone
thyrotropin-releasing hormone
TRH test
triad
Charcot t.
Hoyt-Spencer t.
Hutchinson t.

T

NOTES

triad *(continued)*
    near t.
    t. of retinal cone
trial
    t. case
    t. case and lens
    clinical t.
    t. clip
    Diabetes Control and
      Complications T.
    t. frame
    Ischemic Optic Neuropathy
      Decompression T. (IONDT)
    Optic Neuritis Treatment T.
      (ONTT)
triamcinolone
Triamond
    Fine Finesse T.
triangle
    Arlt t.
    color t.
    fitting t.
    frontal t.
    Wernicke t.
triangular capsulotomy
Tri-Beeled trapezoidal keratome
trichiasis
    t. repair
trichilemmoma
Trichinella spiralis
trichofolliculoma tumor
trichoma
trichomatosis
trichomatous
trichophytosis
trichosis carunculae
trichroic
trichroism
trichromasy
trichromatic, trichromic
    t. color theory
trichromatism
    anomalous t.
trichromatopsia
    anomalous t.
trichromic *(var. of* trichromatic)
tricurve contact lenses
trifacial neuralgia
trifluoperazine hydrochloride
trifluperidol hydrochloride
trifluridine eye drops
trifocal
    executive t.

    t. glasses
    t. lens
trigeminal
    t. nerve (NV)
    t. nerve root section
    t. neuralgia
    t. neuropathic keratopathy
    t. pain
    t. reflex
    t. sensory ganglion
    t. shield
trigemino-oculomotor synkinesis
trigeminus
    nervus t.
    reflex t.
    t. reflex
trigger mechanism
trigone
    Mueller t.
triiodothyronine suppression test
trilamellar
trilateral retinoblastoma
trimethidium methosulfate
trimethoprim and polymyxin B
triopathy
Tri-Ophtho
triparanol
tripeennamine
Tripier
    T. operation
    T. operation throw square knot
    T. operation triple
    T. operation vision
triple
    T. Antibiotic
    t. procedure
    t. symptom complex
    Tripier operation t.
    t. vision
triple facet-tip needle
Triple-Gen
triple-throw square knot stitch
triplokoria
triplopia
Tri-Port sub-tenon anesthesia
    cannula
triptokoria
TripTone Caplets
triradiate line
trisodium phosphonoformate
    hexahydrate
Trisol
tristichia

tritan
    t. axis
tritanomal
tritanomalous
tritanomaly
tritanope
tritanopia
tritanopic
Tri-Thalmic
Tri-Thalmic HC
Triton
trocar
    Veirs t.
trochlea
    t. musculi obliqui superioris bulbi
    t. musculi obliqui superioris oculi
    t. of superior oblique muscle
trochlear
    t. fossa
    t. fovea
    t. hamulus
    t. muscle
    t. nerve (N.IV)
    t. nerve lesion
    t. nerve nucleus
    t. nerve palsy
    t. tubercle
trochlearis
    fossa t.
    fovea t.
    nervus t.
    spina t.
Trokel lens
Trokel-Peyman laser lens
troland
tromethamine
    ketorolac t.
    lodoxamide t.
Troncoso
    T. gonioscope
    T. gonioscopic lens implant
Tropheryma whippelii
trophic
    t. change
    t. defect

t. keratitis
t. keratopathy
t. retinal degeneration
t. ulceration of the cornea
tropia
    alternating t.
    constant monocular t.
    t. deviation
    intermittent t.
    vertical t.
tropica
    Leishmania t.
Tropicacyl
tropical
    t. optic neuropathy
    t. polyhexamethylene biguanide
tropicalis
    Candida t.
tropicamide
    hydroxyamphetamine and t.
tropic deviation
tropometer
troposcope
Trousseau sign
Troutman
    T. bladebreaker
    T. cannula
    T. conjunctival scissors
    T. corneal dissector
    T. corneal knife
    T. forceps
    T. implant
    T. lamellar dissector
    T. lens loupe
    T. microsurgical scissors
    T. needle holder
    T. operation
    T. punch
    T. rectus forceps
    T. suture scissors
    T. tenotomy trephine
    T. trephine
    T. tying forceps
Troutman-Barraquer
    T.-B. corneal fixation forceps
    T.-B. corneal utility forceps

T

NOTES

523

Troutman-Castroviejo
    T.-C. corneal fixation forceps
    T.-C. corneal section scissors
Troutman-Katzin corneal transplant
    scissors
Troutman-Llobera fixation forceps
Troutman-Tooke corneal knife
Truc
    T. flap
    T. operation
true
    t. exfoliation
    t. hemianopsia
    t. image
    t. visual acuity (TVA)
Trump solution
truncated contact lens
trunk
    facial nerve t.
Trupower aspherical lens
TruPro lacrimal cannula
Trusopt
TruVision lens
Trypanosoma
trypanosomiasis
trypsin-digested explant
TSC
    tuberous sclerosis complex
T-sign
TS III ROP
    threshold stage III of retinopathy of
    prematurity
TS-SPCL
    transsclerally sutured posterior
    chamber lens
tsukubaensis
    Streptomyces t.
TT
    transpupillary thermotherapy
t **test**
t-**test**
    Student unpaired t-t.
TTT
    transpupillary thermotherapy
T-tube
    cul-de-sac irrigation T.-t.
    Houser cul-de-sac irrigator T.-t.
    lacrimal duct T.-t.
    polyethylene T.-t.
    Pyrex T.-t.
    Silastic T.-t.
    vinyl T.-t.

tube
    Ahmed glaucoma drainage t.
    Ahmed shunt t.
    angled suction t.
    anterior chamber t.
    Baerveldt glaucoma implant t.
    Baerveldt shunt t.
    Bowman t.
    corneal t.
    Crawford t.
    encircling polyethylene t.
    endotracheal t.
    Eppendorf t.
    fil d'Arion silicone t.
    Frazier suction t.
    fusion t.
    Guibor duct t.
    Guibor Silastic t.
    Houser cul-de-sac irrigator t.
    Jones Pyrex t.
    Jones tear duct t.
    laser t.
    Lester Jones t.
    L.T. Jones tear duct t.
    Luer t.
    Microfuge t.
    Molteno shunt t.
    Moulton lacrimal duct t.
    neural t.
    polyethylene t.
    Pyrex t.
    Questek laser t.
    Quickert-Dryden t.
    Reinecke-Carroll lacrimal t.
    silicone t.
    vinyl t.
tuber
    frontal t.
tubercle
    t. bacillus
    caseating t.
    lacrimal t.
    lateral orbit t.
    lateral orbital t.
    lateral palpebral t.
    optic disk t.
    trochlear t.
    Whitnall t.
tuberculin syringe
tuberculomas
    optochiasmatic t.
tuberculosis
    t. conjunctivitis

intraocular t.
Mycobacterium t.
tuberculous
t. dacryocystis
t. dacryocystitis
t. iritis
t. keratitis
t. phlyctenulosis
t. rhinitis
t. tarsitis
t. uveitis
tuberous
t. sclerosis
t. sclerosis complex (TSC)
tubing
bicanalicular t.
t. introducer forceps
silicone t.
viscodissector t.
Tübinger
T. perimeter
T. perimetry
tubular
t. vision
t. visual field
tuck
iris t.
left superior oblique t.
t. procedure
tucked lid of Collier
tucker
Bishop-Peter tendon t.
Bishop tendon t.
Burch-Greenwood t.
Burch-Greenwood tendon t.
Fink tendon t.
Green muscle t.
Green strabismus t.
Ruedemann-Todd tendon t.
tendon t.
Tudor-Thomas
T.-T. graft
T.-T. operation
tuft
cystic retinal t.
neovascular t.
retinal t.

vitreoretinal t.
zonular-traction retinal t.
Tukey HSD test
tularemia
oculoglandular t.
tularemic conjunctivitis
tularensis
conjunctivitis t.
Francisella t.
Tulevech cannula
Tulio phenomenon
tulle gras dressing
tumbling
t. E cube
t. E test
t. procedure
t. technique
t. technique operation
tumor
anemone cell t.
t. apex
apical t.
benign t.
brain t.
Brooke t.
carcinoid t.
cerebellar astrocytoma t.
cerebellopontine angle t.
choristoma t.
choroidal melanocytic t.
Coerens t.
collision t.
congenital limbal corneal
dermoid t.
conjunctival lymphoid t.
craniofacial fibro-osseous t.
cystic hydrocystoma t.
dermoid t.
embryonal t. of ciliary body
ependymoma t.
epithelial t.
t. of eyelid
eyelid t.
fibro-osseous t.
fossa t.
Grawitz t.
hair follicle t.

T

NOTES

tumor *(continued)*
  histiocytic t.
  interior eye t.
  t. of interior of eye
  intrasellar t.
  Koenen t.
  lacrimal gland epithelial t.
  lymphoid t.
  lymphoproliferative t.
  malignant epithelial t.
  medulloblastoma t.
  melanocytic iris t.
  mesenchymal t.
  metastasis of t.
  t. metastasis
  metastatic choroidal t.
  mixed t.
  mucinous adenocarcinoma t.
  neurogenic t.
  nonepithelial t.
  ocular adnexal t.
  optic nerve t.
  t. of optic nerve
  orbital t.
  Pancoast t.
  papilliform t.
  phakomatous choristoma t.
  pilomatrixoma t.
  pituitary t.
  plasma cell t.
  primitive neuroectodermal t.
    (PNET)
  Rathke pouch t.
  retinal anlage t.
  rhabdoid t.
  Schmincke t.
  spinal canal t.
  spindle-cell t.
  suprasellar t.
  syringoma t.
  trichofolliculoma t.
  vascular t.
  Warthin t.
  waxy t.
  Wilms t.
  Zimmerman t.
tunable dye laser
TUNEL
  in situ DNA nick end labeling
  TUNEL staining
tungsten-halogen lamp
tunic
  Brücke t.

  fibrous t.
  fibrovascular t.
  Ruysch t.
  vascular t.
tunica
  t. adnata oculi
  t. albuginea oculi
  t. conjunctiva
  t. conjunctiva bulbi oculi
  t. conjunctiva palpebra
  t. fibrosa bulbi
  t. fibrosa oculi
  t. interna bulbi
  t. nervea
  t. nervosa oculi
  t. sclerotica
  t. sensoria bulbi
  t. uvea
  t. vascularis oculi
  t. vasculosa bulbi
  t. vasculosa lentis
  t. vasculosa oculi
tunnel
  scleral t.
  t. vision
tunneled implant
turbidity-reducing units
TurboSonic tip
TurboStaltic pump
turbo-tip of phacoemulsification unit
turcica
  sella t.
Turkish saddle
Turk line
turnover
  epithelial t.
  tear t.
Turtle chart
tutamina oculi
TVA
  true visual acuity
Tween
tweezers
  jeweler t.
twelfth nerve palsy
twenty/twenty
  t. argon-fluoride excimer laser
  T. drops
twilight
  t. blindness
  t. vision
twin cone

Twirl
    Spherical T.
twirling method
Twisk microscissors
twist
    t. fixation hook
    scleral t.
    stitch with t.'s
twisted virgin silk suture
twitch
    Cogan lid t.
two-angled polypropylene loop
two-light discrimination
two-plane lens
two-way
    t.-w. cataract-aspirating cannula
    t.-w. syringe
    t.-w. towel clip
Tycos manometer
tying forceps
tying/stitch removal forceps
tyloma
    t. conjunctivae
tylosis ciliaris
tyloxapol
Tyndall
    T. effect
    T. phenomenon

type
    t. 1 diabetes
    t. 2 diabetes
    Jaeger test t.
    t. 1 herpes simplex virus
    point system test t.
    Snellen test t.
typhlology
typhlosis
typhus
    epidemic t.
    scrub t.
typical
    t. achromatopsia
    t. coloboma
typoscope
tyramine hydrochloride
Tyrell iris hook
tyrosinase-negative type
    oculocutaneous albinism
tyrosinase-positive type
    oculocutaneous albinism
tyrosinase test

T

NOTES

UBM
ultrasound biomicroscopy
UCVA
uncorrected visual acuity
UGH
uveitis glaucoma hyphema
UGH syndrome
UGH+ syndrome
Uhthoff
U. phenomenon
U. sign
U. symptom
U. syndrome
UL
upper lid
Ulanday double cannula
ulcer
acne rosacea corneal u.
ameboid u.
annular u.
bacterial infectious corneal u.
catarrhal corneal u.
central corneal u.
chronic serpiginous u.
community-acquired corneal u.
conjunctival u.
corneal u.
dendriform u.
dendritic herpes simplex
corneal u.
fascicular u.
fungal corneal u.
geographic herpes simplex
corneal u.
herpes simplex corneal u.
herpetic u.
hypopyon u.
infectious corneal u.
Jacob u.
marginal catarrhal u.
marginal corneal u.
metaherpetic u.
Mooren corneal u.
noncentral u.
oval-shaped vernal u.
peripheral corneal u.
pneumococcal u.
pneumococcus u.
pyocyaneal u.
ring u.

rodent u.
Saemisch u.
serpiginous corneal u.
shield u.
sterile corneal u.
stromal u.
superior corneal shield u.
suppurative u.
Terrien u.
von Hippel internal corneal u.
xerophthalmic u.
ulceration
catarrhal marginal u.
u. of cornea
frank corneal u.
geographic u.
herpes epithelial tropic u.
indolent u.
necrotizing sclerocorneal u.
(NSU)
perilimbal u.
rheumatoid related u.
ulcerative keratitis
ulcerogranuloma
ulceromembranous
ulcerosa
blepharitis u.
ulcus
u. serpens corneae
ulectomy
ulerythema ophryogene
Ulloa operation
Ullrich syndrome
Ultex
U. bifocal
U. lens
U. lens implant
Ultima
Dioptron U.
U. photocoagulator
U. 2000 photocoagulator
Ultra
U. mag lens
U. Tears
U. Tears Solution
U. view SP slit lamp lens
Ultracaine
Ultra-Care
Ultra-Image A-scan
Ultra-Lase

U

Ultramatic
 U. Project-O-Chart
 U. Project-O-Chart projector
 (UPOC)
 U. Rx Master phoroptor
 U. Rx Master phoroptor
 retractor
Ultrapred
UltraPulse laser
ultrascan
 Digital B System u.
 U. Digital B system
ultrasonic
 u. cataract-removal lancet
 u. cataract-removal lancet
 needle
 u. insonification
 U. lancet needle
 u. micrometer
 U. pachymeter
 u. pachymetry
ultrasonogram
 A-scan u.
 B-scan u.
 Doppler u.
 gray-scale u.
ultrasonography
 A-scan u.
 B-scan u.
 contact B-scan u.
 CooperVision u.
 Doppler u.
 water-bath u.
ultrasound
 Acuson u.
 Alcon Digital B 2000 u.
 Axisonic II u.
 u. biomicroscopy (UBM)
 CooperVision u.
 3D i-Scan ophthalmic u.
 high-gain digital u.
 kinetic u.
 Ocuscan A-scan biometric u.
 u. pachometer
 renal u.
 through-the-lid contact u.
UltraThin surgical blade
ultraviolet
 u. burn
 u. filter
 u. keratoconjunctivitis
 u. light

 u. radiation
 u. ray ophthalmia
ultraviolet-induced injury
Ultravue lens
Ultrazyme enzymatic cleaner
umbilicated cataract
umbra
umbrella
 u. iris
 U. punctum plug
umbrella-like pattern
uncal syndrome
uncinate
 u. procedure
 u. process of lacrimal bone
unconventional outflow
uncorrected visual acuity (UCVA,
 UNCVA)
uncrossed diplopia
uncut spectacle lens
UNCVA
 uncorrected visual acuity
underaction
 congenital superior oblique u.
undercorrection
underlying conus
underwater diathermy unit
undine
 u. dropper
undissociated alkaloid
undulatory nystagmus
unequal retinal image
Unfolder implantation system
ung
 ointment
unguis
 os u.
 pterygium u.
unharmonious ARC
Unicare blue and green all-in-one
 cleaning solution
Unicat knife
unifocal
 u. helioid choroiditis
 u. optic nerve lesion
unilateral
 u. acute idiopathic maculopathy
 u. altitudinal scotoma
 u. arcus
 u. conjunctivitis
 u. hearing loss
 u. hemianopsia
 u. lesion

u. microtremor
u. papilledema
u. proptosis
u. ptosis of eyelid
u. sporadic retinoblastoma
u. strabismus
uniocular
u. hemianopsia
u. strabismus
Uniplanar style PC II lens
UniPulse
U. CO_2 surgical laser system
U. 1040 Surgical CO_2 laser system
Unisol
U. 4
U. Plus
unit
Alcon cryosurgical u.
Alcon irrigating/aspirating u.
Alcon 20,000 Legacy u.
Alcon 10,000 Master u.
Alcon phacoemulsification u.
Aloe reading u.
Amoils cryosurgical u.
Ångström u.
AO Ful-Vue diagnostic u.
AO Reichert Instruments Ful-Vue diagnostic u.
Bishop-Harman irrigating/aspirating u.
Bovie electrocautery u.
Bovie electrosurgical u.
Bovie retinal detachment u.
Bracken irrigating/aspirating u.
Cavitron irrigating/aspirating u.
Cavitron-Kelman irrigating/aspirating u.
Charles irrigating/aspirating u.
Cilco Ultrasound u.
Coburn irrigation/aspiration u.
Cooper I&A u.
Cooper irrigating/aspirating u.
CooperVision irrigating/aspirating u.
CooperVision irrigation/aspiration u.

cryosurgical u.
DeVilbiss irrigating/aspirating u.
diathermy u.
Dougherty irrigating/aspirating u.
Drews irrigating/aspirating u.
Drews-Rosenbaum irrigating/aspirating u.
Empac-Cavitron irrigation/aspiration u.
Fink irrigating/aspirating u.
Fox irrigating/aspirating u.
Frigitronics cryosurgical u.
Gass irrigating/aspirating u.
Gibson irrigating/aspirating u.
Girard ultrasonic u.
Hartstein irrigating/aspirating u.
Holzknecht u.
Hyde irrigating/aspirating u.
Hyde irrigator/aspirator u.
Intermedics Phaco I/A u.
IOLAB irrigating/aspirating u.
irrigation-aspiration u.
Irvine irrigating/aspirating u.
Keeler cryophake u.
Keeler cryosurgical u.
Kelman-Cavitron I/A u.
Kelman-Cavitron irrigating/aspirating u.
Kelman cryosurgical u.
Kelman irrigating/aspirating u.
Kelman phacoemulsification u.
Krymed Cryopexy u.
u. of light
log u.
u. of luminous flux
u. of luminous intensity
McIntyre irrigating/aspirating u.
microcautery u.
Mira diathermy u.
N_2O cryosurgical u.
u. of ocular convergence
Ocutome vitrectomy u.
OMS Empac Irrigation/Aspiration u.
Peczon I/A u.
Peyman vitrectomy u.

U

NOTES

531

unit *(continued)*
- Peyman vitreophage u.
- Phaco Cavitron
  irrigating/aspirating u.
- Phaco Emulsifier Cavitron u.
- Pierce I/A u.
- Premiere irrigation-aspiration u.
- Rollet irrigating/aspirating u.
- Schepens retinal detachment u.
- SITE TXR 2200
  microsurgical u.
- Storz-Walker retinal
  detachment u.
- Surg-E-Trol System
  irrigating/aspirating u.
- Svedberg u.
- Sylva irrigating/aspirating u.
- Talbot u.
- turbidity-reducing u.'s
- turbo-tip of
  phacoemulsification u.
- underwater diathermy u.
- Visitec aspiration u.
- Visitec irrigating/aspirating u.
- Visitec vitrectomy u.
- Vitrophage-Peyman u.

unitas
- oculi u. (both eyes)

United Sonics J shock phaco fragmentor system
unity conjugacy planes
univariate polytomous logistic regression
Universal
- U. conformer
- U. eye shield
- U. II forceps
- U. implant
- U. Pathfinder knife
- U. slit lamp

universale
- angiokeratoma corporis
  diffusum u.

University of Waterloo chart
Univis
- U. bifocal
- U. lens

Univision low-vision microscopic lens
Unna abtropfung theory
unrefined refraction
unstained wet mount
up-and-down staircases procedure

upbeat nystagmus
updrawn pupil
upgaze
UPOC
- Ultramatic Project-O-Chart projector

upper
- u. canaliculus
- u. eyelid
- u. hemianopsia
- u. lid (UL)
- u. punctum
- u. retina
- u. tarsal conjunctiva

upside-down
- u.-d. ptosis
- u.-d. reversal of vision

uptake
- lacrimal gland gallium u.

upward
- u. gaze
- u. squint

URAM E2 compact MicroProbe laser
urate band keratopathy
uratic
- u. conjunctivitis
- u. iritis

urea
Ureaphil Injection
uremic
- u. amaurosis
- u. amblyopia
- u. optic neuropathy
- u. retinitis

Uribe orbital implant
urica
- cornea u.
- keratitis u.

urinary
- u. GAG assay
- u. glycosaminoglycan
  measurement assay

urine refractometry
Urrets-Zavalia retinal surgical lens
Usher syndrome
UTAS 2000 electroretinography instrument
uterque
- oculi u. (each eye) (OU)
- visio oculus u. (vision of both
  eyes) (VOU)

Utrata
- U. capsulorrhexis forceps

U. cutter
U. retriever
Utrata-Kershner capsulorrhexis cystitome forceps
utricular reflex
UV
U. blocking filter
U. Nova Curve lens
uvea
tunica u.
uveae
ectropion u.
entropion u.
sarcomatosum u.
uveal
u. atrophy
u. coat
u. effusion
u. effusion syndrome
u. entropion
u. framework
u. juvenile xanthogranuloma
u. melanocyte
u. melanoma
u. metastasis
u. neurofibroma
u. nevus
u. osteoma
u. staphyloma
u. tissue
u. tract
u. tract hamartoma
u. tract hemangioma
uvealis
pars u.
uveitic
u. band keratopathy
u. glaucoma
uveitides
uveitis, uveitides, pl. **uveitides**
anterior u.
aspergillosis u.
bacterial u.
Behçet u.
bilateral u.

candidal u.
chronic anterior u. (CAU)
endogenous u.
excessive rebound u.
Förster u.
Fuchs u.
fungal u.
u. glaucoma hyphema (UGH)
granulomatous anterior u.
herpes simplex u.
heterochromic u.
intermediate u.
Kirisawa u.
lens-induced u.
LHA-B27-associated u.
nongranulomatous anterior u.
parasitic u.
peripheral u.
phacoanaphylactic u.
phacogenic u.
phacolytic u.
phacotoxic u.
posterior u.
protozoan u.
sarcoid u.
sarcoidosis-associated u.
sympathetic u.
toxoplasmic u.
tuberculous u.
viral u.
vitiligo u.
Vogt-Koyanagi bilateral u.
zoster u.
uveitis-vitiligo-alopecia-poliosis syndrome
uveocutaneous syndrome
uveoencephalitic syndrome
uveoencephalitis
uveolabyrinthitis
uveomeningeal syndrome
uveomeningitis syndrome
uveomeningoencephalitis
uveoneuroaxitis
uveoparotitis

U

NOTES

uveoplasty
uveoretinitis
uveoscleral outflow
uveoscleritis
uveovertex drainage

Uvex lens
uviban
Uyemura
    U. operation
    U. syndrome

V
  volume
    V pattern
    V syndrome
VA
  visual acuity
  VA magnetic orbital implant
vaccinia
  blepharoconjunctivitis v.
  v. gangrenosa
  generalized v.
  v. infection
  keratitis v.
  progressive v.
vaccinial keratitis
vacciniforme
  hydroa v.
vaccinulosa
  keratitis post v.
Vactro
  V. perilimbal suction
  V. perilimbal suction apparatus
vacuolar configuration
vacuole
  autophagic v.
  cortical v.
vacuum-centering guide
vaginae
  v. externa nervi optici
  v. interna nervi optici
  v. nervi optici
  v. oculi
vagus nerve paralysis
Vahlkampfia **cyst**
Vaiser-Cibis muscle retractor
Vaiser sponge
Valilab electrocautery
ValleyLab cautery
valproate sodium
Valsalva
  V. maneuver
  V. retinopathy
value
  C v.
  DK v.
  equivalent oxygen
    percentage v.
  ocular hemodynamic v.
  p v.
  predictive v.

  prismatic dioptric v.
  threshold limit v. (TLV)
valve
  Ahmed glaucoma v.
  Béraud v.
  Bianchi v.
  Foltz v.
  Hasner v.
  v. of Hasner
  Huschke v.
  Krause v.
  Krupin v.
  Krupin-Denver v.
  Rosenmüller v.
  v. of Rosenmüller
  Taillefer v.
  Van Herick v.
van
  v. der Hoeve disease
  V. Herick filtration
  V. Herick modification
  V. Herick valve
  V. Heuven retinopathy
  V. Lint akinesia
  V. Lint anesthesia
  V. Lint-Atkinson lid akinetic
    block
  V. Lint block
  V. Lint flap
  V. Lint injection
  V. Lint modified technique
  V. Milligen eyelid repair
    technique
  V. Milligen operation
vanillism
Vannas
  V. capsulotomy
  V. capsulotomy scissors
  V. iridocapsulotomy scissors
Vantage ophthalmoscope
Vaper Vac II
variabilis
  erythrokeratodermia v. (EKV)
variable strabismus
variance
  analysis of v. (ANOVA)
varians
  metamorphopsia v.
variant
  Miller-Fisher v.

V

variation
coefficient of v.
diurnal v.
v. diurnal
Vari bladebreaker
varicella
v. iridocyclitis
v. keratitis
varicella-zoster
v.-z. ophthalmicus
v.-z. virus (VZV)
varices (*pl. of* varix)
varicoblepharon
varicose ophthalmia
Varigray
V. implant
V. lens
Varilux
V. lens
V. lens implant
varix, pl. **varices**
conjunctival v.
orbital v.
vortex vein v.
vasa
v. sanguinea retinae
Vasco-Posada orbital retractor
vascular
v. abnormality
v. arcade
v. cataract
v. cerebellar disease
v. circle of optic nerve
v. coat of eyeball
v. congestion
v. disorder
v. endothelial cell
v. filling defect
v. frond
v. funnel
v. hamartoma
v. keratitis
v. lamina of choroid
v. loop
v. network
v. occlusion
v. occlusive disease
v. optical disk swelling
without visual loss
v. plexus
v. retinopathy
v. sheathing
v. tree

v. tumor
v. tunic
vascularization
conjunctival v.
corneal v.
v. elsewhere in the retina
(VNE)
stromal v.
vascularized
v. scar
v. tortuosity
vasculature
choroidal v.
disk v.
perimacular v.
retinal v.
spider v.
vasculitis
benign retinal v.
granulomatous v.
idiopathic retinal v.
limbal v.
obstructive retinal v.
orbital v.
v. retinae
retinal v.
vasculonebulous keratitis
vasculopathy
idiopathic polypoidal
choroidal v. (IPCV)
radiogenic v.
vasoactive amine
Vasocidin
V. Ophthalmic
VasoClear
V. Ophthalmic
VasoClear A
Vasocon
V. Regular
V. Regular Ophthalmic
Vasocon-A
V.-A. Ophthalmic
Vasosulf
V. Ophthalmic
vaulting of contact lens
VBIO
Video Binocular indirect
ophthalmoscope
VDTS
video display terminal simulator
Veatch ophthalmic ReSeeVit system
VECP
visual-evoked cortical potential

vectis
    Anis irrigating v.
    anterior chamber irrigating v.
    aspirating/irrigating v.
    cul-de-sac irrigating v.
    Drews-Knolle reverse
      irrigating v.
    irrigating anterior chamber v.
    irrigating/aspirating v.
    Look irrigating v.
    Peczon I/A v.
    Pierce I/A irrigating v.
    Pierce irrigating v.
    plastic disposable irrigating v.
    Sheets irrigating v.
    Snellen v.
vectograph chart
vectographic study
vector
    v. analysis
    v. array transducer
vegetable ophthalmia
veil
    dimple v.
    pigmented v.
    Sattler v.
    vitreal v.
    vitreous v.
veiling glare
vein
    angular v.
    anterior ciliary v.
    anterior conjunctival v.
    aqueous v.
    Ascher v.
    central retinal v. (CRV)
    choroid v.
    choroidovaginal v.
    ciliary v.
    cilioretinal v.
    conjunctival v.
    corticose v.
    endophlebitis of retinal v.
    episcleral v.
    facial v.
    frontal diploic v.
    Galen v.

    inferior nasal v.
    inferior ophthalmic v.
    inferior palpebral v.
    inferior temporal v.
    Kuhnt postcentral v.
    lacrimal v.
    muscular v.
    nasofrontal v.
    nicking of retinal v.
    occlusion of branch v.
    occlusion of retinal v.
    ophthalmic v.
    ophthalmomeningeal v.
    opticociliary shunt v.
    palpebral v.
    posterior ciliary v.
    posterior conjunctival v.
    retinal v.
    superior nasal v.
    superior ophthalmic v.
    superior palpebral v.
    superior temporal v.
    supraorbital v.
    vortex v.
Veinlaser Captured-Pulse laser
Veirs
    V. cannula
    V. trocar
Velcro head strap
velocardiofacial syndrome
velocimeter
    Doppler v.
    laser Doppler v.
velocimetry
    laser Doppler v.
velocity
    v. error
    retinal-slip v.
    saccadic v.
velonoskiascopy, belonoskiascopy
velum
    corneal v.
Velva Kleen
VEM
    vergence eye movement
vena
    v. angularis

V

NOTES

vena *(continued)*
  v. centralis retinae
  v. choroideae oculi
  v. ciliares anteriores
  v. diploica frontalis
  v. facialis
  v. lacrimalis
  v. nasofrontalis
  v. ophthalmica inferior
  v. ophthalmica superior
  v. ophthalmomeningea
  v. vorticosae
venae
  v. anteriores conjunctivales
  v. conjunctivales
  v. episclerale
  v. palpebrales
  v. palpebrales inferiores
  v. palpebrales superiores
  v. posteriores conjunctivales
venography
  orbital v.
venomanometer
  Zeimer v.
venomanometry
venous
  v. beading
  v. congestion
  v. engorgement
  v. hemangioma
  v. loop
  v. occlusive disease
  v. pulsation
  v. sheathing
  v. sheath patch
  v. sinus
  v. stasis
  v. stasis retinopathy (VSR)
  v. stenosis retinopathy
  v. tortuosity
venter frontalis musculi
  occipitofrontalis
ventricle
  cerebral v.
ventriculography
venturi
  V. aspiration vitrectomy device
  v. effect
Venturi-Flo valve system
venula
  v. macularis inferior
  v. macularis superior
  v. medialis retinae

  v. nasalis retinae inferior
  v. nasalis retinae superior
  v. retinae medialis
  v. temporalis retinae inferior
  v. temporalis retinae superior
venule
  v. banking
  macular v.
  retinal v.
  right-angle deflected v.
VEP
  visual-evoked potential
VER
  visual-evoked response
vera
  polycoria v.
Verga lacrimal groove
vergence
  ability v.
  v. eye movement (VEM)
  v. facility
  fusional v.
  v. of lens
  negative vertical v.
  power v.
  reduced v.
  reflux v.
  tonic v.
  vertical v.
  zero v.
vergens
  strabismus deorsum v.
  strabismus sursum v.
Verhoeff
  V. capsule forceps
  V. lens expressor
  V. operation
  V. scissors
  V. streak
  V. suture
Verhoeff-Chandler
  V.-C. capsulotomy
  V.-C. operation
vermiform
  v. contraction
  v. movement
vermis
  cerebellar v.
  dorsal v.
Vernacel
vernal
  v. catarrh

v. conjunctivitis
v. keratoconjunctivitis (VKC)
Vernier
V. optometer
V. stimulus
V. visual acuity
version
ductions and v.'s (D&V)
v.'s and ductions
v. movement
vertebral angiography
vertebrobasilar
v. artery
v. system
v. vascular abnormality
verteporfin
vertex
v. of distance
front v.
v. of power
v. refractionometer
vertexmeter
vertical
v. axis
v. axis of eye
v. axis of Fick
v. comitant deviation
v. diplopia
v. divergence
v. divergence position
v. duction
v. forceps
v. fusional vergence amplitude
v. fusion range
v. gaze
v. gaze center
v. gaze paresis
v. hemianopsia
v. illumination
v. meridian
v. movement
v. muscle
v. myoclonus
v. nystagmus
v. parallax
v. phoria
v. plane

v. prism test
v. retraction syndrome
right gaze v.'s
v. strabismus
v. strabismus fixus
v. stria
v. tropia
v. vergence
v. vertigo
verticillata
cornea v.
corneal v.
vertigo
benign paroxysmal
positional v. (BPPV)
objective v.
ocular v.
sham-movement v.
special sense v.
subjective v.
vertical v.
vertometer
Verwey eyelid operation
vesicle
chorionic v.
clear lid v.
compound v.
cornea v.
lens v.
lenticular v.
lid v.
multilocular v.
ocular v.
ophthalmic v.
optic v.
pinocytotic v.
vesicula ophthalmica
vesicular
v. keratitis
v. keratopathy
vesiculation
eyelid v.
vesiculosus linear endothelial
vessel
v. abnormalities of retina
anomalous v.
choroidal v.

V

NOTES

vessel *(continued)*
  ciliary v.
  collateral v.
  congested v.
  conjunctival v.
  disk neurovascular v.
  disk new v.
  episcleral blood v.
  feeder v.
  frond of v.
  ghost v.
  neovascularization of new v.'s
    elsewhere (NVE)
  opticociliary shunt v.
  orbital v.
  retinal v.
  sheathing of v.
  v. sheathing
  sheathing of retinal v.
  shunt v.
  silver-wire v.
  stromal blood v.
  succulent v.
  tensile strength of v.
  tortuosity of retinal v.
  v. traction
vestibular
  v. cortex
  v. nerve
  v. nucleus
  v. nystagmus
  v. organ
  v. pupillary reaction
  v. system
vestibulocerebellar ataxia
vestibulo-ocular
  v.-o. reflex
  v.-o. response (VOR)
Vexol
  V. 1%
  V. Ophthalmic Suspension
VF
  visual field
VF-14 questionnaire
V-groove gauge
VG slit lamp
VH
  vitreous hemorrhage
VI
  visual impairment
vibrating scissors
vibratory nystagmus
Vickerall round ringed forceps

Vickers
  V. forceps
  V. needle holder
vicrosurgery
Vicryl suture
VID
  visible iris diameter
vidarabine
Vidaurri irrigator
video
  V. Binocular indirect
    ophthalmoscope (VBIO)
  v. display terminal simulator
    (VDTS)
  v. specular microscope
videoendoscope
  fiberoptic v.
videokeratograph
videokeratographic corneal
  steepening
videokeratography
  computerized v. (CVK)
  computerized corneal v.
videokeratoscope
  computer-assisted v.
  EyeSys v.
  PAR-C-Scan v.
  TechnoMed C-Scan v.
videometer
vidian
  v. nerve
  v. neuralgia
Viers
  V. erysiphake
  V. needle
  V. operation
  V. rod
Vieth-Mueller
  V.-M. circle
  V.-M. horopter
view
  axial v.
  Caldwell v.
  Caldwell-Waters v.
  coronal v.
  field of v.
  sweep v.
  Waters v.
Villasenor-Navarro fixation ring
Villasensor ultrasonic pachymeter
villi
  pectinate v.

vinyl
  v. T-tube
  v. tube
violet
  v. haptic
  v. vision
  visual v.
Vira-A
  V.-A. Ophthalmic
viral
  v. blepharitis
  v. capsid antigen
  v. conjunctivitis
  v. keratoconjunctivitis
  v. ocular disease
  v. uveitis
Virchow corpuscle
virgin silk suture
viridans
  Streptococcus v.
VIRIDIS-LITE photocoagulator
VIRIDIS photocoagulator
Viroptic
  V. Ophthalmic
virtual
  v. focus
  v. image
  v. point
virus
  BK v.
  Coxsackie v.
  cytomegalic inclusion v.
  Epstein-Barr v. (EBV)
  herpes simplex v. (HSV)
  herpes zoster v.
  human immunodeficiency v.
  human T-lymphotropic v.
  influenza v.
  JC v.
  molluscum v.
  Newcastle disease v.
  type 1 herpes simplex v.
  varicella-zoster v. (VZV)
Visalens
  V. contact lens cleaning and
    soaking solution
  V. Wetting

VISC
  vitreous infusion suction cutter
  OMS Machemer/Parel VISC
visceral
  v. larva migrans (VLM)
  v. larva migrans syndrome
  v. myopathy
Viscoat
  V. solution
viscocanalostomy
viscodissector tubing
viscoelastic
  v. solution
Visco expression cannula
Viscoflow cannula
Viscolens lens
viscotechnique
viscous
  v. ochre fluid
  v. xanthochromic fluid
Visculose
visibility
  v. acuity
  v. curve
visible
  v. drusen
  v. iris diameter (VID)
  v. spectrum
Visi-Drape
  V.-D. Elite ophthalmic drape
  V.-D. mini aperture drape
  V.-D. mini incise drape
Visiflex drape
visile
Visine
  V. A.C.
  V. Extra
  V. Extra Ophthalmic
  V. L.R. Ophthalmic
  V. Tears
visio
  v. oculus
  v. oculus dextra (vision of
    right eye) (VOD)
  v. oculus sinister (vision of
    left eye) (VOS)

V

NOTES

visio *(continued)*
    v. oculus uterque (vision of
      both eyes) (VOU)
vision
    6/6 v.
    20/20 v.
    achromatic v.
    ambulatory v.
    V. analyzer
    V. Analyzer/Overrefraction
      System
    artificial v.
    best-corrected v.
    binocular single v. (BSV)
    blue v.
    blurred v.
    blurring of v.
    botulism-induced blurred v.
    V. Care enzymatic cleaner
    central island of v.
    central keyhole of v.
    cerebral tunnel v.
    chromatic v.
    color v.
    cone v.
    day v.
    decreasing v.
    v. deprivation myopia
    dichromatic v.
    dimness of v.
    direct v.
    distortion of v.
    double v.
    duplicity theory of v.
    eccentric v.
    extramacular binocular v.
    facial v.
    false v.
    field of v.
    finger v.
    form v.
    foveal v.
    glare v.
    green v.
    half v.
    halo v.
    haploscopic v.
    Helmholtz theory of color v.
    Hering theory of color v.
    indirect v.
    iridescent v.
    keyhole v.
    line of v.

    linear v.
    loss of v.
    low v.
    macular binocular v.
    misty v.
    monocular v.
    motion v.
    multiple v.
    naked v. (Nv)
    near v.
    night v.
    no-light-perception v.
    obscure v.
    organ of v.
    oscillating v.
    peripheral v.
    phantom v.
    photopic v.
    Pick v.
    pinhole v.
    pseudoscopic v.
    rainbow v.
    red v.
    residual v.
    v. rod
    rod v.
    scoterythrous v.
    scotopic v.
    shaft v.
    single binocular v. (SBV)
    solid v.
    stable v.
    stereoscopic v.
    subjective v.
    subnormal v.
    suboptimal v.
    V. Tech lens
    tilted v.
    v. training
    transient obscuration of v.
    Tripier operation v.
    triple v.
    tubular v.
    tunnel v.
    twilight v.
    upside-down reversal of v.
    violet v.
    word v.
    yellow v.
Visi-Spear eye sponge
Visitec
    V. angled lens hook
    V. aspiration unit

V. capsule polisher curette
V. Company lens
V. corneal shield
V. corneal suture manipulating hook
V. cortex extractor
V. double-cutting cystitome
V. intraocular lens dialer
V. iris retractor
V. irrigating/aspirating cannula
V. irrigating/aspirating unit
V. lens pusher
V. manipulator
V. micro double-iris hook
V. microhook
V. microiris hook
V. nucleus removal loupe
V. RK zone marker
V. straight lens hook
V. vitrectomy unit
Visolett
Visometer
  Lotman V.
Vista
  Blue V.
Vistacon
Vistaject-25
Vistaject-50
Vistaquel
Vistaril
Vistazine
Vistech
  V. 6500 contrast test
  V. Multivision Contrast Tester 8000
  V. wall chart
Vistide
visual
  V. Activities Questionnaire
  v. acuity (VA)
  v. acuity decrease
  v. acuity testing
  v. agnosia
  v. allesthesia
  v. angle
  v. aphasia
  v. association area

v. attentiveness
v. axis
v. blackout
v. cell
v. cone
v. confusion
v. corkscrew defect
v. cortex
v. cycle
v. deprivation syndrome
v. development
v. direction
v. discrimination
v. disturbance
v. efficiency
v. extinction
v. field (F, VF)
v. field defect
v. field indices
v. field testing
v. function
v. function evaluation
v. hallucination
v. halo
v. image
v. impairment (VI)
v. inattention
v. line
v. memory
v. orbicularis reflex
v. organ
v. paraneoplastic syndrome
v. pathway
v. pathway disease
v. perception
v. perseveration
v. pigment
v. plane
v. point
v. preservation
v. process
v. prognosis
v. projection
v. psychophysics
v. purple
v. radiations
v. seizure

NOTES

V

visual *(continued)*
  v. sensory system
  v. spread
  v. threshold
  v. tilt
  v. violet
  v. white
  v. yellow
  v. zone
visuale
  organum v.
visual-evoked
  v.-e. cortical potential (VECP)
  v.-e. potential (VEP)
  v.-e. response (VER)
visualization
  contrast v.
  double-contrast v.
visualize
visually evoked potential mapping
visual-spatial agnosia
Visual-Tech machine
visual-vestibulo-ocular response
Visudyne
Visulab System
Visulas
  V. argon C laser
  V. argon/YAG laser
  V. 532 Combi software
  V. InterChange software
  V. Nd:YAG laser
  V. YAG C laser
  V. YAG E laser
  V. YAG S laser
VisuMed MEL60 laser
visuoauditory
visuognosis
visuolexic
visuometer
visuopsychic
visuosensory
visuospatial
  v. disorder
visus
  linea v.
  organum v.
Visuscope
  Cüppers V.
  V. motor
  V. motor test
  V. ophthalmoscope
  V. sensory test
Visuskop

Visutron
VISX
  V. 2020 excimer laser
  V. Refractive Planner
  V. Star excimer laser system
  V. STAR S2 excimer laser
    system
  V. Star S2 laser
  V. Twenty/Twenty excimer
    laser
  V. Twenty/Twenty system
Vit
  V. Commander foot pedal
  V. Commander handpiece
  V. Commander System
Vit-A-Drops
VitaLase Er:YAG laser
vital dye
VitalEyes
Vitallium
  V. implant
  V. miniplate
vitamin
  v. A deficiency
vitamins
  ICaps ocular v.'s
vitelliform
  v. degeneration of macula
  v. dystrophy
  v. macular degeneration
  v. maculopathy
vitelline macular degeneration
vitelliruptive
  v. degeneration
  v. macular dystrophy
vitellirupture
  autosomal dominant v.
vitiliginous chorioretinitis
vitiligo, pl. **vitiligines**
  v. iridis
  perilimbal v.
  v. uveitis
Vitrase
Vitrasert
  V. intravitreal implant
Vitravene
Vitrax
vitrea
  lamina v.
  membrana v.
vitreal
  v. bleed
  v. cell

v. detachment
v. hemorrhage
v. lamina
v. liquefaction
v. membrane
v. veil
vitrectomy
anterior v.
closed-system pars plana v.
core v.
v. instrument
lens-sparing v.
open-sky v.
pars plana v. (PPV)
pars plana Baerveldt tube
  insertion with v.
port v.
3-port pars plana v.
posterior v.
v. prism lens tab
v. for proliferative retinopathy
v. sponge
Weck-cel v.
vitrector
Alcon v.
Cilco v.
CooperVision v.
Frigitronics v.
Kaufman type II v.
mechanical v.
Microvit v.
Peyman v.
Storz Microvit v.
vitrectorhexis
vitrei
synchesis corporis v.
vitrein
vitreitis
dense v.
idiopathic v.
vitreocapsulitis
vitreociliary glaucoma
vitreofoveal
v. separation
vitreolysis
vitreomacular
v. interface

v. separation
v. traction
v. traction syndrome
Vitreon
V. sterile intraocular fluid
vitreopapillary traction
vitreophage
Kaufman v.
vitreoretinal (VR)
v. adhesion
v. aspirate
v. attachment
v. choroidopathy syndrome
v. condensation
v. contusion
v. degeneration
v. disorder
v. dysplasia
v. infusion cutter
v. interface
v. surgeon
v. tag
v. traction
v. traction syndrome
v. tuft
vitreoretinochoroidopathy
vitreoretinopathy
closed-funnel v.
erosive v.
exudative v.
familial exudative v. (FEVR)
proliferative v. (PVR)
release of traction for
  hypotony and v.
vitreo-tapetoretinal dystrophy
vitreous
v. abscess
v. aspirating needle
v. aspiration
v. aspiration biopsy
v. base
v. block
v. block glaucoma
v. blood
v. break-through hemorrhage
v. bulge
v. cavity

V

NOTES

vitreous *(continued)*
v. cell
v. cells as indicator of retinal tears
v. chamber
v. clouding
v. coloboma
coloboma of v.
v. contraction
core v.
cortical v.
v. culture
v. cutter
detached v.
v. detachment
v. face
v. fiber
v. floater
v. fluff
v. fluorophotometry
v. foreign body
v. foreign body forceps
v. gel
v. haze
v. hemorrhage (VH)
v. hemorrhage breakthrough
v. hernia
v. herniation
v. humor
hyperplastic v.
hyperplastic primary v.
v. infusion suction cutter (VISC)
knuckle of loose v.
v. lacuna
v. lamina
liquified v.
v. loss
loss of v.
v. membrane
micelles in v.
v. neovascularization
v. opacity
organized v.
v. pencil
persistent anterior hyperplastic primary v.
persistent hyperplasia of primary v. (PHPV)
persistent hyperplastic primary v.
persistent posterior hyperplastic primary v.

persistent primary hyperplastic v.
posterior v.
primary persistent hyperplastic v.
v. prolapse
puff of loose v.
v. retraction
secondary v.
v. seeding
v. separation
v. skirt
spontaneous extrusion of v.
v. strand
v. strand scissors
v. stroma
v. surgery
v. sweep spatula
syneresis of v.
syneretic v.
v. tap
tertiary v.
v. touch
v. traction
v. transplant needle
v. veil
v. wick syndrome
vitreous-aspirating cannula
vitreum
corpus v.
v. corpus
stroma v.
vitrina
v. ocularis
v. oculi
vitritis
idiopathic v.
senile v.
Vitrophage-Peyman unit
vitrosin
ViVa binocular infrared vision analyzer
Viva-Drops Solution
VKC
vernal keratoconjunctivitis
V-K-H syndrome
V-lance
V.-l. blade
V.-l. blade/knife
V.-l. Sharpoint
V-lancet knife
VLM
visceral larva migrans

VNE
vascularization elsewhere in the retina
VOD
visio oculus dextra (vision of right eye)
Vogt
V. cataract
V. cornea
V. degeneration
V. disease
glaukomflecken of V.
limbal girdle of V.
limbal palisades of V.
V. line
V. operation
palisades of V.
V. stria
V. syndrome
white limbal girdle of V.
V. white limbal girdle
Vogt-Barraquer
V.-B. corneal needle
V.-B. eye needle
Vogt-Koyanagi
V.-K. bilateral uveitis
V.-K. syndrome
Vogt-Koyanagi-Harada
V.-K.-H. disease
V.-K.-H. syndrome (V-K-H syndrome)
Vogt-Spielmeyer
V.-S. disease
V.-S. syndrome
volitantes
muscae v.
Volk
V. aspheric lens
V. conoid lens implant
V. coronoid lens
V. High Resolution aspherical lens
V. Minus non-contact adapter
V. 3 Mirror ANF+ lens
V. 3 Mirror gonio fundus laser lens

V. Plus non-contact adapter cap and equipment
V. Quadraspheric lens
V. retinal scale adapter
V. SuperField aspherical lens
V. Superfield multi-adapter transformer lens set
V. SuperField NC lens
V. SuperQuad 160 contact lens
V. SuperQuad 160 panretinal lens
V. Transequator lens
V. ultra field aspherical lens adapter
V. yellow filter adapter
Voltaren Ophthalmic
volume (V)
choroidal blood v. (ChBVol)
tear v.
voluntary
v. convergence
v. convergency
v. eye movement
v. nystagmus
v. saccadic oscillation
volvulus
Onchocerca v.
von
V. Ammon operation
v. Blaskovics-Doyen operation
v. Frisch theory
v. Gierke disease
v. Graefe cataract knife
v. Graefe cautery
v. Graefe cystitome
v. Graefe electrocautery
v. Graefe fixation forceps
v. Graefe iris forceps
v. Graefe knife needle
v. Graefe muscle hook
v. Graefe operation
v. Graefe prism dissociation method
v. Graefe sign
v. Graefe strabismus hook
v. Graefe syndrome

V

NOTES

von *(continued)*
    v. Graefe technique
    v. Graefe tissue forceps
    v. Helmholtz eye model
    v. Hippel disease
    v. Hippel internal corneal
      ulcer
    v. Hippel-Lindau disease
    v. Hippel-Lindau syndrome
    v. Hippel operation
    v. Mondak capsule fragment-
      clot forceps
    v. Noorden incision
    v. Recklinghausen disease
    v. Recklinghausen syndrome
VOR
    vestibulo-ocular response
vortex, pl. vortices
    v. corneal dystrophy
    Fleischer v.
    v. keratopathy
    v. lentis
    v. pattern
    v. system
    v. vein
    v. vein varix
vortex-like clump

vorticosae
    vena v.
VOS
    visio oculus sinister (vision of left
      eye)
Vossius lenticular ring
VOU
    visio oculus uterque (vision of both
      eyes)
V-pattern
    V.-p. esotropia
    V.-p. exotropia
VR
    vitreoretinal
V-slit lamp
VSR
    venous stasis retinopathy
Vuero meter
V-Y advancement
    myotarsocutaneous flap for upper
    eyelid reconstruction
Vygantas-Wilder retinal drainage
    probe
VZV
    varicella-zoster virus
    VZV dendrite
    VZV disciform lesion

W4D test
Waardenburg-Jonkers
  corneal dystrophy of W.-J.
  dystrophy of W.-J.
Waardenburg-Klein syndrome
Waardenburg syndrome
Wachendorf membrane
Wadsworth lid forceps
Wadsworth-Todd
  W.-T. cautery
  W.-T. electrocautery
Wagener-Clay-Gipner classification
Wagener retinitis
Wagner
  W. disease
  W. hereditary vitreoretinal
    degeneration
  W. hyaloid retinal degeneration
  W. syndrome
  W. vitreoretinal dystrophy
Wagner-Stickler syndrome
Wainstock suturing forceps
waking ptosis
Waldeau fixation forceps
Waldeyer gland
Waldhauer operation
Walker
  W. coagulator
  W. electrode
  W. lid everter
  W. micro pin
  W. scissors
  W. trephine
Walker-Apple scissors
Walker-Atkinson scissors
Walker-Lee sclerotome
Walker-Warburg syndrome
wall
  eye w.
  w. push maneuver
Wallace-Maloney fixation diamond
  knife
Wallach cryosurgical pencil
Wallenberg lateral medullary
  syndrome
Wallerian degeneration
walleye
Walser corneoscleral punch
Walter
  W. Reed implant

W. Reed operation
W. spud
Walton
  W. punch
  W. spud
wand
  Connor w.
  Powell w.
Wang lens
Wan side port splitter
Warburg syndrome
warfarin sodium
warm-same
  cold-opposite, w.-s. (COWS)
warneri
  Staphylococcus w.
warpage
  contact lens-induced w.
  corneal w.
wart
  Hassall-Henle w.
  Henle w.
Warthin tumor
wartlike body
wash
  eye w.
  Irrigate eye w.
  Lavoptik eye w.
  Star-Optic eye w.
washout
  anterior chamber w.
  color w.
water
  w. cell
  w. content
  w. fissure
  w. provocative test
water-bath ultrasonography
water-contact angle
water-drinking test
watered-silk retina
water-silk reflex
Waters view
watery
  w. discharge
  w. eye
Watt stave bender
Watzke
  W. band
  W. cuff

W

549

Watzke *(continued)*
  W. forceps
  W. operation
  W. sleeve
  W. tire
Watzke-Allen
  W.-A. sign
  W.-A. test
wave-edge knife
waveform
  blood flow velocity w.
  (BFVW)
  pendular-jerk w.
wavefront
  convergent w.
waxy
  w. exudate
  w. lesion
  w. tumor
wear
  enzymatic cleaner for
  extended w.
Weaver
  W. chalazion forceps
  W. trocar introducer
Weber
  W. knife
  W. law
  W. paralysis
  W. sign
  W. syndrome
Weber-Elschnig
  W.-E. lens
  W.-E. lens loupe
Weber-Gubler syndrome
Weber-Rinne sign
web eye
Webster needle holder
Weck
  W. astigmatism ruler
  W. eye shield
  W. knife
  W. microscope
  W. sponge
  W. trephine
Weck-cel
  W.-c. sponge
  W.-c. surgical spear
  W.-c. vitrectomy
wedge
  Livingston peribulbar w.
  w. resection
  temporal w.

Wedl cell
Weeker operation
Weeks
  W. bacillus
  W. needle
  W. operation
  W. speculum
weeping eczematous lesion
Wegener granulomatosis
  conjunctivitis
WEH/CHOP
  Wills Eye Hospital/Children's
  Hospital of Philadelphia
Weibel-Palade body
Weigert ligament
weight
  EyeClose external eyelid w.
  gold w.
Weil-Felix reaction
Weil lacrimal cannula
Weill-Marchesani syndrome
Weisinger operation
Weiss
  W. gold dilator
  W. reflex
  W. ring
  W. self-retaining cannula
  W. speculum
Welch
  W. four-drop device
  W. rubber bulb erysiphake
Welch-Allyn
  W.-A. halogen penlight
  W.-A. ophthalmoscope
  W.-A. Pocket scope
welchii
  Clostridium w.
Welcker
  cribra orbitalis of W.
welder's
  w. conjunctivitis
  w. keratoconjunctivitis
Welland test
Wells enucleation spoon
Welsh
  W. cortex extractor
  W. cortex stripper cannula
  W. flat olive-tip
  W. flat olive-tip double
  cannula
  W. iris retractor
  W. olive-tip cannula

W. pupil-spreader forceps
W. silastic erysiphake
Wendell Hughes operation
Werb
W. operation
W. right-angle probe
W. scissors
Werdnig-Hoffmann disease
Wergeland
W. double cannula
W. double needle
Werner
W. syndrome
W. test
Wernicke
W. encephalopathy
W. pupil
W. reaction
W. sign
W. symptom
W. syndrome
W. triangle
WESDR
Wisconsin Epidemiologic Study of
Diabetic Retinopathy
Wesley-Jessen lens
Wessely ring
West
W. gouge
W. Indian amblyopia
W. lacrimal cannula
W. lacrimal sac chisel
W. operation
Westcott
W. conjunctiva scissors
W. stitch scissors
W. tenotomy scissors
W. test
W. utility scissors
Westergren method
Western immunoblotting analysis
Westphal
W. phenomenon
W. pupillary reflex
Westphal-Piltz
W.-P. phenomenon
W.-P. reflex

Westphal-Strümpell disease
wet
w. ARMD
bedewing to w.
w. cell
w. dressing
w. eye
Lens W.
w. mount
Wet-cote
wet-field
w.-f. cautery
w.-f. diathermy
w.-f. electrocautery
Wet-N-Soak
W.-N.-S. Plus
wetting
w. angle
w. angle of contact lens
Liquifilm W.
w. solution
Visalens W.
Weve
W. electrode
W. operation
Weyers-Thier syndrome
WF
wide field
Wharton-Jones operation
Whatman filter
Wheeler
W. blade
W. cyclodialysis system
W. cystitome
W. discission knife
W. eye sphere implant
W. halving repair
W. iris spatula
W. method
W. operation
W. procedure
Wheeler-Reese operation
wheel rotation
whippelii
Tropheryma w.

W

NOTES

Whipple
  W. disease
  W. disk
white
  w. braided silk suture
  calcofluor w.
  w. cell
  w. dot
  w. dot syndrome
  w. of eye
  W. glaucoma pump shunt
  w. laser
  w. laser lesion
  w. light
  w. light tandem-scanning
  confocal microscope
  w. limbal girdle of Vogt
  w. pigment
  w. pupil
  w. pupillary reflex
  w. retinal necrosis
  w. ring
  w. ring of cornea
  w. sclera
  w. spot
  w. stromal infiltrate
  w. tunica fibrosa oculi
  visual w.
  w. without pressure
white-centered hemorrhage
whitening
  ischemic retinal w.
  retinal w.
Whitnall
  W. ligament
  W. sling operation
  W. tubercle
Whitney superior rectus forceps
whole-globe enucleation
whorl lens
whorl-like configuration
Wicherkiewicz eyelid operation
wick
  filtering w.
wicking
  w. glue patch
wide-angle glaucoma
wide field (WF)
wide-field eyepiece
widening
  palpebral fissure w.
Widmark conjunctivitis

Widowitz sign
width
  angle w.
  curve w.
  orbital w.
Wieger ligament
Wiener
  W. corneal hook
  W. keratome
  W. operation
  W. scleral hook
  W. speculum
Wies
  W. chalazion forceps
  W. operation
  W. procedure
  W. spot
Wilbrand prism test
Wilcoxon
  W. matched pairs test
  W. signed rank test
Wild
  W. lens
  W. operating microscope
Wilde forceps
Wilder
  W. band spreader
  W. cystitome
  W. cystitome knife
  W. lacrimal dilator
  W. lens loupe
  W. scleral depressor
  W. scleral retractor
  W. scoop
  W. sign
Wildervanck syndrome
WildEyes costume contact lens
Wildgen-Reck
  W.-R. localizer
  W.-R. locator
Wilkerson intraocular lens-insertion forceps
Willebrandt
  anterior knee of von W.
Williams
  W. pediatric eye speculum
  W. probe
Willis
  circle of W.
Wills
  W. cautery
  W. Eye Hospital

W. Eye Hospital/Children's
Hospital of Philadelphia
(WEH/CHOP)
W. Hospital utility forceps
W. utility eye forceps
Wilmer
W. Cataract Photo-grading
System
W. conjunctival scissors
W. Eye Institute
W. operation
W. Ophthalmological Institute
W. refractor
W. retractor
Wilmer-Bagley expressor
Wilms tumor
Wilson
W. degeneration
W. disease
W. syndrome
Wiltmoser optical arm
Wincor enucleation scissors
wind-blown contaminant
window
clear w.
w. defect
scleral w.
windshield wiper syndrome
wing cell
winking
jaw w.
w. spasm
wink reflex
Winslow star
Wintersteiner rosette
wipe debridement
wipe-out syndrome
Wipes-SPF
Lid W.-S.
wire
cheese w.
w. enucleation snare
w. frame spectacles
Kirschner w.
w. lid speculum
w. mesh implant
wire-loop keratoscope

wiring
copper w.
interosseous w.
Wirt
W. stereopsis test
W. stereo test
W. vision test
Wisconsin
W. age-related maculopathy
grading system
W. Epidemiologic Study of
Diabetic Retinopathy
(WESDR)
Wise
W. iridotomy laser lens
W. iridotomy-sphincterotomy
laser lens
with
w. contact lenses (c̄cl)
w. correction (cc)
w. motion
without correction (s̄c)
with-the-rule astigmatism
W.K. Kellogg Eye Center
Wolfe
W. forceps
W. graft
W. method
W. ptosis operation
Wolff-Eisner
W.-E. prism
W.-E. test
Wölfflin-Krückmann spot
Wolfram syndrome
Wolfring
gland of W.
W. lacrimal gland
Wolf syndrome
Wollaston
W. doublet
W. theory
Wood
W. lamp
W. lens
wooden swab
Woods
W. Concept lens

W

NOTES

Woods *(continued)*
   W. light examination
   W. sign
wool saturated in saline dressing
Wooten needle
word
   w. blindness
   w. vision
Worksheet
   Thill Aniseikonia W.
workstation
   Light Blade laser w.
   Tomey refractive w.
Worst
   W. Claw lens
   W. corneal bur
   W. goniotomy lens
   W. Medallion lens
   W. needle
   W. operation
   W. pigtail probe
   W. Platina iris-fixated lens
   W. suture
Wort circle
Worth
   W. amblyoscope

   W. concept of fusion
   W. four-dot near flashlight test
   W. four-dot test
   W. ptosis operation
   W. strabismus forceps
wound
   w. closure
   w. dehiscence
   w. gape
   open-sky cataract w.
   puncture w.
Wrattan filter
wreath pattern stromal infiltrate
Wright
   W. fascia needle
   W. operation
   W. ophthalmic needle
wrinkling
   macular surface w.
   w. membrane
   retinal w.
Wucherer conjunctivitis
Wullstein-House cup forceps
Wundt-Lamansky law
Wyburn-Mason syndrome
Wydase

χ (*var. of* chi)
X
  exophoria
  X cell
  X chrom contact lens
  X chrom lens
x
  axis of cylindric lens
Xalatan
xanthelasma
  x. around eyelid
  florid x.
xanthelasmatosis
  x. bulbi
  x. iridis
xanthism
xanthochromic fluid
xanthocyanopsia
xanthogranuloma
  juvenile x. (JXG)
  juvenile iris x.
  necrobiotic x.
  uveal juvenile x.
xanthogranulomatosis
xanthokyanopy
xanthoma
  x. elasticum
  x. palpebrarum
  x. planum
xanthomatosis
  x. bulbi
  cerebrotendinous x.
  x. iridis
xanthophane
xanthophyll pigment
xanthopsia, xanthopia
xanthopsin
x axis
X cell
xenon
  x. arc
  x. arc photocoagulation
  x. arc photocoagulator
xenophthalmia
xeroderma
  x. of Kaposi
  x. pigmentosum

xeroma
xerophthalmia
xerophthalmic ulcer
xerophthalmicus
  fundus x.
xerophthalmus
Xeroscope
  X. grid distortion
xerosis
  x. conjunctivae
  conjunctival x.
  x. of cornea
  corneal x.
  Corynebacterium x.
  x. superficialis
xerotic
  x. degeneration
  x. keratitis
X-linked
  X.-l. achromatopsia
  X.-l. blue cone
    monochromatism
  X.-l. cone
  X.-l. cone dystrophy
  X.-l. congenital night blindness
  X.-l. fashion
  X.-l. juvenile retinopathy
  X.-l. juvenile retinoschisis
  X.-l. retinitis
  X.-l. retinitis pigmentosa
    (XLRP)
XLRP
  X-linked retinitis pigmentosa
Xomed Surgical Products
XP
  exophoria
x-ray
  orbital x.-r.
  polytome x.-r.
  stereo x.-r.
x-ray-induced cataract
XT
  exotropia
X(T)
  intermittent exotropia
Xylocaine
  X. with epinephrine

X

Y

Y. cell
Y. hook
Y. suture

YAG

Y. cyclocryotherapy
Y. laser
Y. laser disruption

Yale

Y. Luer-Lok
Y. Luer-Lok needle
Y. Luer-Lok syringe

Yannuzzi fundus laser lens
y axis
Yazujian bur
Y cells
YC 1400 Ophthalmic YAG laser system
yellow

y. blindness
y. dye laser
indicator y.
y. light reflex
y. point
y. spot
y. spot of retina
y. vision
visual y.

yellow-mutant oculocutaneous albinism
yellow-ochre hemorrhage
yellow-white choroidal mass
yoked muscle
yoke movement
Youens lens
Young

Y. operation
Y. theory of light

Young-Helmholtz theory of color vision
yttrium-aluminum-garnet laser (YAG laser)

Y

Z

Z. axis of Fick
Z. band
Z. marginal tenotomy
Z. myotomy
Zaldivar
Z. knife
Z. limbal relaxing incision
system
Z. marker
Zeeman effect
Zeimer venomanometer
Zeis
gland of Z.
Z. gland
zeisian
z. gland
z. sty
Zeiss
Z. carbon arc slit lamp
Z. cine adapter
Z. DAS-1 hydrophobic system
Z. fiberoptic illumination
system
Z. fundus camera
Z. goniolens
Z. gonioscope
Z. LA 110 projection
Lensmeter
Z. lens
Z. OM-3 operating microscope
Z. operating field loupe
Z. ophthalmoscope
Z. OpMi-6 FR microscope
Z. photocoagulator
Z. slit lamp
Z. slit-lamp series
Z. vertex refractionometer
Z. VISULAS 532 laser
Z. VISULAS YAG II laser
Zeiss-Barraquer
Z.-B. cine microscope
Z.-B. surgical microscope
Zeiss-Comberg slit lamp
Zeiss-Gullstrand
Z.-G. lens
Z.-G. loupe
Zeiss-Nordenson fundus camera
Zellballen pattern
Zellweger syndrome

Zephiran
zero
z. optical power
z. power lenses
z. vergence
Ziegler
Z. blade
Z. cautery
Z. cilia forceps
Z. electrocautery
Z. iris knife-needle
Z. knife
Z. knife-needle
Z. lacrimal dilator
Z. operation
Z. probe
Z. puncture
Z. speculum
Zimmerman tumor
zinc
z. bacitracin
bacitracin z.
z. sulfate
z. sulfate solution
Zincfrin
Zinn
annulus of Z.
Z. circle
Z. circlet
Z. corona
Z. ligament
Z. membrane
Z. ring
Z. tendon
zone of Z.
zonule of Z.
Z. zonule
Zinn-Haller arterial circle
zinnii
annulus z.
circulus z.
zipped angle
zipper stitch
Zirm LASIK aspiration speculum
Zöllner
Z. figure
Z. line
Zolyse
zona, pl. zonae

Z

559

zona *(continued)*
  z. ciliaris
  z. ophthalmica
zonal granuloma
zone
  ablation z.
  anterior optical z. (AOZ)
  apical z.
  z. B-cell lymphoma
  blur z.
  Bowman z.
  Boyd z.
  central steep z.
  choroidal watershed z.
  ciliary z.
  z. of contact lens
  z. of discontinuity
  z. 1 disease
  extravisual z.
  fissure z.
  foveal avascular z. (FAZ)
  interpalpebral z.
  junctional z.
  limbal z.
  markers for z.
  neutral z.
  nuclear z.
  null z.
  optical z. (OZ)
  posterior optical z. (POZ)
  pupillary z.
  Z. Quick tear volume testing
  retinal z.
  transition z.
  transitional z.
  visual z.
  z. of Zinn
zonula, pl. zonulae
  z. adherens
  z. ciliaris
  z. occludens
zonular
  z. attachment
  z. band
  z. fiber
  z. keratitis
  z. pulverulent cataract
  z. scotoma
  z. space

  z. stripper
  z. tension
  z. tetany
zonulares
  fibrae z.
zonularia
  spatia z.
zonular-traction retinal tuft
zonule
  ciliary z.
  lens z.
  z. stripper
  Zinn z.
  z. of Zinn
zonulitis
zonulolysis, zonulysis
  Barraquer z.
  enzymatic z.
zonulotomy
zoom system
zoster
  z. ophthalmicus
  z. sine eruptio
  z. uveitis
Zostrix
Z-plasty
  Spencer-Watson Z.-p.
Zuckerkandl dehiscence
zygoma
zygomatic
  z. bone
  z. foramen
  z. foramen of Arnold
  z. fracture
  z. nerve
  z. suture
zygomatici
  facies orbitalis ossis z.
  processus frontosphenoidalis
    ossis z.
zygomaticofacial
  z. canal
  z. foramen
  z. nerve
zygomatico-orbital
  z.-o. artery
  z.-o. foramen
  z.-o. process
  z.-o. process of the maxilla

zygomatico-orbitale
foramen z.-o.
zygomaticotemporal
z. canal
z. foramen
z. nerve

zygomaticus
nervus z.
Zylik operation

NOTES

Z

Appendix 1
Anatomical Illustrations

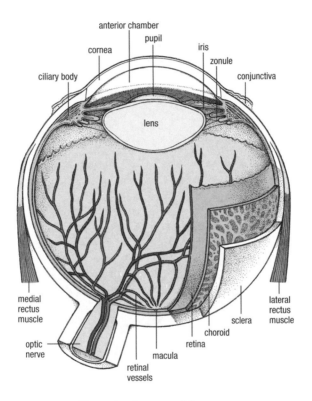

Figure 1. Structure of the eye.

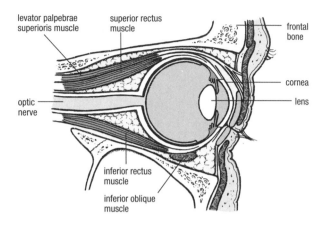

Figure 2. Orbit: containing the eyeball and the ocular muscles.

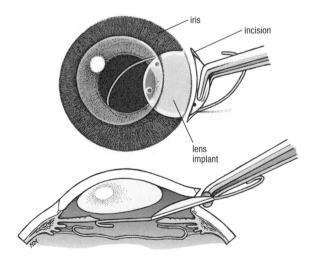

Figure 3. Intraocular lens implant insertion into the anterior chamber of the eye.

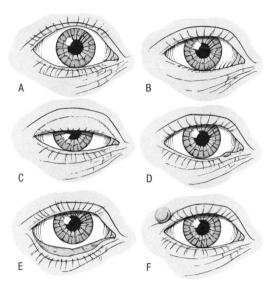

Figure 4. Structural alterations and disorders of the eye: (A) exophthalmos, (B) entropion, (C) ptosis, (D) sty, (E) ectropion, (F) chalazion.

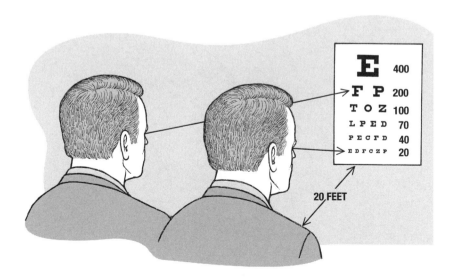

Figure 5. Snellen test of visual acuity.

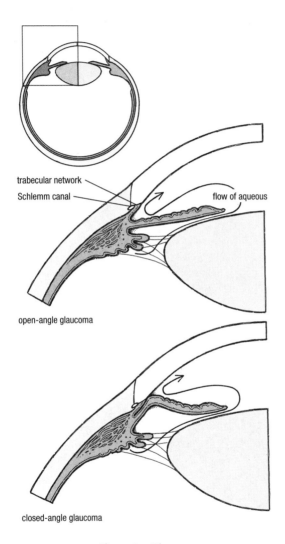

trabecular network

Schlemm canal

flow of aqueous

open-angle glaucoma

closed-angle glaucoma

Figure 6.   Glaucoma.

Appendix 2
Sample Reports

SAMPLE DACRYOCYSTORHINOSTOMY

TITLE OF OPERATION: 1. Dacryocystorhinostomy, left.
2. Silicone intubation, left.

PROCEDURE IN DETAIL: The patient was brought to the operating room, prepped and draped in the usual fashion. A 4% cocaine solution was then used to soak the half-inch nasal packing, which was applied to the left naris into the region of the superior and middle turbinate. The patient then had approximately 5 cc of lidocaine 1% with epinephrine and 1 cc of Wydase injected into the lacrimal sac region and nasal periorbital region on the left side. The patient was then prepped and draped in a sterile fashion, and using a marking pen a vertical incision mark was made approximately 3-4 mm from the medial canthal region approximately 1.5 cm in length. A #15 Bard-Parker blade was then used to make an incision over this marked area down to the depths of the periosteum. At this point, a 4 × 4 was applied to the incision site, and Bovie cautery was used for hemostasis. Once good hemostasis had been achieved at the initial incision, periosteal elevators were used to elevate the periosteum.

Once the lacrimal fossa had been identified, the osteotomy was enlarged with the bone rongeurs to the size of approximately 0.75 × 1 cm in diameter. Next, the punctal dilator was used to dilate the stenotic puncta both superiorly and inferiorly on the left side, and increasingly larger lacrimal probes were passed, up to a #8 lacrimal probe, in through the superior and inferior canaliculi.

Next, after the canaliculi had been dilated appropriately, a large silicone tube was passed through the superior and inferior canaliculi into the area where the lacrimal sac previously was, and in through the osteotomy into the nose. This was tied off leaving adequate loop for the patient's comfort. The wound was checked for hemostasis and a few small bleeders were cauterized and hemostasis was noted to be excellent. The wound was closed with interrupted 4-0 Dexon suture in interrupted fashion in three layers. In the most superficial layer, we used 5-0 Prolene suture to close the skin. After this, the patient had Maxitrol ointment applied to the left eye into the wound area. Nasal dressing was placed. The nasal packing had been removed during the surgery. The patient was taken to the recovery room in good condition.

SAMPLE ENUCLEATION

TITLE OF OPERATION: Enucleation of right eye.

DETAILS OF OPERATION: The patient was brought to the operating room, prepped and draped in the usual fashion. The left eye was approached and a 360-degree conjunctival peritomy was performed with Westcott scissors. Wet-field cautery was used for hemostasis during the procedure. Dissection took place in all four quadrants to loosen the Tenon capsule from the scleral adhesions.

Next, the rectus muscles were isolated in turn and cut with cautery. Finally, the oblique muscles were isolated and cut with cautery, and then a large curved hemostat was placed on the optic nerve. The optic nerve was then cut with curved scissors, and the eye removed from the socket. There was about a 0.25-cm stump of optic nerve attached to the globe, and the clamp was left on the remaining optic nerve segment for hemostasis. After approximately five minutes, this was removed and hemostasis was noted to be excellent. The enucleated eye was sent for pathology.

Finally, the implant ball was placed into the socket and the Tenon capsule was closed with 4-0 Vicryl suture in an interrupted fashion in two different layers. The conjunctiva was closed with 8-0 Vicryl suture in a running fashion with meticulous closure.

A conformer was placed into the conjunctival sac and Maxitrol ointment placed in the socket. The patient had subconjunctival injections of Decadron and gentamicin, and a pad and a Fox shield were placed over the eye.

SAMPLE EXTRACAPSULAR CATARACT EXTRACTION WITH INSERTION OF INTRAOCULAR LENS

TITLE OF OPERATION: Extracapsular cataract extraction with insertion of an intraocular lens, left eye.

DETAILS OF OPERATION: Prior to surgery, a Honan intraocular pressure reducer balloon was placed over the left eye. The balloon pressure was then inflated to 30 mmHg and allowed to remain in place for 45 minutes prior to surgery. The patient was taken to the operating room where local anesthesia was administered with lidocaine 2% with epinephrine for a Nadbath lid block. Retrobulbar anesthesia and akinesia were achieved with an equal mixture of Marcaine 0.75% with epinephrine and lidocaine 4% along with Wydase. The patient was then prepped and draped in the usual sterile ophthalmic manner and attention was directed to the left eye.

A lid speculum was inserted between the lids and the intraocular pressure was measured with a Schiotz tonometer. The remainder of the procedure was conducted through the use of the Weck ophthalmic microscope.

The eye was stabilized with a 4-0 black silk superior rectus traction suture and was subsequently deflected downward. A limbal peritomy was performed with Westcott scissors from 10 o'clock around to 2 o'clock. Eraser bipolar cautery was utilized to effect hemostasis. A scleral incision was made 2 mm superior to the superior limbus with a 6610 Beaver blade to one-half the depth of the sclera for 12 mm in length. The dissection was then carried posteriorly from the base of the incision into clear cornea. A #75 Beaver blade was utilized to create a stab wound into clear cornea at 2 o'clock to provide an access port. A keratome was utilized to enter the anterior chamber through the base of the corneoscleral wound at 10 o'clock.

Healon was injected into the anterior chamber through a cystitome needle. The needle was subsequently used to effect an anterior capsulotomy and capsule forceps were utilized to effect a circular tear capsulorrhexis capsulotomy. Balanced salt solution was injected underneath the capsule to dissect the nucleus free from the capsule.

The 10 o'clock incision was then enlarged with right and left cutting corneoscleral scissors to 12 mm in length. Through the use of a lens loop and Colibri forceps, the nucleus was expressed through the wound. Two interrupted 10-0 nylon sutures were then inserted through the corneoscleral wound, dividing the wound into equal thirds.

A Cavitron irrigation and aspiration tip was inserted through the wound and lens cortical material irrigated and aspirated. Following this, the posterior capsule was noted to be intact and Healon was injected into the anterior chamber.

An Iolab posterior chamber intraocular lens, Model G-708G of 22 diopters lens power had previously been soaked in balanced salt solution. The lens was flushed with fresh balanced salt solution and coated with Healon. Angled McPherson tying forceps were then used to insert the lens through the scleral incision with the inferior foot of the haptic passing beneath the anterior capsule at 6 o'clock. Long-angled McPherson tying forceps were then used to place the superior foot of the haptic through the pupil behind the anterior capsule at 12 o'clock. A Sinskey hook was utilized to rotate the lens and ensure its stability. Miochol was injected into the anterior chamber to constrict the pupil.

Balanced salt solution was then utilized to deepen the chamber and firm up the eye. Additional 10-0 nylon interrupted sutures were utilized to close the corneoscleral wound. At the completion of the maneuver, the wound was watertight. The eye evidenced normal pressure and the pupil was round, central, and lay immediately over the haptic of the posterior chamber lens. The conjunctival wound was coapted with bipolar cautery. Gentamicin and Celestone, 0.5 cc each, were separately injected through the inferior conjunctival cul-de-sac into the sub-Tenon space. The Barraquer lid speculum was removed, Maxitrol ointment instilled, and a patch and Fox shield placed over the eye.

SAMPLE INCISION AND DRAINAGE OF CHALAZION

TITLE OF OPERATION: Chalazion incision and drainage of the right eye.

PROCEDURE IN DETAIL: The patient was brought into the operating room. The right eye was prepped and draped for the procedure. Chalazion forceps were used to grasp the upper eyelid. The pretarsal conjunctival surface of the chalazion was incised. The contents of the chalazion were curetted. Chalazion forceps were removed. Hemostasis was achieved with a modified amount of pressure. Maxitrol ointment was placed in the eye with an overlying eye pad. The patient was reversed from anesthesia and transferred to the recovery area in stable condition.

SAMPLE NASOLACRIMAL DUCT PROBING AND IRRIGATION WITH PUNCTAL DILATION

TITLE OF OPERATION: 1. Nasolacrimal duct probing and irrigation for right eye.
2. Punctal dilation of the right eye.

PROCEDURE IN DETAIL: The patient was brought into the operating room. The operative eye was prepped and draped. A punctal dilator was used to dilate the superior and inferior puncta of the operative eye. A double-0 Bowman probe was passed through one of the puncta and passed into the common canaliculus. The probe was passed into the nasolacrimal sac and down the bony canal of the nasolacrimal duct. The probe was passed into the nasal cavity beneath the inferior turbinate. The probe was removed. A lacrimal cannula attached to a 3-cc syringe filled with fluorescein solution was used to cannulate the nasolacrimal duct. An aspirating catheter was placed in the ipsilateral nasal cavity. Fluorescein was irrigated into the nasolacrimal duct. Fluorescein was aspirated from the nasal cavity following the irrigation. This demonstrated patency of the nasolacrimal drainage system. The lacrimal cannula and aspiration catheter were removed. The patient tolerated the procedure well and was transferred to the recovery room in stable condition.

SAMPLE PARS PLANA VITRECTOMY, MEMBRANE PEELING, SCLERAL BUCKLE, ENDOLASER AND GAS-FLUID EXCHANGE

TITLE OF OPERATION: Pars plana vitrectomy for complex retinal detachment, membrane peeling, scleral buckle, endolaser, and gas-fluid exchange.

PROCEDURE IN DETAIL: Following informed consent and the identification of the patient, the patient was brought into the operating room, alert and in stable condition. Regional anesthesia and akinesia were obtained using a mixture of Marcaine, lidocaine and Wydase given in a retrobulbar block. The patient was then prepped and draped in the usual sterile fashion for ophthalmic procedure. The lid speculum was placed. A conjunctival peritomy was performed to 360 degrees using Westcott scissors and 0.12 forceps. Stevens scissors were used to dissect in each of the four quadrants. A muscle hook was used to grasp the inferior rectus muscle and the muscle was then bridled using 4-0 black silk suture. Each of the four rectus muscles was bridled in a similar fashion. Once all the muscles were isolated and each muscle was cleaned using a Q-tip, 4-0 white silk suture bites were placed in each of the four quadrants in preparation for placing the scleral buckle. A Ruby blade was used to enter the eye 4 mm posterior to the surgical limbus inferotemporally and a trocar cannula infusion system was put into position and the position checked with a light pipe prior to turning the infusion on. Additional sclerotomies were made supratemporally and supranasally using the Ruby blade, also 4 mm posterior to the surgical limbus. The light pipe and ocutome were then inserted through the sclerotomy sites and the cortical vitreous was removed from the posterior surface in the lens to the anterior surface of the retina. The retina was noted to be detached and there was noted to be a large open macular hole present; in addition, there were membranes present on the surface of the retina creating a star-fold inferotemporally. A Michel pick was used to raise membranes from the surface of the retina and peel back the posterior hyaloid to approximately the equator. The ocutome probe was used to remove remaining vitreous from the eye. Subretinal fluid was drained through a macular hole and also through a small retinotomy which was made near the supratemporal arcade. At this time, a 287 scleral buckle element was placed for 360 degrees around the eye and the four pre-placed sutures were then tightened and tied, notch rotated posteriorly. The ends of the buckle were tied together using 4-0 white silk suture. Scleral plugs were placed into the sclerotomy sites prior to placing the buckle. An air-fluid exchange was then performed and the retina was noted to flatten nicely. Additional drainage of fluid was performed through the retinotomy site. Several minutes were allowed to pass for additional fluid to accumulate and this fluid was removed using active suction. Active suction was also used prior to the gas-fluid exchange to raise portions of the posterior hyaloid. Once the retina was completely flattened, endolaser approximately 500 spots, were placed along the buckle and around the retinotomy site. A gas-gas exchange was then performed using SF-6 gas. The sclerotomy sites were closed using 7-0 Vicryl suture material. The conjunctiva was closed using 6-0 plain suture material. All of the bridle sutures were removed prior to closing of the conjunctiva. Subconjunctival injection of Ancef and dexamethasone was performed. Atropine drops were placed topically on the eye and the eye was then patched in closed position with an eye shell placed on top. The patient tolerated the procedure well and was transferred to the recovery room in stable condition.

SAMPLE PENETRATING KERATOPLASTY

TITLE OF OPERATION: Penetrating keratoplasty, 7.75 mm in a 7.5 mm-bed, right eye

DETAILS OF OPERATION: After clearance from the anesthesiologist and topical anesthesia with 0.75% bupivacaine, the right eye was prepped and draped in the usual fashion and massage was done until the bulb and orbit were soft. The Goldman-McNeill blepharostat was inserted and sutured to the episclera with Vicryl suture. The recipient cornea was measured and a 7.75-mm trephine was selected for the donor, which was prepared in the usual fashion. A 7.5-mm trephine was then used for the recipient until penetration occurred. Additional deepening of the outer quadrants was done with a Supersharp. Curved corneal scissors to the right and left were used to completely excise the recipient button. The fluid centrally was cleaned up with cellulose sponges. The pupil was enlarged by first creating snip incisions with Vannas scissors and then extending these, and small amounts of capsule and cortical material were also excised. A very small amount of bleeding occurred but this stopped spontaneously. The Healon was then placed, as well as Miochol, and the donor corneal button was transferred to the operative field, where it was secured in position using four interrupted 10-0 nylon sutures followed by a 10-0 nylon suture in running fashion with the knot superiorly. Prior to tying this, the interrupted sutures were removed, the running suture tension was adjusted, a permanent knot was created and buried in recipient stroma. The suture tension was adjusted further. The intraocular Healon was evacuated and replaced with balanced salt solution, and the wound was assessed with saline sponges and found to be watertight and in good position with a deep anterior chamber and no evidence of vitreous to the wound. The blepharostat was removed and subconjunctival injections of gentamicin, Ancef and Celestone were given and a drop of Betagan 0.5% was instilled. A semi-pressure patch and shield were placed over the operated eye and the patient was brought to the recovery room in good condition.

SAMPLE PHACOEMULSIFICATION WITH POSTERIOR CHAMBER LENS IMPLANT, LEFT EYE

TITLE OF OPERATION: Cataract phacoemulsification with posterior chamber intraocular lens implant, left eye.

DETAILS OF PROCEDURE: After the patient was taken to the operating room, the area of the left eye was prepped and draped in the usual manner. A wire lid speculum was inserted to hold the lids apart. Tetracaine drops were instilled over the inferonasal conjunctiva. Westcott scissors were used to buttonhole conjunctiva and Tenon capsule. A smooth curved cannula was placed through this incision and used to infuse 1.5 ml of 2% plain Xylocaine under Tenon capsule. A temporal limbal groove is made with a crescent blade. A 15-degree blade was used to make a superonasal paracentesis. A 3.0-mm keratome was used to create a corneal tunnel incision, beginning in the temporal limbal groove. Viscoat was placed on the cornea and used to deepen the anterior chamber. A circular tear capsulorrhexis was performed with cystotome and capsulorrhexis forceps. The nucleus was loosened by infusing balanced salt solution around it. The phacoemulsification handpiece was used to remove nucleus, epinuclear shell, and cortex. Viscoat was again used to deepen the anterior chamber. An Alcon Model MA30VA acrylic 22.5 diopter intraocular lens implant was unfolded in the capsular bag. Viscoat was aspirated from the anterior chamber. Balanced salt solution was infused through the paracentesis. The temporal limbal incision was checked and found to be watertight. Half-strength Betadine drops in Pilopine gel were placed in the cul-de-sac. The wire lid speculum was removed. The eye was patched with a soft patch. The patient tolerated the procedure well and left the operating room in satisfactory condition.

SAMPLE PHOTOCOAGULATION

TITLE OF OPERATION: Nd:YAG transscleral contact cycle photocoagulation.

PROCEDURE IN DETAIL: The patient was brought to the operating room. A drop of topical anesthetic was applied. The patient had 4 cc of a mixture of Carbocaine, Marcaine and Wydase in a standard retrobulbar. A wire lid speculum was inserted. The YAG contact probe with sapphire tip was readied, and applications were performed approximately 1 mm from limbus for 360 degrees, sparing the 3 and 9 o'clock positions. The patient tolerated the procedure well and left the operating room with stable vital signs. The settings were 0.7 seconds at 7 watts of energy. Atropine drops and Maxidex drops were instilled. A light patch was applied.

SAMPLE PTERYGIUM EXCISION

TITLE OF OPERATION: Pterygium removal with conjunctival graft.

PROCEDURE IN DETAIL: Local anesthesia was achieved with a 50/50 mixture of 2% Xylocaine and 0.75% Marcaine with Wydase. The eye was prepped and draped in the usual sterile fashion. The lashes were isolated on Steri-Strips and the lids separated with the wire speculum. The pterygium was marked with a marking pen and subconjunctival injection of 1% lidocaine with epinephrine was injected underneath the pterygium. The pterygium was then resected and the body of the pterygium was resected with sharp dissection with Westcott scissors. The head of the pterygium was dissected off the cornea with Martinez corneal dissector. The cornea was then smoothed with an ototome bur. Hemostasis was achieved with bipolar cautery.

A conjunctival graft measuring 10 × 8 mm was harvested from the superior bulbar conjunctiva by marking the area, injecting it with subconjunctival 1% lidocaine with epinephrine. This was dissected with Westcott scissors and sutured in place with multiple interrupted 9-0 Dexon sutures. Subconjunctival Decadron and gentamicin injections were given. A bandage contact lens was placed on the eye. Maxitrol ointment was placed on the eye. A patch was placed on the eye. The patient tolerated the procedure well and was taken to the recovery room in good condition.

SAMPLE OF PTOSIS REPAIR

TITLE OF OPERATION: Repair of ptosis, right and left eyes.

PROCEDURE IN DETAIL: The patient was brought into the operating room. The eyes were prepped and draped for bilateral eyelid surgery. Tetracaine was applied to both eyes. The upper lid crease was demarcated with a marking pen on both upper lids. The excess upper eyelid skin tissue was then demarcated with a marking pen. Intravenous sedation was given. Lidocaine 2% with epinephrine was used to infiltrate both upper eyelids. Adequate anesthesia was achieved.

The right eye was addressed first. Utilizing a #15 Bard-Parker blade, an incision was made along the lid crease. The incision was then carried along through the superior margin of the demarcated upper eyelid excess tissue. Utilizing sharp dissection as well as the unipolar cutting and coagulating Bovie, the eyelid skin and orbicularis were removed. Areas of thinning of the intramuscular septum with prolapsed fat were addressed. The prolapsed fat was excised where indicated. Hemostasis was achieved with unipolar Bovie. A 4 × 4 moistened saline sponge was placed over the right upper eyelid. Attention was then directed to the left upper eyelid. The excess upper lid skin was removed in a similar fashion. Hemostasis was achieved with a Bovie. Closure was then performed of the right upper eyelid. Several supratarsal fixation sutures were placed to address the ptosis. The skin was then closed with a running 6-0 Prolene suture. The left eye was closed in a similar fashion. The patient tolerated the procedure well. The drapes were removed. Maxitrol ointment was placed in each eye. The patient was transferred to the recovery area in stable condition.

SAMPLE RECESSION AND RESECTION

TITLE OF OPERATION: Recession and resection, right eye.

DETAILS OF PROCEDURE: General anesthesia was attained. The patient was prepped and draped in the usual sterile fashion. A lid speculum was placed. A 5-0 silk was placed in a milk pail fashion, anchoring it at six o'clock and twelve o'clock. The eye was reflected laterally, and a conjunctival peritomy and tenotomy was performed between seven o'clock and eleven o'clock. The Stevens scissors were used to spread in the off quadrant, and the two-muscle-hook technique was used until the medial rectus muscle was completely isolated. At this point, the overlying tendons and conjunctiva were elevated, and sharp dissection was used to clear the muscular septal attachments. When the muscle was completely isolated and hemostasis was obtained, a 6-0 Vicryl suture was imbricated and knotted in place. The muscle was cut free from its insertion. The old insertion was cleaned, and the surgical field was rendered dry. A caliper was used to measure off a 5-mm recession, and the double-armed 8-0 Vicryl that had been placed through the muscle was passed in an intrascleral fashion as to form a new insertion 10 mm posterior to the limbus. This was tied and was indeed secure. Closure was obtained with 8-0 collagen. The eye was then reflected medially and similarly a peritomy and tenotomy was performed on the lateral aspect with the muscle being isolated in the same fashion. A muscle clamp was applied to the muscle 8 mm posterior to its insertion. The muscle was cut free from its insertion, and muscle that was distal to the clamp was removed. An 8-0 Vicryl was then imbricated into the muscle and tied in a closure knot. This new muscle was inserted at the old muscle insertion, forming a new head, again with the 6-0 Vicryl that was used to imbricate the muscle. The closure at this side was obtained with 8-0 Vicryl. The patient was then patched with Maxitrol and returned to postanesthesia recovery without event.

SAMPLE TRABECULECTOMY

NAME OF OPERATION: Trabeculectomy.

PROCEDURE IN DETAIL: The patient was brought to the operating room and a mild IV sedative was given. As the patient became sleepy, 3 cc of 2% Xylocaine was given as a peribulbar injection through the skin, carefully following the globe and with the point out. The needle was partly withdrawn and 1 cc more was injected. The barrel was removed and 1 cc of dexamethasone with 1 cc of Indocin was injected. The barrel was again withdrawn and 1 cc of gentamicin was injected. Depo-Medrol 1 cc was then injected. The above 3 cc of half and half 0.75% Marcaine and 2% Xylocaine was placed as a peribulbar.

The eye was almost completely immobile, indicating the block was working. Gentle pressure was applied for 3 minutes. The patient was then prepped and draped in the usual manner. The sterile lid drape applied, slit, and the limbs of the drape were passed under the Jaffe lid speculum to isolate the lids and the lashes.

The microscope was put into position and the conjunctiva was taken down in the area of least scarring in a limbal-based fashion. The episclera was cleaned away with the #57 Beaver blade, and hemostasis was applied. Excess Tenon fascia was removed.

Mitomycin 0.5% was applied for 5 minutes on the sclera under the conjunctival flap. The Beaver blade was then used to make the 1.5 × 4-mm flap of sclera one-third thickness to the limbus.

A Supersharp opening was made to fill the anterior chamber with Ocucoat. The anterior chamber was then entered with a Supersharp blade under the scleral flap. The block of 1 × 2 × 3 mm of trabecular meshwork was removed with the Supersharp blade and the blunt scissors. A generous iridectomy was performed. The trabecular meshwork was then secured with two sutures of 10-0 nylon just under the scleral flap. Two sutures were used on each side to tack down the scleral flap around the slightly protruding trabecular meshwork. A double row of locking stitches of 10-0 Vicryl were used to secure Tenon's and the conjunctiva. The patient tolerated the procedure well and left the operating room in good condition.

Common Terms by Procedure

Sample Dacryocystorhinostomy
4% cocaine solution
Bard-Parker blade
bone rongeurs
canaliculi
dacryocystorhinostomy
lacrimal fossa
lacrimal probe
marking pen
Maxitrol ointment
punctal dilator
Wydase

Sample Enucleation
conformer
conjunctival peritomy
enucleation
implant ball
Tenon capsule
Westcott scissors

Sample Extracapsular Cataract Extraction with Insertion of Intraocular Lens
Barraquer lid speculum
Beaver blade
coapted
eraser bipolar cautery
Fox shield
Honan intraocular pressure reducer
balloon
keratome
limbal peritomy
Maxitrol ointment
Miochol
Nadbath lid block
Schiotz tonometer
Sinskey hook

Tenon space
Weck ophthalmic microscope
Westcott scissors
Wydase

Sample Incision and Drainage of Chalazion
chalazion
chalazion forceps
Maxitrol ointment

Sample Nasolacrimal Duct Probing and Irrigation with Punctal Dilation
aspiration catheter
Bowman probe
canaliculus
lacrimal cannula
nasolacrimal duct
nasolacrimal sac
punctal dilator

Sample Pars Plana Vitrectomy, Membrane Peeling, Scleral Buckle, Endolaser and Gas-Fluid Exchange
0.12 forceps
atropine drops
endolaser
gas-fluid exchange
gas-gas exchange
hyaloid
light pipe
membrane peeling
Michel pick
ocutome probe
pars plana vitrectomy
pre-placed sutures
retinotomy

retrobulbar block
scleral buckle
scleral plugs
SF-6 gas
Stevens scissors
subconjunctival injection
surgical limbus
Westcott scissors

Sample Penetrating Keratoplasty

balanced salt solution
bupivacaine
corneal button
episclera
Goldman-McNeill blepharostat
Miochol
penetrating keratoplasty
stroma
Vannas scissors

Sample Phacoemulsification with Posterior Chamber Lens Implant, Left Eye

15 degree blade
Alcon Model MA30VA acrylic 22.5
    diopter intraocular lens
Betadine drops
capsulorrhexis forceps
circular tear capsulorrhexis
corneal tuneel incision
crescent blade
cul-de-sac
cystotome
epinuclear shell
inferonasal conjunctiva
keratome
paracentesis
phacoemulsification
Pilopine gel
temporal limbal groove
Tenon capsule
tetracaine drops
Viscoat

Westcott scissors
wire lid speculum

Sample Photocoagulation

Maxidex drops
photocoagulation
wire lid speculum
YAG contact probe

Sample Pterygium Excision

conjunctival graft
marking pen
Martinez corneal dissector
ototome bur
pterygium
Westcott scissors

Sample of Ptosis Repair

Bard-Parker blade
intramuscular septum
marking pen
orbicularis
prolapsed fat
supratarsal fixation sutures

Sample Recession and Resection

caliper
conjunctival peritomy
lid speculum
Maxitrol
milk pail fashion
Stevens scissors
tenotomy
two-muscle-hook technique

Sample Trabeculectomy

Beaver blade
episclera
iridectomy
Jaffe lid speculum
peribulbar injection
Supersharp blade
Tenon fascia
trabecular meshwork
trabeculectomy

Appendix 4
Drugs by Indication

ALLERGIC DISORDERS (OPHTHALMIC)
Adrenal Corticosteroid
  HMS Liquifilm®
  medrysone

BLEPHAROSPASM
Ophthalmic Agent, Toxin
  Botox®
  botulinum toxin type A

CATARACT
Adrenergic Agonist Agent
  Mydfrin® Ophthalmic Solution
  Neo-Synephrine® Ophthalmic
    Solution
  phenylephrine

CONJUNCTIVITIS (ALLERGIC) — SEE ALSO OPHTHALMIC DISORDERS
Adrenal Corticosteroid
  HMS Liquifilm®
  medrysone
Antihistamine
  Aller-Chlor® [OTC]
  AllerMax® Oral [OTC]
  AL-R® [OTC]
  Antihist-1® [OTC]
  Anxanil®
  astemizole
  Atarax®
  azatadine
  Banophen® Oral [OTC]
  Belix® Oral [OTC]
  Benadryl® Oral [OTC]
  Bromarest® [OTC]

Brombay® [OTC]
Bromphen® [OTC]
brompheniramine
Brotane® [OTC]
Chlo-Amine® [OTC]
Chlorate® [OTC]
Chlorphed® [OTC]
chlorpheniramine
Chlor-Pro® [OTC]
Chlor-Trimeton® [OTC]
Claritin®
clemastine
Cophene-B®
cyproheptadine
Dexchlor®
dexchlorpheniramine
Diamine T.D.® [OTC]
dimenhydrinate
Dimetabs® Oral
Dimetane® Extentabs® [OTC]
Diphenhist® [OTC]
diphenhydramine
Dormarex® 2 Oral [OTC]
Dormin® Oral [OTC]
Dramamine® Oral [OTC]
E-Vista®
Genahist® Oral
Hismanal®
Hydrate® Injection
hydroxyzine
Hyrexin-50® Injection
Hyzine-50®
levocabastine
Livostin®
loratadine
Nasahist B®
ND-Stat®
Nolahist® [OTC]

olopatadine
Optimine®
Patanol®
PBZ®
PBZ-SR®
Periactin®
Phendry® Oral [OTC]
phenindamine
Poladex®
Polaramine®
QYS®
Seldane®
Siladryl® Oral [OTC]
Tavist®
Tavist®-1 [OTC]
Telachlor®
Teldrin® [OTC]
terfenadine
tripelennamine
TripTone® Caplets® [OTC]
Vistacon®
Vistaject-25®
Vistaject-50®
Vistaquel®
Vistaril®
Vistazine®
Antihistamine/Decongestant
Combination
Biohist-LA®
carbinoxamine and pseudoephedrine
Carbiset® Tablet
Carbiset-TR® Tablet
Carbodec® Syrup
Carbodec® Tablet
Carbodec TR® Tablet
Cardec-S® Syrup
Rondec® Drops
Rondec® Filmtab®
Rondec® Syrup
Rondec-TR®
Nonsteroidal Anti-Inflammatory
Agent (NSAID)

Acular® Ophthalmic
ketorolac tromethamine
Toradol® Injection
Toradol® Oral
Phenothiazine Derivative
Anergan®
Phenazine®
Phenergan®
promethazine
Prorex®

CONJUNCTIVITIS (VERNAL)
Adrenal Corticosteroid
HMS Liquifilm®
medrysone
Mast Cell Stabilizer
Alomide® Ophthalmic
lodoxamide tromethamine

CONJUNCTIVITIS (VIRAL)
Antiviral Agent
trifluridine
Viroptic® Ophthalmic

ESOTROPIA
Cholinergic Agent
Floropryl® Ophthalmic
isoflurophate
Cholinesterase Inhibitor
demecarium
echothiophate iodide
Humorsol® Ophthalmic
Phospholine Iodide® Ophthalmic

EYE INFECTION
Antibiotic/Corticosteroid, Ophthalmic
AK-Cide® Ophthalmic
AK-Neo-Dex® Ophthalmic
AK-Spore H.C.® Ophthalmic
Ointment
AK-Spore H.C.® Ophthalmic
Suspension

AK-Trol®
bacitracin, neomycin, polymyxin B,
  and hydrocortisone
Blephamide® Ophthalmic
Cetapred® Ophthalmic
chloramphenicol and prednisolone
chloramphenicol, polymyxin B, and
  hydrocortisone
Chloroptic-P® Ophthalmic
Cortisporin® Ophthalmic Ointment
Cortisporin® Ophthalmic
  Suspension
Dexacidin®
Dexasporin®
FML-S® Ophthalmic Suspension
Isopto® Cetapred® Ophthalmic
Maxitrol®
Metimyd® Ophthalmic
Neo-Cortef®
NeoDecadron® Ophthalmic
NeoDecadron® Topical
Neo-Dexameth® Ophthalmic
neomycin and dexamethasone
neomycin and hydrocortisone
neomycin, polymyxin B, and
  dexamethasone
neomycin, polymyxin B, and
  hydrocortisone
neomycin, polymyxin B, and
  prednisolone
Neotricin HC® Ophthalmic
  Ointment
oxytetracycline and hydrocortisone
Poly-Pred® Ophthalmic Suspension
Pred-G® Ophthalmic
prednisolone and gentamicin
sulfacetamide sodium and
  fluorometholone
sulfacetamide sodium and
  prednisolone
Terra-Cortril® Ophthalmic
  Suspension

TobraDex® Ophthalmic
tobramycin and dexamethasone
Vasocidin® Ophthalmic
Antibiotic, Ophthalmic
  Achromycin® Ophthalmic
  AK-Chlor® Ophthalmic
  AK-Poly-Bac® Ophthalmic
  AK-Spore® Ophthalmic Ointment
  AK-Spore® Ophthalmic Solution
  AK-Sulf® Ophthalmic
  AKTob® Ophthalmic
  AK-Tracin® Ophthalmic
  Aureomycin®
  bacitracin
  bacitracin and polymyxin B
  bacitracin, neomycin, and
    polymyxin B
  Betadine® First Aid Antibiotics +
    Moisturizer [OTC]
  Bleph®-10 Ophthalmic
  Cetamide® Ophthalmic
  chloramphenicol
  Chloromycetin®
  Chloroptic® Ophthalmic
  chlortetracyline
  Ciloxan™ Ophthalmic
  ciprofloxacin
  Garamycin® Ophthalmic
  Genoptic® Ophthalmic
  Genoptic® S.O.P. Ophthalmic
  Gentacidin® Ophthalmic
  Gentak® Ophthalmic
  gentamicin
  Ilotycin® Ophthalmic
  Isopto® Cetamide® Ophthalmic
  neomycin, polymyxin B, and
    gramicidin
  Neosporin® Ophthalmic Ointment
  Neosporin® Ophthalmic Solution
  Ocusulf-10® Ophthalmic
  oxytetracycline and polymyxin B
  Polysporin® Ophthalmic

Polytrim® Ophthalmic
Sodium Sulamyd® Ophthalmic
Sulf-10® Ophthalmic
sulfacetamide sodium
sulfacetamide sodium and
phenylephrine
Terak® Ophthalmic Ointment
Terramycin® Ophthalmic
Ointment
Terramycin® w/Polymyxin B
Ophthalmic Ointment
tetracycline
tobramycin
Tobrex® Ophthalmic
trimethoprim and polymyxin B
Vasosulf® Ophthalmic
Antibiotic, Topical
silver protein, mild

EYELID INFECTION
Antibiotic, Ophthalmic
mercuric oxide
Pharmaceutical Aid
boric acid

GIANT PAPILLARY CONJUNCTIVITIS
Mast Cell Stabilizer
Crolom® Ophthalmic Solution
cromolyn sodium

GLAUCOMA — SEE ALSO HYPERTENSION (OCULAR)
Adrenergic Agonist Agent
AK-Dilate® Ophthalmic Solution
AK-Nefrin® Ophthalmic Solution
AKPro® Ophthalmic
dipivefrin
Epifrin®
Epinal®
epinephrine

epinephryl borate
Glaucon®
I-Phrine® Ophthalmic Solution
Mydfrin® Ophthalmic Solution
Neo-Synephrine® Ophthalmic
Solution
phenylephrine
Propine® Ophthalmic
Alpha2-Adrenergic Agonist Agent,
Ophthalmic
Alphagan®
apraclonidine
brimonidine
Iopidine®
Beta-Adrenergic Blocker
AKBeta®
Betagan® Liquifilm®
betaxolol
Betimol® Ophthalmic
Betoptic® Ophthalmic
Betoptic® S Ophthalmic
carteolol
Cartrol® Oral
Kerlone® Oral
levobunolol
metipranolol
Ocupress® Ophthalmic
OptiPranolol® Ophthalmic
timolol
Timoptic® Ophthalmic
Timoptic-XE® Ophthalmic
Carbonic Anhydrase Inhibitor
acetazolamide
Daranide®
Diamox®
Diamox Sequels®
dichlorphenamide
dorzolamide
GlaucTabs®
methazolamide
Neptazane®
Trusopt®

Cholinergic Agent
  Adsorbocarpine® Ophthalmic
  Akarpine® Ophthalmic
  carbachol
  Carbastat® Ophthalmic
  Carboptic® Ophthalmic
  E-Pilo-x® Ophthalmic
  Floropryl® Ophthalmic
  isoflurophate
  Isopto® Carbachol Ophthalmic
  Isopto® Carpine Ophthalmic
  Miostat® Intraocular
  Ocusert Pilo-20® Ophthalmic
  Ocusert Pilo-40® Ophthalmic
  Pilagan® Ophthalmic
  Pilocar® Ophthalmic
  pilocarpine
  pilocarpine and epinephrine
  Pilopine HS® Ophthalmic
  Piloptic® Ophthalmic
  Pilostat® Ophthalmic
  PxEx® Ophthalmic
Cholinesterase Inhibitor
  Antilirium®
  demecarium
  echothiophate iodide
  Humorsol® Ophthalmic
  Phospholine Iodide® Ophthalmic
  physostigmine
Diuretic, Osmotic
  Ismotic®
  mannitol
  Osmitrol® Injection
  urea
  Ureaphil® Injection
Ophthalmic Agent, Miscellaneous
  glycerin
  Ophthalgan® Ophthalmic
  Osmoglyn® Ophthalmic
Prostaglandin
  latanoprost
  Xalatan®

GLIOMA

Antineoplastic Agent
  CeeNU®
  lomustine
Biological Response Modulator
  interferon alfa-2b
  Intron® A

GONOCOCCAL OPHTHALMIA NEONATORUM

Topical Skin Product
  Dey-Drop® Ophthalmic Solution
  silver nitrate

HYPERTENSION (OCULAR)

Alpha2-Adrenergic Agonist Agent, Ophthalmic
  Alphagan®
  brimonidine
Beta-Adrenergic Blocker
  AKBeta®
  Betagan® Liquifilm®
  levobunolol

INTRAOCULAR PRESSURE

Ophthalmic Agent, Miscellaneous
  glycerin
  Ophthalgan® Ophthalmic
  Osmoglyn® Ophthalmic

IRIDOCYCLITIS—SEE ALSO OPHTHALMIC DISORDERS

Adrenal Corticosteroid
  HMS Liquifilm®
  medrysone
Anticholinergic Agent
  Isopto® Hyoscine Ophthalmic
  Mydriacyl®

Opticyl®
scopolamine
Tropicacyl®
tropicamide

KERATITIS—SEE OPHTHALMIC DISORDERS
KERATITIS (EXPOSURE)

Ophthalmic Agent, Miscellaneous
  Adsorbotear® Ophthalmic Solution [OTC]
  Akwa Tears® Solution [OTC]
  AquaSite® Ophthalmic Solution [OTC]
  artificial tears
  Bion® Tears Solution [OTC]
  Comfort® Tears Solution [OTC]
  Dakrina® Ophthalmic Solution [OTC]
  Dry Eyes® Solution [OTC]
  Dry Eye® Therapy Solution [OTC]
  Dwelle® Ophthalmic Solution [OTC]
  Eye-Lube-A® Solution [OTC]
  HypoTears PF Solution [OTC]
  HypoTears Solution [OTC]
  Isopto® Plain Solution [OTC]
  Isopto® Tears Solution [OTC]
  Just Tears® Solution [OTC]
  Lacril® Ophthalmic Solution [OTC]
  Liquifilm® Forte Solution [OTC]
  Liquifilm® Tears Solution [OTC]
  LubriTears® Solution [OTC]
  Moisture® Ophthalmic Drops [OTC]
  Murine® Solution [OTC]
  Murocel® Ophthalmic Solution [OTC]

Nature's Tears® Solution [OTC]
Nu-Tears® II Solution [OTC]
Nu-Tears® Solution [OTC]
OcuCoat® Ophthalmic Solution [OTC]
OcuCoat® PF Ophthalmic Solution [OTC]
Puralube® Tears Solution [OTC]
Refresh® Ophthalmic Solution [OTC]
Refresh® Plus Ophthalmic Solution [OTC]
Tear Drop® Solution [OTC]
TearGard® Ophthalmic Solution [OTC]
Teargen® Ophthalmic Solution [OTC]
Tearisol® Solution [OTC]
Tears Naturale® Free Solution [OTC]
Tears Naturale® II Solution [OTC]
Tears Naturale® Solution [OTC]
Tears Plus® Solution [OTC]
Tears Renewed® Solution [OTC]
Ultra Tears® Solution [OTC]
Viva-Drops® Solution [OTC]

KERATITIS (FUNGAL)
Antifungal Agent
  Natacyn®
  natamycin

KERATITIS (HERPES SIMPLEX)
Antiviral Agent
  Herplex® Ophthalmic
  idoxuridine
  trifluridine
  vidarabine

Vira-A® Ophthalmic
Viroptic® Ophthalmic

KERATITIS (VERNAL)

Antiviral Agent
trifluridine
Viroptic® Ophthalmic
Mast Cell Stabilizer
Alomide® Ophthalmic
lodoxamide tromethamine

KERATOCONJUNCTIVITIS (VERNAL)

Mast Cell Stabilizer
Alomide® Ophthalmic
lodoxamide tromethamine

MIOSIS

Alpha-Adrenergic Blocking Agent
dapiprazole
Rev-Eyes™
Cholinergic Agent
acetylcholine
Adsorbocarpine® Ophthalmic
Akarpine® Ophthalmic
carbachol
Carbastat® Ophthalmic
Carboptic® Ophthalmic
E-Pilo-x® Ophthalmic
Isopto® Carbachol Ophthalmic
Isopto® Carpine Ophthalmic
Miochol-E®
Miostat® Intraocular
Ocusert Pilo-20® Ophthalmic
Ocusert Pilo-40® Ophthalmic
Pilagan® Ophthalmic
Pilocar® Ophthalmic
pilocarpine
pilocarpine and epinephrine
Pilopine HS® Ophthalmic
Piloptic® Ophthalmic
Pilostat® Ophthalmic

PxEx® Ophthalmic
Nonsteroidal Anti-Inflammatory
Agent (NSAID)
flurbiprofen
Ocufen® Ophthalmic

MIOSIS (INOPERATIVE)

Nonsteroidal Anti-Inflammatory
Agent (NSAID)
Profenal® Ophthalmic
suprofen

MYDRIASIS

Adrenergic Agonist Agent
hydroxyamphetamine
hydroxyamphetamine and
tropicamide
I-Phrine® Ophthalmic Solution
Mydfrin® Ophthalmic Solution
Neo-Synephrine® Ophthalmic
Solution
Paredrine®
Paremyd® Ophthalmic
phenylephrine
Anticholinergic/Adrenergic Agonist
Cyclomydril® Ophthalmic
cyclopentolate and phenylephrine
Murocoll-2® Ophthalmic
phenylephrine and scopolamine
Anticholinergic Agent
AK-Homatropine® Ophthalmic
AK-Pentolate®
Atropair®
atropine
Atropine-Care®
Atropisol®
Cyclogyl®
cyclopentolate
homatropine
I-Pentolate®
Isopto® Atropine
Isopto® Homatropine Ophthalmic

I-Tropine®
Mydriacyl®
Opticyl®
Tropicacyl®
tropicamide

OCULAR INJURY
Nonsteroidal Anti-Inflammatory
Agent (NSAID)
flurbiprofen
Ocufen® Ophthalmic

OCULAR REDNESS
Adrenergic Agonist Agent
AK-Dilate® Ophthalmic Solution
AK-Nefrin® Ophthalmic Solution
Albalon® Liquifilm® Ophthalmic
Allerest® Eye Drops [OTC]
Clear Eyes® [OTC]
Collyrium Fresh® Ophthalmic
[OTC]
Comfort® Ophthalmic [OTC]
Degest® 2 Ophthalmic [OTC]
Estivin® II Ophthalmic [OTC]
Eyesine® Ophthalmic [OTC]
Geneye® Ophthalmic [OTC]
I-Naphline® Ophthalmic
I-Phrine® Ophthalmic Solution
Mallazine® Eye Drops [OTC]
Murine® Plus Ophthalmic [OTC]
Mydfrin® Ophthalmic Solution
Nafazair® Ophthalmic
naphazoline
Naphcon Forte® Ophthalmic
Naphcon® Ophthalmic [OTC]
Neo-Synephrine® Ophthalmic
Solution
OcuClear® Ophthalmic [OTC]
Opcon® Ophthalmic
Optigene® Ophthalmic [OTC]
oxymetazoline
phenylephrine

Prefrin™ Ophthalmic Solution
Relief® Ophthalmic Solution
tetrahydrozoline
Tetrasine® Extra Ophthalmic
[OTC]
Tetrasine® Ophthalmic [OTC]
VasoClear® Ophthalmic [OTC]
Vasocon Regular® Ophthalmic
Visine® Extra Ophthalmic
[OTC]
Visine® L.R. Ophthalmic [OTC]
Antihistamine/Decongestant
Combination
Albalon-A® Ophthalmic
Antazoline-V® Ophthalmic
naphazoline and antazoline
naphazoline and pheniramine
Naphcon-A® Ophthalmic [OTC]
Vasocon-A® [OTC] Ophthalmic

OPHTHALMIC DISORDERS
Adrenal Corticosteroid
AK-Dex® Ophthalmic
AK-Pred® Ophthalmic
betamethasone
Decadron® Phosphate
dexamethasone
Econopred® Ophthalmic
Econopred® Plus Ophthalmic
Flarex®
fluorometholone
Fluor-Op®
FML®
FML® Forte
hydrocortisone
Inflamase® Forte Ophthalmic
Inflamase® Mild Ophthalmic
Maxidex®
methylprednisolone
paramethasone acetate

Predcor-TBA® Injection
Pred Forte® Ophthalmic
Pred Mild® Ophthalmic
prednisolone
prednisone
triamcinolone

OPHTHALMIC SURGERY

Nonsteroidal Anti-Inflammatory
Agent (NSAID)
diclofenac
Voltaren® Ophthalmic

OPHTHALMIC SURGICAL AID

Ophthalmic Agent, Miscellaneous
Gonak™ [OTC]
Goniosol® [OTC]
hydroxypropyl methylcellulose

OPTIC NEURITIS—SEE OPHTHALMIC DISORDERS RETINOBLASTOMA

Antineoplastic Agent
Cosmegen®
cyclophosphamide
Cytoxan® Injection
Cytoxan® Oral
dactinomycin
Neosar® Injection

STRABISMUS

Cholinergic Agent
Floropryl® Ophthalmic
isoflurophate
Cholinesterase Inhibitor
echothiophate iodide
Phospholine Iodide® Ophthalmic
Ophthalmic Agent, Toxin
Botox®
botulinum toxin type A

UVEITIS—SEE ALSO OPHTHALMIC DISORDERS

Adrenal Corticosteroid
rimexolone
Vexol® Ophthalmic Suspension
Adrenergic Agonist Agent
AK-Dilate® Ophthalmic Solution
AK-Nefrin® Ophthalmic Solution
I-Phrine® Ophthalmic Solution
Mydfrin® Ophthalmic Solution
Neo-Synephrine® Ophthalmic
Solution
phenylephrine
Prefrin™ Ophthalmic Solution
Relief® Ophthalmic Solution
Anticholinergic Agent
AK-Homatropine® Ophthalmic
Atropair®
atropine
Atropine-Care®
Atropisol®
homatropine
Isopto® Atropine
Isopto® Homatropine Ophthalmic
Isopto® Hyoscine Ophthalmic
I-Tropine®
scopolamine

XEROPHTHALMIA

Ophthalmic Agent, Miscellaneous
Adsorbotear® Ophthalmic Solution
[OTC]
Akwa Tears® Solution [OTC]
AquaSite® Ophthalmic Solution
[OTC]
artificial tears
Bion® Tears Solution [OTC]
Comfort® Tears Solution [OTC]
Dakrina® Ophthalmic Solution
[OTC]

Dry Eyes® Solution [OTC]
Dry Eye® Therapy Solution [OTC]
Dwelle® Ophthalmic Solution [OTC]
Eye-Lube-A® Solution [OTC]
HypoTears PF Solution [OTC]
HypoTears Solution [OTC]
Isopto® Plain Solution [OTC]
Isopto® Tears Solution [OTC]
Just Tears® Solution [OTC]
Lacril® Ophthalmic Solution [OTC]
Liquifilm® Forte Solution [OTC]
Liquifilm® Tears Solution [OTC]
LubriTears® Solution [OTC]
Moisture® Ophthalmic Drops [OTC]
Murine® Solution [OTC]
Murocel® Ophthalmic Solution [OTC]
Nature's Tears® Solution [OTC]
Nu-Tears® II Solution [OTC]
Nu-Tears® Solution [OTC]

OcuCoat® Ophthalmic Solution [OTC]
OcuCoat® PF Ophthalmic Solution [OTC]
Puralube® Tears Solution [OTC]
Refresh® Ophthalmic Solution [OTC]
Refresh® Plus Ophthalmic Solution [OTC]
Tear Drop® Solution [OTC]
TearGard® Ophthalmic Solution [OTC]
Teargen® Ophthalmic Solution [OTC]
Tearisol® Solution [OTC]
Tears Naturale® Free Solution [OTC]
Tears Naturale® II Solution [OTC]
Tears Naturale® Solution [OTC]
Tears Plus® Solution [OTC]
Tears Renewed® Solution [OTC]
Ultra Tears® Solution [OTC]
Viva-Drops® Solution [OTC]